Management of
Unintended and
Abnormal Pregnancy
Comprehensive Abortion Care

This book is dedicated to family planning and abortion providers throughout the world whose expertise, courage, and commitment make such a difference in women's lives.

Management of Unintended and Abnormal Pregnancy

Comprehensive Abortion Care

Edited by

Maureen Paul, MD, MPH

E. Steve Lichtenberg, MD, MPH

Lynn Borgatta, MD, MPH

David A. Grimes, MD

Phillip G. Stubblefield, MD

Mitchell D. Creinin, MD

Illustrator: Lisa Peñalver, BA, AMI

WILEY-BLACKWELL

A John Wiley & Sons, Ltd., Publication

Blackwell Publishing was acquired by John Wiley & Sons in February 2007. Blackwell's publishing program has been merged with Wiley's global Scientific, Technical and Medical business to form Wiley-Blackwell.

Registered office: John Wiley & Sons Ltd, The Atrium, Southern Gate, Chichester, West Sussex, PO19 8SQ, UK

Editorial offices: 9600 Garsington Road, Oxford, OX4 2DQ, UK
The Atrium, Southern Gate, Chichester, West Sussex, PO19 8SQ, UK
111 River Street, Hoboken, NJ 07030-5774, USA

For details of our global editorial offices, for customer services and for information about how to apply for permission to reuse the copyright material in this book, please see our website at www.wiley.com/wiley-blackwell.

ISBN: 978-1-4051-7696-5

A catalogue record for this book is available from the British Library.

Set in 9/12pt Meridien by Aptara® Inc., New Delhi, India
Printed and bound in the UK by TJ International

1 2009

Contents

List of contributors

Elisabeth Åhman, MA
Department of Reproductive Health and Research
World Health Organization
Geneva, Switzerland

Anne Baker, MA
Director of Counseling
The Hope Clinic for Women, Ltd.
Granite City, IL USA

Kurt T. Barnhart, MD, MSCE
Associate Director
Penn Fertility Care
Director of Clinical Research for the Department of Obstetrics and Gynecology
Associate Professor of Obstetrics and Gynecology
University of Pennsylvania School of Medicine
Philadelphia, PA USA

Terry Beresford, BA
Consultant
Alexandria, VA USA

Paul D. Blumenthal, MD, MPH
Professor
Department of Obstetrics & Gynecology
Stanford University School of Medicine
Stanford, CA USA

Lori A. Boardman, MD, ScM
Professor of Obstetrics and Gynecology
College of Medicine
University of Central Florida
Orlando, FL USA

Lynn Borgatta, MD, MPH
Associate Professor
Department of Obstetrics and Gynecology
Boston University School of Medicine
Boston, MA USA

David W. Britt, PhD
Department Chair, Professor
Department of Health & Sport Sciences
University of Louisville
Louisville, KY USA

Daniela Carusi, MD, MSc
Instructor in Obstetrics, Gynecology and Reproductive Biology
Harvard Medical School
Brigham and Women's Hospital
Boston, MA USA

Laura Castleman, MD, MPH, MBA
Medical Director
Ipas
Chapel Hill, NC USA
Adjunct Clinical Assistant Professor
Department of Obstetrics & Gynecology
University of Michigan School of Medicine
Ann Arbor, MI USA

Stephen T. Chasen, MD
Associate Professor of Obstetrics and Gynecology
Weill Medical College of Cornell University
New York, NY USA

Mitchell D. Creinin, MD
Professor
Department of Obstetrics, Gynecology & Reproductive Sciences
Division of Gynecologic Specialties
University of Pittsburgh School of Medicine
Professor of Epidemiology
University of Pittsburgh Graduate School of Public Health
Pittsburgh, PA USA

Jennifer Dalven, JD
Deputy Director
Reproductive Freedom Project
American Civil Liberties Union Foundation
New York, NY USA

Anne Davis, MD, MPH
Assistant Clinical Professor of Obstetrics and Gynecology
Columbia University College of Physicians and Surgeons
Columbia Presbyterian Medical Center
New York, NY USA

Jeffrey S. Dungan, MD
Associate Professor
Division of Reproductive Genetics
Department of Obstetrics and Gynecology
Northwestern University Feinberg School of Medicine

NMH/Prentice Women's Hospital
Chicago, IL USA

Thomas Easterling, MD
Professor MFM
Department of Obstetrics & Gynecology
University of Washington School of Medicine
Seattle, WA USA

Carla Eckhardt, CPHQ
Co-founder
bdi Consulting
Executive Director
Advancing New Standards in Reproductive Health (ANSIRH)
and Program on Reproductive Health and the
Environment (PRHE)
University of California, San Francisco
San Francisco, CA USA

Eve Espey, MD, MPH
Associate Professor
General Obstetrics & Gynecology
University of New Mexico School of Medicine
Albuquerque, NM USA

Mark I. Evans, MD
President
Fetal Medicine Foundation of America
Director
Comprehensive Genetics
Clinical Professor
Obstetrics, Gynecology and Reproductive Science
Mt. Sinai School of Medicine
New York, NY USA

Kristina Gemzell Danielsson, MD, PhD
Professor
Department of Obstetrics and Gynecology
Karolinska University Hospital
Karolinska Institutet
Stockholm, Sweden

Clifford Gevirtz, MD, MPH
Medical Director
Somnia Pain Management
Adjunct Associate Professor of Anesthesiology
Louisiana State University - New Orleans
New York, NY USA

Alisa B. Goldberg, MD, MPH
Director of Clinical Research and Training
Planned Parenthood League of Massachusetts, Inc.
Assistant Professor of Obstetrics, Gynecology and Reproductive Biology
Harvard Medical School
Director
Division of Family Planning
Brigham and Women's Hospital
Boston, MA USA

Robert C. Goldstein, MD
Chief Medical Officer
Somnia, Inc.
New Rochelle, NY USA

Steven R. Goldstein, MD
Professor
Department of Obstetrics and Gynecology
New York University School of Medicine
New York, NY USA

David A. Grimes, MD
Clinical Professor
Department of Obstetrics & Gynecology
Division of Women's Primary Healthcare
University of North Carolina School of Medicine
Chapel Hill, NC USA

Glenna Halvorson-Boyd, PhD, RN
Co-Director
Fairmount Center
Dallas, TX USA

Cassing Hammond, MD
Director
Section and Fellowship in Family Planning & Contraception
Associate Professor of Obstetrics and Gynecology
Northwestern University Feinberg School of Medicine
Chicago, IL USA

David Healow, MD
Associate Medical Director for Surgical Services
Intermountain Planned Parenthood
Billings, MT USA

Stanley K. Henshaw, PhD
Senior Fellow
Guttmacher Institute
New York, NY USA

Carol J. Rowland Hogue, PhD, MPH
Terry Professor of Maternal and Child Health
Director
Women's and Children's Center
Professor of Epidemiology
Rollins School of Public Health
Robert W. Woodruff Health Sciences Center
Emory University
Atlanta, GA USA

Carole Joffe, PhD
Professor
Department of Sociology
University of California, Davis
Davis, CA USA

Bonnie Scott Jones, JD
Deputy Director
U.S. Legal Program
Center for Reproductive Rights
New York, NY USA

Nathalie Kapp, MD, MPH
Medical Officer
Department of Reproductive Health and Research
World Health Organization
Geneva, Switzerland

Beth Kruse, MS, CNM, ARNP
Associate Director of Clinical Services
National Abortion Federation
Washington, DC USA

Jennifer L. Kulp, MD
Women's Health Clinical Research Center
University of Pennsylvania Medical Center
Philadelphia, PA USA

E. Steve Lichtenberg, MD, MPH
Medical Director
Family Planning Associates Medical Group, Limited
Assistant Professor in Clinical Obstetrics and Gynecology
Northwestern University Feinberg School of Medicine
Chicago, IL USA

Laura MacIsaac, MD, MPH
Director
Division of Family Planning
Beth Israel Medical Center
Assistant Professor
Department of Obstetrics & Gynecology and Women's Health
Albert Einstein College of Medicine
New York, NY USA

Karen Meckstroth, MD, MPH
Associate Clinical Professor
Department of Obstetrics, Gynecology & Reproductive Sciences
Director
UCSF Family Planning at Mt. Zion
University of California, San Francisco
San Francisco, CA USA

Mark Nichols, MD
Professor
Department of Obstetrics and Gynecology
Oregon Health & Science University School of Medicine
Portland, OR USA

Maureen Paul, MD, MPH
Chief Medical Officer
Planned Parenthood of New York City
Associate Clinical Professor
Department of Obstetrics, Gynecology & Reproductive Science
Mt. Sinai School of Medicine
New York, NY USA

Matthew F. Reeves, MD, MPH
Assistant Professor
Department of Obstetrics, Gynecology & Reproductive Sciences
University of Pittsburgh School of Medicine
Pittsburgh, PA USA

Neil J. Sebire, MD
Consultant in Pediatric Pathology
Department of Histopathology
Great Ormond Street Hospital
Consultant Pathologist to the Trophoblastic Disease Unit,
Charing Cross Hospital
London, United Kingdom

Michael J. Seckl, MD, PhD
Professor of Molecular Cancer Medicine
Imperial College School of Medicine
Director
Gestational Trophoblastic Disease Centre
Department of Cancer Medicine
Charing Cross Hospital
London, United Kingdom

Iqbal H. Shah, PhD
Coordinator
Preventing Unsafe Abortion
UNDP/UNFPA/WHO/ World Bank Special Programme in Human Reproduction
Department of Reproductive Health and Research
World Health Organization
Geneva, Switzerland

Lee P. Shulman, MD
Anna Ross Lapham Professor in Obstetrics and Gynecology
Chief
Division of Reproductive Genetics
Northwestern University Feinberg School of Medicine
Chicago, IL USA

Nada Stotland, MD, MPH
Professor
Department of Psychiatry
Rush Medical College of Rush University
Chicago, IL USA

Phillip G. Stubblefield, MD
Professor
Department of Obstetrics and Gynecology
Boston University School of Medicine
Boston, MA USA

Helena von Hertzen, MD, DDS
Medical Officer
Department of Reproductive Health and Research
World Health Organization
Geneva, Switzerland

Melissa Werner, MPH, MAT
Reproductive and Women's Health Consultant
Washington, DC USA

Carolyn Westhoff, MD
Columbia University Medical Center
New York, NY USA

Beverly Winikoff, MD, MPH
President
Gynuity Health Projects
New York, NY USA

Foreword

Allan Rosenfield MD

No topic engenders more heated controversy in the USA and elsewhere in the world than induced abortion, and this conflict is not likely to be resolved in the foreseeable future. Those who feel that life begins at fertilization or implantation, and that abortion at any stage of development is the equivalent of murder, will not compromise their strong views. Similarly, those who defend a woman's right to control her body and to decide whether to continue or terminate a pregnancy will not moderate their strong views. Other than supporting better programs to prevent unwanted pregnancies (and even here, a subset of those opposed to abortion also objects to all modern forms of contraception), no real common ground exists between these opposing points of view, despite many attempts to search for some means of communication between the two.

Notwithstanding prevailing religious, moral, or cultural attitudes toward abortion, women who do not wish to be pregnant for whatever reason will attempt to terminate the pregnancy, regardless of the risks involved [1]. Worldwide, approximately 42 million abortions occur annually, and 20 million or more are performed under unsafe, usually illegal, circumstances [2]. Furthermore, the World Health Organization estimates that between 65,000 and 70,000 women die each year from unsafe abortion, and 5 million more suffer from complications of hazardous or botched abortions, most taking place in the developing world and primarily in those countries in which abortion is illegal [2].

In the USA in the late 1980s, data from the National Survey of Family Growth (NSFG) showed that nearly 60% of all pregnancies were unintended at the time of fertilization [3]. Thus, over 3 million pregnancies per year were unintended and 45% of these pregnancies, or 1.4 million, ended in abortion. Approximately half of all unintended pregnancies in the USA still end in abortion, resulting in approximately 1.2 million induced abortions each year. Moreover, the most recent NSFG data from 2002 demonstrated a notable increase in the proportion of births to women who wanted no more children (approximately 14% as compared to 9% in the 1995 data) [4]. According to Finer and Henshaw, "between 1994 and 2001, the rate of unintended pregnancy declined among adolescents, college graduates, and the wealthiest women, but increased among poor and less educated women" [5]. Thus, women with the least resources bear a disproportionate burden of unintended pregnancy and its consequences. Although many assume that teenagers have the majority of abortions in the USA, they actually account for less than one-fifth of all abortions, the remainder taking place among women over age 20.

In close to half of those women experiencing an unintended pregnancy, the woman or her partner regularly used a contraceptive method, but for a variety of reasons, it was not used on that occasion or it failed. Similarly, approximately 54% of US women who had an abortion in 2000–2001 had been using a contraceptive method during the month they conceived [6]. Despite the relatively large number of highly effective reversible contraceptive methods on the market, none meets the needs of all couples. The most effective ones (intrauterine devices, injectables, and implants, which have failure rates essentially equal to a sterilization procedure) all have drawbacks or are associated with misperceptions that limit their use. Oral contraceptives, the most widely used reversible method of contraception, carry failure rates of 6 to 8% in actual practice. The advent of emergency contraception is an important advance, providing an option for those women who have unexpected mid-cycle intercourse.

Clearly, a need for abortion services in the USA and worldwide will continue. Nonetheless, those who provide abortion care are subject to harassment and violence, as well as subtle condemnation from many of their medical colleagues. Since 1993 in North America seven people have been murdered in connection with their work at reproductive health clinics, and five more were shot and wounded, some in their homes.

Over the past decade, training of obstetrics and gynecology residents has increased due to various advocacy effects and to guidelines established in 1996 by the Accreditation Council for Graduate Medical Education (ACGME) that direct ob-gyn residency programs to include experience with induced abortion [7]. A recent survey, however, indicates that only about half of the obstetrics and gynecology residency programs in the USA offer abortion training as a routine component of their curricula. Compared to residents in programs that offer only optional training, those in programs with routine training are more likely to learn a variety of abortion techniques and to perform a greater number of procedures [8]. Given the "graying" of experienced abortion providers in the USA, continued efforts to enhance training opportunities for a range of practitioners will be crucial to ensuring that women have the means of exercising their right to safe abortion care.

Due to myriad factors, including the shortage of abortion providers and state and federal restrictions on abortion, many areas of the USA lack abortion services. As a result, many women travel considerable distances in order to obtain abortions. In some states, services are severely limited, and a few dedicated clinicians travel by plane to different clinic settings on a regular, repeating schedule. This situation is extraordinary in a country in which abortion is legal and in which over 40,000 obstetrician-gynecologists practice.

Access to safe abortion services is an urgent need in the developing world as well, particularly in countries throughout Asia, Africa, and Latin America, where an estimated 68,000 deaths occur each year due to unsafe abortion procedures. Many more women (20 to 50% of those undergoing unsafe abortion) suffer from life-threatening complications [9]. All too often, those who survive are permanently scarred by these procedures that take place in hazardous and unsanitary conditions.

Globally, many developing world nations are characterized by limited resources, few physicians, and almost no obstetricians. In these areas where need is greatest, abortion service providers and their patients are unfairly stigmatized and subjected to violence and coercion. These threats to reproductive freedom are exacerbated by the persistence of laws banning abortion procedures throughout much of the developing world. Unfortunately, laws denying reproductive freedom are not unique to developing countries, as evidenced by the recent US Supreme Court decision upholding a ban on certain second-trimester procedures [10].

Violence against women is another area of serious global concern, affecting one in three women and girls worldwide. In sub-Saharan Africa, Asia, and Latin America, teenage women are at particular risk; they are often subject to forced sexual intercourse, which can result in unwanted pregnancies and the transmission of sexually transmitted infections and HIV/AIDS. Many women who are subject to forced sex seek abortion in order to avoid carrying resulting pregnancies to term. Women confronted by these circumstances all too often lack the resources to access safe abortion services, or they face a legal system in which abortion is denied. Women are subsequently forced to self-induce or seek out unsafe and illegal abortion providers, placing their lives at serious risk.

Global advocacy efforts must focus on changing laws and formulating national policies that respect reproductive freedom and a woman's right to choose as a matter of basic human rights. In rural areas where access to services is scarce and few obstetricians are available, training community health workers in manual vacuum aspiration and early medical abortion is critical. Even in the case of India, where abortion services are generally legal, the lack of trained personnel remains a critical public health challenge.

If we are to attempt to increase the availability of abortion services, we need an up-to-date and comprehensive guide for clinicians who will be providing medical or surgical abortion services. This publication is an outstanding response to this need. It is edited by a group of committed physicians, all of whom have extensive experience in the provision of abortion services. The opening chapter offers a rich historical review and an analysis of the role of mainstream medicine in abortion care. Chapter 2 introduces a new and critical addition to the revised text, providing a comprehensive overview of the global public health implications of unsafe abortion. Chapters 3 and 4 address fundamental public health, legal, and policy-related issues associated with abortion provision in the USA. The book is then divided into sections on preprocedure care; abortion methods and techniques, which includes five chapters covering all aspects of medical and surgical abortion procedures; postprocedure care; management of abnormal pregnancies; and abortion service delivery.

Chairs and residency program directors in obstetrics and gynecology and family medicine, as well as other leaders in the field, are increasingly recognizing the need to increase the training of residents in family planning and abortion care. Moreover, where the law allows, efforts are under way to enhance training and utilization of nonphysician clinicians in early abortion provision. This new and revised text can have a truly significant impact on training, providing clinicians and educators with the means, clearly and simply presented, to develop effective training opportunities for diverse practitioners. In addition, new chapters on the global restrictions and implications of abortion broaden this critical subject matter to include an often-overlooked dimension of women's health and rights in resource-poor countries. I hope that those in charge of residency programs and other health profession educators, both domestically and globally, will review and use this most important text as they strive to prepare future generations of providers to meet the health care needs of women.

References

1 Rosenfield A. Abortion and women's reproductive health. *Int J Gynaecol Obstet* 1994; **46**: 173–179.

2 Sedgh G, Henshaw SK, Singh S, Åhman E, Shah I. Induced abortion: estimated rates and trends worldwide. *Lancet* 2007; **370**: 1338–1345.

3 Forrest JD. Epidemiology of unintended pregnancy and contraceptive use. *Am J Obstet Gynecol* 1994; **170**: 1485–1489.

4 Chandra A, Martinez GM, Mosher WD, Abma JC, Jones J. Fertility, family planning, and reproductive health of U.S. women:

data from the 2002 National Survey of Family Growth. *Vital Health Stat* 23. 2005 Dec (25): 1–160.

5 Finer L, Henshaw SK. Disparities in rates of unintended pregnancy in the United States, 1994 and 2001. *Perspect Sex Reprod Health* 2006; **38**: 90–96.

6 Jones RK, Darroch JE, Henshaw SK. Contraceptive use among U.S. women having abortions in 2000–2001. *Perspect Sex Reprod Health* 2002; **34**: 294–303.

7 Accreditation Council for Graduate Medical Education [Online]. Chicago: Accreditation Council for Graduate Medical Education; 2008. Obstetrics/Gynecology Program Requirements; 2008 Jan [cited 2008 Sep 25]. Available from: URL:http://www.acgme.org/acWebsite/RRC_220/220_prIndex.asp

8 Eastwood KL, Kacmar JE, Steinauer J, Weitzen S, Boardman LA. Abortion training in United States obstetrics and gynecology residency programs. *Obstet Gynecol* 2006; **108**: 303–308.

9 Grimes DA, Benson J, Singh S et al. Unsafe abortion: the preventable pandemic. *Lancet* 2006; **368**: 1908–1919.

10 Partial-Birth Abortion Ban Act of 2003. 18 U.S.C. §1513 (2003).

Foreword

Malcolm Potts, MB, BChir, PhD, FRCOG

Think outside the box, or perhaps more accurately, inside the pouch. Let us suppose that the big-brained, technically competent mammal ruling the globe was not a hairless primate but a marsupial. No laws on abortion would exist. The female who wanted to end an early pregnancy would look into her pouch and simply remove an unintended early embryo. Alternatively, perhaps more plausibly, suppose that rhubarb were a totally effective abortifacient without side effects. Then every farm since the dawn of civilization and every contemporary window box would grow the plant, and women would make an appropriate brew whenever they decided against continuing an early pregnancy.

Worldwide women do attempt to terminate their own pregnancies with mechanical or chemical means, but commonly at great danger of perforation and infection. In part the laws, guidelines, attitudes, and controversy that surround abortion derive from the fact that a woman who wishes to end a pregnancy must seek the assistance of a second party, a health professional who is appropriately trained in safe abortion techniques. Although there is still a long way to go, technology is moving closer to putting the abortion decision where it belongs – in the hands of the woman.

Management of Unintended and Abnormal Pregnancy: Comprehensive Abortion Care achieves two goals. First, it spells out the scale of safe and unsafe abortion, both in the USA and globally. Second, it reviews the best surgical and medical practices for managing ectopic and other abnormal pregnancies, for inducing a safe abortion, or treating the complications of abortion. In each case, it does so in a humane, sensitive, woman-centered context. The editors and many of the authors also produced *A Clinician's Guide to Medical and Surgical Abortion* [1], published in 1999. A comparison of the two books reveals an important overarching theme, namely that best practices have moved much nearer to the ultimate goal of enabling a woman to decide, safely and responsibly, if and when to terminate an unintended pregnancy.

In the preface to *A Clinician's Guide,* I expressed fear about the rising mean age of US physicians providing abortion care. Today, although the problem has not totally disappeared, a new generation of abortion providers has emerged. This change is due in large part to the Kenneth J. Ryan Residency Training Program in Abortion and Family Planning, which provides support for residency training in these areas, and the Fellowship in Family Planning, which is producing a new cadre of physician leaders with clinical and research expertise in contraception and abortion. The older generation of providers in North America and Western Europe was largely male, often motivated to provide safe abortion by the hypocrisy, exploitation, pain, death, and damage they had witnessed when abortion was illegal. Most new providers are women. Fortunately, they know the central role abortion plays in the autonomy of women without ever having to care for a patient with a fulminating infection following an attempt to induce an abortion by pushing a stick through the cervix, or having had to reanastomose a small intestine that had been pulled through a uterine perforation sustained during a clandestine abortion. This new cohort of abortion providers simply respects the decisions of those they have the privilege to care for; shares objective information about the risks and benefits of the various options available; and then, if requested, completes a safe abortion with skill and the least discomfort possible. The intelligent marsupial will of course remain a fantasy, but step by step, we are approaching a reality in which a woman can terminate a pregnancy in the most straightforward way possible.

Manual vacuum aspiration continues to be an exceptionally safe and simple way of performing a first-trimester abortion. Ten years ago, medical abortion was still a novelty; but as this book documents, a large and compelling evidence base now exists on the effectiveness and safety of mifepristone and misoprostol for inducing an early abortion, and on the use of misoprostol alone for treating incomplete abortion or fetal demise. Both mifepristone and misoprostol are now off patent, making high-quality generic products increasingly available in many developing countries. In low-resource settings, misoprostol also has a life-saving potential in the treatment and prevention of postpartum hemorrhage and its availability is bound to increase. An effective abortifacient may not be growing in every window box, but it is becoming closer to reality.

Do technological simplifications trump all ethical considerations surrounding abortion? Personally, I do not think so. As a physician who has provided abortions, but also as a one-time research embryologist, I am awed by the development of the early embryo yet impressed by the frequency of developmental errors. If, as is pharmacologically plausible, someone invented a pill to prevent spontaneous abortion, then 15 to 30% of all term deliveries would involve severe and often fatal anomalies. In many such cases, spontaneous abortion is a natural healing process. In a similar way, the option of a safe induced abortion can change the future life course of a 17-year-old student in Chicago with an unintended pregnancy, or ameliorate a social inequity when a family in Addis Ababa, Ethiopia, who can just afford to keep two children in school, would have collapsed into poverty if they had had a third child.

Most countries still view abortion as a medical procedure where the provider, not the woman, is the ultimate decision-maker, as did the reform of the British abortion law in 1967, which requires two doctors to agree that a woman needs an abortion. Politically, the British legislation has proved less controversial than the 1973 US Supreme Court ruling in *Roe v. Wade*, but it is still a patriarchal position. Philosophically, *Roe v. Wade* is a more profound judgment because it gives the woman a right to decide on an abortion based upon her Constitutional right to privacy. The US Supreme Court did not say abortion is right or wrong. What it did assert is that a law "need not resolve the difficult question of when life begins. When those trained in the respective disciplines of medicine, philosophy, and theology are unable to arrive at any consensus, the judiciary, at this point in the development of man's knowledge, is not in a position to speculate as to the answer" [2]. Dignitatis humanae (1965) stated that the "right to religious freedom has its foundation in the very dignity of the human person" [3]. Bernard Haring, who has been called "the foremost Catholic moral theologian of the 20th century," wrote "The moment of ensoulment . . . does not belong to the data of revelation" [4]. If, "the moment of ensoulment" is indeed a matter of faith, then religious freedom must encompass different interpretations of abortion. In short, in any society that separates church and state, the status of the embryo-fetus is a matter of personal, usually religious assertion; and like other religious assertions, it must remain a matter for tolerance. Logically, any pluralistic society built on religious tolerance must permit safe abortion.

Access to safe abortion is as essential to modern living as the internal combustion engine or silicon chip. No woman can be free until she can control her fertility. Lowering maternal mortality without safe abortion is impossible. No society has achieved replacement-level fertility without the use of abortion. In short, women's medical, social, and family health depends on having access to safe abortion.

We are not marsupials and rhubarb is not an abortifacient. As *Management of Unintended and Abnormal Pregnancy: Comprehensive Abortion Care* illustrates, however, medical and surgical abortion techniques are getting simpler, provider attitudes are less patriarchal, and the locus of decision-making is passing more and more to the pregnant woman. If we were to seek a metric to measure the health of any civilization and its respect for women, given the frequency of induced abortion and the scale of suffering when it is not legal, then perhaps access to safe abortion could prove a robust and practical measure of a truly civilized society.

References

1 Paul M, Lichtenberg ES, Borgatta L, Grimes DA, Stubblefield PG, eds. *A Clinician's Guide to Medical and Surgical Abortion*. Churchill Livingstone, New York, 1999.

2 410 U.S. at 159 (1973).

3 Pope Paul VI. Declaration of Religious Freedom - Dignitatis humanae. On the right of the person and of communities to social and civil freedom in matters religious. Second Vatican Council, 1965 Dec 7.

4 Ford NM. *When did I begin? Conception and the Human Individual in History, Philosophy, and Science*. Cambridge University Press, Cambridge (MA), 1988.

Preface

Maureen Paul MD, MPH

Tremendous advances have occurred since the publication of the National Abortion Federation's (NAF) first textbook on abortion care in 1999 [1]. Contraceptive methods have expanded to include new delivery systems and highly effective long-acting methods. The increasing dissemination of mifepristone and misoprostol offers women new safe and effective early abortion options, as well as improved regimens for cervical preparation, second-trimester induction abortion, and management of spontaneous abortion. The resurgence of manual vacuum aspiration provides a simple and cost-effective means of inducing abortion or treating incomplete abortion in ambulatory facilities ranging from modern emergency departments to low-resource settings. Technologies for pregnancy termination have extended into other areas of women's health as well, such as the multifetal pregnancy reduction techniques used to improve outcomes in women undergoing infertility therapy. In addition, innovative educational initiatives launched over the last decade are honing a new generation of academic leaders in family planning and abortion and expanding the types of practitioners involved in abortion care.

Notwithstanding these impressive strides, the past decade also has brought numerous challenges. Notably, little progress has been made in reducing rates of unintended pregnancy. More than one-third of the 205 million pregnancies that occur annually worldwide are unintended [2], as are nearly half of all pregnancies in the USA [3]. In contrast to the trend toward liberalization of abortion laws worldwide [4], women's reproductive rights in the USA have suffered major setbacks in recent years. The clinic protesters of the 1990s have been joined by pharmacists who refuse to dispense birth control or emergency contraception, the US Supreme Court justices who upheld a federal ban on certain abortion procedures without regard for women's health, pseudo-scientists who allege that abortion causes long-lasting psychological trauma despite incontrovertible evidence to the contrary, and a conservative White House administration that has left a legacy of hostility to women's rights that will take many years to undo. Indeed, these countercurrents embody one of the great moral contradictions of our time: that is, while we have simple, safe, and effective technologies to provide women with the means to control their fertility, millions of women across the globe lack access to family planning services and one woman continues to die every 8 minutes from an unsafe abortion.

Reflecting this breadth of progress and challenge, *Management of Unintended and Abnormal Pregnancy: Comprehensive Abortion Care* is not simply an update of the previous textbook, but essentially a new work with an expanded purpose. Divided into six sections, the textbook addresses unintended pregnancy and abortion from historical, legal, public health, clinical, and quality care perspectives. Although much of the book focuses on medical practice in the USA, it also features an expanded roster of international contributors and new chapters on the global health challenge of unsafe abortion and abortion provision in low-resource settings. A dedicated section on management of abnormal pregnancy includes chapters on pregnancy loss, ectopic pregnancy, gestational trophoblastic disease, multifetal pregnancy reduction, and pregnancy termination for maternal or fetal indications. Each chapter is written by eminent experts in women's health with the goal of providing information that is both evidence-based and clinically practical.

This book is written for every practitioner who provides health care to women of reproductive age and for those educators who teach others to do so. May it honor and assist the courageous work of family planning and abortion providers around the world who strive to meet the needs of women, often against great odds. May it inform the practice of clinicians who do not provide abortions themselves, but who play critical roles in counseling and referring women with unintended or abnormal pregnancies. May it serve as an important resource to the growing number of residency programs that are integrating family planning and abortion care into their curricula. And in the words of our cherished colleague, the late Dr. Felicia Stewart, may it "tell why as well as how" [5] to the thousands of young students in the health professions who never knew firsthand the horrific consequences of illegal, unsafe abortion.

Producing this book was a massive collaborative undertaking, and I have many people to thank. First and foremost, NAF under the leadership of Vicki Saporta launched this project and provided steadfast support during the many months of its development. I appreciate the guidance of the editors at John Wiley & Sons who were consistently professional, gracious, and helpful. This book would not have been possible without the tireless dedication of my five coeditors and the 50 chapter contributors whose unparalleled expertise fill its pages. I am deeply indebted to the leadership of Melissa Fowler and the NAF team who spent hour upon hour preparing the manuscript for submission: Lisa Brown, Bill Falls, Tanya Holland, Andrea Irwin, Jen Mraz, Laura Galloway, Beth Kruse, Ashley Washington, Dawn Fowler, Hannah Spector, Sophia Axtman, Heron Greenesmith, Sarah Runels, and Melissa Sepe. In addition, Melissa Werner from NAF assembled the informative appendix with photographic assistance from David Keough of Boston University, Dr. Konia Trouton of Vancouver Island Women's Clinic, and Rosemary Codding and her staff at Falls Church Health Care Center, LLC. Lisa Penalver's talent and artistry are once again reflected in several of the medical illustrations throughout the book. A number of experts provided insightful review and commentary including Talcott Camp of the American Civil Liberties Union Reproductive Freedom Project and Cathy Mahoney and Jennifer Blasdell of NAF. I acknowledge and appreciate the foundation that anonymously gave generous support for this book project, and I thank all of my colleagues at Planned Parenthood of New York City who so willingly covered for me during my "textbook days" away from the office. Finally and perhaps most profoundly, I thank and honor the women who entrust their health to our care every day and whose experiences form the heart and soul of this book.

References

1 Paul M, Lichtenberg ES, Borgatta L, Grimes DA, Stubblefield P. (eds.) *A Clinician's Guide to Medical and Surgical Abortion*. Churchill Livingstone, New York, 1999.

2 Guttmacher Institute [Online]. New York: Gutmacher Institute; 2008. Facts on induced abortion worldwide; Oct 2008 [cited 2008 Nov 12]. Available from: URL:http://www.guttmacher.org/pubs/fb_IAW.html

3 Finer LB, Henshaw SK. Disparities in rates of unintended pregnancy in the United States, 1994 and 2001. *Perspect Sex Reprod Health* 2006; **38**: 90–96.

4 Boland R, Katzive L. Developments in laws on induced abortion: 1998–2007. *Int Fam Plan Perspect* 2008; **34**: 110–120.

5 Stewart FH, Darney PD. Abortion: teaching why as well as how. Perspect Sex Repord Health 2003; **35**:37–39.

1

CHAPTER 1

Abortion and medicine: A sociopolitical history

Carole Joffe, PhD

LEARNING POINTS

- Abortion was apparently widely practiced in the ancient world, with mention of the procedure in some of the earliest known medical textbooks.
- Physicians, as well as lay advocates, have always played an active role in social movement activity concerning abortion, sometimes promoting legal abortion, and less often, opposing it.
- Today about two-thirds of the world's women live in societies where abortion is legal, but the bare fact of legality per se masks considerable differences among countries as to the availability of abortion services and the social climate in which they exist.
- Compared to other advanced industrialized societies, the contemporary USA is the extreme example of a society in which an antiabortion movement arose in response to legalization and ultimately managed to become a leading force in domestic politics.
- Currently, the movement for safe, legal, and accessible abortion has assumed a transnational character, with joint activities of physicians from both developing and developed countries having an important impact.

Introduction

"(T)here is every indication that abortion is an absolutely universal phenomenon, and that it is impossible even to construct an imaginary social system in which no woman would ever feel at least compelled to abort [1]." So concluded an anthropologist after an exhaustive review of materials from 350 ancient and preindustrial societies.

Beyond the stark fact of its universality, abortion throughout history exhibits a number of other distinctive features. First is the willingness on the part of women seeking abortion and those aiding them to defy laws and social convention; in every society that has forbidden abortion, a culture of illegal provision has emerged. Second, to a far greater degree than is the case with most other medical procedures, the status of abortion has been inextricably bound up with larger social and political factors, such as changes in women's political power or in the population objectives of a society. Finally, the mere fact of legality does not necessarily imply universal access to abortion services. Crucial factors in the availability of abortion include the structure of health care services, and especially the willingness of the medical profession to provide abortion.

With these points in mind, this chapter presents a brief historical overview of abortion provision, including the role of social movements among physicians and other clinicians in both facilitating and impeding the availability of abortion services.

Abortion in the past

Throughout recorded history, populations have risen and declined in ways that cannot be attributed solely to natural events such as plagues or famines. For example, a marked decline in population occurred in the early Roman Empire, despite prosperity and an apparently ample food supply [2]. Such events suggest that individuals in past societies vigorously sought to regulate their fertility; they did so by use of abortion and contraception, and also by practices of child abandonment and infanticide [3].

To give some sense of the ubiquity of abortion in the premodern world, consider the following: Specific information about abortion appears in one of the earliest known medical texts, attributed to the Chinese emperor Shen Nung (2737

Management of Unintended and Abnormal Pregnancy, 1st edition. By M Paul, ES Lichtenberg, L Borgatta, DA Grimes, PG Stubblefield, MD Creinin
 ISBN: 9781405176965.

to 2696 BC); the Ebers Papyrus of Egypt (1550 to 1500 BC) contains several references to abortion and contraception; during the Roman Empire numerous writers mention abortion, including the satirist Juvenal who wrote about "our skilled abortionists"; and the writings of the 10th-century Persian physician Al-Rasi include instructions for performing an abortion through instrumentation [2, 4].

Most interesting, perhaps, is the reinterpretation that some scholars have given to the famed Hippocratic Oath (400 BC), which has long been used by abortion opponents to argue that the so-called Father of Medicine opposed abortion. These scholars argue that the passage commonly translated as "Neither will I give a woman means to procure an abortion" is rendered more correctly as "Neither will I give a suppository (also translated as 'pessary') to cause an abortion." According to this view, Hippocrates was urging a ban on one form of abortion that he considered dangerous to women, but was not condemning the practice generally. Indeed works ascribed to Hippocrates describe a graduated set of dilators that could be used for abortions, as well as prescriptions for abortifacients [2, 5].

The rise of the Christian era brought more public regulation of sexual life, including increased condemnation of abortion. Open discussion of abortion techniques lessened, as did direct abortion provision by physicians. Until the 18th century, therefore, abortion and contraception became largely contained within a women's culture. Midwives in particular became key providers of abortion and family planning services, for which they were periodically persecuted as "witches [2, 6]."

Despite shifting opinion about abortion and organized medicine's reluctance to engage with the issue, early monotheistic traditions did not hold the strong, unified position against abortion that is now associated with the contemporary Roman Catholic church. While early Islamic teachings prohibited abortion after the soul enters the fetus, religious scholars disagreed about when this event occurred, with estimates ranging from 40 to 120 days after conception [7]. Early Christian thought was divided as to whether abortion of an early "unformed fetus" actually constituted murder [5]. The Catholic church tacitly permitted earlier abortions, and it did not take a highly active role in antiabortion campaigns until the 19th century.

In Europe and the USA, the 17th through the 19th centuries were an especially interesting period in abortion history. On one hand, advances in gynecology, such as the discovery (or more correctly, rediscovery) of dilators and curettes, meant that physicians could offer safer and more effective abortions. On the other hand, the conservatism of the medical profession regarding reproductive issues prevented widespread discussion and dissemination of abortion techniques. As three longtime scholars of abortion have noted, "The combination of medicine with anything concerning sex appears to have a particularly paralytic effect upon human resourcefulness. This has been especially true in the field of abortion... [8]."

At the same time that the medical profession responded ambivalently to patients' requests for abortions, a widespread culture of abortion provision by others flourished. Abortion providers, including midwives, homeopaths, and other self-designated healers, as well as some physicians, advertised freely of their willingness to help with "female problems" and of potions and pills that would "bring on the menses [5, 9]." This commercial provision of abortion remained largely unregulated by law until the 19th century. Under the prevailing standard, abortions performed before "quickening" were not regulated at all, and attempts to police later abortions were minimal. In England, it was only during Queen Victoria's reign that the Offences against the Person Act of 1861 passed, which made surgical abortion at any stage of pregnancy a criminal act [7]. In the USA, a vigorous antiabortion campaign was launched around 1850, and by the 1870s, all states had criminalized abortion.

Notwithstanding involvement on the part of Catholic and Protestant clergy and others, physicians were the leading force in the campaign to criminalize abortion in the USA. The American Medical Association (AMA), founded in 1847, argued that abortion was both immoral and dangerous, given the incompetence of many practitioners at that time. According to a number of scholars, the AMA's drive against abortion formed part of a larger and ultimately successful strategy that sought to put "regular" or university-trained physicians in a position of professional dominance over the wide range of "irregular" clinicians who practiced freely during the first half of the 19th century [5, 9].

What followed was a "century of criminalization" characterized by a widespread culture of illegal abortion provision. Thousands of women died or sustained serious injuries at the hands of the infamous "back alley butchers" of that period, and encountering these victims in hospital emergency rooms became a nearly universal experience for US medical residents [10]. However, safe abortions were available to some women, performed by highly skilled laypersons [11] and physicians with successful mainstream practices who were motivated primarily by the desperate situations of their patients. These "physicians of conscience" were instrumental in convincing their medical colleagues of the necessity to decriminalize abortion. By 1970, the AMA reversed its earlier stance and called for the legalization of abortion [10].

This overview of the history of abortion suggests several themes. Besides the omnipresence of the desire for abortion, the record of very early understanding of abortion techniques and actual abortion provision by some sectors of the medical profession are striking. This knowledge, however, was willfully forgotten as abortion became socially controversial and the medical profession avoided the issue for the most part. Consequently, until quite recently in the developed world (and continuing today in many developing nations), two parallel streams of abortion provision emerged: a minimalist one, by physicians, only to selected patients under narrowly specified conditions, and a broader extralegal one, in which a variety of providers with widely ranging skill levels offered abortion services.

What is less clear to contemporary scholars is the degree of safety and effectiveness of abortion provision before the widespread legalization that started in the latter half of the 20th century. Ample documentation attests to the many injuries and deaths that occurred before legalization in the USA and elsewhere, and that continues today where abortion remains illegal. However, given the historical record that points to the persistent search for abortions in all cultures and at all times, without death records to match this volume of abortion, some observers suggest that many illegal abortions were relatively safe, although probably painful and unpleasant [2, 3, 6]. What remains indisputable is the greatly improved safety record once abortion is legalized. In the USA, abortion-related mortality declined dramatically after nationwide legalization, eventually reaching 0.6 deaths per 100,000 procedures between 1979 and 1985, "more than 10 times lower than the 9.1 maternal deaths per 100,000 live births between 1979 and 1986 [12]."

New technologies, new organizational forms

Around the period of legalization in the USA, technological advances in the field of abortion care facilitated new models of abortion delivery. Specifically, development of the vacuum aspirator, cervical anesthesia methods, and the Karman cannula all improved the safety of abortion and permitted its provision in nonhospital settings.

The vacuum aspirator, introduced to US physicians in 1968 at a landmark conference on abortion sponsored by the Association for the Study of Abortion, lessened blood loss and lowered the risk of uterine perforation compared to the older method of dilation and sharp curettage [13, 14]. Cervical anesthesia techniques allowed clinicians to manage procedural pain using local injections rather than the more risky general anesthesia. The Karman cannula, invented by a California psychologist who had been involved in illegal abortion provision in the 1960s, was composed of plastic rather than metal. This soft flexible cannula facilitated provision of early abortion using local anesthesia and made perforation less likely [8]. The widespread adoption of the Karman cannula represents a vivid example of a larger phenomenon: the extent to which, as abortion services rapidly expanded after legalization, the medical profession was compelled to seek the advice of a number of illegal abortionists, both lay and physician [10].

Taken together, these innovations in abortion methods catalyzed the creation of the freestanding abortion clinic, which was pioneered in the USA. Washington, DC, and New York City had liberalized their abortion laws several years before the *Roe v. Wade* decision, and clinics in these cities attracted women from all over the country. These clinics were able to offer safe outpatient abortion services at lower cost, and often in a more supportive manner, than hospital-based facilities. The creation of the role of the "abortion counselor"—someone specifically trained to discuss the abortion decision with the patient, explain the procedure, and support her throughout the process—was a distinctive contribution of this early period in legal abortion [15]. These clinics also were instrumental in pioneering a model of ambulatory surgery that became widely adopted by the medical profession.

Freestanding clinics remain the dominant form of abortion delivery in the USA, while in Europe and Canada, abortions are more evenly spread between clinics and hospitals. Notwithstanding the many benefits of the freestanding clinic model, it also has contributed to the marginalization of abortion services from mainstream medicine in the USA and left clinics more vulnerable to attacks from antiabortion extremists. In contrast, those European countries where abortions are delivered as part of national health care systems have experienced less difficulty in finding providers and far less antiabortion activity at service sites.

Medical abortion (Chapter 9) is another technological innovation that has permitted new categories of abortion providers to emerge in many parts of the world. Mifepristone, approved in France in 1988 but not in the USA until 2000, is gradually taking hold and bringing a number of primary care practitioners to abortion care. In 2005, a national survey of US abortion providers by the Guttmacher Institute revealed that medical methods comprised 21% of abortions provided at 8 weeks' gestation or less [16]. Midlevel clinicians (also referred to as advanced practice clinicians) deliver mifepristone medical abortion services in many states in the USA and in certain developing countries where abortion is legal, such as South Africa. Finally, misoprostol, the drug commonly used in conjunction with mifepristone for early medical abortion, has received increasing attention within the medical community for its ability to terminate a pregnancy when used alone. Evidence suggests that access to misoprostol has reduced morbidity and mortality from illegal abortions in the developing world (Chapters 2 and 22) [17].

Abortion in sociopolitical context

By the early 1950s only a handful of countries had legalized abortion; however, in the last half of the 20th century, an "abortion revolution" of sorts occurred. As a result, nearly three-fourths of the world's women now live in countries where abortion is legal either in all circumstances (up to a certain point in pregnancy) or when specific medical or social conditions are present [18]. Major forces leading to this liberalization included recognition of the health costs of illegal abortion, with the medical profession often acting as key advocates for legalization; the rising status of women, and especially the entry of women into the paid labor force, which led feminist groups to mobilize on behalf of abortion and improved contraceptive services; and, to a lesser degree, various countries' explicit interests in limiting population growth.

However, the bare fact of legality per se masks considerable differences among countries as to the availability of abortion services and the social climate in which they exist. The contemporary USA is the extreme example of a society in which an antiabortion movement arose in response to legalization and ultimately managed to become a leading force in domestic politics. However, abortion remains controversial in many other countries as well, with periodic attempts by both abortion rights supporters and their opponents to modify existing arrangements.

Europe and North America

Nearly all the countries of Western Europe that did not already have liberal abortion laws underwent progressive abortion reform in the 1970s and 1980s. Following unification of East and West Germany in the early 1990s, Germany became the one case of a European Community (EC) member that adopted more restrictive laws than had existed previously [19]. In the contemporary EC, Ireland and Poland represent the only countries that do not permit abortion, presenting baffling issues about how to reconcile their strict antiabortion policies with the more liberal policies of the others. Although EC member countries are free to devise their own abortion policies, they theoretically give free access to citizens who wish to travel to other member nations. The conflict between these two principles has emerged periodically, as exemplified by several notorious cases in which the Irish government attempted to prevent women in dire circumstances from traveling to England for an abortion. In a 2007 case, "Miss D.," a 17-year-old carrying a fetus with anencephaly, had her passport confiscated in order to prevent such travel. After numerous court hearings (and litigation estimated to cost 1 million euros), she was finally permitted to go to England [20].

In general, Western Europe has had a quite stable abortion environment. In contrast to the situation in the USA, access to abortion-providing facilities in Western European countries (with a few exceptions) is substantially easier, with most offering subsidized abortions for health indications and many for elective abortions as well. Moreover, abortion provision in these countries is largely free from the extremes of violence and controversy that have characterized abortion care in the USA. Such differences testify to the important role that national health care systems play in assuring access to abortion care. The European and US comparison also reveals that the centrality of abortion in US political culture is almost unique among advanced Western democracies.

Eastern Europe

In 1920, Russia was the first country in the world to legalize abortion (although it reversed its stance in 1936 and then later reestablished legalization). By the 1950s, all the countries of Eastern Europe had legalized abortion. This reform occurred primarily because of the various regimes' needs for women to enter the paid labor force, rather than as a response to women's demands for reproductive freedom or concerns about the consequences of illegal abortion. In the absence of adequate contraception in most Eastern bloc countries, abortion became an accepted method of fertility control, and abortion rates were among the highest in the world [21].

After the fall of communism in 1990, a number of Eastern European countries experienced pressures to reevaluate abortion policies. Contributing factors included the renewed power of the Catholic church in some cases, as well as the association of abortion with the discredited policies of the old Communist regimes and the corresponding "sentimental perceptions of a pre-Communist world where home and family were paramount [19]." Hungary and Slovakia restricted their abortion policies somewhat, and they continue to have conflicts about this issue. However, the most dramatic reversal took place in Poland, which moved from a policy of abortion on demand to one that permitted abortion only in cases of severe fetal malformation or serious threat to the life or health of the pregnant woman [21]. The new legislation, strongly advocated by the Catholic church, called for imprisonment of doctors who performed unauthorized abortions. Not surprisingly, as pointed out in a recent publication by a reproductive rights group in Poland tellingly titled *Contemporary Women's Hell: Polish Women's Stories* [22], women in that country have an extraordinarily difficult time obtaining a legal abortion. The group estimates that only about 150 legal abortions take place in the country each year. "This is mainly because doctors do not want to take responsibility for consenting to a legal abortion. Women are sent from one doctor to another, referred for tests that are not legally required, and misinformed about their health...For doctors...such women represent problems that need to be eliminated as quickly as possible [22]."

As is typical in all societies that restrict abortion, Polish women who can afford it travel to clinics in other countries or find doctors within Poland who are willing to provide illegal abortions (often costing as much as US $1,000) [22]. Those without such resources often resort to attempts at self-abortion; abandonment of newborns in maternity hospitals; illegal adoptions; and in some instances, according to press reports, infanticide [23].

Although Poland has the most visible antiabortion movement in Eastern Europe, the former Soviet Union also has experienced a backlash against abortion and family planning efforts. At the same time, abortion supporters (both medical and lay) in Poland and various republics of the former

Soviet Union are part of the global reproductive rights movement, from which they gain resources and the support of colleagues. The Polish publication cited earlier, for example, was translated and printed with financial aid from Ipas and the International Women's Health Coalition, organizations that are based in the USA but whose focus is international. Similarly, various US foundations have funded training programs in medical abortion and manual vacuum aspiration for physicians in various parts of the former Soviet Union.

Canada

Historically, Canada's abortion reform centered largely on the activities of one individual, Henry Morgentaler, a physician who has repeatedly challenged that country's abortion laws since 1968. Morgentaler's crusade culminated in the 1988 Canadian Supreme Court decision, *R. v. Morgentaler*, which removed abortion from Canada's criminal code [24, 25]. However, abortion policies still differ considerably from province to province, with various restrictions put forward by antiabortion legislators and some provinces (especially in the Maritimes) having a shortage of providers. Although in no way approaching the level of US antiabortion activity, Canada has experienced several incidents of violence directed against abortion providers, as well as destructive acts at clinic sites. Canada has not yet approved mifepristone, but methotrexate regimens are used for early medical abortion.

USA

The 1973 *Roe v. Wade* decision that legalized abortion throughout the USA resulted in large part from mobilization among the medical community and feminist groups [26]. This ruling quickly gave rise to an antiabortion movement, which in its degree of political power and its willingness to engage in violence and intimidation makes the US abortion situation unique. As of 2007, some seven members of the abortion-providing community (physicians, receptionists, a volunteer, and an off-duty police officer employed as a clinic security guard) have been murdered, and thousands of others have been harassed at their workplaces and homes [27]. Due to stiffened federal penalties for antiabortion violence and disruption established during the Clinton presidency in the 1990s, these incidents have diminished in number, if not in seriousness.

During the two presidential terms of George W. Bush (2000–2008), the climate for legal abortion in the USA worsened considerably. Acting on the recommendations of religious right leaders, the President appointed two new conservative justices to the US Supreme Court. In 2007 these two justices provided the margin needed in *Gonzales v. Carhart* to uphold the federal Partial-Birth Abortion Ban Act of 2003, the first ever federal ban on certain abortion procedures. The actions of Congress and the Court were unprecedented in their willingness to ignore the best judgment of the medical community: the American College of Obstetricians and Gynecologists (ACOG), the National Abortion Federation, and Planned Parenthood Federation of America all had decried the ban, arguing that banned procedures were the safest option in certain circumstances [28]. Adding to the dismay of abortion rights supporters, the majority in this case for the first time found constitutional an abortion restriction that did not have an exception for women's health. The federal ban adds to the massive number of restrictions that already exist at the state level to curtail women's access to abortion, especially for the most vulnerable (Chapter 4).

The Bush presidency also brought the spread of abortion politics to other issues, as the religious right gained enormous political leverage within the administration. Attacks on stem cell research, promotion of discredited "abstinence only" sex education programs, and cutbacks in contraceptive funding, both domestically and internationally, were only some of the steps taken by President Bush to satisfy his right-wing base. The Bush administration was noteworthy as well for making inappropriate, ideologically driven appointments to important governmental posts. For example, the credentials of the physician selected as head of all government-funded contraceptive programs included his service as medical director of an agency that declared birth control to be "degrading"; similarly, prospective appointees for both domestic positions on scientific panels and assignments to the Coalition Provision Authority in Iraq were vetted on the basis of their opinions of *Roe v. Wade* [29].

Enhanced mobilization among health care providers associated with the religious right also occurred during the Bush years. Groups such as the Christian Medical and Dental Associations, Pharmacists for Life, and "pro-life" caucuses within ACOG and other medical associations worked in various ways to impede access to abortion and contraception. A number of individual pharmacists and some pharmaceutical chains, for example, have refused to fill prescriptions for emergency contraception; some pharmacists have even refused to fill prescriptions for regular oral contraceptives, on the alleged grounds that these medications constitute abortifacients [30]. Moreover, the large number of mergers between Catholic and secular hospitals that have occurred in the USA has compromised delivery of abortion care and other reproductive health services, such as family planning, sterilization, and assisted reproduction [31, 32].

The abortion rights medical community in the USA has mobilized as well, particularly since the mid-1990s, in reaction to growing evidence of an abortion provider shortage and the unacceptable level of violence occurring at clinics. The formation of Medical Students for Choice (MSFC) in 1994 represents a particularly important development. The group has chapters on most US medical school campuses, as well as physician activists in more than 200 residency programs in obstetrics and gynecology and other fields (Backus, personal communication, 2008). One of the group's first activities was to successfully help pressure the Accreditation

Council for Graduate Medical Education (ACGME) and the Council on Resident Education in Obstetrics and Gynecology to mandate abortion training in obstetrics and gynecology residency programs (with opt-out provisions for those with religious or moral objections) [33]. This positive step was nullified in part by the US Congress when, in an unprecedented intrusion into medical affairs, it stipulated that those residency programs that failed to conform to this standard would not lose federal funding. Nonetheless, the revised ACGME guidelines have substantially increased abortion training in the USA [34, 35].

Other health care professionals, particularly primary care practitioners, have spearheaded efforts to expand abortion training and access. Family practice and other primary care physicians have organized to increase abortion training opportunities [36] and legitimatize abortion provision within primary care medical institutions. Groups similar to MSFC have emerged among advanced practice clinicians (nurse practitioners, nurse midwives, and physician assistants) committed to safe and legal abortion care. Not all of these health professionals will necessarily become abortion providers themselves, but one can reasonably assume that they will be supportive of their colleagues who do (Fig. 1.1).

The establishment of the Kenneth J. Ryan Residency Training Program and the Fellowship in Family Planning (see Appendix) also has been pivotal in assuring the vibrancy of the abortion provider community in the USA. By offering technical and financial assistance, the Ryan Program helps obstetrics and gynecology and family medicine residency programs integrate abortion training into their curricula. The Fellowship in Family Planning, established in 1991 at the University of California at San Francisco, offers postgraduate training (including clinical and research experience, as well as an international component) to physicians who are committed to abortion and contraceptive work. Numerous graduates from this fellowship have assumed positions as faculty and directors of family planning divisions in leading medical institutions, thereby increasing the visibility of abortion in US medical culture [37].

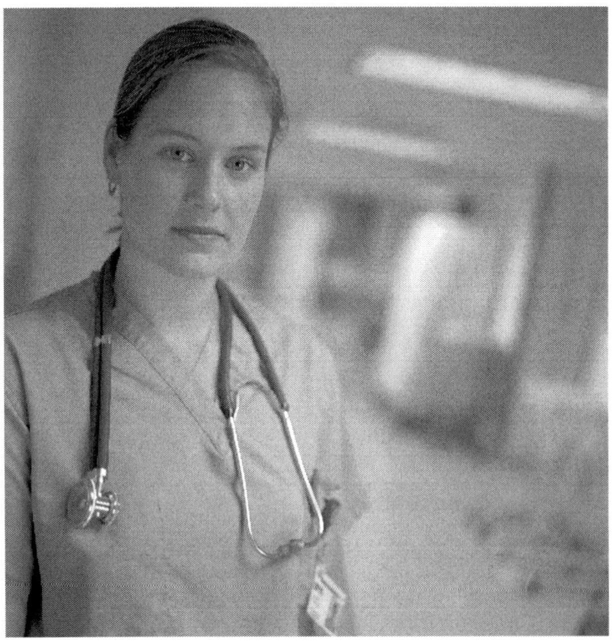

Figure 1.1 Efforts to increase abortion training opportunities and legitimatize abortion provision within primary care medical institutions and the emergence of groups like Medical Students for Choice (MSFC) have been pivotal in assuring the vibrancy of the abortion provider community in the USA.

Professional organizations such as the Association of Reproductive Health Professionals and Physicians for Reproductive Choice and Health, comprised of both individuals who provide abortion and those who do not, also have been important advocates for safe and accessible abortion. Both groups have argued forcefully that reproductive health practice and policy must be based on scientific evidence, not on personal or religious beliefs. The National Abortion Federation, the professional association of abortion providers in the USA and Canada, establishes evidence-based guidelines for abortion care and offers its members continuing medical education as well as opportunities for community building (Fig. 1.2) (Appendix).

Developing countries

Except in a few countries such as China and India, most women in the developing world do not have access to legal abortions, although changes are under way in a number of places. In some situations of formal illegality, women can still obtain safe abortions, as in certain large cities of Latin America or in the menstrual regulation clinics in Bangladesh, Malaysia, and Indonesia. Nonetheless, some 65,000 to 70,000 women die each year from unsafe abortion, primarily in developing countries, and thousands of others are seriously injured (Chapter 2).

Two United Nations (UN) conferences, the International Conference on Population and Development held in Cairo in 1994 and the Fourth World Conference on Women held in Beijing in 1995, were noteworthy for the centrality of debates over abortion and reproductive rights. In spite of vigorous opposition from the Vatican and a few Catholic and Muslim nations, a coalition of feminists from both developed and developing countries managed to push the final conference documents in a far more progressive direction than had previously been the case. Language was approved that acknowledged the right of women to control their fertility and that called for greatly expanded family planning services. The documents also recognized that abortions take place, whether legal or not; that in those countries in which it is legal, abortion should be safe; and that women who have unsafe abortions should not be prosecuted and should have access to adequate health care services to manage

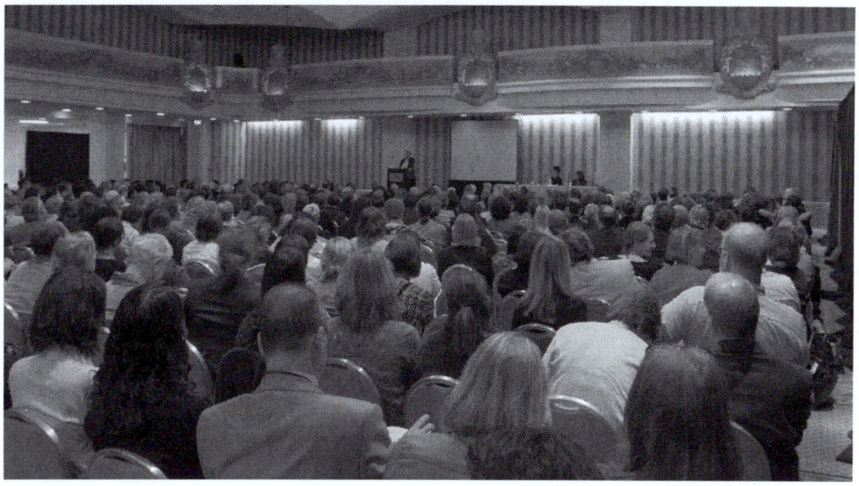

Figure 1.2 Members of the National Abortion Federation, the professional association of abortion providers in the USA and Canada, benefit from continuing medical education as well as opportunities for community building.

complications [38, 39]. The Cairo and Beijing conferences did not create any mechanisms for implementing these recommendations, and the 10-year follow-up discussions at the UN brought similar political cleavages [40]; nonetheless, these conferences established a critical precedent in the international community by situating abortion and reproductive health in the context of basic human rights.

In the decade that has passed since these two crucial meetings, a number of countries in the developing world have liberalized their abortion policies, including Nepal, Colombia, and various Caribbean nations, as well as Mexico City. In the summer of 2007 leaders of ten African nations, including the Vice-President of Kenya, called for the legalization of abortion as a response to unacceptably high mortality rates among African women from unsafe abortion [41]. At the same time, however, other countries have regressed in their abortion policies. Nicaragua and El Salvador, for example, have instituted strict policies prohibiting abortion, even to save a woman's life [42, 43].

Conclusion

In considering the contemporary status of abortion, we can speak of a "cup half full, half empty" quality to this highly controversial issue. On the negative side, too many women still suffer injury or death from unsafe abortion, and too many women are forced to carry unwanted pregnancies to term. Too many abortion providers face unacceptable threats of violence and intimidation, as well as restrictive legislation that may include criminal penalties. On the positive side, some countries where abortion has been previously illegal are starting to liberalize their laws. Recent developments in abortion care, such as medical abortion and the return of manual vacuum aspiration, have made abortion care safer in various developing countries and have enlarged the pool of abortion providers in developed countries, including the USA.

The history of the relationship of abortion and the medical profession reveals an inescapable connection between abortion provision and social movement activity on both sides of the issue. This connection will only intensify in the foreseeable future. Clinicians who support abortion rights, along with their lay allies from the reproductive justice movements, will continue to mobilize in various ways to establish or expand abortion care, while antiabortion activists will attempt to thwart them at every turn.

More so than in the past, however, the activities of these social movements within medicine are assuming a transnational character. As patients, medications, and Internet information have crossed borders, abortion-related activism has globalized as well. Physicians affiliated with the US-based antiabortion movement engage in numerous international campaigns against abortion and contraception. One recent campaign, for example, warned of the coming "demographic winter" of too many Muslim births and not enough Caucasian ones in European countries [44].

Within pro-choice medical circles, groups such as the International Federation of Professional Abortion and Contraception Associates and the International Federation of Gynecologists and Obstetricians focus on the medical aspects of abortion care, and International Planned Parenthood Federation has long worked on issues of access as well. Global Doctors for Choice (GDC) is a particularly promising recent addition to these international efforts on behalf of safe and legal abortion. A loose confederation of physicians in various countries, GDC activities integrate medicine and advocacy directed at governmental bodies, transnational policy makers, and organized medical institutions. In a number of countries where abortion is contested or remains illegal, GDC-affiliated physicians have engaged in various advocacy efforts: they testified on human rights issues at international tribunals (Ireland); participated in coalitions that organized successfully for liberalized abortion laws (Mexico City; Portugal); and worked on innovative ways to reduce mortality from unsafe abortion (e.g., the "harm reduction model" pioneered by doctors in Uruguay) (Chavkin, personal communication, 2008). Many of the physicians who participate in these transnational movements speak of gaining a sense of community and solidarity with colleagues worldwide, which is no small benefit for those who work in such a contested area of medicine.

In sum, significant obstacles to abortion access, safety, and services persist in many parts of the world. Nonetheless, the steadfast commitment of pro-choice physicians and other clinicians offers hope that the goal of normalizing abortion as part of women's reproductive health care is gradually drawing closer.

References

1 Devereux G. A typological study of abortion in 350 primitive, ancient and pre-industrial societies. In: Rosen H, ed. *Therapeutic Abortion*. Julian Press, New York, 1954: 98.

2 Riddle JM. *Contraception and Abortion from the Ancient World to the Renaissance*. Harvard University, Cambridge (MA), 1992.

3 Petchesky R. *Abortion and Women's Choice: The State, Sexuality and Reproductive Freedom*. Northeastern University, Boston, 1990, 48–50.

4 Himes NE. *Medical History of Contraception*. Gamut Press, New York, 1936.

5 Luker K. *Abortion and the Politics of Motherhood*. University of California, Berkeley, 1984.

6 Gordon L. *The Moral Property of Women: A History of Birth Control Politics in America*. University of Illinois, Urbana, 2002.

7 David H. Abortion policies. In: Hodgson JE, ed. *Abortion and Sterilization: Medical and Social Aspects*. Academic Press, London, 1981: 1–38.

8 Potts M, Diggory P, Peel J. *Abortion*. Cambridge University, Cambridge (MA), 1977.

9 Mohr J. *Abortion in America: The Origins and Evolution of National Policy, 1800–1900*. Oxford University, New York, 1978.

10 Joffe C. *Doctors of Conscience: The Struggle to Provide Abortion Before and After Roe v. Wade*. Beacon Press, Boston, 1995.

11 Solinger R. *The Abortionist: A Woman Against the Law*. Free Press, New York, 1994.

12 American Medical Association, Council on Scientific Affairs. Induced termination of pregnancy before and after *Roe v. Wade*: trends in the mortality and morbidity of women. *JAMA* 1992; **268**: 3231–3239.

13 Novac F. Experience with suction curettage. In: Hall R, ed. *Abortion in a Changing World*. Colombia University, New York, 1970: 74–84.

14 World Health Organization. *Safe Abortion: Technical and Policy Guidance for Health Systems*. World Health Organization, Geneva, 2003.

15 Joffe C. *The Regulation of Sexuality: Experiences of Family Planning Workers*. Temple University, Philadelphia, 1986.

16 Jones R, Zolna M, Henshaw S, Finer L. Abortion in the United States: incidence and access to services, 2005. *Perspect Sex Reprod Health* 2008; **40**: 6–16.

17 Harper C, Blanchard K, Grossman D, Henderson J, Darney P. Reducing maternal mortality due to elective abortion: potential impact of misoprostol in low-resource settings. *Int J Gynaecol Obstet* 2007; **98**, 66–69.

18 Boland R, Katzive L. Developments in laws on induced abortion: 1998–2007. *Int Fam Plann Perspect* 2008; **34**, 110–120.

19 Githens M. Reproductive rights and the struggle with change in Eastern Europe. In: Githens M, Stetson DM, eds. *Abortion Politics: Public Policy in Cross-Cultural Perspective*. Routledge, New York, 1996: 55–70.

20 Abortion Review [Online]. 2007 May 24 [cited 2008 6 August]; Warwick, UK: British Pregnancy Advisory Service. Ireland's Miss D: a bizarre dispute. Available from: URL: http://www.abortionreview.org/index.php/site/article/186/

21 Gal S, Kligman G. *Reproducing Gender: Politics, Publics and Everyday Life After Socialism*. Princeton University, Princeton (NJ), 2000.

22 Polish Federation for Women and Family Planning. *Contemporary Women's Hell: Polish Women's Stories*. Polish Federation for Women and Family Planning, Warsaw, 2005.

23 David HP, Titkow A. Abortion and women's rights in Poland, 1994. *Stud Fam Plann* 1994; **25**: 239–242.

24 Morgentaler H. My struggle for abortion rights in Canada. *Relig Humanism* 1992; **26**: 159–175.

25 Morton F. Morgentaler v. Borowski*: Abortion, the Charter, and the Courts*. McClelland and Stewart, Toronto, 1992.

26 Joffe C, Weitz T, Stacey C. Uneasy allies: pro-choice physicians, feminist health activists and the struggle for abortion rights. In: Brown P, Zavestocki S, eds. *Social Movements in Health*. Blackwell, Oxford, 2005: 94–115.

27 National Abortion Federation [Online]. 2008 Mar 31 [cited 2008 August 8]; Washington (DC): National Abortion Federation; 2008. NAF violence and disruption statistics: incidents of violence and disruption against abortion providers in the U.S. and Canada. Available from: URL: http://www.prochoice.org/pubs_research/publications/downloads/about_abortion/violence_statistics.pdf

28 Joffe C. The abortion procedure ban: Bush's gift to his base. *Dissent* Fall 2007; 57–61.

29 DiMauro D, Joffe C. The religious right and the reshaping of sexual policy: an examination of reproductive rights and sexuality education. *Sexuality Research and Social Policy* 2007; **4**: 67–92.

30 Stein R. Health workers' choice debated. *Washington Post*, 2006 January 30: Sect. A:1.

31 Donovan P. Hospital mergers and reproductive health care. *Fam Plann Perspect* 1996; **28**: 281–284.

32 Uttley L, Pawelko R. No strings attached: Public funding of religiously sponsored hospitals in the United States [Online]. New York: The Merger Watch Project; 2002 [cited 2008 June 2]. Available from: URL: http://www.mergerwatch.org/pdfs/bp_no_strings.pdf

33 Joffe C, Anderson P, Steinauer J. The crisis in abortion provision and pro-choice medical activism in the 1990s. In: Solinger R, ed. *Abortion Wars: A Half-Century of Struggle, 1950–2000*. University of California, Berkeley, 1998: 320–334.

34 Foster A, van Dis J, Steinauer J. Educational and legislative initiatives affecting residency training in abortion. *JAMA* 2003; **290**: 1777–1778.

35 Eastwood KL, Kacmar JE, Steinauer J, Weitzen S, Boardman LA. Abortion training in United States obstetrics and gynecology residency programs. *Obstet Gynecol* 2006; **108**: 303–308.

36 Dehlendorf C, Brahmi D, Engel D, Grumbach K, Joffe C, Gold M. Integrating abortion training into family medicine residency programs. *Fam Med* 2007; **39**: 337–342.

37 Fellowship in Family Planning [Online]. San Francisco: Fellowship in Family Planning [cited 2008 Aug 6]. Available from: URL: http://www.familyplanningfellowship.org/

38 United Nations Population Fund. *Programme of Action Adopted at the International Conference on Population and Development, Cairo, 5–13 September 1994*. United Nations Population Fund, New York, 1995.

39 World Conference on Women. The Beijing declaration and the platform for action on women and health. *Popul Dev Rev* 1995; **21**: 907–913.

40 International Women's Health Coalition [Online]. New York: International Women's Health Coalition; 2004. Beijing at 10; 2005 [cited 2008 Aug 6] Available from: URL: http://www.iwhc.org/index.php?option=com_content&task=view&id=3385&Itemid=824

41 Barasa L. Kenya: Awori roots for safe abortion. *The Nation* [Online]. 2007 Jun 27 [cited 2008 Aug 6]. Available from: URL: http://allafrica.com/stories/200706270082.html

42 McKinley J. Nicaragua eliminates last exception to strict antiabortion law. *New York Times* [Online]. 2006 Nov 20 [cited 2008 Jun 2]; Available from: URL: http://www.nytimes.com/2006/11/20/world/americas/20nicaragua.html.

43 Hitt J. Pro-life nation. *New York Times Magazine* [Online]. 2006 Apr 9 [cited 2008 Aug 6]. Available from: URL: http://www.nytimes.com/2006/04/09/magazine/09abortion.html

44 Joyce K. Wanted: more white babies. *The Nation* [Online]. 2008 Mar 3 [cited 2008 Aug 6]. Available from: URL: http://www.thenation.com/doc/20080303/joyce_video

2

CHAPTER 2

Unsafe abortion: The global public health challenge

Iqbal H. Shah, PhD, and Elisabeth Åhman, MA

LEARNING POINTS

- The World Health Organization defines unsafe abortion as a procedure for terminating an unintended pregnancy either by individuals without the necessary skills or in an environment that does not conform to the minimum medical standards, or both.
- Each year approximately 20 million unsafe abortions occur, primarily in developing countries, and they account for 20% of all pregnancy-related deaths and disabilities.
- A woman's likelihood of having an induced abortion is almost the same whether she lives in a developed country or a developing country. The main difference is safety: abortion is primarily safe in the former and mostly unsafe in the latter.
- Legal restrictions do not eliminate abortion; instead, they make abortions clandestine and unsafe.
- Most induced abortions follow unwanted or unintended pregnancies, which in turn often result from non-use of contraception; method or user-failure of contraception; rape; or such contextual factors as poor access to quality services and gender norms that deprive women of the right to make decisions about their sexual and reproductive health.
- Unsafe abortion and related deaths and suffering are entirely preventable.

Introduction

Each year throughout the world, approximately 205 million women become pregnant and some 133 million of them deliver live-born infants [1]. Among the remaining 72 million pregnancies, 30 million end in stillbirth or spontaneous abortion and 42 million end in induced abortion. An estimated 22 million induced abortions occur within the national legal systems; another 20 million take place outside this context and by unsafe methods or in suboptimal or unsafe circumstances.

When faced with unwanted or unintended pregnancies, women resort to induced abortion irrespective of legal restrictions. In contrast to other medical conditions, ideologies and laws restrict access to safe abortion services, especially in developing countries and among the poorest of poor countries. Information on the incidence of induced abortion, whether legal and safe or illegal and unsafe, is crucial for identifying policy and programmatic needs aimed at reducing unintended pregnancy and addressing its consequences. Understanding the magnitude of unsafe abortion and related mortality and morbidity is critical to addressing this major yet much neglected public health problem.

This chapter focuses on induced unsafe abortions, which carry greater risks than those performed under legal conditions. It provides the latest estimates of the magnitude of the problem including rates, trends, and differentials in unsafe abortion. The links between contraceptive prevalence, unmet need for family planning, and unsafe abortion are described, as well as the mortality and morbidity as a result of unsafe abortion. The chapter concentrates on developing countries, where 97% of unsafe abortions and nearly all related deaths occur. Finally, the chapter describes the international discourse on addressing unsafe abortion.

Definitions and context

The World Health Organization (WHO) defines *unsafe abortion* as a procedure for terminating an unintended pregnancy either by individuals without the necessary skills or in an environment that does not conform to the minimum medical standards, or both [2]. With the advent and expanding use of early medical abortion, this definition may need to be

Management of Unintended and Abnormal Pregnancy, 1st edition. By M Paul, ES Lichtenberg, L Borgatta, DA Grimes, PG Stubblefield, MD Creinin
 ISBN: 9781405176965.

modified to incorporate standards appropriate to these less technical methods of pregnancy termination.

Induced abortions may take place within or outside of the prevailing legal framework. When performed within the legal framework, the safety of the procedure depends on the requirements of the law and the resources and medical skills available. In countries that lack human and technical resources, abortions may not be sufficiently safe by international standards although they meet the legal and medical requirements of the country. Legal authorization is, therefore, a necessary but insufficient remedy for unsafe abortion.

Induced abortions outside of the legal framework are frequently performed by unqualified and unskilled providers, or are self-induced; such abortions often take place in unhygienic conditions and involve dangerous methods or incorrect administration of medications. Even when performed by a medical practitioner, a clandestine abortion generally carries additional risk: medical backup is not immediately available in an emergency; the woman may not receive appropriate postabortion attention and care; and, if complications occur, the woman may hesitate to seek care. The risk of unsafe abortion differs by the skills of the provider and the methods used, but it is also linked to the de facto application of the law [3].

More than 60% of the world's population lives in countries where induced abortion is allowed for a wide range of reasons [3]. Nevertheless, some of these countries have a high incidence of unsafe abortion. Current estimates indicate that only 38% of women aged 15 to 44 years live in countries where abortion is legally available and where no evidence of unsafe abortion exists. A number of countries allow abortion on broad grounds, but unsafe abortions still occur outside the legal framework. Abortion has been, for example, legal on request in India since 1972; however, many women are unaware that safe and legal abortion is available. Even those who know of its legality may not have access to safe abortion because of poor quality of services and/or economic and social constraints. Reports also suggest that unsafe abortions may be increasing in several of the newly independent states, formerly part of Russia, as a result of increased fees and fewer services for legal abortions.

Global and regional levels and trends of induced abortion

In 2003, about 3% of all women of reproductive age worldwide had an induced abortion. Overall, the number of induced abortions declined from 46 million in 1995 to 42 million in 2003 (Table 2.1). Most of the decline occurred in developed countries (10.0 million to 6.6 million), with little change evident in developing countries (35.5 million to 35 million).

Induced abortion rates are, however, surprisingly similar across regions (Table 2.1). A woman's likelihood of having an induced abortion is almost the same whether she lives in a developed country (26 per 1,000) or a developing country (29 per 1,000). The main difference is safety: abortion is primarily safe in the former and mostly unsafe in the latter. Latin America, which has some of the world's most restrictive induced abortion laws, has the highest abortion rate (31 per 1,000), but other regions have similar rates: Africa and Asia (29), Europe (28) and North America (21), and Oceania (17).

Induced abortion rates vary by subregion, however (Table 2.2). Eastern Africa and South-East Asia show a rate of 39 per 1,000 women, while other subregions in Africa and Asia

Table 2.1 Global and regional estimated number of all (safe and unsafe) induced abortions and abortion rates, 2003 and 1995.

	Number of abortions (millions)		Induced abortion rate[a]	
	2003	1995	2003	1995
World	41.6	45.6	29	35
Developed countries[b]	6.6	10.0	26	39
Excluding Eastern Europe	*3.5*	*3.8*	*19*	*20*
Developing countries[b]	35.0	35.5	29	34
Excluding China	*26.4*	*24.9*	*30*	*33*
Africa	5.6	5.0	29	33
Asia	25.9	26.8	29	33
Europe	4.3	7.7	28	48
Latin America	4.1	4.2	31	37
North America	1.5	1.5	21	22
Oceania	0.1	0.1	17	21

[a] Induced abortions per 1,000 women aged 15 to 44 years.

[b] Developed regions were defined to include Europe, North America, Australia, Japan, and New Zealand; all others were classified as developing. Australia, Japan, and New Zealand are nevertheless included in their respective regions.

Table 2.2 Estimated number of safe and unsafe induced abortions and abortion rates by region and subregion, 2003[a].

Region and Subregion	Number of abortions (millions)			Abortion rate[b]		
	Total	Safe	Unsafe	Total	Safe	Unsafe
World	41.6	21.9	19.7	29	15	14
Developed countries[a]	6.6	6.1	0.5	26	24	2
Developing countries	35.0	15.8	19.2	29	13	16
Africa	5.6	0.1	5.5	29	∧∧	29
Eastern Africa	2.3	∧	2.3	39	∧∧	39
Middle Africa	0.6	∧	0.6	26	∧∧	26
Northern Africa	1.0	∧	1.0	22	∧∧	22
Southern Africa	0.3	0.1	0.2	24	5	18
Western Africa	1.5	∧	1.5	27	∧∧	28
Asia[a]	25.6	15.8	9.8	29	18	11
Eastern Asia[a]	9.7	9.7	∧	29	29	∧∧
South-Central Asia	9.6	3.3	6.3	27	9	18
South-East Asia	5.2	2.1	3.1	39	16	23
Western Asia	1.2	0.8	0.4	24	16	8
Europe	4.3	3.9	0.5	28	25	3
Eastern Europe	3.0	2.7	0.4	44	39	5
Northern Europe	0.3	0.3	∧	17	17	∧∧
Southern Europe	0.6	0.5	0.1	18	15	3
Western Europe	0.4	0.4	∧	12	12	∧∧
Latin America and the Caribbean	4.1	0.2	3.9	31	1	29
Caribbean	0.3	0.2	0.1	35	19	16
Central America	0.9	∧	0.9	25	∧∧	25
South America	2.9	∧	2.9	33	∧∧	33
North America	1.5	1.5	∧	21	21	∧∧
Oceania[a]	0.02	∧	0.02	11	∧∧	11

[a] Japan, Australia, and New Zealand have been excluded from the regional estimates, but are included in the total for developed countries. Numbers, rates, and ratios of Asia, Eastern Asia, and Oceania therefore show results only including developing countries of those regions. The calculations of these regions differ from Table 2.1.

[b] Abortions per 1,000 women aged 15 to 44 years.

∧ Less than 0.05.

∧∧ Less than 0.5.

exhibit rates between 22 and 28 per 1,000. The Caribbean and South America subregions have high rates of 35 and 33 per 1,000. However, the highest abortion rate of all subregions remains in Eastern Europe (44 per 1,000), while the lowest rate is found in the other subregions of Europe (12 to 18 per 1,000). In Europe, most induced abortions are safe and legal and the abortion incidence has been low for decades. The abortion rate has fallen substantially in recent years in Eastern Europe, as contraceptives have become increasingly available. Nevertheless, women continue to rely on induced abortion to regulate fertility to a greater extent in this region than elsewhere.

The distinction among regions becomes more marked when one compares the incidence and proportion of safe and unsafe abortions. In 2003, 48% of all abortions worldwide were unsafe, and more than 97% of these unsafe abortions occurred in developing countries. In Africa and Latin America abortions are almost exclusively unsafe; so are almost 40% of abortions in Asia. Unsafe abortion is rare in Europe. Legal restrictions on abortions have little effect on women's propensity to terminate an unintended pregnancy. Restrictions do, however, lead to clandestine abortions, which, in turn, injure and kill many women.

Estimating unsafe abortions

Since 1990, WHO has been collecting data and estimating the incidence of unsafe abortion [4–7] (Box A). However, estimating the magnitude of unsafe abortion is complex for several reasons. Induced abortion is generally stigmatized and frequently censured by religious teaching or ideologies, which makes women reluctant to admit to having had an induced abortion. Surveys show that underreporting occurs even where abortion is legal [8–12]. This problem is exacerbated in settings where induced abortion is restricted and largely inaccessible, or legal but difficult to obtain. Little information is available on abortion practice in these circumstances, and abortions tend to be unreported or vastly underreported. Moreover, clandestine induced abortions may be misreported as spontaneous abortion (miscarriage) [13,14]. The language used to describe induced abortion reflects this ambivalence: terms include "induced miscarriage" (*fausse couche provoquée*) [15], "menstrual regulation," and "regulation of a delayed or suspended menstruation [16]." In spite of these challenges, estimates of the frequency of unsafe abortion can be made mainly by using hospital data on abortion complications or abortion data from surveys and validated against the legal context of induced abortion, contraceptive prevalence, and total fertility rate (the average number of children a woman is likely to have by the end of her reproductive years).

Globally, WHO estimates that some 19 to 20 million unsafe abortions occurred each year between 1993 and 2003 [7]. This figure has remained relatively constant despite an increase in contraceptive prevalence during the same period. Although the transition to low fertility with smaller families has become a norm in most countries, family planning has not been able to entirely meet the need of couples to regulate fertility.

Recently published research from sub-Saharan Africa, Southern Asia, and Latin America has improved the precision of the estimates. Although the estimate of the global number of unsafe abortions is close to earlier figures, the regional estimates have changed. For example, the recent estimates for Africa are higher than the previous cautious estimates, better reflecting the actual situation and suggesting that earlier estimates were too low.

Regional differentials in unsafe abortion

Globally, an estimated 1 in 10 pregnancies ended in an unsafe abortion in 2003, giving a ratio of 1 unsafe abortion to about 7 live births [7] (Table 2.3). The unsafe abortion rates or ratios for each region are estimated by dividing the number of unsafe abortions in that region by the regional number of all women aged 15 to 44 years or by the regional number of live births, respectively, in the same reference year (Box A).

Table 2.3 provides the average rates and ratios, that is, relative to women and to births of *all* countries of a subregion, region, or globally, whether unsafe abortion is known to take place (e.g., Kenya) or not (e.g., China) or takes place in parallel to abortions within the framework of the law (e.g., India). However, measures that consider only those countries with reported incidence of unsafe abortion describe its magnitude more adequately. This approach correctly links both numerator (unsafe abortions) and denominator (number of women or number of live births) to the same set of countries in the region or globally. Therefore, Table 2.3 also reports, in parentheses, rates and ratios restricted to *affected* countries (i.e., those with evidence of unsafe abortion), with the number of unsafe abortions, women aged 15 to 44 years and live births referring to the same set of countries. The resultant rates and ratios are higher than those using all countries, better illustrating the

Table 2.3 Global and regional estimates of annual incidence of unsafe abortion in 2003 (Rates and ratios are calculated for all countries and, in parentheses, only for countries with evidence of unsafe abortion.[a])

	Number rounded[b]	Incidence rate per 1000 women aged *15 to 44* years	Incidence ratio per *100* live births
World	19 700 000	14 (22)	15 (20)
Developed countries[c]	500 000	2 (6)	3 (13)
Developing countries	19 200 000	16 (24)	16 (20)
Least developed countries	4 000 000	25	15
Other developing countries	15 300 000	15 (23)	17 (22)
Sub-Saharan Africa	4 700 000	31	16
Africa	5 500 000	29	17
Eastern Africa	2 300 000	39	20
Middle Africa	600 000	26	12
Northern Africa	1 000 000	22 (23)	20 (21)
Southern Africa	200 000	18	18
Western Africa	1 500 000	28	14
Asia[c]	9 800 000	11 (20)	13 (18)
Eastern Asia[c]	°	°	°
South-Central Asia	6 300 000	18	16
South-East Asia	3 100 000	23 (27)	27 (31)
Western Asia	400 000	8 (13)	7 (10)
Europe	500 000	3 (6)	6 (13)
Eastern Europe	400 000	5 (6)	13 (14)
Northern Europe	2 000	0.1 (1)	0.1 (2)
Southern Europe	100 000	3 (6)	7 (14)
Western Europe	°	°	°
Latin America and the Caribbean	3 900 000	29 (30)	33 (34)
Caribbean	100 000	16 (28)	19 (26)
Central America	900 000	25	26
South America	2 900 000	33	38
North America	°	°	°
Oceania[c]	20 000	11	8

[a] Rates, ratios, and percentages are calculated for all countries of each region, except Asia (which excludes Japan) and Oceania (which excludes Australia and New Zealand). Rates, ratios, and percentages in parentheses were calculated exclusively for countries with evidence of unsafe abortion. Where the difference between the two calculations was less than one percentage point, only one figure is shown.

[b] Figures may not exactly add up to totals because of rounding.

[c] Japan, Australia, and New Zealand have been excluded from the regional estimates, but are included in the total for developed countries.

° No estimates are shown for regions where the incidence is negligible.

Box A Measurement Indicators

Absolute numbers of unsafe abortions cannot be compared meaningfully across different regions and subregions or over time because of differing size of populations at risk. The choice of a particular descriptive measure is dictated by the purpose of presentation and discussion. The following standardized measures are often used for comparison.

Unsafe abortion rate: The estimated annual number of unsafe abortions per 1,000 women aged 15 to 44 years. This summary measure describes the level (new cases) of unsafe abortion in a given population in a specified time interval. It shows how many women of reproductive age (15 to 44 years) have an unsafe abortion per 1,000 in the same age range during a particular year. Further decomposition of this overall rate by 5-year age-groups allows for ascertainment of age patterns of unsafe abortion as well as the indicator *total unsafe abortion rate*, which describes the average number of unsafe abortions a woman is likely to experience by the end of her reproductive life (generally assumed at 45 years) if the current age-specific rates persist.

Unsafe abortion ratio: The estimated annual number of unsafe abortions per 100 live births. The indicator shows the relative propensity of unsafe abortions compared to live births in a population. By extension, substituting live birth as a proxy for pregnancy, this measure roughly indicates the likelihood that a pregnancy will end in unsafe abortion rather than a live birth.

Unsafe abortion mortality ratio: The estimated annual number of maternal deaths due to unsafe abortion per 100,000 live births. This indicator is a subset of the maternal mortality ratio (number of maternal deaths per 100,000 live births) and measures the risk of a woman dying due to unsafe abortion relative to 100,000 live births.

Unsafe abortion case-fatality rate: This measure refers to the estimated number of maternal deaths per 100,000 unsafe abortion procedures; it is sometimes expressed per 100 procedures. The case-fatality rate shows the mortality risk associated with unsafe abortion.

Percentage of maternal deaths due to unsafe abortion: This measure indicates the estimated number of unsafe abortion deaths per 100 maternal deaths. When maternal mortality is relatively low and where other causes of maternal death have already been substantially reduced, a small number of unsafe abortion deaths may account for a significant percentage of maternal deaths. This measure is, therefore, not particularly suitable for comparison, especially across countries with different levels of maternal mortality.

severity of the public health problem in the countries of a region where unsafe abortions occur.

Unsafe abortion rates close to 30 per 1,000 women aged 15 to 44 years are seen in both Africa and Latin America and the Caribbean; however, because of the higher numbers of births, the unsafe abortion ratio for Africa is only half that for Latin America (Table 2.3). According to recent estimates, the number of unsafe abortions in South America may have reached a peak and begun to decline. If Cuba, where abortion is legally available upon request, is excluded from the calculation, the rate for the Caribbean falls between that for Central America (25 per 1,000) and South America (33 per 1,000). The range of estimates for Africa is wide: eastern Africa has the highest rate of any subregion, at 39 per 1,000, whereas South Africa has among the lowest, at 18 per 1,000 (not counting legal abortions of 5 per 1,000 women). The 1996 law liberalizing abortion in South Africa has clearly reduced the number of unsafe abortions in the subregion. Half of all unsafe abortions take place in Asia; however, rates and ratios are generally lower. Only in South-East Asia are rates and ratios similar to those of Africa and Latin America. South-Central Asia has the highest number of unsafe abortions of any subregion, owing to the sheer size of its population.

The differences in the estimates based on countries *at risk* as compared to all countries in the region (Table 2.3) are particularly marked for Asia. When the populous region of eastern Asia (with abortion available upon request) is excluded from the denominator, the rate rises from 11 to 20 unsafe abortions per 1,000 women aged 15 to 44 years. This pattern is also apparent for the Caribbean (28 vs. 16 per 1,000) when Cuba is excluded. On the other hand, the exclusion of Cuba makes little difference for the rates for Latin America as a whole (30 vs. 29 per 1,000). The differences in South-East Asia (27 vs. 23 per 1,000) and western Asia (13 vs. 8 per 1,000) are the result of excluding Singapore and Vietnam, and Turkey, respectively, from the calculations.

The ratio of unsafe abortion generally ranges from 10 to 20 unsafe abortions per 100 births (Table 2.3). However, when declining fertility results in fewer and fewer births without an accompanying major shift from unsafe abortion to modern contraceptive uptake, ratios become high. Also, where the motivation is stronger to end an unwanted or unintended pregnancy through abortion rather than unwanted birth, the ratio would be higher. Such is the case in South America (38 per 100), Central America (26 per 100), the Caribbean (26 per 100 for all countries vs. 19 per 100 for countries at risk) and South-East Asia (31 per 100 for all countries vs. 27 per 100 for countries at risk).

The global figures in Table 2.3 show the full effect of restricting the analysis appropriately only to the relevant countries with evidence of unsafe abortion. The 19.7 million unsafe abortions that occurred worldwide in 2003 correspond to an unsafe abortion rate of 22 per 1,000 women aged 15 to 44 years when only countries with unsafe abortion are considered versus 14 per 1,000 when the rate is based on all countries. The respective change in the abortion ratio is 20 versus 15 per 100 live births. For developing countries, the rate increases from 16 to 24 per 1,000 women of reproductive age when only countries at risk are considered. The few developing countries with liberal abortion laws and no evidence of unsafe abortion (e.g., China, Cuba, Turkey, and Singapore) all fall in the group of "other developing countries," leading to a marked difference in the incidence rate and ratio. The least developed countries show a high unsafe abortion rate of 25 per 1,000 women.

In short, the alternative figures presented in parentheses in Table 2.3 reveal where unsafe abortion is clearly a major public health concern. These figures are alarming and require urgent attention by policy makers and program managers.

Unsafe abortion trends by region

Rates and ratios of unsafe abortion vary widely by region (Fig. 2.1). For the sake of comparability with the previous estimates, the rates are for women aged 15 to 49 years and for all countries of each region. The comparisons are illustrative of trends, but 1993 estimates are less credible than 2003 estimates; for example, the latest research evidence from Africa shows higher rates of unsafe abortion than previously believed probable. The 2003 estimates more accurately reflect the current situation in Africa; thus, the increases may be less accentuated than those indicated in Fig. 2.1. Eastern, middle, and western Africa show separate patterns in a high fertility setting. The rate for eastern Africa is notable, increasing to more than 35 per 1,000 women aged 15 to 49 years as use of contraception has remained low (around 20%) in the region; the ratio has decreased because of a less significant increase in unsafe abortion than in births. Aside from Africa, the rates mostly show a slow decline while ratios have increased; however, the trend in ratios is less marked.

The interpretation of trends in unsafe abortion ratios is not straightforward because it is a composite index of the degree of motivation to terminate an unwanted pregnancy by induced abortion as well as the trends in unsafe abortion relative to live births. With the increasing motivation to regulate fertility, the unsafe abortion ratio increases.

Notwithstanding the complex relationship between trends in fertility and trends in unsafe abortion ratios, two main patterns emerge (Fig. 2.1). The first is represented by South America, and also includes Central America, the Caribbean, and South Africa, where fertility has declined to around 2.5 children per woman. South Africa nevertheless is distinct with legal, safe abortion increasingly replacing unsafe abortion. However, the case of South America is striking: the unsafe abortion ratio is still very high in spite of a rise in the prevalence of modern contraceptives from 50 to 65%, with more than half of the modern method use attributable to

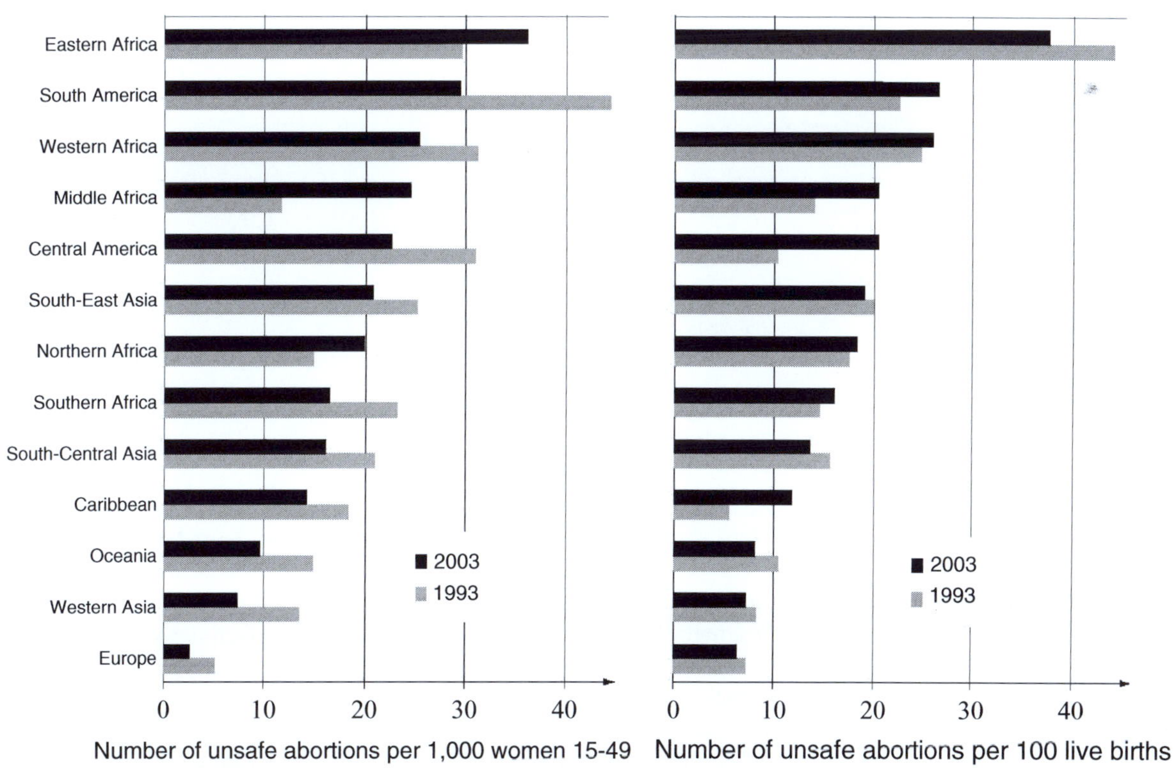

Figure 2.1 Trends in unsafe abortion rate (per 1,000 women aged 15 to 49 years) and ratio (per 100 births), 1993 and 2003 (From WHO, 1994 [4], WHO, 2007 [7].)

Table 2.4 Percent of women using a contraceptive method by type of method used in 2005 and unsafe abortion rate and ratios in 2003. (Unsafe abortion rates and ratios are calculated for all countries of each region.[a])

	Contraceptive use (% of women in union)					Unsafe abortion incidence	
	Any method	Any modern method	Reversible modern methods	Female and male sterilization	Any traditional method	Rate per 1,000 women 15 to 44	Ratio per 100 live births
World	61	54	30	24	7	14	15
Developed countries	69	55	40	15	13	2[b]	3[b]
Developing countries	59	54	28	26	6	16	16
Africa	27	20	18	2	7	29	17
Eastern Africa	22	17	15	2	5	39	20
Middle Africa	23	5	4	1	18	26	12
Northern Africa	47	42	40	2	5	22	20
Southern Africa	53	51	36	16	1	18	18
Western Africa	15	8	7	0	7	28	14
Asia	63	58	30	29	5	11[b]	13[b]
Eastern Asia	82	81	43	38	1	°	°
South-Central Asia	48	41	13	28	7	18	16
South-East Asia	57	49	42	8	8	23	27
Western Asia	47	28	25	3	19	8	7
Europe	67	49	42	7	18	3	6
Eastern Europe	61	35	33	3	26	5	13
Northern Europe	79	74	50	25	5	0	0
Southern Europe	67	46	38	8	21	3	7
Western Europe	74	71	65	6	4	°	°
Latin America and the Caribbean	71	62	29	32	9	29	33
Caribbean	60	57	35	22	4	16	19
Central America	64	55	27	28	9	25	26
South America	74	65	30	35	9	33	38
North America	76	71	33	38	5	°	°
Oceania	62	57	28	29	4	3[b]	4[b]
Australia/New Zealand	76	72	35	37	4	°	°
Melanesia	27	21	13	8	6	10	8

[a] See footnotes and text with Table 2.3.

[b] Japan, Australia, and New Zealand have been excluded from the regional estimates of unsafe abortion, but are included in the total for developed countries.

° No estimates are shown for regions where the incidence is negligible.

sterilization to terminate childbearing (Table 2.4). Nonetheless, an unmet need for spacing births appears to be met through unsafe abortion. The decline in regional numbers of births is because of the increasing tendency to regulate fertility by either contraceptive use or unsafe abortion. The speed of decline in fertility has outstripped the decline in unsafe abortion, thus accounting for relatively higher ratios.

South-East Asia and South-Central Asia (and to some extent western Asia and Oceania) represent the other pattern of moderately high fertility of around three children per woman and less than 50% modern contraceptive method use. A moderate decline in the unsafe abortion rate is noticed with little change in the ratio relative to live births. The trend in western Asia is less clear, because available data are generally limited.

Who is more likely to have an unsafe abortion?

All sexually active (including sexually coerced) fertile women face some risk of unintended pregnancy and, consequently, of induced abortion or unwanted birth. Contrary to the commonly held view, most women seeking abortion are married or live in stable unions and already have several children. Some have an induced abortion to limit family size and some to space births [17–22]. Where abortion is highly restricted, educated affluent women can often successfully obtain an abortion from a qualified provider, whereas poor women or those who have little or no education lack this option [23,24]. Policy makers and program managers often need to know if certain groups require particular attention for prevention of unplanned pregnancy and unsafe abortion. Because of the limited data, however, socioeconomic and demographic differentials in unsafe abortion by marital status, education, income, work participation, type of occupation, urban-rural place of residence, ethnicity, and parity are difficult to document.

Contraceptive methods remain inaccessible or limited in choice for married women in some countries. However, access to contraception is worse for unmarried women, particularly adolescents. The age patterns of unsafe abortion reveal these most vulnerable groups. A recent review found that two-thirds of unsafe abortions occur among women aged 15 to 30 years [25]. More importantly from a public health perspective, 2.5 million, or almost 14%, of all unsafe abortions in developing countries occur among women younger than 20 years of age.

Unsafe abortions show a distinct age pattern by region (Fig. 2.2). The proportion of women aged 15 to 19 years in Africa who have had an unsafe abortion is higher than in any other region; almost 60% of unsafe abortions in Africa occur among women younger than 25 years old, and almost 80% are among women younger than 30 years of age. This situation contrasts with Asia, where 30% of unsafe abortions occur among women less than 25 years old and 60% are among women less than 30 years old. In Latin America and the Caribbean, women aged 20 to 29 years account for more than half of all unsafe abortions, with almost 70% of unsafe abortions occurring among women younger than 30 years old, demonstrating an age pattern between those for Africa and Asia. Interventions need to be tailored to the specific regional age pattern of unsafe abortion, although prevention of unsafe abortion at all ages should remain a high priority.

Contraceptive use, unmet need for family planning, unplanned pregnancy, and unsafe abortion

Induced abortion is linked to the level and pattern of contraceptive use, unmet need for family planning, and, consequently, to the level of unplanned pregnancy. Nearly 40% of pregnancies (or about 80 million) worldwide are unplanned, the result of non-use of contraceptives, ineffective contraceptive use, method failure, or lack of pregnancy planning. Indeed, one in four of the world's 133 million births is reported to be "unwanted" or mistimed.

Unintended pregnancy and induced abortion can be reduced by expanding and improving family planning services and choices and by reaching out to communities and underserved population groups, including sexually active teenagers and unmarried women. Furthermore, any abortion, whether initiated within or outside the official health system, should be accompanied by appropriate family planning services.

Even when people are motivated to regulate their fertility, unplanned pregnancies will occur if effective contraception is largely inaccessible or not consistently or correctly used. Many married women in developing countries do not have access to the contraceptive methods of their choice [26–29]. The situation is even more difficult for unmarried women, particularly adolescents, who rarely have access to information and counseling on sexual and reproductive health and are frequently excluded from contraceptive services. An estimated 123 million women have an unmet need for family planning [30]; that is, they want to limit or space childbearing but are not using any method of contraception.

The reasons for the continuing high level of unmet need are numerous and complex. They range from such contextual factors as gender norms that deprive women

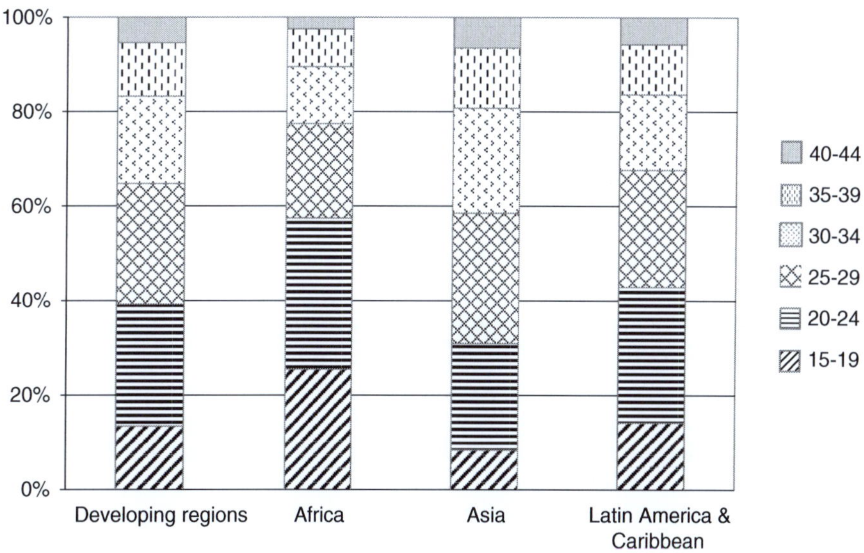

Figure 2.2 Percent distribution of unsafe abortion by age-group (years), by region (From WHO [7].)

of the decision-making power to use contraceptives and poor access to quality services to side effects and health concerns perceived or experienced by using a certain method.

As countries transition from high to low fertility, contraceptive services are often unable to meet the growing demand of couples for fertility regulation [31]. This situation results in an increased number of unplanned pregnancies, some of which are terminated by induced abortion. Also, where less effective family planning methods (e.g., withdrawal or fertility awareness-based methods) are commonly used, unplanned pregnancies are likely to result. Each year an estimated 27 million unintended pregnancies occur as a result of method failure or ineffective use; of these, about 6 million occur although the contraceptive method has been used correctly and consistently [32].

Increases in contraceptive prevalence and in the use of effective contraceptive methods are associated with a reduced incidence of induced abortion over time [33]. Using the time series data from developed countries, Marston and Cleland [34] noted that the onset of fertility decline in some countries was characterized by simultaneous increases in both abortion and contraceptive use. Contraceptive use alone was not sufficient to meet the growing demand for fertility regulation and, therefore, recourse to induced abortion increased. In other countries, abortion declined with an increase in contraceptive use. More recently, the increases in contraceptive use in Eastern Europe have resulted in falling abortion rates. Thus, with expanding and sustained high levels of contraceptive use, abortion rates fall. Current estimates of unsafe abortion and contraceptive use by fertility level in developing countries demonstrate similar trends [35].

Table 2.4 shows the percentage of women using contraceptive methods by type of method and abortion rate and ratios globally and by region. No clear pattern emerges between contraceptive prevalence and unsafe abortion rate or ratio by region because of the varying types of methods used with their associated risks of contraceptive failure and the contraceptive options available.

For example, Middle, Western, and Eastern Africa all have a contraceptive prevalence of less than 25%, with heavy reliance on traditional methods that are associated with high failure rates. In Southern and Northern Africa, contraceptive prevalence among married women is around 50% and more couples rely on reversible modern methods (36% and 43%, respectively). This difference explains the moderate abortion rates of around 20 per 1,000 women in Southern and Northern Africa, as compared to 26 to 39 per 1,000 in other parts of Africa.

In Latin America, the prevalence of modern contraceptives ranges from 57 to 65%; however, 40 to 54% of use is attributable to female sterilization (male sterilization is low). The moderate (around 30%) prevalence of reversible method use could mean that women rely on unsafe abortion for spacing purposes before achieving the desired level of fertility and opting for sterilization. Improved access to a range of birth-spacing methods could, therefore, reduce the number of unintended pregnancies and hence the need for unsafe abortion for spacing childbearing.

Use of modern contraceptive methods among married women is modest (41%) in South-Central Asia, and sterilization represents two-thirds of this use. Given the low prevalence of spacing methods, the high number of unsafe abortions in the region may be a response to the desired spacing of childbearing. Nevertheless, among Asia's subregions, South-East Asia has the highest unsafe abortion rate, at 27 per 1,000 women aged 15 to 44 years (excluding countries with no evidence of unsafe abortion); this rate is similar to those of the Caribbean and Central America. South-East Asia has a 49% prevalence of modern family planning methods, almost exclusively of reversible methods (42%). It appears, though, that abortion is used to keep fertility low.

Unsafe abortion-related mortality and morbidity

Each year more than 5 million women having an unsafe abortion (about one in four) experience complications, placing heavy demands on scarce medical resources [36]. Mortality because of unsafe abortion is estimated from the total maternal mortality level. The estimated number of maternal deaths as a result of unsafe abortion ranges between 65,000 and 70,000 deaths per year. This corresponds to one woman dying because of a botched abortion approximately every 8 minutes.

The most recent estimate (for 2003) shows that nearly all deaths attributable to unsafe abortion occur in developing countries (Table 2.5). In eastern, western, and middle Africa, where maternal mortality is high, the unsafe abortion-related mortality ratio is higher than anywhere else, double that of Asia and more than five times that of Latin America. Morbidity is an even more frequent consequence of unsafe abortion; the disease burden for Africa is exceptionally high, threatening women's lives and health and straining scarce resources.

An estimated 2,000 deaths from unsafe abortion occurred in Latin America in 2003, approximately 20 per 100,000 births. This mortality ratio is the lowest among the developing regions and is attributable to both the methods used to initiate an abortion and to the relatively well-functioning health services. The widespread use of misoprostol to induce abortion in Latin America has been associated with fewer complications and relatively safer, although illegal, induced abortion in the region [37,38]. The unsafe abortion-related mortality for Asia is two to three times that for Latin America but less than half that for Africa, reflecting the relative standards of health services and infrastructure.

Table 2.5 Global and regional estimates of mortality as a result of unsafe abortion in 2003. (Percentages and ratios are calculated for all countries of each region.[a])

	Mortality due to unsafe abortion		
	Number of deaths rounded[b]	**% of all maternal deaths**	**Mortality ratio per 100,000 live births rounded[b]**
World	66,500	13	50
Developed countries*	<60	4	°
Developing countries	66,400	13	60
Least developed countries	24,000	10	90
Other developing countries	42,400	15	50
Sub-Saharan Africa	35,600	14	120
Africa	36,000	14	110
Eastern Africa	17,600	17	160
Middle Africa	5,000	10	100
Northern Africa	1,100	11	20
Southern Africa	300	9	20
Western Africa	11,900	13	110
Asia[c]	28,400	12	40
Eastern Asia[c]	°	°	°
South-Central Asia	24,300	13	60
South-East Asia	3,200	14	30
Western Asia	1,000	11	20
Europe	<60	6	1
Eastern Europe	<50	6	2
Northern Europe	°	3	°
Southern Europe	°	11	1
Western Europe	°	°	°
Latin America and the Caribbean	2,000	11	20
Caribbean	200	12	30
Central America	300	11	10
South America	1,400	11	20
North America	°	°	°
Oceania[c]	<100	10	20

[a] See footnotes and text with Table 2.3.
[b] Figures may not exactly add up to totals because of rounding.
[c] Japan, Australia, and New Zealand have been excluded from the regional estimates of unsafe abortion, but are included in the total for developed countries.
° No estimates are shown for regions where the incidence is negligible.

Table 2.6 Case-fatality rate of unsafe abortion per 100,000 unsafe abortion procedures, 2003.

	Estimated number of deaths per 100,000 unsafe abortion procedures (rounded)
World	300
Developed countries	10
USA	<1
Developing countries	350
Least developed countries	600
Other developing countries	300
Sub-Saharan Africa	750
Africa	650
Asia	300
Latin America and the Caribbean	50
Oceania	300

Case fatality rates by region

The estimated case-fatality rates of unsafe abortion [7] range from a high of 750 per 100,000 procedures in sub-Saharan Africa to 10 in developed regions, with an average of 350 for developing regions (Table 2.6). The risk of death as a result of unsafe abortion procedures is the highest in Africa at 650 per 100,000, followed by Asia at 300 per 100,000. The global case-fatality rate associated with unsafe abortion is some 550 times higher than the rate associated with legal and safe induced abortions in the USA (0.7 per 100,000 procedures) [39]; in sub-Saharan Africa, the rate is more than 1,000 times higher.

The high risk of death from unsafe abortion in Africa (Table 2.6 and Fig. 2.3) reflects the procedures used and the poor availability, accessibility, and quality of services for management of complications. In middle, western, and eastern Africa, dangerous abortion methods, failing infrastructure, and poor public health facilities result in estimated case-fatality rates of around 800 per 100,000 procedures. In contrast, South and Central America have case-fatality rates lower than 100 per 100,000 as a result of better infrastructures for health services and wider use of misoprostol [37,38]. For Southern and Northern Africa and South-East Asia, the rates appear low but are still almost 200 times higher than that associated with a legal and safe abortion in the USA.

The global health burden of unsafe abortion: death and disability

For each woman who dies, many others suffer infections, bleeding, damage to bowel and reproductive tract organs, and secondary infertility. Investigators recently measured the disease burden using disability-adjusted life years (DALYs) (Åhman E, Mathers CD, Shah IH (2005) *Death and Disability Due to Unsafe Abortion: Global and Regional Estimates* [unpublished]). The DALY combines years of life lost from premature death and years of life lived with disabilities in a single indicator, allowing assessment of the total loss of health from different causes. One lost DALY can be thought of as one lost year of "healthy" life. The burden of disease is evident in the gap between the current health of a population and an ideal situation where everyone in the population lives to old age in full health [40]. DALYs for a disease or health condition are calculated as the sum of the years of life lost as a result of premature mortality (YLL) in

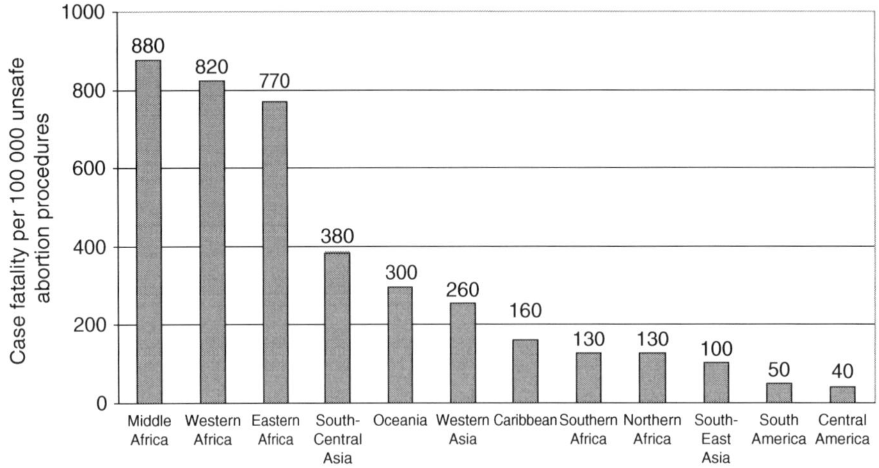

Figure 2.3 Number of deaths as a result of unsafe abortion per 100,000 unsafe abortion procedures, by subregion, 2003.

the population and the equivalent healthy years lost as a result of disability (YLD) for incident cases.

Although unsafe abortion accounts for 13% of maternal deaths, it causes one-fifth of the total burden of the consequence of pregnancy and childbirth complications (Fig. 2.4). The DALY of 100 per 1,000 unsafe abortions in Latin America and the Caribbean is estimated to be the lowest among developing regions (Table 2.7). The DALYs in Africa, Asia, and Oceania are six times, four times, and three times higher, respectively. These disparities reflect the risks because of abortion methods as well as access to health services in case of complications.

The most common causes for women to seek hospital care following an unsafe abortion are sepsis, hemorrhage, and trauma. However, for every woman who seeks medical care, many more have chronic pelvic or back pain and other complications. Women may attempt to remedy these problems by homemade cures or by consulting a pharmacist or an untrained person. Chronic or repeat infection as well as uterine trauma may lead to secondary infertility. In some cases, an emergency hysterectomy is needed to save the woman's life. Using the methodology outlined in the Global Burden of Disease series [41], each year 1.7 million women are estimated to experience secondary infertility, while more than 3 million are estimated to suffer from pelvic inflammatory disease or reproductive tract infections as a consequence of unsafe abortion.

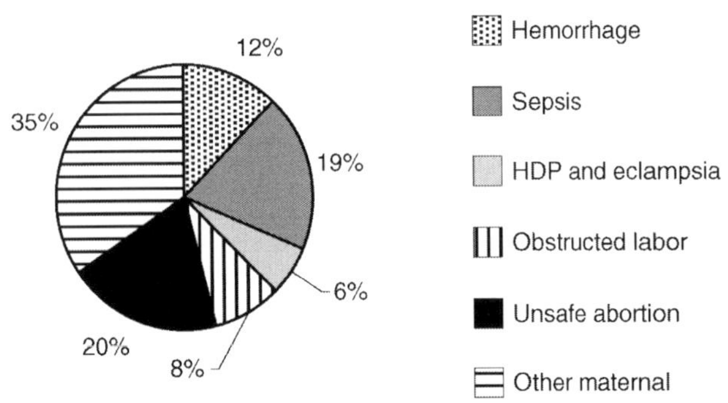

Figure 2.4 Percentage distribution of Disability-Adjusted-Life-Years (DALYs) by pregnancy and childbirth related causes, 2002. *Note:* "Other maternal" includes direct obstetric causes of death and sequelae not among the five mentioned and all indirect obstetric causes of sequelae and death. HDP = hypertensive disorders of pregnancy.

Legal context of abortion

Legal restrictions do not eliminate abortion; instead, they make abortions clandestine and unsafe. Unsafe abortion carries high risk of death and disability. Unsafe abortion and related mortality are consistently higher in countries with increasing restrictions on legal abortion [3].

Abortion is permitted on several grounds in most countries. However, in five countries (Holy See, Chile, El Salvador, Malta, and Nicaragua) induced abortion is not permitted even to save the life of the woman [42]. While 67% of developed countries permit abortion on request, the corresponding figure is 15% for developing countries

Table 2.7 Disability-Adjusted Life Years (DALYs) per 1,000 unsafe abortions by major geographical regions, 2002.

	DALYs per 1000 abortions (rounded)
World	350
Developed countries	100
Developing countries	400
Sub-Saharan Africa	650
Africa	550
Asia	400
Latin America and the Caribbean	100
Oceania	300

Table 2.8 Grounds on which abortion is permitted (United Nations [42].)

	To save the woman's life	To preserve physical health	To preserve mental health	Rape or incest	Fetal impairment	Economic or social reasons	On request
				% of countries			
All countries	97	67	64	48	45	34	28
Developed countries	96	88	86	84	84	78	67
Developing countries	97	60	57	37	32	19	15
				% of population			
World population	99	78	75	72	64	61	40

(Table 2.8). Abortion is permitted solely to save the woman's life in 22 countries in Africa, 15 in Asia, 3 in Europe, 11 in Latin America, and 7 in Oceania. During the last decade, abortion laws have been liberalized in Guyana, South Africa, Nepal, and most recently, in Mexico City. The positive health impact of these changes has been documented for South Africa [43]. In Benin, Bhutan, Burkina Faso, Chad, Colombia, Ethiopia, Guinea, Mali, Saint Lucia, Swaziland, and Togo, grounds for legal abortion have been expanded, although abortion is not permitted on request.

The global discourse addressing unsafe abortion

As early as 1967, the World Health Assembly identified unsafe abortion as a serious public health problem [44]. The 1994 International Conference on Population and Development (ICPD) highlighted the concept of reproductive rights and established goals and targets, including universal access to reproductive health (services) by 2015. The ICPD Programme of Action called for all parties to address the health impact of unsafe abortion and improve family planning services:

> In circumstances where abortion is not against the law, such abortion should be safe. In all cases, women should have access to quality services for management of complications arising from abortion. Postabortion counselling, education, and family planning services should be offered promptly, which will also help to avoid repeat abortion [45].

In June to July 1999, the Special Session of the United Nations General Assembly urged access to safe abortion services:

> In circumstances where abortion is not against the law, health systems should train and equip health service providers and should take other measures to ensure such abortion is safe and accessible [46].

In 2004, the World Health Assembly approved the Reproductive Health Strategy of the World Health Organization, noting:

> As a preventable cause of maternal mortality and morbidity, unsafe abortion must be dealt with as part of the Millennium Development Goal on improving maternal health and other international development goals and targets [47].

In September 2006, the Special Session of the African Union Conference of Ministers of Health [48] held in Maputo agreed on a Plan of Action to:

- enact policies and legal frameworks to reduce the incidence of unsafe abortion
- prepare and implement national action plans to reduce the incidence of unwanted pregnancies and unsafe abortion
- provide safe abortion services to the fullest extent of the law
- educate communities on available safe abortion services as allowed by national laws
- train health providers in preventing and managing unsafe abortion.

Consensus is established on a number of points. For example, unsafe abortion is generally accepted as being an important and preventable cause of maternal death. Most international resolutions signed by countries note the agreement that safe abortion services should be provided to the full extent of the law and that postabortion care should be provided in all cases. Expansion of access to family planning services for prevention of unsafe abortion is universally supported. However, reducing legal restrictions on access to safe abortion services remains a highly contentious issue.

To identify reducing maternal mortality as a public health priority while failing to prevent unsafe abortion that kills tens of thousands of women each year is paradoxical. Although much emphasis is placed on providing postabortion care, too little is directed toward preventing unwanted pregnancy and unsafe abortion. The public health impact of unsafe abortion has long been recognized, but more needs to be done to remove the strategic and policy barriers to saving women's lives.

Conclusion

Induced abortion is arguably the most important human rights and equity issue of our time. Induced abortion exists in all parts of the world. Legal restrictions, mostly in developing countries, make abortion clandestine. The persistence of unsafe abortion continues to exert a heavy toll on women's lives, especially in poor regions of the world and among the most disadvantaged. In sub-Saharan Africa, the health burden of unsafe abortion is exceptionally high when compared to any other region. Sub-Saharan Africa is also the region with the highest levels of maternal mortality.

To meet the Millennium Development Goal to improve maternal health, countries and the global community will have to aggressively address women's family planning needs, provide services to manage complications arising from unsafe abortion, and provide postabortion care as agreed at the 1994 ICPD in Cairo. Governments will have to reduce the burden of unintended pregnancy through expanded and improved family planning services and social policies that promote equity and empowerment for women. Abortion laws and policies should reflect our current commitment to women's health and well-being rather than criminal codes and punitive measures left over from past centuries. Prevention of unwanted pregnancies must be given highest priority, and all attempts should be made to eliminate the need for unsafe abortion. Women seeking abortion deserve ready access to compassionate counseling, skilled medical care, family planning services, and prompt management of complications should they occur.

Acknowledgment

The views expressed are those of the authors and may not necessarily reflect those of the Special Programme of Research, Development, and Research Training in Human Reproduction (HRP) or of its cosponsors UNDP/UNFPA/WHO/World Bank.

References

1 Sedgh G, Singh S, Henshaw S, Åhman E, Shah I. Induced abortion: estimated rates and trends worldwide. *Lancet* 2007; **370**: 1338–1345.

2 World Health Organization. *The Prevention and Management of Unsafe Abortion: Report of a Technical Working Group*. World Health Organization, Geneva, 1992.

3 Berer M. National laws and unsafe abortion: the parameters of change. Abortion law, policy, and practice in transition. *Reprod Health Matters* 2004; **12**: 1–8.

4 World Health Organization. *Abortion: A Tabulation of Available Data on the Frequency and Mortality of Unsafe Abortion*, 2nd edition. World Health Organization, Geneva, 1994.

5 World Health Organization. *Unsafe Abortion: Global and Regional Estimates of Incidence of and Mortality due to Unsafe Abortion with a Listing of Available Country Data*, 3rd edition. World Health Organization, Geneva, 1998.

6 World Health Organization. *Unsafe Abortion: Global and Regional Estimates of the Incidence of Unsafe Abortion and Associated Mortality in 2000*, 4th edition. World Health Organization, Geneva, 2004.

7 World Health Organization. *Unsafe Abortion: Global and Regional Estimates of the Incidence of Unsafe Abortion and Associated Mortality in 2000*, 5th edition. World Health Organization, Geneva, 2007.

8 Wilcox AJ, Horney LF. Accuracy of spontaneous abortion recall. *Am J Epidemiol* 1984; **120**: 727–733.

9 Udry RJ, Gaughan M, Schwingl PJ, van den Berg BJ. A medical record linkage analysis of abortion underreporting. *Fam Plann Perspect* 1996; **28**: 228–231.

10 Jones EF, Forrest JD. Underreporting of abortion in surveys of U.S. women: 1976 to 1988. *Demography* 1992; **29**: 113–126.

11 Anderson BA, Katus K, Puur A, Silver BD. The validity of survey responses on abortion: evidence from Estonia. *Demography* 1994 ; **31**: 115–132.

12 Lindefors-Harris BM, Eklund G, Adami HO, Meirik O. Response bias in a case-control study: analysis utilizing comparative data concerning legal abortion from two independent Swedish studies. *Am J Epidemiol* 1991; **134**: 1003–1008.

13 Canto de Cetina TE, Colven CE, Hernández Cano JM, Vera Gamboa L. Aborto incompleto: caracteristicas de las pacientes tratadas en el Hospital O'Horan de Merida, Yucatán. *Salúd Pública Méx* 1985; **27**: 507–513.

14 Osis MJ, Ardí E, Faúndes A, Rodrigues T. Dificuldades para obtener informações da população de mulheres sobre aborto ilegal. *Rev Saúde Pública* 1996; **30**: 444–451.

15 Ravolamanana Ralisata L, Rabenjamina FR, Razafintsalama DL, Rakotonandrianina E, Randrianjafisamindrakotroka NS. Postabortum peritontitis pelvipertonitis at the Androva Mahajanga University Hospital: 23 cases. *J Gynecol Obstet Biol Reprod* 2001; **30**: 282–287.

16 Nations MK, Misago C, Fonseca W, Correia LL, Campbell OM. Women's hidden transcripts about abortion in Brazil. *Soc Sci Med* 1997; **44**: 1833–1845.

17 Remez LC. Confronting the reality of abortion in Latin America. *Internacional Family Planning Perspectivas* 1995; **21**: 287–289.

18 Pardo F, Uriza G. Estudio de morbilidad y mortalidad por aborto en 36 instituciones de Bolivia, Colombia, Perú y Venezuela. *Revista Colombiana de Obstetricica y Ginecología*, 1991.

19 Encuentro de investigadores sobre aborto inducido en América Latina y el Caribe. *Representaciones sociales y movimientos sociales.* Satafé de Bogotá, DC Colombia: Universidad Externado de Colombia, 1994.

20 Barrère M. Avortement. In: Demographic and Health Surveys (DHS), and Direction Générale de Statistique et de la Études Économiques (DGSEE, Gabon) and ORC Macro. *Enquête*

démographique et de santé Gabon 2000. DGSEE, UNFPA, ORC Macro International, Inc., Calverton, MD, 2001.

21 National Statistical Office of Mongolia and United Nations Population Fund. *National Report: Mongolia, Reproductive Health Survey 1998*. National Statistical Office, Ulaanbaatar, Mongolia, 1999.

22 Serbanescu F, Morris L, Nutsubidze N, Imnadze P, Shaknazarova M. *Women's Reproductive Health Survey Georgia, 1999–2000*. National Center for Disease Control, Republic of Georgia and U.S. Centers for Disease Control and Prevention, Atlanta, GA, 2001.

23 Alan Guttmacher Institute. *Sharing Responsibility: Women, Society, and Abortion Worldwide*. Alan Guttmacher Institute, New York, 1999.

24 Nduny L. Induced abortion amongst women in Kenya. *Loyola Journal of Social Science* 2007; **21**: 9–28.

25 Shah IH, Åhman E. Age patterns of unsafe abortion in developing country regions. *Reprod Health Matters* 2004; **12**(24 Suppl): 9–17.

26 Westoff CF, Ochoa LH. *Unmet Need and the Demand for Family Planning (Comparative Studies No.5)*. Institute for Resource Development/Macro International Inc., Columbia, MD, 1991.

27 Westoff CF. *Unmet Need at the End of the Century (Comparative Reports No. 1)*. ORC Macro, Calverton, MD, 2001.

28 Westoff CF, Bankole A. *Unmet Need: 1990–1994 (Comparative Studies, No.16)*. Macro International Inc., Calverton, MD, 1995.

29 Korra A. *Attitudes Toward Family Planning and Reasons for Non-Use Among Women with Unmet Need for Family Planning in Ethiopia (Further Analysis No. 40)*. ORC Macro, Calverton, MD, 2002.

30 Ross JA, Winfrey WL. Unmet need for contraception in the developing world and the former Soviet Union: an updated estimate. *Int Fam Plann Perspect* 2002; **28**: 138–143.

31 Govindasamy P, Boadi E. *A Decade of Unmet Need for Contraception in Ghana: Programmatic and Policy Implications*. Macro International Inc., Calverton, MD, National Population Council Secretariat, Accra, Ghana, 2000.

32 World Health Organization. *Safe Abortion: Technical and Policy Guidance for Health Systems*. World Health Organization, Geneva, 2003.

33 Bongaarts J, Westoff CF. The potential role of contraception in reducing abortion. *Stud Fam Plann* 2000; **31**: 193–202.

34 Marston C, Cleland J. *Relationships Between Contraception and Abortion: A Review of the Evidence*. Centre for Population Studies, London School of Hygiene and Tropical Medicine, London, 2002.

35 Åhman E, Shah IH. Contraceptive use, fertility, and unsafe abortion in developing countries. *Eur J Contracept Reprod Health Care* 2006; **11**: 126–131.

36 Singh S. Hospital admissions resulting from unsafe abortion: estimates from 13 developing countries. *Lancet* 2006; **368**: 1887–1892.

37 Faúndes A, Santos LC, Carvalho M, Gras C. Post-abortion complications alter interruption of pregnancy with misoprostol. *Adv Contracept* 1996; **12**: 1–9.

38 Miller S, Lehman T, Campbell M et al. Misoprostol and declining abortion-related morbidity in Santo Domingo, Dominican Republic: a temporal association. *BJOG* 2005; **112**: 1291–1296.

39 Gold RB. *Abortion and Women's Health. A Turning Point for America?* The Alan Guttmacher Institute, New York, 1990.

40 Murray CJL, Salomon JA, Mathers CD. A critical examination of summary measures of population health. *Bull World Health Organ* 2000; **78**: 981–994.

41 Abou-Zahr C, Åhman E. Unsafe abortion and ectopic pregnancy. In: Murray CJL, Lopez AD, eds. *Health Dimensions of Sex and Reproduction*. Harvard School of Public Health on behalf of the World Health Organization and the World Bank, Cambridge, MA, 1998.

42 United Nations Department for Economic and Social Affairs, Population Division. *World Abortion Policies 2007*. United Nations, New York, 2007.

43 Jewkes R, Brown H, Dickson-Tetteh K, Levin J, Rees H. Prevalence of morbidity associated with abortion before and after legalisation in South Africa. *BMJ* 2002; **324**: 1252–1253.

44 World Health Organization. *World Health Assembly Resolution: Health Aspects of Family Planning*. World Health Organization, Geneva, 1967.

45 United Nations Population Fund. *Programme of Action Adopted at the International Conference on Population and Development, Cairo, 5–13 September 1994*. United Nations Population Fund, New York, 1995.

46 United Nations Population Fund. *Key Actions for the Further Programme of Action of the International Conference on Population and Development, Adopted by the Twenty-first Special Session of the General Assembly, New York, 30 June–2 July 1999*. United Nations Population Fund, New York, 1999.

47 World Health Organization: Documentation. Reproductive health strategy to accelerate progress towards the attainment of international goals and targets. [Online]. 2004 May 22 [cited 2008 6 August]; Geneva: World Health Organization. Available from: URL:http://www.who.int/gb/e/e_wha57.html

48 Special Session of the African Union Conference of Ministers of Health. Maputo, Mozambique: The African Union Commission [Online]. 2006 18–22 September [cited 2008 8 August]; Available from: URL:http://www.africa-union.org/root/au/Conferences/Past/2006/September/SA/Maputo/CAMH2.htm

3

CHAPTER 3

Unintended pregnancy and abortion in the USA: Epidemiology and public health impact

Stanley K. Henshaw, PhD

LEARNING POINTS

- Unintended pregnancy occurs frequently in the USA, especially among women who are young, have low income, are Black or Hispanic, or have had a prior unintended pregnancy.
- Unintended pregnancy and abortion result about equally from non-use of contraception and imperfect use, which in turn are related to chance-taking, problems with contraceptive methods, not expecting to have sex, and barriers to access to contraception.
- Women with unwanted pregnancies have many reasons for choosing abortion, the most common of which are inadequate finances, lack of partner support, desire to continue education or career, not wanting more children, and feeling too immature.
- The US abortion rate has been falling in recent years, especially among teenagers.
- Although repeat abortion is often a source of concern, the data provide no justification for prejudicial attitudes.

Introduction

Couples in all developed countries want to control the timing and number of their children. Women typically initiate sexual activity long before they want children and continue long after they have their desired number, leaving them to rely on contraception during the majority of their reproductive lives. Failure of contraception results in abortion and unwanted births, and these outcomes occur more frequently in the USA than in most other Western developed countries. This chapter describes the reasons for unintended pregnancy in the USA, its relation to contraceptive use, the frequency and epidemiology of abortion utilization, the accessibility of services, the frequency with which various abortion procedures are used, and the public health effects of abortion legalization.

Unintended pregnancy

In 2001, 49% of pregnancies in the USA were unintended [1]. For this figure, all abortions as estimated by the Guttmacher Institute were considered to result from unintended pregnancies, as were 35% of births, as reported in the 2002 National Survey of Family Growth (NSFG) [2]. A pregnancy is considered to be unintended if the woman says that at the time she became pregnant she wanted no more children or did not want to become pregnant until later.

Many unintended pregnancies come to be wanted, and some women report being happy to find themselves accidentally pregnant. Attitudes toward pregnancy form a continuum from extremely unwanted to welcome, even among women who did not plan to become pregnant. Some women decide whether a pregnancy is wanted only after it occurs and the degree of social support for a birth and its other implications become apparent.

A majority of unintended pregnancies, however, were unwanted in 2001: 48% (excluding miscarriages) ended in induced abortion; undoubtedly many of the women who continued their pregnancies would have preferred not to give birth. Approximately 35% of births during the five years before the 2002 NSFG resulted from unintended pregnancies [2].

In 2001 the unintended pregnancy rate in the USA, including unintended pregnancies that miscarried, was 51 per 1,000 women aged 15 to 44 years (Table 3.1) [1,3]. This rate

Management of Unintended and Abnormal Pregnancy, 1st edition. By M Paul, ES Lichtenberg, L Borgatta, DA Grimes, PG Stubblefield, MD Creinin
 ISBN: 9781405176965.

Table 3.1 Unintended pregnancy rate of all women and exposed women, per cent ending in abortion, and unintended birthrate, by demographic characteristics, 2001 (Finer et al [1], Mosher et al [3].)

Characteristic	Unintended pregnancy rate[a]	Unintended pregnancy rate among exposed women[b]	Per cent of unintended pregnancies ending in abortion[c]	Unintended birthrate[a]
All women	51	109	48%	22
Age at pregnancy outcome				
<15	3	n.a.	51%	1
15–19	67	174	40%	34
15–17	40	n.a.	39%	21
18–19	108	n.a.	41%	53
20–24	104	157	49%	46
25–29	71	113	50%	32
30–34	44	87	49%	20
35–39	20	51	60%	6
≥40	6	21	56%	3
Marital status at pregnancy outcome				
Currently married	32	69	27%	20
Unmarried	67	140	58%	24
Cohabiting	138	229	54%	54
Unmarried and not cohabiting	52	117	61%	18
Income as a percentage of the poverty level				
<100%	112	266	42%	58
100–199%	81	187	50%	35
≥200%	29	58	54%	11
Education[d]				
Not HS graduate	76	221	36%	40
HS graduate/GED	54	119	46%	25
Some college	47	91	60%	16
College graduate	26	48	55%	10
Race/ethnicity				
White non-Hispanic	35	73	44%	17
Black non-Hispanic	98	223	58%	35
Hispanic	78	176	43%	40

Note: n.a. = not available.

[a] Per 1,000 women aged 15–44 or in age-group.

[b] Per 1,000 women exposed to risk of unintended pregnancy.

[c] Excluding spontaneous fetal loss.

[d] Among women aged 20 and older.

and the proportion of pregnancies that were unintended remained virtually unchanged from 1994. However, the proportion of unintended pregnancies that ended in abortion declined from 54 to 48%, and the unintended birthrate increased from 20 to 22 per 1,000 women. Three possible explanations for these changes are that social acceptance of nonmarital childbearing has increased along with the proportion of births to unmarried mothers [4], that attitudes toward abortion have become less favorable, or that access to abortion services has decreased.

Although comparative data are not readily available, the unintended pregnancy rate in the USA appears to be higher than those of most other developed countries. Both the abortion rates and the unintended birthrates are lower in most Western European countries [5]. Because women in those countries are as likely to be sexually active as US women, the explanation of their lower rates lies in the use of more effective contraceptive methods, especially oral contraceptives and the intrauterine device (IUD), less non-use of contraception, and more effective use of the methods.

The unintended pregnancy rate varies widely according to demographic characteristics of the women. In 2001, the latest year with available data, the rate was higher than 100 per 1,000 of the age-group among older teenagers and women aged 20 to 24 years, meaning that 1 in 10 accidentally became pregnant during the year (Table 3.1). The rate declined with age, reflecting reduced fecundity and more effective contraceptive practice. Use of contraceptive sterilization increases with age, thereby reducing the risk of pregnancy among older women.

The rate of unintended pregnancy was highest among unmarried cohabiting women (138 per 1,000) and was also higher among other unmarried women than among those who were married, in part because of the younger age of unmarried women. The rate was almost three times as high among women with incomes below the federal poverty level as among those with income twice the poverty level, and it was also strongly associated with low education. Non-Hispanic Black women were almost three times as likely as non-Hispanic White women to have an unintended pregnancy, with Hispanic women in between.

These findings understate the problems couples have with unintended pregnancy because many women are not actually at risk of an unintended pregnancy. Rates are higher when women not at risk are removed from the denominator. Rates of unintended pregnancy based on women at risk of unintended pregnancy are shown in the second column of Table 3.1, where the denominator is limited to women who are sexually active, not infecund or surgically sterilized, and not pregnant or seeking pregnancy. The overall rate was 109 pregnancies per 1,000 women at risk of unintended pregnancy, which means that 11% of these women experienced a pregnancy in 2001. Among teenagers, 17% became pregnant, as did 16% of women aged 20 to 24 years. The rate of unintended pregnancy was highest among poor women (27%), cohabiting women (23%), Black women (22%), and women who had not graduated from high school (22%).

Surprisingly, the percentage of teenagers' unintended pregnancies terminated by abortion (about 40%) was lower than that among US women generally (48%). Teenagers may have been less motivated than older women to avoid childbearing but unwilling to admit an openness to having a baby. Also, they may have been more opposed to abortion on principle. The percentage was elevated (56 to 60%) among women aged 35 years and older, perhaps because these women were less willing to accept an unplanned pregnancy than were younger women. It was low (only 27%) among married women, who may have found an unexpected child less disruptive to their lives compared with unmarried women, who terminated 58% of their unintended pregnancies. Women with low income or low education were less likely than other women to resolve an unintended pregnancy by abortion, while Black women were more likely to do so.

Because of the high rate of unintended pregnancy combined with moderate use of abortion, the unintended birthrate was 22 per 1,000 women and 35% of births resulted from unintended pregnancies. The unintended birthrate was 40 per 1,000 or higher among women aged 18 to 24 years, cohabiting women, poor women, those without a high school degree, and Hispanics.

Contraceptive use

The rate of unintended pregnancy, in turn, depends on the amount of exposure and on the extent and effectiveness of contraceptive use. According to NSFG data, 11% of sexually active US women who were not seeking pregnancy were using no method in 2002, up from 7% in 1995 [3]. Women not using a method accounted for 52% of the unintended pregnancies that ended in 2001 [1].

According to a 2001 survey of 10,683 women having abortions at 100 facilities in the USA [6], about 46% did not use contraception during the month they became pregnant. Of these women, 83% had used a method in the past; in many cases, the women had recently discontinued a method and become pregnant before starting a new method. The most common reasons for non-use were as follows:

- believing the risk of pregnancy was low (33%);
- problems with methods in the past and fear of side effects (32%);
- not expecting to have sex (27%); and
- problems obtaining contraception, mainly because of financial barriers (12%).

Those who perceive a low risk of pregnancy probably know they are taking a chance but see the risk as low for a single act of intercourse.

Of the 54% of abortion patients who had been using contraception during the month they became pregnant, 51% had been using condoms, 25% oral contraceptives, 14% withdrawal, 4% periodic abstinence, and 6% other methods. Fourteen per cent of the condom users said they had used the method correctly at every exposure, 49% said they had not used the method consistently, and 42% said a condom had slipped or broken. (Some said that both their use had been inconsistent and that a condom had broken or slipped.) The most frequent reasons for inconsistent use were believing the risk of pregnancy was low (41%), not having a condom available (29%), and not expecting to have sex (26%). Twelve per cent cited attitudes and behavior of partners as reasons for inconsistent use [6].

Only 13% of the pill users said they had used the method correctly. Among the inconsistent users, 50% said they had forgotten to take pills, 21% reported that they had been away from home and did not have pills available, and 14% said they ran out of supplies [6].

Similar barriers to contraceptive use were found in a population telephone survey of US women at risk of unintended pregnancy. About one-fourth reported that they had experienced a gap in contraceptive use in the past year. Forty per cent of these women cited problems accessing or using methods, including:

- problems or side effects of a method (17%);

- difficulties paying for a method (5%);
- lack of time for medical visits to obtain a method (5%); and
- not liking any available method (5%).

Nineteen per cent reported infrequent sexual activity as the main reason for non-use [7]. All methods fail occasionally, however; even when used perfectly, between 2,000 and 3,000 abortions in 2000 were obtained by women who had relied on their own or their partners' surgical sterilization or on an IUD [6].

Although contraceptive use is often imperfect, any use is more effective than none at all. Overall, averaging together all methods and both effective and less effective users, contraceptive use has been found to reduce the probability that a woman will have an abortion by 85% [8].

Pill scares that occurred in England and Wales illustrate the importance of contraceptive use in preventing abortion. In 1977, 1983, and again in 1995, popular press reports of harmful side effects of oral contraceptives were followed by sudden increases in the abortion rate. Many pill users switched to less effective methods or temporarily stopped using any method when they became concerned that pill use might be dangerous. In October 1995, the popular press gave extensive coverage to reports that two third-generation pill formulations pose higher risk of thromboembolism than the earlier pills [9]; in 1996, the number of abortions in England and Wales jumped 8% over the 1995 number [10].

Repeat abortion

Although contraceptive use increases after abortion, women remain at elevated risk of having another abortion because they are sexually active, willing to terminate an unintended pregnancy by abortion, have difficulty using contraceptive methods effectively, and probably become pregnant more easily than other women. In 2004, 47% of US women obtaining abortions had had a prior induced abortion: 27% had had one, 12% two, and 8% three or more prior abortions. From 1973 until reaching a high of 49% in 1997, this percentage increased each year along with the proportion of women in the population who had had abortions and were therefore at risk of an additional abortion [11]. In 1994, about 30% of all US women aged 15 to 44 years had had one or more induced abortions [12],and the abortion rate among the women who had had a previous abortion was about twice that of women who had never had an abortion. Canadian statistics show that approximately 25% of teenage abortion patients will have another abortion within the next four years [13]. An analysis of the NSFG found that 42% of US women who had a repeat abortion did so within two years of the prior abortion [14].

The high rate of repeat abortion does not mean that large numbers of women are relying on abortion as their primary means of birth control. A woman who used only abortion to limit her number of children to two would have more than 30 abortions during her lifetime [15]. No evidence indicates that American women have such large numbers of abortions.

On the contrary, women tend to improve their contraceptive use after having an abortion. According to the 2001 Guttmacher Institute survey of 10,683 abortion patients [6], 46% of women having a first abortion had used no contraceptive method during the month they became pregnant. If they had continued to use no method, on the order of 85 to 90% of second abortions would have occurred among women who had used no method because of the high pregnancy rate of non-users. In fact, the distribution of method use was similar to that of women having a first abortion, indicating that women who have an abortion improve their contraceptive use to about the same level as the women generally [16]. The Guttmacher Institute analysis found little difference between first and subsequent abortions in the reasons for non-use or inconsistent use of contraception [14].

A number of studies have sought risk factors for repeat abortion but few have been identified. The best predictors of repeat abortion are factors that reflect exposure to risk, most notably age; the older a woman is, the more opportunity she has had to experience two unintended pregnancies that end in abortion. A logistic regression analysis of the Guttmacher patient survey found that women having second or higher order abortions are also more likely to have existing children, controlling for age and other demographic variables [14]. An analysis of the NSFG in the same report found that almost half (47%) of women who have multiple abortions also have unintended births, another consequence of unintended pregnancy and therefore a risk factor for abortion. Other studies have found that women who have a second or higher order abortion engage in more frequent sexual intercourse than women having a first abortion [17,18].

The Guttmacher regression analysis of the 2001 abortion patient survey also found that women having a second or subsequent abortion were more likely than first abortion patients to be Black, enrolled in Medicaid, and cohabiting or never married. These groups include a high proportion of women in the population who have had a first abortion and are therefore at risk of another. Other studies have compared the psychological characteristics of first and repeat abortion patients but have found few differences. One of these studies concluded that the two groups do not "differ in any important ways in any of 15 measures of personality adjustment, in the length of their relationship with their partner, in their contraceptive practice, in their reasons for failing to use a contraceptive method or for seeking an abortion, or in their own feelings about their abortion decision [17]."

Reasons for terminating a pregnancy

About half of US women with unintended pregnancies choose to resolve them by abortion. In general these women believe that, given their life circumstances, taking responsibility for a new baby would be a mistake. The demographic characteristic most associated with the decision to terminate an unintended pregnancy is marital status: in 2001, 58% of unmarried women with unintended pregnancies decided on abortion, whereas only 27% of married women did so. Evidently the security of having a committed partner and the financial resources of a marriage allow most married women to continue their unplanned pregnancies.

A recent survey of 1,209 women having abortions in 11 clinics in the USA sheds more specific light on the thinking of women who have decided to end a pregnancy [19]. Most women (89%) gave more than one reason for choosing abortion, with the median number of reasons being four. The most common reason, mentioned by 73%, was financial. Many of these women indicated that their lack of resources resulted from:

- being unmarried (42% of all the respondents);
- having inadequate support from their husband or partner (14%); or
- having a husband or partner who was unemployed (12%).

Other reasons given for not being able to support a baby were that they:

- could not afford child care (28%);
- were students and presumably did not have a good source of income (34%);
- could not afford the basic necessities of life (23%);
- were unemployed (22%);
- would need more living space (19%); or
- were receiving public assistance (8%).

Almost half (48%) said they had relationship problems and did not want to be a single mother. Eleven per cent said they were not currently in a relationship, and 2% reported that their husband or partner abused them or their children. Other frequently mentioned reasons included the following:

- they have completed their childbearing (38%);
- a baby would interfere with their education (38%) or their job or career (38%) or their responsibilities for other children or dependents (32%);
- they were not ready for an(other) child (32%); and/or
- they did not feel mature enough (22%).

One per cent reported that they were the survivors of rape.

The reasons for deciding on abortion are likely to be similar in any developed country. For example, a study in Norway found that, compared with women who continued unintended pregnancies, those choosing abortion were much more likely to be single and not cohabiting, to be a student or unemployed, and/or to have a crowded living situation [20].

A study based on in-depth interviews with 38 women in four US clinics concluded that a primary concern of women having abortions is the desire to be the best possible parent for their existing children and any future children: "The women believed that children were entitled to a stable and loving family, financial security, and a high level of care and attention [21]."

Abortion epidemiology

Abortion incidence can be measured as the rate of abortions in relation to the size of a population or as a ratio of abortions to live births or pregnancies. The discussion here will rely mainly on the rate per 1,000 women aged 15 to 44 years, which directly reflects the proportion of women exposed to the risks and benefits of abortion.

In 2005, the latest year for which data are available, 1,204,500 induced abortions were obtained by women in the USA, for an abortion rate of 19.4 per 1,000. About 22% of pregnancies (excluding miscarriages) were terminated by abortion in that year [22].

The US abortion rate is similar to those of Australia, New Zealand, and Sweden but higher than those of other Western European countries (Fig. 3.1). It is lower than the rates in most of the former Soviet bloc countries and most developing countries where abortion is legal [23]. The US abortion rate has fallen one-third from its peak rate in 1981 and 9% since 2000.

Demographic patterns

A woman's probability of having an unintended pregnancy and abortion is strongly influenced by her stage in life and her socioeconomic status. Likelihood is highest around age 20 to 22 years, when most women are sexually active, highly fecund, and not seeking pregnancy. Thereafter, the abortion rate falls sharply with age.

Table 3.2 shows the abortion rate by age-group for US women in 1994. The highest abortion rate, 40 abortions per 1,000 women in the age-group, occurred among women aged 20 to 24 years. Approximately 18% of abortions were obtained by teenagers, with the abortion rate considerably higher among women aged 18 to 19 years than among younger teenagers. The abortion rate has fallen significantly among teenagers in recent years, more than among older women [24].

Another measure of abortion utilization, the ratio of abortions to births (not shown in Table 3.2), shows a somewhat different pattern with age than the abortion rate. The abortion ratio is high among teenagers, among which about 33% of pregnancies (excluding miscarriages) are terminated by abortion. The abortion ratio declines to 16% at ages 30 to 34 years, and then rises with age to 26% [24].

Among non-Hispanic White women in the USA, the abortion rate was approximately 11 per 1,000 in 2004, which

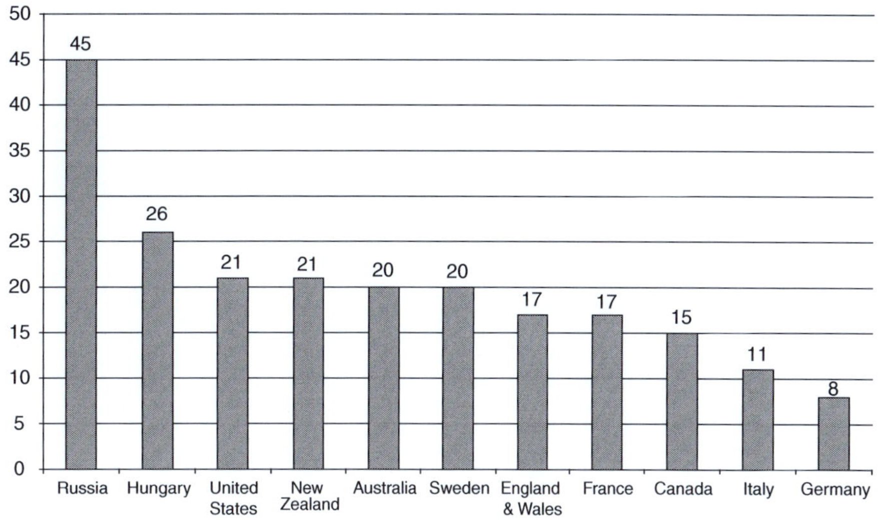

Figure 3.1 Abortion rate per 1,000 women aged 15–44, selected countries, 2003. (From Sedgh et al [23].)

is in the mid-range of the rates in other Western industrialized countries (Table 3.2). The rate among Black women (52) is more than four times as high, and that of Hispanic women (28) lies between that of Black and White women. Among both Black and Hispanic women, low income and high rates of unintended pregnancy help to explain the high abortion rates. Asian and Native American women have a moderate abortion rate; this category includes a mixture of ethnic groups with widely varying abortion patterns.

Occasional large-scale surveys of abortion patients have provided demographic information that is not available from abortion reporting forms. The most recent study was conducted by the Guttmacher Institute in 2000 and 2001 and involved 10,683 abortion patients in 100 US abortion facilities. Patients were asked to complete self-administered questionnaires at the time of the abortion. Most of the information in the rest of this section derives from the survey results and is illustrated in Table 3.2 [25].

Women of all education levels have occasion to seek abortion services, but college graduates have a lower abortion rate than less-educated women. Some 41% of abortions are obtained by women with some post-high school education but who are not college graduates.

Never-married women obtain the bulk of abortions (67%); married women account for only 17%. The abortion rate is higher among never-married women (35 per 1,000) than among previously married (29) or currently married women (8). The high rate among never-married women results partly from their young age compared with the other marital groups.

Women living with a partner to whom they are not married account for 25% of abortions but only about 10% of women in the population. Their abortion rate is almost two times that of other unmarried women. Thus, cohabiting is one of the strongest risk factors for abortion.

A majority (61%) of women having abortions in 2004 had had at least one birth, and one-third had had two or more. When age is taken into account, women who have children are substantially more likely than women without children to have an abortion, and the highest abortion rate is found among women with four or more children. Such women may have difficulty using contraception and thus may have unplanned children as well as abortions. A large majority of abortion patients with children is unmarried (76%), and more than half (56%) of the unmarried abortion patients have children (not shown).

The abortion rate among Protestants (18 per 1,000) is somewhat lower than that of all women (21 in the year 2000), while that of Catholics (22) is about the same. Women of other religions, including Russian and Greek Orthodox as well as Islam and others, and those who claim no religious identification appear to have somewhat higher abortion rates (30–31). The rate among women who name no religion is somewhat uncertain, because answers to questions on religious identification vary according to the context and wording of the question.

The higher abortion rate of Catholics compared with Protestants is confirmed by a comparison of their rates after excluding women from minority groups with high abortion rates, namely Black and Hispanic women. As expected, excluding Black and Hispanic women reduces the abortion rates of both Protestants and Catholics but that of Catholics remains higher (not shown). Possible reasons for the higher rate among Catholics include that Catholics use less effective methods of contraception, are more opposed to childbearing outside marriage, and are concentrated in cities and geographic areas with high abortion rates.

Household income is strongly associated with abortion utilization. Women whose income is below the federal poverty level are over four times as likely to have an

Table 3.2 Percentage distribution of abortions and abortion rate per 1,000 women aged 15–44, by selected characteristics, USA, 2000[a] (Jones et al [25], Ventura et al [24].)

Characteristic	%	Rate
Total[a]	100	20
Age years[a]		
<15[b]	1	3
15–17	6	12
18–19	11	32
20–24	33	40
25–29	23	30
30–34	15	18
35–39	8	10
≥40[c]	3	3
Race/ethnicity[a]		
White non-Hispanic	33	11
Black non-Hispanic	37	52
Other non-Hispanic	8	23
Hispanic	22	28
Education[d]		
Not HS graduate	13	23
HS graduate/GED	30	20
Some college	41	26
College graduate	16	13
Marital status		
Married	17	8
Previously married	16	29
Never-married	67	35
Cohabiting[e]		
Unmarried, cohabiting	25	55
Unmarried, not cohabiting	58	29
Number of live births		
0	39	19
1	27	32
2 or more	34	18
Religion[f]		
Protestant	43	18
Catholic	27	22
Other	8	31
None	22	30
Income as a percentage of the poverty level		
<100%	27	44
100–199%	31	38
200–299%	18	21
≥300%	25	10
Has Medicaid coverage		
Yes	24	57
No	76	18
County of residence		
Metropolitan	88	24
Nonmetropolitan	12	12

[a] Total, age, and race/ethnicity are for 2004.
[b] Denominator is women aged 14.
[c] Denominator is women aged 40–44.
[d] Among women aged 20 and older.
[e] Based on single women only.
[f] Limited to women over 17.

abortion as are those with income three or more times the poverty standard.

The high relative abortion rate of low-income women is reflected in the abortion rate according to Medicaid coverage. Twenty-four per cent of abortion patients say they are covered by Medicaid (although not necessarily for the abortion per se, except in the states that allow Medicaid to pay for abortion services), while only 9% of all US women of reproductive age have Medicaid coverage (as of 2000). Thus, the abortion rate of women with Medicaid coverage is three times as high as that of other women.

Women covered by Medicaid have a number of attributes that may contribute to their relatively high risk of abortion: they are disproportionately non-White, unmarried, and poor, all characteristics associated with high abortion rates. In addition, many women on Medicaid are covered by that program because of a prior accidental pregnancy that they carried to term and are prone to unplanned pregnancy.

Gestational age and procedure

Gestational age

More than half (62%) of all induced abortions in the USA occur at eight weeks' gestation or earlier, counting from the first day of the last menstrual period (LMP) or two weeks before the estimated date of conception (Table 3.3). Approximately 12% of abortions are performed past 12 weeks LMP, including 1.4% past 20 weeks LMP [26]. In most developed countries other than England and Wales, somewhat fewer abortions take place after 12 weeks LMP, probably because women respond more promptly to unwanted pregnancies and because restrictions in some countries make later abortions more difficult to obtain. Moreover, most other countries provide universal health insurance that covers abortion services. In contrast, women in the USA may be delayed by difficulty gaining access to abortion services and acquiring money to pay for the procedure [19,22].

In all countries with relevant statistics, teenagers obtain abortions later in gestation on average than do older women. In the USA in 2004, 27% of abortions obtained by women younger than age 15 years were past 12 weeks LMP as were 17% among women aged 15 to 19 years, compared with 11% among women aged 20 and older (Fig. 3.2). Abortions generally occur earlier with age until age 40, after which a few women are delayed because they mistake pregnancy for the menstrual changes of menopause [27].

The delay among younger women probably reflects their inexperience in recognizing the symptoms of pregnancy, their reluctance to accept the reality of their situation, lack of knowledge of where to seek advice and services, and their hesitation to confide in adults. In addition, teenagers may have more difficulty paying for abortions, and minors may be affected by parental consent or notification requirements (Chapter 4). In the USA, laws requiring minors to either

Table 3.3 Percentage distribution of reported legal abortions, by weeks of gestation and type of procedure – USA, 2005[a] (From Gamble et al [26].)

	Weeks of Gestation						
	≤8	9–10	11–12	13–15	16–20	>20	Total
Type of Procedure	%	%	%	%	%	%	%
Curettage (suction or sharp)[b]	82.4	97.3	98.7	98.6	95.4	85.1	88.0
Intrauterine instillation	0.1	0.1	0.1	0.1	0.7	1.1	0.1
Medical (nonsurgical)[c]	15.1	2.0	0.5	0.4	2.1	4.7	9.9
Other[d]	2.5	0.6	0.7	0.9	2.0	9.1	2.0
Total[e]	100.0	100.0	100.0	100.0	100.0	100.0	100.0
Percent of all abortions	62.1	17.2	9.3	6.3	3.8	1.4	100.0

[a] Based on 587,607 abortions reported to state health agencies.
[b] Primarily vacuum aspiration; includes D&C and dilation and evacuation.
[c] Procedures at ≤8 weeks were primarily by mifepristone or methotrexate with misoprostol; later abortions were primarily by vaginal prostaglandins.
[d] Includes hysterotomy/hysterectomy and procedures reported as "other."
[e] Percentages may not add to 100.0 because of rounding.

consult their parents or obtain a court order permitting the abortion cause some teenagers to experience delay in obtaining abortions [27,28,29].

Procedure

As shown in Table 3.3, approximately 88% of abortions in the USA in 2005 were accomplished by suction or sharp curettage (primarily suction), which includes dilation and evacuation (D&E). During the first trimester, vacuum aspiration represented the most frequently used method, although early medical abortions utilizing mifepristone or methotrexate followed by a prostaglandin accounted for at least 15% of abortions before 9 weeks LMP. (Some early medical abortions were probably classified as "other" in states whose reporting forms have no separate category for nonsurgical procedures.) According to the Guttmacher survey of US abortion providers, 161,000 early medical abortions were provided in 2005, accounting for about 21% of abortions before 9 weeks LMP [22]. Provision of suction abortion before 7 weeks LMP represents another recent trend, because use of sensitive pregnancy tests and vaginal ultrasound have reduced the risk of failing to end an early pregnancy or to detect an ectopic pregnancy (see Chapter 18). The proportion of US abortions occurring before 7 weeks LMP increased from about 16% in 1995 to 30% in 2005 [26].

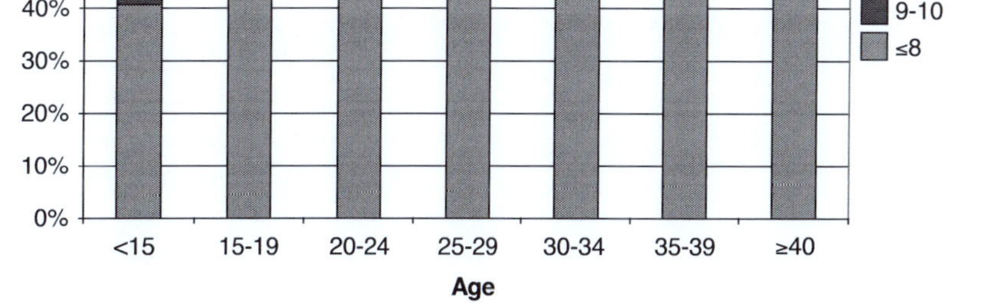

Figure 3.2 Gestation by woman's age, 2004. (From Strauss et al [26].)

Of all US abortions past 12 weeks LMP, the vast majority (96%) are performed by D&E (Table 3.3). Even after 20 weeks LMP, this method was used for 85% of abortions. D&E is at least as safe as labor induction abortion and has other advantages: It is preferred by most women, because it is fast and avoids the pain and stress of labor [30]; it can be performed outside of hospitals; and it is less expensive than induction abortion (see Chapter 11). Second trimester induction abortion using prostaglandin administered by various routes has almost completely replaced saline instillation. (Some prostaglandin induction procedures may have been reported as "other" in states where the reporting form makes no provision for this method.) Abortions by hysterotomy or hysterectomy involve higher risk of morbidity and mortality than do other methods, and these methods have almost disappeared in the USA.

Setting

Both first and second trimester abortions can be provided safely in clinics and physicians' offices [31,32]. The proportion of US abortions performed in hospitals has declined from more than 50% in 1973 to 5% in 2005 [22]. The number of hospitals where abortions are performed has dropped sharply, as has the average number of abortions per hospital provider. A tabulation of data on approximately 300,000 abortions in 14 states in 1992 indicates that, even after 20 weeks LMP, 83% were performed outside of hospitals. Near universal agreement as to the safety of second trimester abortion outside of hospitals is further demonstrated by the finding that in 2001 about 55% of abortion clinics offered the service at 18 weeks LMP or later [33].

Accessibility of abortion services

Despite the large number of women who need abortion care, services are less available than for other common medical conditions. A significant but unknown number of women continue unwanted pregnancies because of lack of access to an abortion provider.

Distance

The number of large nonhospital abortion providers (those that provided 400 or more abortions per year) in the USA fell from 668 in 2000 to 616 in 2005, continuing a long-term decline in the number of facilities where abortions are provided. Although some 604 hospitals and 367 physicians' offices offered abortion services in 2005, the large nonhospital facilities accounted for 91% of abortions provided during the year [22].

Abortion providers are concentrated in large and medium-size metropolitan areas, leaving many smaller cities and rural areas without services. Of the 362 metropolitan areas defined by the US government, 134 (37%) have no abortion provider. In 2005, 35% of women lived in counties without a provider, and 42% lived in counties without a provider of 400 or more abortions. The size of the provider affects access because facilities with small abortion caseloads charge more on average and are unlikely to advertise or make their services widely known in the community. As a consequence of the absence of abortion services in many areas, 8% of abortion patients in 2005 traveled more than 100 miles for services and 19% traveled 50 to 100 miles, according to providers' estimates [22]. The abortion rate of nonmetropolitan women is about half that of women who live in metropolitan counties, possibly because of access problems [25].

The task of finding an abortion provider is more difficult for a woman whose pregnancy has advanced into the second trimester. At each additional week of gestation, fewer providers are available to terminate the pregnancy. In 2005, 20% of US providers offered abortions after 20 weeks LMP and only 8% did so at 24 weeks LMP [22].

Cost

Cost represents a barrier for women of limited means, who constitute a majority of abortion patients. In 2001, 57% of US women obtaining abortions had family income less than two times the federal poverty level [25]. In that year, 74% paid in cash; of the remainder, half had Medicaid coverage in states where Medicaid pays for all or most medically necessary abortions, and half had private insurance that was accepted by the provider [33]. In states where Medicaid does not cover abortion except in extremely limited circumstances, 91% of women paid out of pocket. An unknown but probably small proportion of these women received reimbursement from private insurance, and some chose not to use insurance because of concerns about confidentiality.

Some poor women without insurance are unable to secure funds to pay for an abortion. Studies have found that public funding of abortion makes services accessible to women who would otherwise carry unintended pregnancies to term. Between one-fifth and one-third of eligible women who would seek abortion continue their pregnancies in the absence of Medicaid or other public funding [34,35]. In a 1995 survey of abortion patients, in states where Medicaid paid for abortions the abortion rate of women covered by Medicaid was 3.9 times that of women who were not covered; while in nonfunding states, Medicaid recipients were 1.6 times as likely to have abortions as were non-Medicaid women [8]. Similar patterns were found in the 2001 patient survey. This difference indicates that Medicaid coverage of abortion has an important impact on the ability of poor women to end unwanted pregnancies.

Another effect of the cost barrier is that the time required to secure the necessary funds causes women to delay their abortions to later points in gestation. One recent study found that 26% of women having abortions said they were delayed by the time needed to raise money to have the abortions. For women having second trimester abortions, the percentage was 36%. Poor women were delayed 11 days on average [36]. A study of the impact of the discontinuation of Medicaid coverage of abortion in one clinic found that 22% of Medicaid-eligible women who had second trimester abortions would have had their abortions in the first trimester if they had not been delayed by the need to find money to pay for the procedure [37].

Other barriers

Harassment by antiabortion activists adds to the difficulty women experience in accessing abortion services and the challenges of providing services. In 2000, 80% of large non-hospital facilities (400 or more abortions a year) in the USA experienced picketing. Picketing was much less common among low-volume providers; only 10% of providers that performed fewer than 30 abortions reported being picketed. Other forms of harassment were also fairly common. Of large providers, 28% reported one or more incidents of picketing with physical contact or blocking of patients, and 18% reported vandalism [33]. These activities impede access for women who might be intimidated by aggressive protesters.

The stigmatization of abortion also undoubtedly affects many women, although this factor is difficult to measure. Fear of the disapproval of relatives or others in the community may inhibit many women who would choose to end their pregnancies. Some women in the USA remain unaware that abortion services are legal and available.

Public health effects of abortion legalization

The legalization of abortion in the USA, which began in several states in 1967 and culminated in the *Roe v. Wade* Supreme Court decision in 1973, brought significant health and social benefits. Before the laws changed, illegal abortions had been common. From a survey in North Carolina in 1967, researchers estimated that 829,000 abortions were occurring in the country as a whole, which is about 80% of the number of legal abortions that took place in 1975, when legal abortion services were available in all states [38]. Other studies based on the change in the birthrate after legalization suggest that the number of illegal abortions was around 600,000 to 700,000 per year [39,40]. Legalization converted those abortions to safe procedures and allowed additional women, some at high risk of complications of pregnancy and childbirth, to avoid unwanted childbearing.

Over the decade spanning 1958 through 1967, more than 3,400 women died from induced abortions, almost all illegal [41][1]. The number rose during the 1950s and reached at least 430 in 1961, then fell during the 1960s when more physicians started providing abortions. The number of deaths fell rapidly after abortion was legalized, from 251 in 1966 to 14 in 1976. In recent years, the number of deaths has ranged between 4 and 12 per year according to the Centers for Disease Control and Prevention (CDC) [26]. During the five years from 2000 to 2004, only 43 deaths were related to legal abortion and two to illegal abortion, for a mortality rate of 0.7 per 100,000 legal abortions[2].

In the 10 years between 1970 and 1980, legal abortion in the USA is estimated to have prevented 1,500 pregnancy-related deaths and thousands of other complications [42]. The deaths prevented were from both unsafe abortions and from childbirth, which has higher mortality and morbidity than induced abortion. Abortions tend to be obtained by women for whom childbirth involves above-average risk (women over aged 35, minorities, low-income women, and women with health problems), so more maternal deaths are prevented than would otherwise be the case.

For each death from unsafe abortion, many other women suffered complications. Several hospital studies of the number of women treated for abortion complications found sharp decreases after legalization. For example, in municipal hospitals in New York City, for each 1,000 births, 234 admissions for incomplete abortion occurred in 1969 compared to 130 such admissions in 1971 after the repeal of abortion restrictions [43].

The availability of safe abortion carries other benefits as well. A study by economists associated with the National Bureau of Economic Research found that the increase in the abortion rate was the most important factor explaining the reduction in neonatal mortality between 1964 and 1977. The abortion rate dominated other public policies, including Medicaid, subsidized family planning services, and maternal and infant care projects, in explaining the mortality decline among both White and Black women [44,45]. Another economist found that abortion also reduced the rate of low-birth-weight and preterm births. This economist attributed these results to a reduction in births among the most high-risk women, specifically the very young, the very old, and women in poor health. The data also suggest that women with wanted pregnancies have healthier children [46]. Also, it is well established that births that are spaced too closely pose health risks for both the children and the mothers.

---

[1] The number of deaths reported by the National Center for Health Statistics has been adjusted to include deaths *associated* with abortion as well as those *attributed* to abortion so they will be comparable to legal abortion mortality statistics compiled by the CDC.

[2] Calculated from the number of deaths reported by Gamble, Strauss, Parker et al 2008 [26], and the number of abortions estimated by Jones, Zolna, Henshaw et al 2008 [22].

One component of infant mortality is infanticide. The homicide rate for infants in the first hour of life decreased from 1.41 per 100,000 during 1963 to 1972 to 0.44 per 100,000 during 1974 to 1983. The rates for children in the first week of life and the first month of life also declined, whereas the overall homicide rate for all ages increased from 7.0 to 9.7 per 100,000 [47]. Moreover, in Kings County Hospital, Brooklyn, the rate of abandonment of newborn infants fell by 56% in the year beginning six months after the change in the law [48].

Studies spanning the period in which abortion was legalized found that birthrates fell, especially among groups without the resources to terminate pregnancies illegally. The most thorough study examined the period between 1970 and 1973 and compared the four states that repealed their abortion laws with all other states [39]. The study found that overall, birthrates in the repeal states fell by 6% compared with those in the nonrepeal states. Over the longer term the effect on birthrates would be less, because a majority of women who have abortions intend to have children in the future [8]. Abortion, like contraception, allows women to postpone childbearing to a time when their life circumstances are more suitable. The groups whose birthrates were most affected were those who currently experience the highest proportion of unintended pregnancies and who tended to have less access to illegal abortion. These groups included teenagers, whose birthrate fell by 12%; non-White women, also 12%; women over age 35 years, 8%; and unmarried women, whose birthrate had been increasing at an accelerating rate until 1970, then fell 6% until 1974, when it resumed its rise.

The birthrate among couples who know they are at risk of giving birth to children with genetic abnormalities is actually higher when abortion services are available. For example, each child of carriers of Tay-Sachs disease has a 25% chance of inheriting a genetic condition that causes death by age 5 years. With prenatal testing and abortion, these couples can have a full and healthy family and avoid having a child who will inevitably die at an early age. Without prenatal testing and second trimester abortion, many such couples would not dare to have children [42].

Conclusion

The prevention of unintended pregnancy avoids both unwanted births and abortions. Nevertheless, contraceptive services receive low priority in many US medical settings, including some facilities that provide abortions. Unnecessary barriers to contraception, including cost, insurance inadequacies, and misconceptions on the part of patients and staff, prevent many couples from receiving optimal contraceptive services. Although the perfect health care system may not exist, most other industrialized countries make contraception more available and have lower rates of unintended pregnancy and abortion.

The groups most at risk of unintended pregnancy are minorities and families with low income. These groups also may have difficulty accessing abortion care because of cost, distance from a provider, and unavailability of second trimester services. If they do overcome these barriers, many teenagers and low-income women experience delay, with the result that their abortions occur later in pregnancy than necessary.

Women who have an unwanted birth or abortion are at high risk of another unintended pregnancy because they are sexually active, fecund, not seeking pregnancy, and have proven difficulties using contraception. Women should be offered the full range of contraceptive methods with special attention to methods such as the IUD, implant, and sterilization that are effective over a long period without attention on the part of the user (see Chapter 14). Both contraception and abortion are remarkably safe–safer than pregnancy and childbirth. Better access to contraceptive and abortion services would benefit public health.

References

1 Finer LB, Henshaw SK. Disparities in rates of unintended pregnancy in the United States, 1994 and 2001. *Perspect Sex Reprod Health* 2006; **38**: 90–96.

2 Chandra A, Martinez GM, Mosher WD, Abma JC, Jones J. Fertility, family planning, and reproductive health of US women: data from the 2002 National Survey of Family Growth. *Vital and Health Statistics* 2005; Series 23, No. 25, Table 21.

3 Mosher WD, Martinez GM, Chandra A, Abma JC, Willson SJ. Use of contraception and use of family planning services in the United States: 1982–2002. *Adv Data* 2004; No. 350.

4 Martin JA, Hamilton BE, Ventura SJ, Menacker F, Park MM, Sutton PD. Births: final data for 2001. *Natl Vital Stat Rep* 2002; **51**: No. 2.

5 Jones EF, Forrest JD, Henshaw SK, Silverman J, Torres A. *Pregnancy, contraception, and family planning services in industrialized countries*. Yale University Press, New Haven, 1989.

6 Jones RK, Darroch JE, Henshaw SK. Contraceptive use among US women having abortions in 2000–2001. *Perspect Sex Reprod Health* 2002; **34**: 294–303.

7 Frost JJ, Singh S, Finer LB. US women's one-year contraceptive use patterns, 2004. *Perspect Sex Reprod Health* 2007; **39**: 48–55.

8 Henshaw SK, Kost K. Abortion patients in 1994–1995: characteristics and contraceptive use. *Fam Plann Perspect* 1996; **28**: 140–147, 158.

9 Office for National Statistics. Legal abortions: September quarter 1996. *Population and Health Monitor* 1997; AB 97/2.

10 Office for National Statistics. Legal abortions in England and Wales 1996. *Population and Health Monitor* 1997; AB 97/4.

11 Tietze C. Repeat abortions – why more? *Fam Plann Perspect* 1978; **10**: 286–288.

12 Henshaw SK. Unintended pregnancy in the United States. *Fam Plann Perspect* 1998; **30**: 24–29, 46.

13 Millar WJ, Wadhera S, Henshaw SK. Repeat abortions in Canada, 1975–1993. *Fam Plann Perspect* 1997; **29**: 20–24.

14 Jones RK, Singh S, Finer LB, Frohwirth LF. Repeat abortion in the United States. New York: Guttmacher Institute, Occasional Report No. 29, 2006.

15 Kost K, Forrest JD, Harlap S. Comparing the health risks and benefits of contraceptive choices. *Fam Plann Perspect* 1991; **23**: 54–61.

16 Henshaw SK. Observation: contraceptive method use following an abortion. *Fam Plann Perspect* 1984; **16**: 75–77.

17 Berger C, Gold D, Andres D, Gillett P, Kinch R. Repeat abortion: is it a problem? *Fam Plann Perspect* 1984; **16**: 70–75.

18 Howe B, Kaplan HR, English C. Repeat abortions: blaming the victims. *Am J Public Health* 1979; **69**: 1242–1246.

19 Finer LB, Frohwirth LF, Dauphinee LA, Singh S, Moore AM. Reasons US women have abortions: quantitative and qualitative perspectives. *Perspect Sex Reprod Health* 2005; **37**: 110–118.

20 Skjeldestad FE. When pregnant – why induced abortion? *Scand J Soc Med* 1994; **22**: 68–73.

21 Jones RK, Frohwirth LF, Moore AM. "I would want to give my child, like, everything in the world.": how issues of motherhood influence women who have abortions. *J Fam Issues* 2008; **29**: 79–99.

22 Jones RK, Zolna MRS, Henshaw SK, Finer LB. Abortion in the United States: incidence and access to services, 2005. *Perspect Sex Reprod Health* 2008; **40**: 6–16.

23 Sedgh G, Henshaw SK, Singh S, Bankole A, Drescher J. Legal abortion worldwide: incidence and recent trends. *Int Fam Plan Perspect* 2007; **33**: 106–116.

24 Ventura SJ, Abma JC, Mosher WD, Henshaw SK. Estimated pregnancy rates by outcome for the United States, 1990–2004. *Natl Vital Stat Rep* 2008; vol. 56, No. 15.

25 Jones RK, Darroch JE, Henshaw SK. Patterns in the socioeconomic characteristics of women obtaining abortions in 2000–2001. *Perspect Sex Reprod Health* 2002; **34**: 226–235.

26 Gamble SB, Strauss LT, Parker WY, Cook DA, Zane SB, Hamdan S. Abortion surveillance – United States, 2005. MMWR, *Surveill Summ* 2008; **57**: No. SS-13.

27 Strauss LT, Gamble SB, Parker WY, Cook DA, Zane SB, Hamdan S. Abortion surveillance – United States, 2004. MMWR, *Surveill Summ* 2007; **56**: No. SS-9.

28 Joyce T, Kaestner R. The impact of mandatory waiting periods and parental consent laws on the timing of abortion and state of occurrence among adolescents in Mississippi and South Carolina. *J Policy Anal Manage* 2001; **20**: 263–282.

29 Joyce T, Kaestner R, Colman S. Changes in abortions and births and the Texas parental notification law. *N Engl J Med* 2006; **354**: 1031–1038.

30 Kaltreider NB, Goldsmith S, Margolis AJ. The impact of midtrimester abortion techniques on patients and staff. *Am J Obstet Gynecol* 1979; **135**: 235–238.

31 Cates W, Grimes DA. Deaths from second trimester abortion by dilatation and evacuation: causes, prevention, facilities. *Obstet Gynecol* 1981; **58**: 401–408.

32 Grimes DA, Cates W, Selik RM. Abortion facilities and the risk of death. *Fam Plann Perspect* 1981; **13**: 30–32.

33 Henshaw SK, Finer LB. The accessibility of abortion services in the United States, 2001. *Perspect Sex Reprod Health* 2003; **35**: 16–24.

34 Cook PJ, Parnell AM, Moore MJ, Pagnini D. The effects of short-term variation in abortion funding on pregnancy outcomes. *J Health Econ* 1999; 18: 241–257.

35 Trussell J, Menken J, Lindheim BL, Vaughan B. The impact of restricting Medicaid financing for abortion. *Fam Plann Perspect* 1980; 12: 120–130.

36 Finer LB, Frohwirth LF, Dauphinee LA, Singh S, Moore AM. Timing of steps and reasons for delays in obtaining abortions in the United States. *Contraception* 2006; **74**: 334–344.

37 Henshaw SK, Wallisch LS. The Medicaid cutoff and abortion services for the poor. *Fam Plann Perspect* 1984; **16**: 170–172, 177–180.

38 Abernathy JR, Greenberg BG, Horvitz DG. Estimates of induced abortion in urban North Carolina. *Demography* 1970; **7**: 19–29.

39 Levine PB, Staiger D, Kane TJ, Zimmerman DJ. *Roe v. Wade* and American fertility. *Am J Public Health* 1999; **89**: 199–203.

40 Tietze C. Two years' experience with a liberal abortion law: its impact on fertility trends in New York City. *Fam Plann Perspect* 1980; **5**: 36–41.

41 Hilgers TW, O'Hare D. (1981) Abortion-related maternal mortality: an in-depth analysis. In: Hilgers TW, Horan DJ & Mall D, eds. *New Perspectives on Human Abortion*. University Publications of America, Inc., Frederick, MD, 1981: 69–91.

42 Tietze C. The public health effects of legal abortion in the United States. *Fam Plann Perspect* 1984; **16**: 26–28.

43 Institute of Medicine, National Academy of Science. *Legalized Abortion and the Public Health:* report of a study by a committee of the Institute of Medicine. National Academy of Sciences, Washington, DC, 1975.

44 Grossman M, Jacobowitz S. Variations in infant mortality rates among counties of the United States: the roles of public policies and programs. *Demography* 1981; **18**: 695–713.

45 Corman H, Grossman M. Determinants of neonatal mortality rates in the US: a reduced form model. *J Health Econ* 1985; **4**: 213–236.

46 Joyce T. The impact of induced abortion on black and white birth outcomes in the United States. *Demography* 1987; **24**: 229–244.

47 Lester D. *Roe v. Wade* was followed by a decrease in neonatal homicide (letter to the editor). *JAMA* 1992; **267**: 3027–3028.

48 Lanham JT, Kohl SG, Bedell JH. Changes in pregnancy outcome after liberalization of the New York State abortion law. *Am J Obstet Gynecol* 1974; **118**: 485–492.

4 CHAPTER 4

Abortion law and policy in the USA

Bonnie Scott Jones, JD, and Jennifer Dalven, JD

LEARNING POINTS

- The constitutionality of US abortion laws is measured by standards set forth in Supreme Court decisions.
- Abortion practice is currently governed by an array of legal requirements that vary state by state.
- Many abortion restrictions hinder clinicians' ability to provide, and women's ability to obtain, abortions.
- Prior to initiating the provision of abortions, clinicians should become familiar with the applicable legal requirements in their area and should seek individualized legal advice as needed.

Introduction

Although modern induced abortion is one of the safest medical procedures available, it is regulated like no other area of medicine in the USA. The procedure is currently subject to a multitude of federal and state laws and regulations. This situation was not always the case. From the country's inception up through the first half of the 19th century, abortion prior to "quickening" was legal and largely unregulated in the USA [1]. Beginning in the mid-1800s, various movements worked to outlaw both abortion and contraception (see Chapter 1). By the early 1900s, most of the states banned abortion with only limited exceptions [2]. As a result of the US Supreme Court's 1973 decision in *Roe v. Wade* [3], the states' bans were invalidated, and abortion services became safer and more accessible to women throughout the country.

Since *Roe*, however, many states have adopted a variety of abortion restrictions that have the effect of impeding women's access to abortion without banning the procedure outright. Because abortion politics influence the government's involvement in abortion provision, those politics, rather than science and medical evidence, often shape the laws in this area. Given the US Supreme Court's recent decision in *Gonzales v. Carhart*, which gave the states greater latitude to regulate abortion and to do so on the basis of ideological concerns about abortion "harming" women, governmental regulation of abortion may well increase. Indeed, recent years have brought renewed attempts to ban abortion altogether. In South Dakota, for example, the legislature passed an abortion ban in 2006 that the state's voters promptly rejected in a referendum [4]. A ballot initiative to ban abortion was then placed on the South Dakota ballot, but the voters defeated it in November 2008 [5]. In addition, four states (Louisiana, Mississippi, North Dakota, and South Dakota) have enacted state laws that will ban abortion if *Roe* is overturned [6].

This chapter sets forth the standards that the courts use to examine governmental actions that hinder a woman's access to abortion in the USA, describes the kinds of restrictions that governments have imposed on abortions, and explains the extent to which the courts have upheld or invalidated these restrictions. It also discusses legislative efforts to protect women's access to abortion.

Overview and timeline of US constitutional protections and Supreme Court abortion jurisprudence

In the 1973 decision *Roe v. Wade*, the US Supreme Court recognized that a woman's right to terminate a pregnancy is protected by the US Constitution. Since *Roe*, the Supreme Court has evaluated the constitutionality of government actions that restrict a woman's right to choose an abortion in a series of major decisions. The Court has thus far refused to overturn *Roe*, but it has weakened considerably the constitutional protection for the right to an abortion. This section traces the history of federal constitutional protection for abortion by examining four key decisions: *Roe v. Wade*; *Planned Parenthood v. Casey*; *Stenberg v. Carhart*; and *Gonzales v. Carhart*.

Management of Unintended and Abnormal Pregnancy, 1st edition. By M Paul, ES Lichtenberg, L Borgatta, DA Grimes, PG Stubblefield, MD Creinin
 ISBN: 9781405176965.

Roe v. Wade

In a series of decisions in the half-century leading up to *Roe*, the US Supreme Court recognized a constitutional right of privacy that protects intimate and personal decisions (including those affecting childrearing, procreation, marriage, family relationships, and the use of contraception) from government interference [7]. The Court explained, "If the right of privacy means anything, it is the right of the *individual*, married or single, to be free from unwanted governmental intrusion into matters so fundamentally affecting a person as the decision whether to bear or beget a child [8]."

In *Roe*, the Supreme Court held that the right to privacy encompasses "a woman's decision whether or not to terminate her pregnancy [9]," and it struck down a Texas law that made it a crime to provide an abortion unless the woman's life was in danger. The Court characterized the right to abortion as "fundamental" to a woman's "life and future," and it accorded the right the highest level of constitutional protection: the government could not prohibit or interfere with abortion without a "compelling" reason to do so [10]. The Court established a trimester framework based on its balancing of the interests involved at each of the three stages of pregnancy. In the first trimester, the Court found no interest sufficiently compelling to permit governmental restrictions on abortion. Beginning in the second trimester, however, the Court held that the government has a sufficiently compelling interest in protecting women's health to permit regulations designed to further that interest. After viability, the Court held that the government has a sufficiently compelling interest in protecting potential life to justify banning abortions, if it so chooses. However, the Court also held that, even after viability, the protection of women's health must remain paramount; any ban on postviability abortions must contain an exception for abortions necessary to preserve the life or health of the woman [11].

Roe rendered state abortion bans unconstitutional, setting the groundwork for making abortion services safer and more accessible to women throughout the country. In response to the decision, however, many state and local governments began passing new restrictions on abortion. During the subsequent two decades, the Supreme Court invalidated many of these laws, including requirements that a woman obtain the consent of her spouse prior to an abortion [12]; that any abortion after the first trimester of pregnancy be provided in a hospital [13]; and that a woman receive information designed to discourage abortion and then wait at least 24 hours after receiving the information before obtaining an abortion [14]. At the same time, the Supreme Court interpreted *Roe* in ways that severely limited access to abortion for poor women and minors: the Court upheld bans on Medicaid coverage of abortion for poor women [15], as well as requirements that minors involve a parent or go to court prior to obtaining an abortion [16].

Planned Parenthood v. Casey

In 1992, in *Planned Parenthood v. Casey*, the Supreme Court considered the constitutionality of several Pennsylvania abortion restrictions [17]. Changes in the makeup of the Supreme Court had led many to believe that the Court might use *Casey* as a vehicle to overturn *Roe*. Those predictions did not materialize. The *Casey* Court reaffirmed *Roe*'s central holdings that a woman has a constitutional right to choose abortion before viability and that, even after viability, any ban on abortion must provide an exception when the woman's life or health is at stake [18]. The Court's refusal to overrule *Roe* was based, in part, on its recognition that the right to choose abortion is critical to women's autonomy and equality. As the Court explained, "[t]he ability of women to participate equally in the economic and social life of the Nation has been facilitated by their ability to control their reproductive lives [19]."

Casey nonetheless represented a substantial shift in the level of constitutional protection for the right to choose abortion. In *Casey*, the Court significantly scaled back that protection, thus making it easier for laws restricting abortion access to survive court challenges. Specifically, the Court abandoned *Roe*'s trimester framework and its use of the most stringent level of constitutional review in favor of a weaker test. Under this new test, regulations of abortions prior to viability are constitutional unless they impose an "undue burden" on abortion. An "undue burden" is one that has the "purpose or effect" of placing a "substantial obstacle in the path of a woman seeking an abortion" of a nonviable fetus [20].

The adoption of the "undue burden" test had significant and immediate consequences. In particular, despite previously striking down similar laws, the Court upheld Pennsylvania's requirement that doctors provide women seeking abortions with information designed to discourage them from having the procedure. The Court held that the requirement did not constitute an "undue burden" because the information was "truthful and not misleading" [21] and because the state is permitted to express a preference for childbirth over abortion [22]. In addition, the Court upheld a mandatory delay law (also similar to laws that had been previously struck down) that required women to wait at least 24 hours after receiving the state-mandated information before obtaining an abortion. Despite evidence that the regulation increased the cost and risk of abortions, the Court reasoned that the delay period did not amount to a "substantial obstacle [23]." The Court held that "[t]he fact that a law which serves a valid purpose, one not designed to strike at the right itself, has the incidental effect of making it more difficult or expensive to procure an abortion cannot be enough to invalidate it [24]." Following *Casey*, numerous states have passed, and many courts have upheld, a variety of abortion restrictions that make it more difficult and expensive for women to obtain abortions. These laws include counseling requirements intended to express a government's preference for childbirth over abortion, mandatory delay periods, and abortion facility licensing requirements.

Applying the undue burden standard, the *Casey* Court did strike down Pennsylvania's requirement that women notify their husbands before getting an abortion. The Court reached that result based largely on its finding that, for women who are victims of spousal abuse, a requirement that they notify their husbands before an abortion is tantamount to an abortion ban [25].

Stenberg v. Carhart

In the 2000 *Stenberg v. Carhart* ruling, the Supreme Court considered the constitutionality of Nebraska's so-called "partial-birth abortion" ban [26]. "Partial-birth abortion" is not a medical term, but a phrase coined by abortion opponents to define a broad range of acts that they sought to criminalize. This legislative initiative, fueled by opposition to the intact variant of dilation and evacuation ("D&E") (see Chapter 11), led to far-reaching bans. Many states, including Nebraska, passed laws that effectively made it a crime for an abortion provider to continue removing a fetus from the uterus if the provider had brought an undefined "substantial portion" of the fetus into the vagina prior to the occurrence of fetal demise.

Applying the *Casey* standard, the Supreme Court struck down Nebraska's ban for two reasons. First, the Court concluded that, contrary to the claims of the ban's proponents, the legislation did not prohibit only the intact variant of D&E, but also encompassed standard[1] D&E procedures. Because D&E procedures in general account for more than 95% of abortions between 12 and 20 weeks of pregnancy, the Court concluded that the ban placed a substantial obstacle in the path of women seeking second-trimester abortions [27]. It was, therefore, an undue burden and unconstitutional.

Second, the Court held that, even if the ban were read narrowly to prohibit only the intact variant of D&E, it would still be unconstitutional because it lacked an exception that would permit a doctor to perform a banned procedure to protect a woman's health [28]. In striking down the law, the Court reaffirmed that the government may not impose abortion restrictions that endanger women's health. The Court also held that, as long as sound medical opinion supports the safety of a particular procedure (regardless of dissenting voices in the medical community), the treating physician must retain the discretion to choose the method most appropriate for the patient's health [29].

[1] While the authors here adopt the term "standard D&E" as the court used it in *Gonzales v. Carhart*, 127 S. Ct. 1610 (2007), to refer to non-intact D&Es, the term is not medical, and the authors in no way suggest that any one variation of D&E is more or less standard than another.

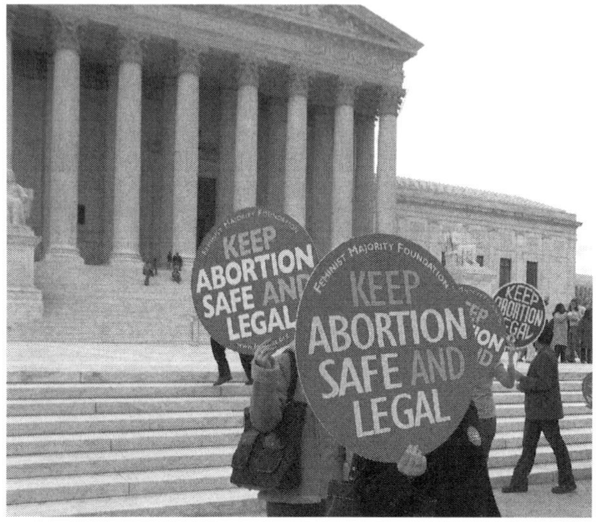

Figure 4.1 Activists protest as the US Supreme Court hears oral arguments on the constitutionality of the federal ban in *Gonzales v. Carhart*.

Gonzales v. Carhart

In response to *Stenberg*, the US Congress passed the Partial-Birth Abortion Ban Act of 2003, the first-ever federal ban on abortion methods [30]. The federal law defined "partial-birth abortion" somewhat differently than did the Nebraska statute; but its broad terms still threatened to criminalize some D&Es, and it still lacked a health exception. Accordingly, the National Abortion Federation (NAF), Planned Parenthood, and a number of individual physicians challenged the federal ban in court. In 2007, when the Supreme Court considered the constitutionality of the federal ban in *Gonzales v. Carhart*, the Court's composition and its decision were different than in *Stenberg* (Fig. 4.1).

In the new case, the Court, with two new Justices, upheld the ban [31]. First, the Court held that the ban was not as broad as Nebraska's, and that it "excludes most D&E procedures in which the fetus is removed in pieces [32]." Second, the Court held that a health exception was unnecessary. In a seeming reversal from its ruling in *Stenberg* about the need to protect women's health, the Court held that where disagreement exists about the safety advantages of a medical procedure, the government can decide to ban the procedure without providing an exception for instances in which a doctor believes it is safer for the patient [33].

Gonzales was the first decision in which the Court rejected a challenge to an abortion restriction that lacked a health exception. It thus undermined the core principle of abortion jurisprudence, dating back to *Roe*, that women's health must remain paramount. Indeed, under *Gonzales*, a "[s]tate's interest in promoting respect for human life at all stages in the pregnancy" can, in some circumstances, outweigh a woman's interest in protecting her own health [34].

The *Gonzales* decision is also unprecedented for its endorsement of the antiquated stereotype that women are unable to make fully informed, intelligent decisions. Indeed, the Court's approval of the ban rests in part on its acceptance of the notion that women require protection from making decisions they may later come to regret. Despite acknowledging the lack of any "reliable data to measure the phenomenon," the Court stated that it "seems unexceptionable to conclude some women come to regret their choice to abort the infant life they once created and sustained.... Severe depression and loss of esteem can follow [35]."

The *Gonzales* decision invites politicians to pass additional restrictions on abortion. The decision also suggests that the right to abortion itself may be in jeopardy. Unlike in *Stenberg*, where the Court *reaffirmed* the central holdings of *Roe* and *Casey*, in *Gonzales* the Court only "*assume[d]*" that the standards set forth in *Casey* were the applicable law [36]. As Justice Ginsburg noted in an impassioned dissent, "[t]he Court's hostility to the right *Roe* and *Casey* secured is not concealed. [37]"

Specific areas of abortion regulation

Restrictions on the use of public funding, facilities, and employees in connection with abortion

After the *Roe* decision, abortion, now a legal medical service, was covered by Medicaid. Abortion opponents, however, quickly sought to end this coverage that had provided access to abortions for Medicaid-eligible women. In 1976, Congress passed the Hyde Amendment, which forbids the use of federal money to pay for almost any abortion under the Medicaid program [38]. Currently, the only exceptions to the ban on the use of federal funds for abortion are where the woman's life is endangered by a physical disorder, illness or injury, or where the pregnancy is a result of rape or incest [39].

In 1980, in a case called *Harris v. McRae*, the US Supreme Court upheld the Hyde Amendment, stating that the US Constitution permits the government to withhold Medicaid funds for virtually all abortions, while continuing to fund all other medically necessary services, including prenatal care and childbirth. The Court reasoned that the discrimination was permissible because, in its view, women's inability to exercise their "constitutionally protected freedom of choice" was caused by their own poverty, and not by the government's skewed funding of pregnancy-related care, but not abortion. Moreover, the Court held that the government could constitutionally encourage childbirth over abortion by funding one but not the other [40].

The denial of Medicaid coverage for abortion has a profound impact on low-income women's access to abortion. Studies estimate that when public funding is unavailable, 18 to 35% of Medicaid-eligible women who want abortions are instead forced to continue their pregnancies [41]. Other women manage to obtain the procedure, but often only after considerable personal sacrifices that affect themselves and their families.

Congress has added restrictions similar to the Hyde Amendment to an array of health care programs on which millions of women rely. In addition to poor women on Medicaid, those who are denied access to federally funded abortions include Native Americans, federal employees and their dependents, Peace Corps volunteers, low-income residents of Washington, DC, federal prisoners, military personnel and their dependents, teenagers covered under the Children's Health Insurance Program (CHIP), and disabled women insured under Medicare [42].

Since *Harris* was decided, advocates have worked to restore Medicaid coverage for abortions. For example, advocates have brought numerous state court challenges arguing that the states' constitutions provide greater protection for women's rights than does the federal Constitution. These efforts have achieved a fair degree of success. As of 2008, lawsuits have resulted in 13 states restoring Medicaid coverage for abortions (Alaska, Arizona, California, Connecticut, Illinois, Massachusetts, Minnesota, Montana, New Jersey, New Mexico, Oregon, Vermont, and West Virginia) [43]. Four other states (Hawaii, Maryland, New York, and Washington) voluntarily cover abortions in their state Medicaid programs [44]. Most other states restrict coverage in line with the Hyde Amendment, only covering abortions in cases of life-endangerment or rape or incest [45] (Fig. 4.2). A handful of states also cover abortions in cases of fetal impairment or where the pregnancy threatens "severe" health problems.

The lack of public funding for abortions also resulted in the establishment of numerous funds to assist women in obtaining abortions they need, but cannot afford. For information about funding options, providers and their patients can contact the National Abortion Federation Hotline at 800-772-9100 or visit the National Network of Abortion Funds' website at www.nnaf.org (see Appendix).

The Supreme Court also has extended the rationale of the *Harris* decision to permit tight government control over the performance of abortions at facilities that receive public funds. In 1989, the Court upheld a Missouri statute that outlawed the use of any public facility for, or the participation of public employees acting in the course of their employment in, the performance of an abortion not necessary to save the life of the woman [46]. In addition to Missouri, to date nine other states have passed similar laws that prohibit the use of some or all public facilities for abortions [47]. At the same time, courts in New Jersey and Alaska have held that their state constitutional protections for reproductive choice forbid hospitals that serve the public and that receive substantial government support from barring the use of their facilities for abortions [48].

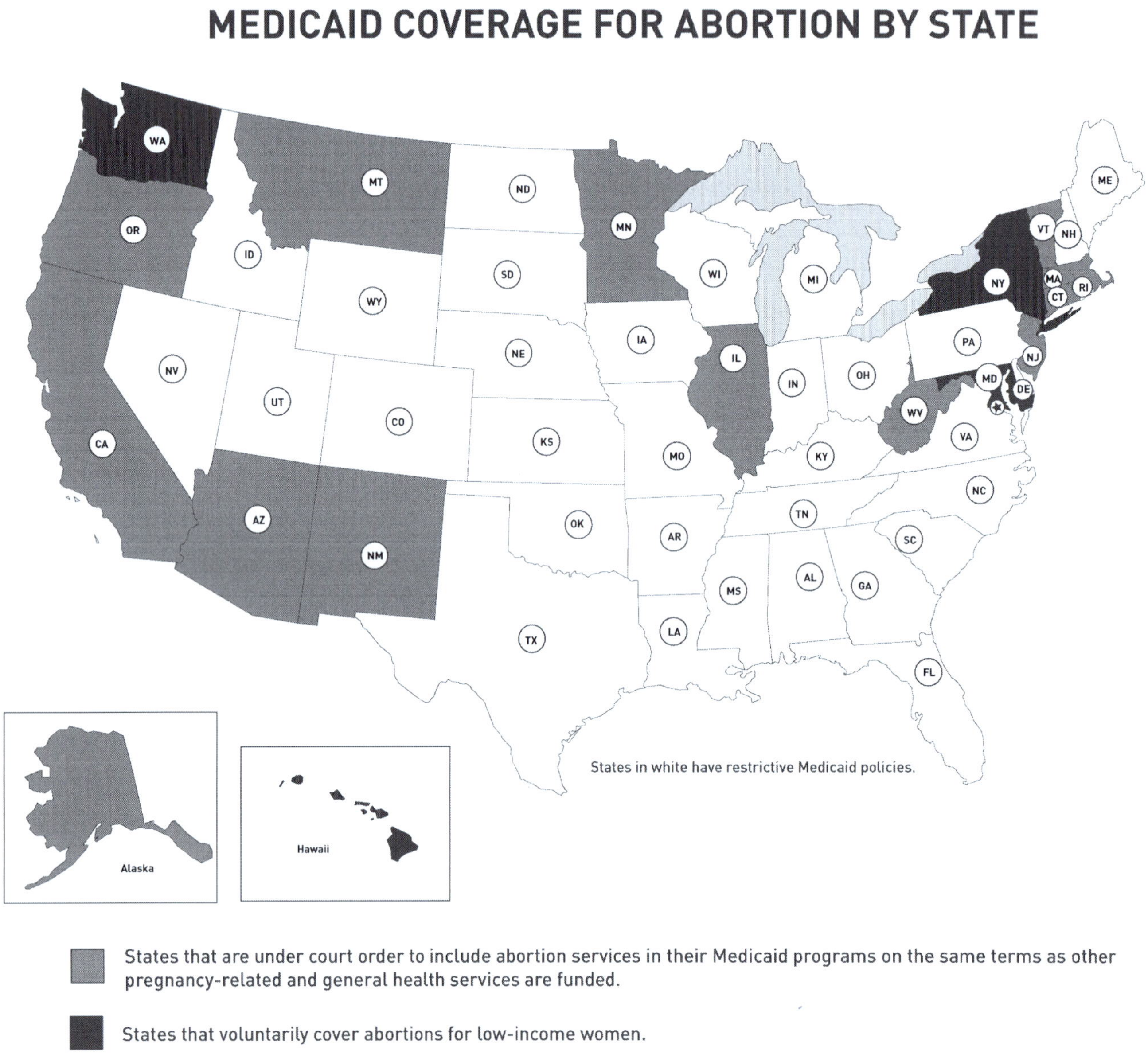

Figure 4.2 Medicaid coverage for abortion by state, USA, 2008.

Laws affecting minors' access to abortion

As of 2008, more than 30 states were enforcing laws that prohibit a physician from providing an abortion for a minor unless the minor has involved one or both of her parents in her decision [49]. Some of these laws require that the minor notify her parent(s) prior to the abortion, whereas others require that the minor actually obtain consent for the procedure from one or both parents. The US Supreme Court has held that such laws are constitutional as long as they contain an exception for medical emergencies and provide a confidential and expeditious alternative to parental involvement. In most states, that alternative takes the form of a court proceeding known as a judicial bypass. To obtain a judicial bypass of the parental involvement requirement, a minor must go to court and prove to a judge either that she is sufficiently mature and well-enough informed to make her own decision about whether to have an abortion, or that obtaining the abortion is in her best interest [50]. The major medical organizations in the USA, including the American Medical Association, the American College of Obstetricians and Gynecologists, the American Academy of Pediatrics, and the American Public Health Association, oppose these laws on the grounds that they put minors' health and safety at risk without increasing family communication [51].

Despite the Supreme Court's approval of these types of laws, advocates had been able to challenge many of them successfully based on deficiencies in their judicial bypass proceedings and medical emergency exceptions. In the last several years, however, states have drafted the laws more carefully to ensure compliance with the federal Constitution.

With fewer federal remedies available, advocates have pursued two other strategies in an attempt to protect minors. First, in some states that provide greater constitutional protections for reproductive choice than does the federal Constitution, advocates have successfully challenged these laws under the states' constitutions. Thus, for example, state courts have struck down parental involvement laws in California, Montana, and New Jersey [52].

Second, in states where no legal challenge is possible, abortion providers and advocates have devised systems to help minors obtain bypasses as efficiently as possible. In many states, providers refer minors to lawyers who have agreed, and in many instances have been specially trained, to represent minors in bypass proceedings. Advocates in some states also have worked with court personnel to devise systems that ensure that the bypass process functions as quickly and smoothly as possible. Abortion clinics in many states help to connect minors with lawyers or otherwise help to guide them through the process. Providers also may contact the American Civil Liberties Union office in their state for information about their state's parental involvement law or assistance with the bypass process.

In addition to parental involvement laws, antichoice advocates have also sought in recent years to use child abuse reporting laws to impede minors' access to abortion and other reproductive health care, as well as to intimidate abortion providers. These advocates have argued that, in states where consensual sex among young people is a crime, it must be reported as child abuse by health care providers and others who are legally obligated to report such abuse. Although in many cases these claims are greatly exaggerated, health care providers serving minors need to understand their state's child abuse reporting obligations, including whether their state requires reporting of some consensual sex among minors.

Restrictions on which medical personnel may provide abortions

Physician-only laws

The vast majority of states permit only physicians to provide abortions, and they apply these restrictions ("physician-only" laws) to both medical and surgical abortions [53]. Only a handful of states lack physician-only laws. As of April 2008, these states were Arizona, Kansas, Montana, New Hampshire, Oregon, Vermont, and West Virginia [54].

Unfortunately, many areas of the country have few or no physicians who provide abortions, and the number of abortion providers continues to decrease [55]. Physician-only laws prevent properly trained nonphysician clinicians from responding to this shortfall by providing abortions. Empirical evidence does not support prohibitions on abortion provision by trained nonphysician clinicians. For example, studies demonstrate that complication rates do not differ for aspiration abortions provided by physician assistants and those performed by physicians [56]. Accordingly, major medical organizations have endorsed the provision of abortion by properly qualified advanced practice clinicians [57].

Nonetheless, the US Supreme Court has consistently upheld physician-only requirements [58]. Most recently, in *Mazurek v. Armstrong* in 1997, the Supreme Court upheld Montana's physician-only requirement against a challenge by a trained physician assistant who had provided abortions safely under supervision for nearly 17 years. Applying the undue burden test, the Court held that evidence was insufficient to establish that the regulation posed a substantial obstacle to women seeking abortions [59].

Given these unfavorable rulings of the US Supreme Court, courts in those states where the state constitution provides broader protections than the federal Constitution offer the primary potential avenue for striking down physician-only laws at this time. This strategy proved successful in Montana, where the law upheld by the US Supreme Court in *Mazurek* was subsequently struck down by the Montana Supreme Court under the state constitution's more stringent protections [60].

Qualified and trained advanced practice clinicians (nurse practitioners, certified nurse midwives, and physician assistants) also provide abortions in Vermont and New Hampshire, which have no physician-only laws [61], and in New York, where the state department of health has construed the state's physician-only law and physician assistant practice act to permit physician assistants to provide first-trimester abortions [62]. In other states, such as California, Connecticut, New Mexico, Rhode Island, and Washington, certain nonphysician clinicians provide medical abortion as a result of various legal mechanisms, including legislation, lawsuits, regulation, and attorney general opinions [63].

Special training and qualification requirements for physicians who provide abortions

Some states have gone beyond physician-only laws by imposing requirements on the qualifications and training of *physicians* who provide abortions. For example, in Louisiana, a state medical board investigator ordered a physician to cease performing abortions because she lacked formal training in obstetrics and gynecology, although she had received comprehensive training from an experienced provider [64], and one-third of first-trimester abortion providers in the USA are not obstetrician-gynecologists [65]. The medical board's action was challenged in a federal court action, which was settled in 2008 [66]. Additionally, Alabama has promulgated regulations that require abortion providers to demonstrate their competency through abortion training in a residency or fellowship program, hospital privileges to provide abortions, or certification by a "properly trained disinterested physician" who has observed the provider performing abortions [67]. Alabama does not require such proof of competency for a physician's performance of any other outpatient medical procedure. Instead, like all other states, it monitors the competence of physicians through licensing boards, professional organizations, insurers, and malpractice liability.

How these new types of "training and qualification" requirements for physicians who provide abortions will fare in court is not yet known. Decisions of the US Supreme Court from the *Roe* era strongly suggest that these requirements are unconstitutional [68]. Since that time, however, the Supreme Court has become increasingly tolerant of laws that subject abortion providers to unique requirements and burdens.

Regulation of facilities in which abortions are provided (TRAP laws)

The term "TRAP" stands for targeted regulation of abortion providers, and it refers to laws that single out abortion providers and impose on them burdensome requirements that are different and more stringent than those applied to providers of comparable medical procedures. TRAP regulations can make it prohibitively expensive for an abortion provider to continue offering abortion services or substantially increase the cost of procedures for the patient. Abortion opponents claim that TRAP laws protect women's health by making abortion safer. Proponents of abortion access claim that TRAP laws impose burdens on abortion without providing any corresponding health benefit and exceed accepted medical standards.

TRAP laws typically take three different forms: (1) health facility licensing schemes that apply only to abortion providers; (2) requirements that abortion facilities be licensed as ambulatory surgical centers (ASCs); and (3) laws requiring that all second-trimester abortions (or abortions after a specified gestational age in the second trimester) be provided in a hospital. A number of states impose more than one of these types of TRAP laws.

Nearly half the states have a TRAP law of the first type, but these health facility licensing schemes vary considerably in terms of their burdens [69]. Additionally, while some such schemes apply to *any* clinician who provides even a single surgical or medical abortion, other schemes: (1) exempt abortion providers who perform less than a specified number of abortions in a given time period; (2) apply only to providers of abortions after the first trimester; (3) exempt private physicians' offices; or (4) apply only to providers of surgical abortions [70]. By way of example, these measures typically include physical plant specifications, such as doorway widths, minimum room sizes, and air circulation systems; requirements for training and qualification of personnel, such as requiring that various functions be performed by registered nurses; burdensome administrative and recordkeeping policies; expensive licensing fees; and authorization for state agencies to review and copy confidential patient records [71].

Approximately 10 states have a TRAP law of the second type, requiring providers of abortion (typically after a specified gestational age) to become licensed as ambulatory surgical centers and comply with ASC regulations [72]. Regulations for ASCs usually include all of the types of burdensome requirements imposed by health facility licensing schemes, as well as more stringent physical plant requirements. The regulations generally cannot be met by doctors' offices or outpatient clinics, and they go far beyond the recommendations of recognized medical guidelines [73].

Hospitalization requirements, the third type of TRAP law, are on the books in many states; however, the vast majority of these laws has been declared unconstitutional by a court ruling or state official, or has been invalidated by another law [74]. One notable exception is Alaska, which has an unchallenged statute that limits second trimester abortion provision to hospitals [75]. In addition, three other states (Arkansas, Nevada, North Carolina) have unchallenged hospitalization laws that apply to abortions after 20 or 24 weeks of gestation [76].

Prior to the US Supreme Court's decision in *Casey* in 1992, the courts regularly invalidated TRAP laws on the grounds that they failed to advance maternal health or that they improperly treated abortion providers differently than providers of comparable medical services [77]. Under *Casey*'s less restrictive "undue burden" standard, however, several challenges to TRAP laws have not succeeded in striking down the schemes [78]. Nevertheless, courts have recognized that "a significant increase in the cost of abortion or the supply of abortion providers can, at some point, constitute a substantial obstacle" to abortion [79]. Whether any TRAP law will be invalidated under this standard remains to be seen.

Biased counseling and mandatory delay requirements

Almost half the states enforce laws that require providers to give a woman information intended to dissuade her from having an abortion and then prohibit the abortion for a specified period of time (most often 24 hours) after the woman receives the information [80]. These laws, which are designed to express the states' preference for childbirth over abortion and to persuade the woman to continue her pregnancy, are commonly referred to as "biased counseling" and "mandatory delay" laws. Some states' biased counseling laws mandate that the required information be given in person, rather than via telephone, mail, or Internet, which results in women needing to make two trips to the provider [81]. A few additional states have biased counseling provisions that do not require a delay before the abortion procedure [82]. The counseling provisions vary, but they typically require abortion providers to inform the woman about the risks of abortion and childbirth; notify the woman that the man with whom she became pregnant is responsible for child support; provide the woman with a list of agencies that offer adoption or other abortion alternatives; and offer her materials published by the state that describe normal embryonic and fetal development and include images of embryos and fetuses at various stages of development [83]. Although these laws are passed under the guise of ensuring that a woman's consent to abortion is informed, existing laws already require informed consent; in addition, these provisions give women biased and, in some cases, inaccurate or incomplete information [84]. Moreover, no laws require that health care providers give comparable information to women planning to continue their pregnancies.

As explained previously, the US Supreme Court upheld the constitutionality of Pennsylvania's mandatory delay and biased counseling laws in *Casey*, holding that states may compel abortion providers to give women state-mandated information designed to discourage abortion, so long as the information is "truthful and not misleading [85]." Since *Casey*, court challenges to similar laws have been largely unsuccessful in both state and federal courts [86].

Mandatory delay laws make obtaining an abortion more difficult and costly for many women, particularly those with the fewest resources, such as poor women, minors, rural women, working women without insurance or sick leave, and battered women. Study data indicate that the costs and logistical barriers posed by the second-trip requirement can be prohibitive for many women. For example, Mississippi's "two-trip" requirement, which was the first of its kind to be enforced, reduced the abortion rate for Mississippi residents by over 15% in the first 12 months after the law took effect; it also caused many Mississippi women to delay their procedures, increasing the proportion of second-trimester abortions provided to residents in the state by almost 40% during that first year [87].

In recent years, some states have undertaken new efforts to influence women's decisions with additional types of biased information. For example, several states have enacted legislation requiring abortion providers to inform women (verbally or through the provision of state-drafted materials) that substantial scientific evidence suggests that the fetus may be able to feel pain at a specific point during the pregnancy (usually at 20 weeks' gestation, but even earlier in some states) [88]. The current medical data on this issue are inconclusive, at best [89]. These measures also typically require providers to give women information about administering anesthesia to the fetus [90], despite the fact that fetal anesthesia poses health risks to the woman [91] and is not widely available. In still other states, legislatures have enacted various measures steering women to view an ultrasound image as a means of discouraging abortions [92].

Opponents of abortion also have sought to require doctors to give women value-laden speeches lacking in medical fact. For example, the New Jersey Supreme Court recently dismissed a lawsuit brought by a woman who claimed that her abortion provider's failure to inform her that the embryo was a "complete, separate, unique, and irreplaceable human being" with whom she had an "existing relationship" constituted malpractice. The Court rejected the notion that these were medical facts that a doctor must disclose rather than moral, philosophical, or religious beliefs [93]. South Dakota has passed a law that compels physicians to make a similar speech before an abortion. Although a federal appeals court has rejected certain claims on a preliminary basis, the litigation challenging the law is ongoing [94]. Such efforts to discourage women from having abortions through biased counseling requirements may increase in light of the US Supreme Court's suggestion in *Gonzales* that women need governmental assistance in order to avoid making abortion decisions that they will later regret [95].

Restrictions on abortion methods

In the 1990s, after the *Casey* Court refused to overturn *Roe*, opponents of abortion began a campaign to enact restrictions on abortion methods. This campaign resulted in the passage of more than two dozen state bans on so-called "partial-birth abortion." No medical procedure known as "partial-birth abortion" exists, and these bans were written in broad terms that encompassed D&E procedures of any variant (as well as other abortions). The Supreme Court struck down Nebraska's "partial-birth abortion" ban in 2000 in *Stenberg v. Carhart*, and that decision had the effect of invalidating all similar state bans.

In response to *Stenberg*, however, the US Congress enacted the Partial-Birth Abortion Ban Act of 2003. The law bans abortions in which the physician deliberately and intentionally vaginally delivers a living fetus to: (1) in the case of a head-first presentation, the point at which the entire fetal head is outside the woman's body; or (2) in the case of a breech presentation, the point at which any part of the fetal trunk above the navel is outside the woman's body, *and*, after the fetus reaches the specified point in either presentation, the physician performs an overt act, separate from delivery, that kills the fetus [96]. As a result of the Supreme Court's 2007 decision in *Gonzales v. Carhart* that upheld the federal ban, the ban went into effect in all 50 states. According to the Court, the ban does not apply to "most" non-intact D&Es; providing less than clear guidance, the Court also stated that it does not apply to abortions in which the doctor intends at the outset to perform a standard[1] D&E [97]. Doctors who intend to remove a fetus as intact as possible during a D&E, however, "must adjust their conduct to the law [98]." Because medical practice varies so much from practitioner to practitioner, there is no single or best way of making sure to comply with the federal ban while still providing the safest possible care. Physicians have adopted many different combinations of strategies, which include using digoxin or potassium chloride injections to ensure fetal demise before evacuation, varying dilation protocols in light of the Court's comments, and documenting the intent to comply with the law. Consultation with legal counsel is critical for US physicians embarking on second trimester practice, particularly a practice that includes abortions at approximately 18 weeks' gestation or later.

Restrictions on postviability abortions

Most states have laws severely limiting or banning abortions after viability. The US Supreme Court has held that these measures are constitutional if they apply only postviability and contain adequate exceptions for abortions necessary to protect the woman's life or health. Accordingly, the viability or nonviability of a fetus often determines whether or not a legal abortion is available to a pregnant woman. The Supreme Court has made clear that the legislatures must leave the viability determination to a woman's physician, and may neither define viability at a specific point in pregnancy nor specify that one element of the viability assessment is determinative [99]. The Court has held, however, that states may require that physicians perform tests to determine viability beginning at 20 weeks of gestation [100].

States may also mandate that a physician who provides an abortion after viability take all reasonable steps to preserve the life and health of the viable fetus, so long as the physician determines that doing so will not increase the risks to the woman's health [101]. Accordingly, the Supreme Court has held that states may not mandate that physicians use the abortion method most likely to result in fetal survival if that requirement poses a greater medical risk to the woman [102]. Moreover, a state may require the attendance of a second physician at postviability abortions to provide neonatal care in the case of a live birth. However, the state must provide an exception for medical emergencies to ensure that the delay caused by the attendance of a second physician will not endanger the woman's health [103].

Laws protecting access to abortion

Efforts to codify abortion protections

In recent years, abortion rights advocates on the state and the federal levels have sought legislation that would protect the right to choose ("Freedom of Choice" acts). These laws essentially codify the protections of *Roe v. Wade* by prohibiting government interference with abortion prior to viability. To date, seven states have enacted such protections [104] and other states are considering them. These state laws grant the right of abortion the protections it enjoyed before *Casey*. A similar law also has been introduced in the US Congress [105]. If passed, the federal law would ensure that women throughout the USA would be able to decide whether to terminate a pregnancy free of government interference.

Legal mechanisms for addressing antiabortion violence and intimidation

Since the US Supreme Court's decision in *Roe*, blockades, invasions, and violence have been directed against abortion providers and abortion-related medical facilities (see Chapter 3). Both federal and state legislatures have passed laws to create mechanisms for addressing this violence and intimidation. A 1994 federal law, the Freedom of Access to Clinic Entrances Act (FACE), makes it a crime to use force or the threat of force to injure, intimidate, or interfere with reproductive health care providers or women seeking their services [106]. The Department of Justice took an active role in enforcing FACE when it was passed [107], and clinic violence has decreased considerably since the law took effect [108].

In addition, state laws provide mechanisms that have been used widely to address clinic violence and intimidation. Many states and localities have enacted laws that bar blockades and create protective zones (known as "buffer zones" or "bubble zones") around women's health clinics and people seeking access to those clinics [109]. Courts have also granted critical injunctive relief and monetary damages to abortion providers under various other state laws, including civil rights acts, trespass statutes, and tort theories [110].

Conclusion

Numerous legal issues affect the practice of abortion in the USA. Because abortion is governed by an often complex interplay of federal, state, and local laws that are subject to change, practitioners need to remain informed about the legal requirements governing abortion provision. Practitioners are encouraged to obtain legal advice prior to incorporating abortion provision into their practices and consistently thereafter. Both the American Civil Liberties Union Reproductive Freedom Project (ACLU RFP) and the Center for Reproductive Rights (CRR) offer pro bono legal advice and support to abortion providers [111]. In addition, online resources of the ACLU RFP [112], CRR [113], the Guttmacher Institute [114], and NARAL Pro-Choice America [115] (see Appendix) provide general information about abortion restrictions applicable in particular states.

Acknowledgment

The authors would like to thank Carrie Y. Flaxman, JD, for her invaluable assistance with the drafting of this chapter.

References

1 See The Emma Goldman Clinic [Online]. Iowa City (IA): The Emma Goldman Clinic; c2008. A brief history of reproductive rights; [cited 2008 Aug 5]. Available from: URL:http://www.emmagoldman.com/publications/Winter06History.htm; National Abortion Federation [Online]. Washington (DC): National Abortion Federation; c2008. History of abortion fact sheet; [cited 2008 Aug 5]. Available from: URL:http://www.prochoice.org/about_abortion/history_abortion.html

2 Id.

3 410 U.S. 113 (1973).

4 H.R. 1215, 2006 Leg., 81st Sess. (S.D. 2006); South Dakota Ban Rejected, *USA Today*, Nov. 11, 2006.

5 URL:http://www.sdsos.gov/electionsvoteregistration/electvoterpdfs/2008/2008regulateperformanceofabortions.pdf; Ballot initiatives to curtail abortions rejected. LA Times, Nov. 5, 2008.

6 La. Rev. Stat. Ann. §§40:1299.30, 14:87; Miss. Code Ann. §414-41-32; N.D. Cent. Code §12.1–31; S.D. Codified Laws §22–17–5.1.

7 *Meyer v. Nebraska*, 262 U.S. 390 (1923); *Pierce v. Soc'y of Sisters*, 268 U.S. 510 (1925); *Skinner v. Oklahoma*, 316 U.S. 535 (1942); *Griswold v. Connecticut*, 381 U.S. 479 (1965); *Loving v. Virginia*, 388 U.S. 1 (1967); *Eisenstadt v. Baird*, 405 U.S. 438 (1972).

8 *Eisenstadt*, 405 U.S. at 453.

9 410 U.S. at 153.

10 Id. at 153–55.

11 Id. at 162–64.

12 *Planned Parenthood v. Danforth*, 428 U.S. 52, 69–72 (1976).

13 *Akron v. Akron Ctr. for Reprod. Health*, 462 U.S. 416, 431–33 (1983).

14 *Thornburgh v. Am. Coll. of Obstetricians & Gynecologists*, 476 U.S. 747, 760 (1986); *Akron*, 462 U.S. at 449-50.

15 *Harris v. McRae*, 448 U.S. 297 (1980).

16 *Bellotti v. Baird*, 443 U.S. 622 (1979).

17 505 U.S. 833 (1992).

18 Id. at 846.

19 Id. at 856.

20 Id. at 878.

21 Id.

22 Id. at 882.

23 Id. at 885–87.

24 Id. at 874.

25 Id. at 893–94.

26 530 U.S. 914 (2000).

27 Id. at 924, 938–39, 945–46.

28 Id. at 930–38.

29 Id. at 937–38.

30 18 U.S.C. §1531 (2003).

31 127 S. Ct. 1610 (2007).

32 Id. at 1629.

33 Id. at 1636–37.

34 Id. at 1636.

35 Id. at 1634.

36 Id. at 1626 (emphasis added).

37 Id. at 1650 (Ginsburg, J., dissenting).

38 See *Harris*, 448 U.S. at 297.

39 Pub. L. No. 109–149, §§507, 508, 119 Stat. 2833.

40 448 U.S. at 314–18.

41 Henshaw SK, Finer LB. The accessibility of abortion services in the United States, 2001. *Perspect Sex Reprod Health* 2003; **35**: 16–24.

42 Boonstra H, Sonfield A. Rights without access: revisiting public funding of abortion for poor women. *The Guttmacher Report on Public Policy* 2000; **3**: 8–11; Boonstra H. The heart of the matter: public funding of abortion for poor women in the United States. *Guttmacher Policy Review* 2007; **10**: 12–16.

43 See *Alaska v. Planned Parenthood*, 28 P.3d 904 (Ak. 2001); *Simat Corp. v. Az. Health Care Cost Containment Sys.*, 56 P.3d 28 (Az. 2002); *Comm. to Defend Reprod. Rights v. Myers*, 625 P.2d 779 (Cal. 1981); *Doe v. Maher*, 515 A.2d 134 (Conn. Super. Ct. 1986); *Doe v. Wright*, No. 91 CH 1958 (Ill. Cir. Ct. Dec. 2, 1994); *Moe v. Sec'y of Admin. & Fin.*, 417 N.E.2d 387 (Mass. 1981); *Women of Minn. v. Gomez*, 542 N.W.2d 17 (Minn. 1995); *Jeannette R. v. Ellery*, No. BDV-94-811 (Mont. Dist. Ct. May 22, 1995); *Right to Choose v. Byrne*, 450 A.2d 925 (N.J. 1982); *N.M. Right to Choose/NARAL v. Johnson*, 975 P.2d 841 (N.M. 1998); *Planned Parenthood Ass'n, Inc. v. Dep't of Human Res.*, 663 P.2d 1247 (Or. Ct. App. 1983), *aff'd on statutory grounds*, 687 P.2d 785 (Or. 1984); *Doe v. Celani*, No. S81-84CnC (Vt. Super. Ct. May 26, 1986); *Women's Health Ctr. of W. Va., Inc. v. Panepinto*, 446 S.E.2d 658 (W. Va. 1993).

44 State Policies in Brief: State Funding of Abortion Under Medicaid [Online]. New York: Guttmacher Institute; 2008 Aug 1 [cited 2008 Aug 5]. Available from: URL:http://www.guttmacher.org/statecenter/spibs/spib_SFAM.pdf

45 Id.

46 *Webster v. Reprod. Health Svs.*, 492 U.S. 490, 507-08 (1989).

47 See URL:http://www.naral.org/choice-action-center/in_your_state/who-decides

48 *Doe v. Bridgeton Hosp. Ass'n, Inc.*, 366 A.2d 641 (N.J. 1976); *Valley Hosp. Ass'n v. Mat-su Coal. for Choice*, 948 P.2d 963 (Ak. 1997).

49 State Policies in Brief: Parental Involvement in Minors' Abortions [Online]. New York: Guttmacher Institute; 2008 Aug 1 [cited 2008 Aug 5]. Available from: URL:http://www.guttmacher.org/statecenter/spibs/spib_PIMA.pdf

50 *Bellotti*, 443 U.S. at 643-644.

51 American Medical Association, Council on Ethical and Judicial Affairs. Mandatory parental consent to abortion. *JAMA* 1993; **269**: 82–86; American Academy of Pediatrics. The adolescent's right to confidential care when considering abortion. *Pediatrics* 1996; **97**: 746–751; American College of Obstetricians

and Gynecologists. *Guidelines for Women's Health Care*. American College of Obstetricians and Gynecologists, Washington, DC, 1996; American Public Health Association. Adolescent access to comprehensive, confidential, reproductive healthcare. *Am J Public Health* 1991; **81**: 241.

52 *Am. Acad. of Pediatrics v. Lungren*, 940 P.2d 797 (Cal. 1997); *Wicklund v. State*, No. ADV-97-671 (Mt. Dist. Ct. Feb. 25, 1999); *Planned Parenthood of Cent. N.J. v. Farmer*, 762 A.2d 620 (N.J. 2000).

53 For the laws of individual states, visit URL:http://www.naral.org/choice-action-center/in_your_state/who-decides

54 See id.

55 Jones RK, Zolna MRS, Henshaw SK, Finer LB. Abortion in the United States: incidence and access to services, 2005. *Perspect Sex Reprod Health* 2008; **40**: 6–16.

56 Freedman MA, Jillson DA, Coffin RR, Novick LF. Comparison of complication rates in first trimester abortions performed by physician assistants and physicians. *Am J Public Health* 1986; **76**: 550–554; Goldman MB, Occhiuto JS, Peterson LE, Zapka JG, Palmer RH. Physician assistants as providers of surgically induced abortion services. *Am J Public Health* 2004; **94**: 1352–1357.

57 See National Abortion Federation [Online]. Washington (DC): National Abortion Federation; c2008. Resource center: statement of ACOG's Executive Board, January 1994; 2008 [cited 2008 Aug 5]. Available from: URL:http://www.prochoice.org/cfc/resources/professional_organizations.html.

58 *Roe*, 410 U.S. at 150, 163; *Connecticut v. Menillo*, 423 U.S. 9 (1975); *Mazurek v. Armstrong*, 520 U.S. 968 (1997).

59 *Mazurek*, 520 U.S. at 971.

60 *Armstrong v. State*, 989 P.2d 364, 380 (Mt. 1999).

61 National Abortion Federation [Online]. Washington (DC): National Abortion Federation; c2008. Clinicians for Choice: Legal practice issues-timeline of events; 2008 [cited 2008 Aug 5]. Available from: URL:http://www.prochoice.org/cfc/legal_practice.html

62 Id.; Letter from Peter J. Millock, General Counsel, State of New York Department of Health, to Donna Lieberman, New York Civil Liberties Union (Dec. 20, 1994).

63 Cal. Bus. & Prof. Code §2253; Conn. Op. Att'y Gen. No. 2001–015 (July 2, 2001); Planned Parenthood v. State, No. CV-200604230 (N.M. Dist. Ct. Oct. 10, 2007); R.I. Code R. 14 000 009, §§1.4, 1.5, 5.1; Wash. Op. Att'y Gen. No. 2004–1 (Jan. 5, 2004).

64 See *Hope Med'l Group for Women v. LeBlanc*, No. 2:06-cv-09176-ILRL-KWR (E.D. La.).

65 O'Connell K, Jones H, Simon M, Saporta V, Paul M, Lichtenberg ES. First trimester surgical abortion practices: a survey of National Abortion Federation members. *Contraception* in press.

66 See *supra* note 64.

67 Ala. Admin. Code r. 420–5–1–.02(d).

68 See *Doe v. Bolton*, 410 U.S. 179, 199 (1973).

69 See Center for Reproductive Rights [Online]. New York: Center for Reproductive Rights; c2008. Targeted regulation of abortion providers (TRAP): avoiding the TRAP; 2007 Nov [cited 2008 Aug 5]. Available from: URL:http://www.reproductiverights.org/en/document/targeted-regulation-of-abortion-providers-trap-avoiding-the-trap.

70 Id.

71 Id.

72 See id.

73 See id.

74 Id.

75 Id.; see Ak. Stat. Ann. §§18.16.010(a)(2), 08.64.105; Ak. Admin. Code tit. 7, §12.370.

76 Center for Reproductive Rights, *supra* note 69.; see also Ark. State Bd. of Health, Rules and Regulations for Abortion Facilities, §3; Nev. Rev. Stat. Ann. §442.250.2; N.C. Gen. Stat. Ann. §14–45.1(b).

77 See,e.g., *Ragsdale v. Turnock*, 841 F.2d 1358, 1370 (7th Cir. 1988); *Birth Control Ctrs., Inc. v. Reizen*, 743 F.2d 352 (6th Cir. 1984).

78 See, e.g., *Greenville Women's Clinic v. Bryant*, 222 F.3d 157 (4th Cir. 2000); *Women's Med. Ctr. v. Bell*, 248 F.3d 411 (5th Cir. 2001).

79 *Tucson Woman's Clinic v. Eden*, 379 F.3d 531, 541 (9th Cir. 2004).

80 State Policies in Brief: Mandatory Counseling and Waiting Periods for Abortions [Online]. New York: Guttmacher Institute; 2008 Aug 1 [cited 2008 Aug 5]. Available from: URL:http://www.guttmacher.org/statecenter/spibs/spib_MWPA.pdf

81 Id.

82 Id.

83 Id.

84 Richardson CT, Nash E. Misinformed consent: the medical accuracy of state-developed abortion counseling materials. *Guttmacher Policy Review* 2006; **9**: 6–11.

85 505 U.S. at 822.

86 E.g., *Woman's Choice-East Side Women's Clinic v. Newman*, 305 F.3d 684 (7th Cir. 2002); *Clinic for Women, Inc. v. Brizzi*, 837 N.E.2d 973 (Ind. 2005); *Barnes v. Moore*, 970 F.2d 12 (5th Cir. 1992); *Pro-Choice Miss. v. Fordice*, 716 So. 2d 645 (Miss. 1998); but see,e.g., *Planned Parenthood of Middle Tenn. v. Sundquist*, 38 S.W.3d 1 (Tenn. 2000).

87 Joyce T, Henshaw SK, Skatrud JD. The impact of Mississippi's mandatory delay law on abortions and births. *JAMA* 1997; **278**: 653–658.

88 See Ark. Code Ann. §20-16-1102 *et seq.*; Ga. Code Ann. §31-9A-3 *et seq.*; La. Rev. Stat. Ann. § 40:1299.35.6(C)(1)(a)(ii); Minn. Stat. Ann. §§145.4242(a)(2)(iii), 145.4243; Okla. Stat. Ann. tit. 63, §1-738.8 *et seq.*

89 Richardson & Nash, *supra* note 84, at 11.

90 See Ark. Code Ann. §20-16-1104; La. Rev. Stat. Ann. §40:1299.35.6(B)(1)(g); Minn. Stat. Ann. § 145.4242(a)(1)(iv); Okla. Stat. Ann. tit. 63, §1-738.9.

91 Richardson & Nash, *supra* note 84, at 11.

92 Ala. Code §26-23A-1 to -13; Miss. Code Ann. §41-41-34; Ark. Code Ann. §20-16-602; Idaho Code Ann. §18-609(3); Ind. Code Ann. §§16–18–2–69, 16–34–2–1, 16–34–2–1; Mich. Comp. Laws Ann. §§333.17014, 333.17015; Okla. Stat. Ann. tit. 63, §§1–738.1 to .5 & 1–738.6 to .12; Utah Code Ann. §§76–7–305 – 767–7–305.5; Wis. Stat. Ann. §253.10.

93 *Acuna v. Turkish*, 930 A.2d 416, 418 (N.J. 2007).

94 S.D. Code Ann. §34–23A–10.1 (2003); *Planned Parenthood Minn. v. Rounds*, 530 F.3d 724 (8th Cir. 2008).

95 127 S. Ct. at 1634.

96 18 U.S.C. §1531(b).

97 127 S. Ct. at 1629.

98 Id. at 1632.

99 *Danforth*, 428 U.S. at 64; *Colautti v. Franklin*, 439 U.S. 379, 388-90 (1979); *Webster*, 492 U.S. at 517.

100 *Webster*, 492 U.S. at 519–20.

101 *Planned Parenthood v. Ashcroft*, 462 U.S. 476, 485–86 (1983).

102 *Thornburgh*, 476 U.S. at 768–70; see also *Colautti*, 439 U.S. at 400–01.

103 *Thornburgh*, 476 U.S. at 770–71.

104 Cal. Health & Safety Code §§123462, 123466; Conn. Gen. Stat. ch. 368y, §19a-609; Hawaii Rev. Stat. §453-16; Me. Rev. Stat. Ann. tit. 263-B, §1598; Md. Code Ann., Health-General §20-209; Nev. Rev. Stat. Ann. §442.250; Wash. Rev. Code Ann §9.02.100 *et seq.*; see also Vt. H.R. Res. 4 (resolving every Vermont woman has a right to privacy in making personal decisions about reproduction).

105 Freedom of Choice Act, S. 1173, H.R. 1964, 110th Cong. (2007).

106 18 U.S.C. §248 (2007).

107 National Abortion Federation [Online]. Washington (DC): National Abortion Federation; c2008. Freedom of access to clinic entrances (FACE) act fact sheet; 2006 [cited 2008 Aug 5]. Available from: URL:http://www.prochoice.org/pubs_research/publications/downloads/about_abortion/face_act.pdf; United States Department of Justice [Online].Washington (DC): National Task Force on Violence Against Health Care Providers. Report on federal efforts to prevent and prosecute clinic violence 1998–2000; [cited 2008 Aug 5]. Available from: URL:http://www.usdoj.gov/crt/crim/tfreppub.htm

108 Id.

109 State Policies in Brief: Protecting Access to Clinics [Online]. New York: Guttmacher Institute; 2008 Aug 1 [cited 2008 Aug 5]. Available from: URL:http://www.guttmacher.org/statecenter/spibs/spib_PAC.pdf

110 See,e.g., *Madsen v. Women's Health Ctr., Inc.*, 512 U.S. 753 (1994); *Schenck v. Pro-Choice Network of W. N.Y.*, 519 U.S. 357 (1997).

111 To contact these organizations, visit URL:http://www.aclu.org/contact/index.html or URL:http://www.reproductiverights.org/ab_contact.html

112 URL:http://www.aclu.org/reproductiverights/index.html

113 URL:http://www.reproductiverights.org/wn_abortion.html

114 URL:http://www.guttmacher.org/statecenter/abortion.html

115 URL:http://www.naral.org/choice-action-center/in_your_state/who-decides/

5

CHAPTER 5

Informed consent, patient education, and counseling

Anne Baker, MA and Terry Beresford, BA

LEARNING POINTS

- Providing proficient patient education and informed consent protects both the provider and the patient.
- Effective communication between provider and patient helps to optimize the outcome of the procedure.
- The patient's history, circumstances, and feelings may need exploration and counseling intervention for adequate decision-making, acceptance, and management of the procedure, as well as coping afterwards.
- Studies of psychological adjustment to abortion help providers differentiate between women who need preabortion counseling intervention and those who simply require patient education and informed consent.

Introduction

Women who seek services from abortion care providers present with varying needs. Many patients are sure about their decision to have an abortion, and they primarily want information about the abortion methods available and what to expect. Other women may wish to explore their pregnancy options more fully and obtain help in making a decision. For some women, having an abortion may be as much an emotional experience as it is physical because of personal circumstances, ambivalence, or intense and perhaps conflicting feelings the decision evokes.

This chapter addresses three separate yet overlapping components of abortion provision: informed consent, patient education, and counseling. Informed consent is a legal and ethical obligation defined by state laws, malpractice standards, and the professional standards governing medical practice; it applies to all patients. Patient education is an integral part of the informed consent process, but many patients benefit from provision of other types of health-related information as well. Counseling in the abortion care setting provides an opportunity for a woman to explore the circumstances, emotions, expectations, and beliefs that may influence her abortion experience. Not all women who seek abortion care need or desire counseling intervention. When needed, however, effective counseling interventions may occur prior to, during, or following the abortion. Attending appropriately and skillfully to the emotional needs of patients is an important component of patient-centered care.

Informed consent

To avoid both civil and criminal liability, obtaining the "informed consent" of a patient prior to an induced abortion or any other medical procedure is imperative. According to the US President's Commission for the Study of Ethical Problems in Medicine and Biomedical and Behavioral Research, informed consent must include three elements [1]:

1 patients must have the *capacity to make decisions* about their care;
2 their participation in these decisions must be *without coercion or manipulation*; and
3 patients must *be given appropriate information* germane to making the particular decision.

The goal of the informed consent process is to protect personal well-being and individual autonomy by providing information on the procedure, risks, and alternatives to the medical intervention being considered.

Management of Unintended and Abnormal Pregnancy, 1st edition. By M Paul, ES Lichtenberg, L Borgatta, DA Grimes, PG Stubblefield, MD Creinin

Regarding abortion, many state legislatures in the USA have mandated scripts for abortion providers to read to patients, and videos, photographs, and/or ultrasounds that patients must view prior to their abortion (Chapter 4). A comprehensive analysis by the Guttmacher Institute found that these materials contained assertions of physical and emotional risks unsupported by scientific research, as well as descriptions of fetal development and pain and procedures not germane to first- or second-trimester abortion [2]. The abortion provider has an ethical responsibility to ensure that the patient receives *accurate* information while following the law.

Informed consent includes informing the patient about her medical condition, available treatment options, and the benefits and risks of these alternatives. The risks of surgical abortion commonly described in the consent form include failed abortion, incomplete abortion, hematometra, infection, hemorrhage, cervical laceration, uterine perforation, anesthesia reactions, and the rare occurrence of hysterectomy or death. For medical abortion, the typical risks include drug side effects and potential teratogenicity, hemorrhage, infection, failed abortion, and the possible need to have a surgical abortion if the medical abortion is not successful. Addressing the risks of morbidity and mortality from continued pregnancy and childbirth, which are considerably higher than those from legal induced abortion, is also important. The patient has the responsibility to weigh the risks and benefits of abortion versus continuing the pregnancy and choose the option that is most appropriate in light of her medical condition and personal values, relationships, and goals.

Whereas most women seeking abortion have already considered the options of parenting or making an adoption plan, the patient must acknowledge these alternatives to abortion. Although some women want their husbands or partners to attend the patient preparation session, the woman should initially be questioned *alone* about her decision and afforded an opportunity to disclose coercion. If a patient expresses doubts or misgivings, her options and feelings warrant more extensive exploration.

Similarly, if the patient is a minor, the provider should seek assurance that she is not being coerced by her parent(s). Only when it is clear that parental coercion is not a factor should the provider obtain any government-mandated parental consent or notification or the consent of a court (Chapter 4) and secure the appropriate forms for the medical record.

Providers may designate trained staff members to obtain informed consent from patients, except where law mandates *clinicians only* may conduct the informed consent process. Ways in which patients receive information vary among abortion providers and may include written material, verbal instruction, or audiovisual media.

Provision of informed consent

In general, the process of informed consent includes the following:

- providing the patient with the information she needs in order to make a voluntary, informed decision about her pregnancy options and, if she chooses abortion, about the methods of abortion available to her;
- answering the patient's questions, such as those pertaining to how the procedure is performed, the length of time required, and issues of pain and safety;
- adhering to all state mandated protocols;
- in cases of illiteracy or language barriers, helping the patient understand the information through audiovisuals, translators, and if possible, written materials in the patient's language;
- postponing the procedure if drug or alcohol use or other conditions have impaired the patient's comprehension and ability to consent;
- obtaining the signature of the legal guardian/parent if the patient has mental or developmental disabilities that prevent comprehension;
- requiring documentation of competency from a psychiatrist if the patient has a history of psychotic episodes; and
- co-signing consent forms that include all the elements of informed consent.

Patient education related to abortion provision

In addition to the patient education that is integral to the informed consent process, the abortion visit may include the following:

- educating the patient about contraceptive options and helping her to choose an appropriate method, if she so desires (Chapter 14);
- educating the patient about prevention of sexually transmitted diseases;
- having a counselor on-site or providing referrals for preabortion counseling in cases of extreme ambivalence, perception of coercion, or other sources of severe emotional upset;
- providing empowering literature, referrals, or websites for postabortion emotional well-being; and
- providing referrals for continued gynecological care in her geographic area.

Nonprocedural counseling

Some patients may have emotional or personal needs that require attention prior to and after the abortion procedure. To assess each patient's potential need for counseling, the informed consent session may include a written or verbal inquiry about:

Table 5.1 Elements of Informed Consent Prior to Abortion

- The gestational age of the pregnancy
- Options available to the woman (i.e., continuing the pregnancy and parenting or placing for adoption) or terminating the pregnancy
- Potential benefits and risks of continuing or terminating the pregnancy
- The voluntary nature of the patient's decision
- The abortion procedure(s) appropriate to the duration of her pregnancy
- Advantages and possible complications of her chosen method of abortion: medical or surgical
- Available anesthesia options and their benefits and risks
- Tests that may be performed to diagnose or treat the patient's condition (e.g., pregnancy tests, ultrasound, hemoglobin, Rh status)
- Any ancillary tests or procedures (e.g., government reporting requirements for sexually transmitted infections)
- Permission to treat the patient in the event of a complication or emergency
- If the patient is a minor and if required by law, notifying the parent(s) or obtaining permission of the parent(s) or court (judicial bypass) prior to providing abortion care (Chapter 4)
- Her understanding of the forms

- her level of certainty about the decision;
- her feelings about her decision;
- her beliefs about abortion, including spiritual beliefs;
- sources of anxiety and ways of decreasing her level of anxiety; and
- her support system.

If this inquiry identifies counseling needs that the person obtaining informed consent is not trained to address, then he or she should seek assistance from a colleague with the requisite counseling skills. Although not essential for counseling, a bachelor's degree in social work or psychology provides excellent background. Counseling may include:

- exploration of negative beliefs about abortion and spiritual fears;
- her expectations for coping with feelings and/or unsupportive significant others;
- effective strategies for coping;
- referrals for domestic violence or rape crisis counseling, or relevant mental health conditions such as depression; and
- intervention if the patient feels coerced.

The individual counseling session should occur in a private setting and be neither rushed nor prolonged beyond the individual's needs. Guidelines in this chapter will help to identify patients who are struggling with their decision or feelings and may need more time before making their final decision.

Potential benefits of preabortion counseling

Little if any research can be found on the specific models of preabortion counseling that exist in clinics. However, when counseling interventions serve to decrease stigma, increase patients' beliefs in their ability to use effective coping skills, and decrease anxiety before or after the procedure, physical and/or emotional outcomes can be positively affected (Littman 2007, unpublished thesis) [3].

Clinical experience shows that when fear and other emotional distress surrounding an abortion are not addressed, patients can experience heightened anxiety, intensified pain during and after the abortion, misdirected anger toward the provider, or dissatisfaction afterwards. In addition, research indicates that a woman's appraisal of her abortion experience guides how she is likely to cope postabortion [4]. In addition to providing supportive care, time spent on preabortion counseling can save time and money in the long run because of the potential benefits to both the patient and provider.

Assessing patients' preabortion emotional needs

The literature on the predictors for psychological adjustment to abortion offers guidance about issues that are relevant to patients' well-being [5–9]. Assessing for warning signs and adequately addressing these issues beforehand are likely to enhance the patient's satisfaction and coping ability on the day of and after her abortion.

During the informed consent session, use of a needs assessment form (Fig. 5.1) can sometimes assist in determining the patient's emotional status. Such forms are designed to reveal indicators for positive or negative postabortion reactions.

Promoting effective communication

Appropriate, sensitive communication that recognizes and responds to the needs of each patient is fundamental to quality gynecological care [10,11]. Even during brief interactions, clinicians using basic counseling skills and motivational interaction techniques can produce a positive impact [12–14].

Table 5.2 Potential Benefits of Preabortion Counseling

Potential Benefits for the Patient
- Decreases anxiety
- Provides emotional support
- Strengthens her belief in her ability to manage physical discomfort
- Fortifies her coping ability
- Helps reduce shame and stigma
- Decreases distress provoked by protesters or other antichoice influences
- Prevents coercion
- Provides patient education about the procedure, aftercare, possible complications, and her contraceptive choice
- Increases potential for a positive memory of the day of her abortion

Potential Benefits for the Provider
- Increases patient satisfaction with her care
- Combats inaccurate social perceptions perpetuated by those opposed to abortion (e.g., abortion providers as money-centered rather than patient-centered)
- Decreases the (already small) chance that the patient will change her mind during the abortion procedure
- Increases the likelihood that the patient will be:
  - > less anxious
  - > more confident in the provider's and nurses' expertise
  - > more knowledgeable about what to expect
  - > equipped with strategies for managing any fear or pain
- Gives the provider:
  - > documentation of the patient's emotional state, certainty about her decision, denial of coercion, her expectation for coping, and any referrals given
  - > an added layer of protection against legal claims

> Studies of physician–patient communication and patient health outcomes reveal a significant correlation between the quality of communication and patients' emotional health, physiologic measures (blood pressure and blood sugar levels), symptom resolution, and pain control [10].

Reflecting

Reflecting the thoughts and feelings the patient expresses is an effective way of showing that the provider is listening to her. It builds trust between clinician and patient. Examples:
- "I'm hearing that you're angry with yourself for not using a more effective birth control method."
- "Sounds to me that these past few weeks have been very stressful to you."

Asking questions

Sometimes a simple pause after a reflective comment elicits a response from the patient. If not, asking *open-ended questions* will prompt a narrative rather than a simple "yes" or "no." Examples:
- "When you're feeling angry with yourself for getting pregnant, what are you saying to yourself?"
- "Of all the stress you've been managing, what is the most stressful part of this experience for you?"

Closed-ended questions are effective when it is desirable to elicit information quickly. Such questions usually elicit one-word answers, such as yes or no, but they can lead to further explanation. Examples:
- "Did you have any physical problems after your first abortion?"
- "Do you have someone you can talk to after the abortion?"

Normalizing

Normalizing occurs when the clinician or counselor lets the patient know that her thoughts, feelings, or questions are *not* stupid or uncommon. Examples:
- "Many women have expressed the same mixture of feelings you're talking about."
- "This is a question many people have asked, and it's important to find out the answer."

Examining consequences

Using "If... then..." statements and questions prompts the patient to think for herself and examine what outcomes she wants and how to achieve them. Examples:
- "If you want to help the doctor keep this procedure very safe, then you'll want to lie still."
- "If you want the birth control pill to be as effective as possible, then remembering to take it at the same time every day will be important to you."

Too many closed-ended questions in succession can feel like an interrogation, inhibit communication, and may also convey the feeling of being rushed.

NEEDS ASSESSMENT FORM **The Hope Clinic for Women**

Patient's Name____________________Date__________Age______

To participate with you in an abortion, we want to know if the following statements are true or false for you. Please answer the questions *in all honesty* in a spirit of cooperation with your emotional and physical care. All is kept *confidential.*

Check the box that best describes you, so we'll know how to better serve you today.

Your Decision	**True**	**Kind of**	**False**
1. I am SURE of my decision to have an abortion.	☐	☐	☐
2. I'm here for an abortion because ***someone else*** is pushing me into it. **(Circle all who are pressuring you.)**	☐	☐	☐

My Mom Boyfriend Husband The partner in the pregnancy
My Dad

Anyone else?____________________

	True	**Kind of**	**False**
3. I want to have the baby and keep it instead of abortion.	☐	☐	☐
4. I want to place the baby for adoption instead of an abortion.	☐	☐	☐

5. How You're Feeling Today: (Check off as many as are true for you)

Very scared ☐ A little nervous ☐ Pretty calm ☐ Confident ☐ Relieved ☐ Angry ☐
Very sick ☐ A little guilty ☐ Very guilty ☐ Ashamed ☐ Very sad ☐
A little sad ☐ Other____________________

6. How Do You View Abortion?

	True	**Kind of**	**False**
At my stage of pregnancy, it's the same as killing a baby that's already born.	☐	☐	☐
Abortion is a better choice for me at this time than having the baby.	☐	☐	☐

Any Comment____________________

7. I have *or* have had: (Check all that are true)

Depression ☐ Anxiety ☐ Panic attacks ☐ Bipolar ☐ ADD ☐
Posttrauma stress ☐ Bulimia ☐ Schizophrenia ☐ Borderline Personality Disorder ☐
Anorexia ☐

8. Who are the people who know you're having an abortion?
(Please check off all that are true for you):

Who knows?	**Is this person supportive to you in what you want to do?**		
☐ Boyfriend	Yes ☐	Not much ☐	No ☐
☐ Ex-boyfriend	Yes ☐	Not much ☐	No ☐
☐ Husband	Yes ☐	Not much ☐	No ☐
☐ Ex-husband	Yes ☐	Not much ☐	No ☐
☐ The father	Yes ☐	Not much ☐	No ☐
☐ Friend	Yes ☐	Not much ☐	No ☐
☐ My mom	Yes ☐	Not much ☐	No ☐
☐ My dad	Yes ☐	Not much ☐	No ☐

Is there anyone else you told? (Who?)____________________

	True	**False**
9. *This* pregnancy is a result of being forced to have sex (rape).	☐	☐

Figure 5.1 Needs Assessment Form (Courtesy of the Hope Clinic for Women; reprinted with permission).

10. If you've had one or more abortions in the past, then answer (a) and (b) please. If not, go on to #11 and answer questions about spiritual concerns.

		True	Kind of	False
a.	I did well emotionally afterwards.	☐	☐	☐
b.	I had a hard time dealing with it afterwards.	☐	☐	☐

11. If you have any belief in God (or a Higher Power), please answer these questions.

		True	Kind of	False
a.	I have some spiritual concerns about abortion.	☐	☐	☐
b.	I'm afraid God won't forgive me.	☐	☐	☐
c.	Spiritually, I'm at peace with this decision.	☐	☐	☐

Comments____

12. Coping Emotionally After the Abortion

Women report a range of feelings afterwards. Some women cope well no matter what feelings come up, and others have a hard time.

How do you think you may feel after having this abortion? (Check all that apply.)

Confident in the decision ☐ Relieved ☐ Happy ☐ A little guilty ☐ A little sad ☐

Very guilty ☐ Very sad ☐ Ashamed ☐ Angry ☐

I'll wish I never went through with the abortion ☐ Other_______________________

13. How do you think you'll deal with the feelings you checked?

☐ I'll deal with my feelings fine afterwards.

☐ It might be a little hard at first, but then I'll be fine and won't regret my decision.

☐ It will probably be VERY hard for me afterwards.

☐ I'll wish I never went through with the abortion.

☐ I believe I will be able to cope with this decision better than having and keeping it or adoption at this time.

14. I have answered this form truthfully, in the spirit of cooperation with my care.

_______________________________ _______________

Signature of Patient **Date**

Figure 5.1 *(Continued)*

> Words such as "should" or "ought" and phrases that begin with "why didn't you" trigger defensiveness, withdrawal, and mistrust.

Reframing

Reframing is looking at something from a new perspective. One of the powerful ways people cope with difficult life challenges is to shift from a negative to a positive perspective [4]. Examples:

- A patient expresses guilt about getting her education first before having a baby because she sees it as "selfish." One way of helping her reframe this perception is by supporting the view that her education will enable her to provide well for any child she has in the future.
- A patient expresses guilt because she "has always been against abortion until now." If she has made exceptions for rape or life endangerment, then she can see herself as having kept an open mind on abortion for certain circumstances, and is now expanding her acceptance of other circumstances.

Communicating nonjudgmental attitudes

Fostering a respectful clinician–patient relationship can pose a challenge when patient behaviors trigger critical judgments. Patients coping with issues related to sexuality and abortion are especially sensitive to censure, and they may avoid surgical abortion for fear of judgmental staff [15]. Even when critical attitudes are unintentionally expressed through the clinician's facial expression, gestures, or word choice, patients notice and react negatively.

A number of patient behaviors may trigger critical judgments (Table 5.3). Examining one's own attitudes toward such behaviors helps the clinician maintain a supportive relationship with the patient.

One of the behaviors that frequently triggers critical judgment is recurrent abortion. The focus of reproach from society is almost always on the woman. She is accused of being "irresponsible" or of "using abortion as birth control." Many patients themselves adopt these cultural views; they regard more than one abortion as reprehensible, blame only themselves, and forget that pregnancy takes *two*. Oddly, the sense of "irresponsibility" is placed on the action of abortion and not on the action of having an unintended pregnancy. If two women each had three unintended pregnancies, and one of the women continued all the pregnancies while the other had three abortions, the underlying issue of responsibility related to birth control still remains relevant.

Table 5.3 Patient Behaviors that May Trigger Critical Judgments

Pregnancies resulting from not using or misusing contraception
Multiple unplanned pregnancies, abortions, or births
Abusive relationships
Preadolescent or adolescent sex and pregnancy
Adolescents not wanting to tell parents
Reasons for the abortion other than what the clinician believes is justifiable
Second-trimester abortion because of patient's denial of pregnancy
Patient being loud and uncooperative on the table or when approached with a needle

> The key to achieving effective clinician–patient communication is the ability to give the clear, comforting message that one is not judging the patient but shares with her a common bond of humanity.

A woman has approximately 37 years of potential fertility, or 444 months in which she could become pregnant. Laws of probability alone account for multiple pregnancies over the course of a lifetime. Most people sustain the required effort to stay in control of some parts of their lives some or most of the time, but not 100% of the time.

Empathy hinges on awareness of how one's own life struggles are similar to those of the patient. Clinicians, nurses, and counselors might recall examples of repeated risk-taking with their own well-being and recurrent failures to control particular areas of their lives such as:

- maintaining a healthy diet;
- exercising;
- drinking in moderation;
- avoiding tobacco use;
- leaving damaging relationships;
- balancing work life and home life;
- practicing emotional self-care; or
- using contraceptives perfectly.

By reviewing the behaviors in Table 5.3 and uncovering parallels in one's own life, the clinician can better understand and relate to patients.

A powerful message of empathy for a patient who presents with a history of abortions is: "I will be here for you and treat you respectfully no matter how many times you need this service. I'll also do my best to help you with future contraception. I know only too well that none of us is perfect!" Trust is also promoted by using a normalizing statement followed by a personal question, such as: "Many women struggle with their fertility and contraception. What experiences have you had?"

Feelings on the day of the abortion

For many women, feelings of relief and confidence in the decision predominate on the day of the abortion, mixed with manageable levels of anxiety. For others, feelings of fear, anxiety, guilt, sadness, anger, or shame are prominent [16]. These feelings may be expressed not in words but in tears. When a patient cries, the clinician can pause, and then seek to understand the source of her tears. For example:

- "Crying is not uncommon at times like this, and people cry for different reasons. I don't want to *assume*—can you help me understand what your tears are about?"
- "You don't have to tell me anything you don't want to. Whatever you *can* tell me, though, will help me understand."

Common fears

Fear of pain, needles, doctors, and medical procedures

The most common fear is fear of pain and needles. Fear of doctors and medical instrumentation, including the speculum, is not uncommon, and sometimes patients express fear of what they might see and hear during the abortion. Showing sensitivity and making whatever accommodations are safe and feasible are part of patient-centered, quality care.

Fear of becoming sterile or dying

Patients may be frightened by antiabortion protesters and websites falsely claiming that sterility and death are commonplace. Giving patients facts and valid sources of information usually eliminates these fears. If not, the fear of dying in particular is sometimes prompted by shame and fear of punishment or unmanaged panic disorder; in these cases, facts will have little effect. If general anesthesia is used, and the patient fears "going to sleep and not waking up," then the clinician can provide realistic estimates of risk or offer other pain management options.

Fear of breached confidentiality

This fear is most frequently voiced if antichoice protesters are taking patients' pictures or filming them as part of their scare tactics on the day of the abortion. The provider can assure them of confidentiality *only* on the part of the staff.

Fear of dire emotional aftermath

Antichoice activists spread misinformation via multiple forms of media about physical *and* emotional aftermath they attribute to abortion, such as high risks of depression, psychiatric admissions, suicide, cancer, trauma, and drug addiction [17] (Chapter 16). Patients sometimes bring up frightening warnings they have heard about how women will feel postabortion. Letting the woman know what factors predict positive and negative outcome and asking how *she* thinks she will cope help to affirm her own judgment.

Fear of God's disapproval, withholding forgiveness, or punishment

Clinicians and counselors can help empower patients who express spiritual fears. Asking the following questions, reflecting on her responses, and giving her appropriate resources can be strengthening. Examples:

- "Do you believe in a merciful God who understands what's in our hearts?"
- (If she believes she needs forgiveness): "What is necessary to receive God's forgiveness, from your viewpoint and that of your faith?"
- "If you fear punishment, what are you afraid will happen?"
- "What are some positive consequences that could come from this experience?"

Effective resources for patients who need spiritual support can be found at www.faithaloud.org, cath4choice.org, www.hopeclinic.org, and www.pregnancyoptions.info (Appendix).

Guilt

The following statements demonstrate possible responses to patients who express guilt:

- "People feel guilty about different things when they have an abortion. Would you help me understand what you're feeling guilty about?"
- If she is feeling guilty about getting pregnant and says she was "stupid," some helpful responses are:
  - "You don't have to explain to *me*, but privately you can ask yourself, 'What were the circumstances that led me to take a risk with my well-being? What are examples of ways I usually take care of myself? How can I protect myself in the future"'?
- If she is feeling guilty about "killing a baby":
  - "Some people consider abortion as killing a baby; others believe it's kind of like killing a baby and kind of not, depending on how developed the pregnancy is. At your stage of pregnancy, how does it feel for you? If you have the abortion, how do expect you'll feel about the decision? About yourself?"
  - If she responds unfavorably, then, "How would you feel about adoption?"
- If she insists abortion is more manageable than any other option, then "What can you tell yourself and do for yourself when you have times of guilt afterwards?"
- If she states she doesn't know or will probably wish she never had the abortion, then the provider needs to decide whether or not to participate in an abortion with her at that time and convey the caring that underlies the decision.

Sadness and loss

Some women experience a sense of loss. It may be the loss of a relationship, a dream, their innocence, a future, a child, or other kinds of loss. In these situations, encouraging the patient to verbalize what the sadness is about can be beneficial. For example:

- "Even when people know they are making the best decision, it's natural to have some sad feelings as well."
- "When you think about other losses you've felt in your life, what did you tell yourself and do for yourself that helped?"

Shame

An important distinction exists between shame and guilt. Guilt is feeling badly about specific behavior; shame is a total condemnation of self. When people feel shame, they are likely to blame others, become hostile and aggressive, withdraw, hide, run away, judge others and themselves harshly, and feel powerless and out of control [18].

Some people are prone to shame (e.g., abuse survivors, those with addictions and other disorders) and are sensitive to external judgment. They are more likely to be upset by what they see and hear from antiabortion websites, protesters, and other sources of judgment. Helping these patients recognize and change shame-producing thoughts offers them ways to shift perspective. For example:

- From "I'm a bad mother because I'm having an abortion" to "Good mothers have to make hard choices, including having an abortion."
- From "I should have known better" to "It's human to make mistakes; all humans have the ability to learn from their mistakes."

Shame-prone individuals habitually criticize themselves, and having an abortion may represent one more piece of distorted evidence of their "unworthiness." A referral for psychological counseling before or after the abortion may be appropriate.

Anger

Some people deny their anger, misdirect it, and alienate their caregivers. They state they just want to get everything over with and go home. Appropriate responses may be:

- "I can see you want to get this over with. I'll try to make things happen as fast as possible. At the same time I don't want to ignore whatever is aggravating to you because it could make the physical procedure harder for you."
- (To the patient who readily admits she is angry): "There can be a number of things to feel angry about today. Can you tell me what *your* feelings are about?"

Request to view the products of conception

Most women do not ask to see the pregnancy tissue. When a patient does ask to view the pregnancy tissue, her reasons may range from curiosity (perhaps about the accuracy of the protesters' posters or website pictures), to wanting forgiveness or punishment, or to say good-bye. To help her understand what underlies the request, the clinician or counselor might ask:

- What do you expect it to look like? (How big, how developed)
- Would you like to see a picture at your stage of pregnancy? The ultrasound picture?
- In what ways do you think viewing it after the abortion will or won't help you cope afterwards?
- How do you feel about what you're seeing? (whether picture or pregnancy tissue)

If the patient has stated she fears God won't forgive her, and she won't be able to forgive herself, then it is appropriate to ask, "Some women think they should see it to punish themselves. How is it for you?"

To date, research is lacking on the emotional effects of viewing the pregnancy tissue at various stages of pregnancy. Clinical experience indicates that respecting the wishes of a woman who chooses to view the tissue may promote her postabortion well-being, as long as the abortion care provider takes the necessary preparatory time and allows the woman to talk about it before and after as needed.

Some state laws mandate that providers show each woman who seeks abortion pictures of embryo-fetal development, even if she prefers not to see them. A woman may prefer not to view these illustrations because they will not change her reasons for the abortion, and she may experience the viewing as punishing. However, some women ask to see the ultrasound screen or picture and want to know about embryo-fetal development. It is important to respond to a patient's requests about seeing what is meaningful to her and to process with her what she sees.

Reactions to ineligibility for an abortion

When a patient is told that she is unable to obtain an abortion because of the advanced stage of the pregnancy or other reasons, she may experience shock, anger, and grief. An appropriate response is to stay physically and emotionally present for a time, without talking, and give the patient the opportunity to cry or otherwise express the intensity of her emotions. Once she seems able to listen, the clinician or counselor can reflect, "This can be upsetting and difficult to accept. Would you like to have the person who came with you join us?" The support person is usually able to comfort the patient and help her process the information about remaining options. Offering them adoption and prenatal care referrals and a copy of the patient's ultrasound, if desired, help them consider their next step. In the absence of a support person, helping the patient identify and contact someone to talk to once she leaves the office is important. If she threatens suicide, which sometimes happens, an assessment is warranted. She may need to go to an emergency department for evaluation.

Recommendations for preabortion care

Factors affecting postabortion emotional outcome and coping

Negative emotional sequelae

Although the predominant emotional response to induced abortion is relief for the vast majority of women, negative

Table 5.4 Risk Factors for Negative Emotional Sequelae

Appraisal of abortion as extremely stressful before it occurs
Experiencing social stigma and antiabortion demonstrators on the day of the abortion
An existing emotional disorder or mental illness prior to the abortion
Significant ambivalence about the decision
Perceived coercion to have the abortion
Intense guilt and shame before the abortion
Belief that abortion is the same act as killing a newborn infant
Lack of emotional support and receiving criticism from significant people in their lives
Fetal abnormality or other medical indications for the abortion
Commitment and attachment to the pregnancy
Advanced stage of pregnancy
Putting great effort into keeping the abortion a secret for fear of stigma
Usual coping style is denial and repressing thoughts
Unresolved past losses and perception of abortion as a loss
Past or present sexual, physical, or emotional abuse
Preexisting experience of trauma
Expecting depression, severe grief or guilt, and regret after the abortion
Disbelief in their ability to do what it takes to produce a positive outcome

reactions can include extreme grief, guilt, shame, anger, regret, increased symptoms of emotional disorders the patient has or has had in the past, and inability to cope [7,19]. Research has identified a number of psychosocial predictors for negative emotional sequelae [5]. Providers are wise to use the list of risk factors to assess the level of care a patient may need preabortion (Table 5.4). Patients with risk factors may require more time to reconsider options or make a plan for coping strategies.

Positive postabortion reactions

Positive reactions can include confidence, certitude, peace, and relief with or without a manageable level of sadness or guilt and positive expectations for coping. Research on coping after abortion shows that the less stressful a woman's appraisal of the abortion experience before it occurs, the more likely she is afterwards to feel satisfied with the decision and confident in her ability to cope, as well as to use more effective coping strategies [8]. Using an Emotional Needs Assessment Form (Fig. 5.1) developed by experienced abortion counselors can help identify patients who do or do not need preabortion counseling for emotional well-being.

> With some patients, it becomes apparent that they need more time to reconsider options or make a plan for effective coping before going through an abortion. Providers have an ethical responsibility to themselves and patients when deciding whether to participate in the provision of an individual's abortion that day.

Potential consequences of inadequate preabortion assessment

Clinical experience shows that inattention to the risk factors for negative sequelae can result in the following patient behaviors on the day of the abortion:

- unexpected displays of emotions;
- crying that does not stop;
- lack of emotional expression;
- little or no communication;
- expressions of hostility;
- demands to "just get this over with"; or
- yelling and an inability to lie still on the table, even with adequate pain medications.

Many patients readily voice their concerns as soon as they are alone with a staff member. Others may not be able to put feelings into words without help from someone skilled in engaging the patient in dialogue about feelings.

Effect of stigma on coping

Stigma is defined as a mark of disgrace; social disapproval. Research on abortion and stigma shows that stigma and secrecy initiate the process of suppressing and experiencing intrusive thoughts [8]. The more a patient feels the need to avoid stigma, the more likely she is to block out feelings and suffer intrusive thoughts. Disclosing feelings safely can improve outcome. Studies of women's expectations for coping, stigma, social support, and self-efficacy (Littman 2007, unpublished thesis)[3,20] indicate that the provider can potentially support effective coping by helping patients:

- decrease their perceived level of stress before the abortion;
- increase their sense of empowerment;
- increase their expectations for coping well afterwards; and
- increase their knowledge of effective coping strategies postabortion.

Supporting patients' coping ability

Counseling staff should be trained to address the patient's feelings and sources of abortion-related stress, the reactions of people whom she has told, the effects of their reactions on her, and her expectations for how she will cope after the abortion [12,16,21,22]. Staff can reinforce the patient's positive expectations and help her reframe her negative thinking by:

- validating positive feelings and manageable feelings of sadness, guilt, or anger;
- exploring other difficult past events with which the patient has coped well;
- identifying and acknowledging her coping strengths:
  - ways she has reached out to trustworthy, supportive people;
  - ways she has coped with other difficult decisions, losses, or events;

- examples of her viewing past abortion or other events in a positive light;
- examples of using her spiritual beliefs to strengthen and comfort herself;
- examples of positive self-talk she is using; and
- compliance with medication or other treatment for mood disorders.

• offering appropriate handouts and referrals and acknowledging her receptivity to them.

When a patient has a history of depression or other emotional disorders, it is important to explain possible hormonally induced symptoms of those disorders and document her agreement to continue or resume proper treatment for optimal postabortion adjustment.

Effects of significant others' reactions on patients' coping

Both opposition and emotional support from a patient's partner, parent, or close friend can affect her emotional state on the day of the abortion and her adjustment afterwards. Research shows that a woman's belief in her ability to cope and her well-being are enhanced when she perceives that she has social support for the abortion, and they are diminished when she does not [3,4,6].

If a woman has a male partner, his reactions can affect her emotional response to the abortion experience positively or negatively [23]. A male partner's low expectation for postabortion coping affects the patient negatively if her own expectation is also low. A patient's strong expectation for coping effectively mitigates a partner's negative expectation. When a patient has received opposition from those she has told, the following questions offer ways of finding sources of support:

- "Of the people you know, who would probably be an understanding listener?" Encourage the patient to consider friends from the present or past, pastor, teacher, counselor, extended family members, and others.
- "Have you ever heard this person's opinion on abortion in general?" If not, ask the patient how it would feel to approach the subject in conversation by bringing up something she saw or heard about abortion in general.
- "Has this person ever betrayed your trust?"

> Asking the patient about her support persons, reflecting on her feelings about the reactions she has received from them, and demonstrating support for her decision and feelings all serve to reduce stress on the day of her procedure.

If the patient can identify no one she can trust, then offering her a referral for postabortion phone counseling can supply accessible, confidential, and nonjudgmental support (www.4exhale.org or www.yourbackline.org) (Appendix).

Adolescents' coping

Although some studies suggest that adolescence is a potential risk factor for negative emotional sequelae after abortion, longitudinal research shows that adolescents do not have a higher incidence of negative reactions, such as long-term regret or depression [24]. In the short term, teens may be more likely to engage in avoidant coping methods such as denial and mental disengagement and have lower expectations for coping ability.

For adolescents, the reactions of parents can significantly increase or reduce emotional distress. Research has found that negative, antagonistic, or conditional support from parents is more detrimental to a young woman's postabortion psychological adjustment than the absence of disclosure [25]. When someone other than the adolescent herself discloses the pregnancy to her parents, the likelihood of negative outcome increases [3]. Furthermore, the patient who chooses not to tell her parents but *believes* they would be supportive of her decision copes better after abortion than the patient who tells her parents but receives less than full support [3].

The provider can often help the adolescent patient plan an optimum way of telling her parent(s) that may include the mediating presence of another family member. The website http://www.MomDadIMpregnant.com is a helpful resource. When an adolescent predicts severe repercussions or is otherwise unable or unwilling to involve a parent, the provider can help the patient navigate the judicial bypass process (Chapter 4). Providers in the USA, as well as local attorneys, can contact the American Civil Liberties Union Reproductive Freedom Project for guidance on the judicial bypass process (Appendix).

Challenging scenarios

Sexually victimized women

Research indicates that 18 to 44% of US women have suffered some form of sexual violation in their lifetime [26]. The National Violence Against Women Survey found that 1 in every 15 US women has been raped, and that 54% of these women were raped before age 18 [27]. Given the high incidence of sexual victimization, most clinicians have more contact with such patients than they realize.

Wording of inquiries about potential sexual victimization can influence patients' responses. For example, consider the following question on the medical history sheet: "Is this pregnancy a result of rape or having been forced to have sex?" Using this kind of wording will probably elicit more accurate responses, because many women do not consider themselves "raped" if the perpetrator was someone with whom they had previously had sex or if they were intoxicated.

When the abortion process takes more than one day, as in some second-trimester procedures or medical abortions, it is important to find out if the patient is being abused by her supposed "support" person. The risk of medical noncompliance is potentially increased for the patient whose abuser will be with her during the abortion process. If trust has been established in the patient–provider relationship, then she is more likely to reveal the truth when asked, "Have you ever been hit, or forced to have sex, or mentally abused by the person who will be with you overnight (if second trimester) or who will be with you during the medical abortion?" If a minor reveals abuse, then the provider must follow the laws for mandated reporting of child abuse. Providing referrals for domestic violence and/or rape crisis counseling would be appropriate for these patients.

Potential anxiety about the clinician's or nurse's gender

Some patients (who may or may not be abuse or rape survivors) express a strong preference for female clinicians/attendants [28]. Other patients are not affected by the provider's gender, or they silently submit to whomever is in attendance. Providing abortion care for the patient whose pregnancy resulted from rape or who has suffered sexual violation in the past can present additional challenges for the clinician, especially if male. If a patient has been violated by a male perpetrator, then she may reject (verbally or nonverbally) being touched by a male clinician, ultrasound technician, or nurse. The key is to find out if gender is an issue for *her* and to offer choices and ways in which she can feel more in control, such as offering a female presence in the room.

Clinician strategies for optimum care

The effectiveness of preabortion preparation is enhanced when clinicians of either gender engage in the following:

- building trust by using effective communication skills with the patient and believing what she says;
- being prepared for very little or much emotion from the patient;
- giving the patient some sense of control in the clinical setting to help increase her awareness that she is in a safe place;
- being extra gentle when inserting the speculum, vaginal probe, or fingers; and
- exercising patience and avoiding being rushed.

> A clinician can create a sense of respectful partnership with the patient by simply stating, "I want you to know I am going to do this procedure *for* you, not *to* you. Together we're going to make this a safe procedure for you. Okay?"

Second-trimester patient

Understanding the reasons that a woman may seek an abortion after the first trimester can help the clinician offer compassionate care. Most women who present for second-trimester abortion care would have preferred to have the procedure earlier in gestation [29]. Recent studies of women having second-trimester abortions in US facilities found that the most common reasons for delay were [29,30]:

- delays in detecting pregnancy;
- indecision about the abortion; and
- difficulties making financial or logistical arrangements for the abortion.

Less common reasons included relationship problems; fears about telling parents (particularly for minors) or others; and/or time restraints because of work, school, or family obligations. In addition, because of the typical timing of prenatal diagnostic testing, a woman may not learn that she is carrying a fetus with serious or fatal congenital anomalies until the second trimester; moreover, some women develop medical or pregnancy complications as the gestation advances, and abortion is advised to preserve their health or lives (Chapter 20).

Although ambivalence may be an issue for some women at any gestational age, ambivalence on the first day of a multiple-day second-trimester abortion is a risk factor for noncompliance with completing the procedure. Exploring the patient's decision and establishing certainty about it enhances her safety as well as her emotional well-being.

Fear of pain can also increase the risk of a patient's unwillingness to complete the abortion, especially if she experiences pain during cervical preparation or dilation. Where deep sedation or general anesthesia is not used, the patient may need preparation time to learn strategies to manage her anxiety before the procedure starts. Appropriate counseling can make the difference between a safe procedure and one that is fraught with difficulty.

If the abortion process will occur over more than one day, covering the following in the patient education or counseling session helps to maximize the likelihood of compliance with safety measures:

- ensuring that she has reliable plans for transportation to the clinic;
- assessing the potential for physical abuse from her "support person";
- providing information to both her and her support person about possible complications that could occur overnight and what to do;
- cautioning the support person to stay with the patient; and
- stressing the importance of staying within a certain distance of the clinic, having access to a telephone, and returning to the clinic for the required number of days to complete the procedure.

> One of the most important aspects of second-trimester counseling is impressing upon both the patient and whomever is staying with her overnight (if indeed someone is) the importance of following *all* the overnight instructions and returning on time to complete the procedure.

Cultural differences

Women seeking abortions come from diverse cultures and communities that shape their attitudes, beliefs, and styles of communication. Differences in health care experiences and expectations are likely to affect interactions between clinicians and patients. Breaking taboos surrounding bodily exposure to male clinicians or nurses or discussing sexual topics in mixed company violates some cultures' norms and causes the woman (and her husband, if she has one) embarrassment or even shame [31].

Honoring the values of family and ancestors may conflict with some recent immigrant women's attempts to adapt to acquired norms in a new country. For example, a woman from a culture where pregnancy out of wedlock brings disgrace upon the whole family may feel shame or fear of being shunned despite now living in a country that accepts single parenthood. Likewise, a woman intending to return to her country may express fear of being killed if she is not an intact virgin at the time of marriage, and she may plan on surgery to reconstruct her hymen.

Acceptable reasons for aborting a pregnancy may vary from culture to culture. For instance, some abortion care providers may find it difficult to accept sex selection as a valid reason for an abortion, whereas a married patient, her husband and both sets of parents may believe that aborting a female fetus is a rational act for the future good of the family.

Some cultures hold the norm of married women deferring decision-making to their husbands and allowing the husband to speak for them. It is also common for both husband and wife to expect the man to take charge of contraception by using condoms. Some cultures fear hormonal contraceptives or distrust pharmaceutical medications in general.

Provision of culturally and linguistically appropriate health care services enhances communication and trust, which in turn leads to improved health outcomes and patient satisfaction [32,33]. Abortion care providers can further these goals by learning about and respecting the cultural perspectives and expectations of their patients, remaining aware of how their own cultural perspectives and biases may influence their interactions with patients, providing information in a language and at a literacy level appropriate for the patient, and continually striving to deliver care that meets her needs. A full discussion of this topic is beyond the scope of this textbook, but numerous resources are available to assist providers in these endeavors (Appendix).

Medical abortion

Giving women an informed choice in the method of abortion enhances their postabortion satisfaction [34]. Staff can improve patient compliance and satisfaction by providing:

- appropriate screening for eligibility for medical abortion;
- comparisons of surgical and medical abortion (Chapters 9 and 10);
- written and verbal instructions about the process [35]; and
- adequate time to present the realities of the process, answer questions, and address emotional concerns.

Making the choice

To ensure that the patient is basing her choice on facts, it helps to ask, "Because both procedures are available to you, I'm wondering what appeals to *you* about the medical abortion?"

Clinical experience supports the research [15] showing that women who choose medical abortion are often those who:

- want to be at home instead of on the table in a procedure room;
- prefer a noninvasive procedure, if possible;
- prefer what seems like a more natural process, similar to a miscarriage;
- want a very early abortion; or
- have the time to go through the multistep process.

One major reason patients choose vacuum aspiration rather than medical abortion is *time*. They may state that they:

- want the abortion to be completed in one day;
- cannot arrange the time to come back to the provider for follow-up;
- do not have the time on the appropriate day to go through the abortion process; or
- want to curtail pregnancy sickness and fatigue.

Miscarriage or abortion?

Sometimes a patient chooses medical over surgical abortion because she is morally opposed to abortion [36]. Some patients report that they prefer the medical abortion because it seems like a heavy period or a miscarriage rather than an abortion. If the issue is her moral opposition to abortion, then the counseling needs to shift the focus onto her beliefs and feelings. It is important for the patient's postabortion well-being that she does not fool herself and that the provider does not participate in her self-deception.

Other times a patient explains that the medical abortion process carries less negative connotation for her. Not uncommonly, a patient will explain, "I know it's an abortion, but I'll just feel better because of the way it's carried out." However, all patients need to know that they *may* need a surgical procedure if the medication regimen fails, and they need to consent to both.

Importance of clear, detailed instructions

Thorough preparation helps clarify each step of the medical abortion process and helps the patient understand what is and is not normal. Instructions should include the following:

- what each medication does and possible side effects;
- when and how to use the medications;

- the range of time it takes to abort;
- the possible intensity of the cramping and pain-relief measures;
- possible amount of bleeding and size of clots;
- access to emergency care;
- length of postabortion bleeding;
- importance of follow-up; and
- risk of failed abortion and the possible need for aspiration.

Postabortion counseling

During recovery

Sensitive care before and during any medical procedure can help diminish the incidence of emotional and physical distress during recovery [10]. Occasionally, however, a patient may become upset in the recovery room and need counseling intervention.

Sources of distress in recovery

A patient may feel distressed immediately following an abortion procedure for one or more of the following reasons:

- perception of clinician's or nurse's insensitivity during the abortion;
- more pain than expected;
- sense of emptiness and loss;
- reactions to drugs administered, such as involuntary crying or panicky feelings; and/or
- shame and/or fear that God won't forgive her for "killing a baby."

Supportive interventions

The following recommendations may help to calm patients who appear upset in recovery:

- if possible, have the same person who already established rapport with the patient beforehand be with her in recovery;
- see the patient in private, if possible;
- help the patient to reframe negative thoughts:
  - from "I'm a bad person who killed my baby" to "I'm one of many good women worldwide who have had to make a hard decision about a pregnancy."
  - from "God is a harsh judge who abandons women in their time of need" to "God is all-merciful and all-compassionate and understands what's in our hearts."
  - from "I shouldn't have done it!" to "I have reasons why I felt this was necessary, which are…"
- help the patient shift her focus from "I'm feeling miserable now" to "What can I (or my support person) do to take care of myself the rest of today? Tomorrow?"

After the day of the abortion

In those rare instances when a woman expresses troubled feelings months or years after an abortion, the following issues often underlie the distress [9,37,38,39]:

- relationship dissatisfaction with her partner;
- conflicts with one or both parents;
- unacknowledged sense of loss;
- significant losses subsequent to the abortion;
- failed outcome of a wanted pregnancy;
- preexisting disorders, such as depression, obsessive-compulsive, bipolar, panic, or personality disorders, and/or previous trauma that may be undiagnosed or untreated;
- prone to shame and sensitive to stigma, and thinking abortion is killing a baby;
- events that trigger troubled memory of the abortion;
- perception of insensitive treatment by the abortion provider;
- joining a church that condemns abortion and emphasizes judgment;
- exposure to antiabortion messages that foster feelings of victimization and shame;
- isolation, lack of social support; and/or
- loneliness, feeling unloved.

The resolution of some of these issues requires professional counseling and possibly medical treatment. Other sources of distress can be relieved by trained secular or pastoral postabortion counselors or self-help resources and social support (Appendix).

Conclusion

Obtaining informed consent, addressing the contraceptive needs of women, and attending to any emotional needs that may arise are essential to providing high-quality abortion care. The use of effective communication skills and needs assessment to discern patients' concerns provides important benefits to both the patient and the abortion care provider.

References

1 Benson Gold R, Nash E. State abortion counseling policies and the fundamental principles of informed consent. *Guttmacher Policy Review* 2007; **10**: 6–13.

2 Richardson C, Nash E. Misinformed consent: the medical accuracy of state-developed abortion counseling materials. *Guttmacher Policy Review* 2006; **9**: 2–8.

3 Major B, Cozzarelli C, Sciacchitano A, Cooper M, Testa M, Mueller P. Perceived social support, self-efficacy, and adjustment to abortion. *J Pers Soc Psychol* 1990; **59**: 452–463.

4 Major B, Richards C, Cooper M, Cozzarelli C, Zubeck J. Personal resilience, cognitive appraisals, and coping: an integrative model of adjustment to abortion. *J Pers Soc Psychol* 1998; **74**: 735–752.

5 Adler N, David H, Major B, Roth S, Russo N, Wyatt G. Psychological factors in abortion: a review. *Am Psychol* 1992; **47**: 1194–1204.

6 Cozzarelli C. Personality and self-efficacy as predictors of coping with abortion. *J Pers Soc Psychol* 1993; **65**: 1224–1236.

7 Major B, Cozzarelli C. Psychosocial predictors of adjustment to abortion. *J Social Issues* 1992; **48**: 121–142.

8 Major B, Gramzow R. Abortion as stigma: cognitive and emotional implications of concealment. *J Pers Soc Psychol* 1999; **77**: 735–745.

9 Rubin L, Russo N. Abortion and mental health: what therapists need to know. *Women & Therapy* 2004; **27**: 69–90.

10 Stewart MA. Effective physician–patient communication and health outcomes: a review. *CMAJ* 1995; **152**: 1423–1433.

11 Brann M, Mattson M. Reframing communication during gynecological exams. In: Buzzanell P., Sterk H., Turner L, eds. *Gender in Applied Communication Contexts.* Sage Publications, Thousand Oaks, CA, 2004: 147–168.

12 Beresford T. *Short-term Relationship Counseling.* Planned Parenthood of Maryland, Baltimore, 1988.

13 Garrity J, Castle M. *A Physician's Guide to Patient-centered Abortion Care: Providing Support to Women During First-trimester Abortion Procedures.* Planned Parenthood of New York City, New York, 1996.

14 Rollnick S, Miller W, Butler C. *Motivational Interviewing in Health Care: Helping Patients Change.* Guilford Press, New York, 2008.

15 Fielding S, Edmunds E, Schaff E. Having an abortion using mifepristone and home misoprostol: a qualitative analysis of women's experiences. *Perspect Sex Reprod Health* 2002; **34**: 34–40.

16 Baker A. *Abortion and Options Counseling: A Comprehensive Reference.* The Hope Clinic for Women, Granite City, IL, 1995.

17 Major B. Commentary: psychological implications of abortion–highly charged and rife with misleading research. *Can Med Assoc J* 2003; **168**: 1257–1258.

18 Price Tangney J, Dearing R. *Shame and Guilt.* Guilford Press, New York, 2002.

19 Major B, Cozzarelli C, Cooper ML et al. Psychological responses of women after first-trimester abortion. *Arch Gen Psychiatry* 2000; **57**: 777–784.

20 Baluk U, O'Neill P. Health professionals' perceptions of the psychological consequences of abortion. *Am J Community Psychol* 1980; **8**: 67–75.

21 Harris A. Supportive counseling before and after elective pregnancy termination. *J Midwifery Women's Health* 2004; **49**: 105–112.

22 Needle R, Walker L. *Abortion Counseling: A Clinician's Guide to Psychology, Legislation, Politics, and Competency.* Springer Publishing Company, New York, 2008.

23 Major B, Cozzarelli C, Testa M. Male partners' appraisals of undesired pregnancy and abortion: implications for women's adjustment to abortion. *J Appl Social Psychol* 1992; **22**: 599–614.

24 Quinton W, Major B, Richards C. Adolescents and adjustment to abortion: are minors at greater risk? *Psychol Public Policy and Law* 2001; **7**: 491–514.

25 Griffin-Carlson M, Schwanenflugel P. Adolescent abortion and parental notification: evidence for the importance of family functioning on the perceived quality of parental involvement in US families. *J Child Psychol Psychiatry* 1998; **39**: 543–553.

26 Russell DEH, Bolen RM. *The Epidemic of Rape and Child Sexual Abuse in the United States.* Sage Publications, Thousand Oaks, CA, 2000.

27 Basille KC, Chen J, Black MC, Saltzman LE. Prevalence and characteristics of sexual violence victimization among US adults, 2001–2003. *Violence and Victims* 2007; **22**: 437–448.

28 Zuckerman M, Navizedeh N, Feldman J, McCalla S, Minkoff H. Determinants of women's choice of obstetrician/gynecologist. *J Women's Health & Gender-Based Medicine* 2002; **11**: 175–180.

29 Finer LB, Forhwirth LF, Dauphinee LA, Singh S, Moore AM. Timing of steps and reasons for delays in obtaining abortions in the United States. *Contraception* 2006; **74**: 334–344.

30 Drey EA, Foster DG, Jackson RA, See SJ, Cardenas LH, Darney PD. Risk factors associated with presenting for abortion in the second trimester. *Obstet Gynecol* 2006; **107**: 128–135.

31 Hammoud M, White C, Fetters M. Opening cultural doors: providing culturally sensitive healthcare to Arab American and American Muslim patients. *Am J Obstet Gynecol* 2005; **193**: 1307–1311.

32 Betancourt JR, Green AR, Carrillo JE. Cultural competence in health care: emerging frameworks and practical approaches [Online]. New York: The Commonwealth Fund; 2002 [cited 2008 Aug 7]. Available from: URL:http://www.commonwealthfund.org/usr_doc/betancourt_culturalcompetence_576.pdf

33 American College of Obstetricians and Gynecologists [Online]. Washington, DC: American College of Obstetricians and Gynecologists; 2008. Cultural competence; 2008 [cited 2008 Aug 7]. Available from: URL:www.acog.org/departments/dept_notice.cfm?recno=18&bulletin=1059

34 Slade P, Heke S, Fletcher J, Stewart P. A comparison of medical and surgical termination of pregnancy: emotional impact and satisfaction with care. *Br J Obstet Gynaecol* 1998; **105**: 1288–1295.

35 National Abortion Federation. *NAF Protocol for Mifepristone/Misoprostol in Early Abortion.* National Abortion Federation, Washington, DC, 2008.

36 Wiebe ER, Trouton KJ, Fielding SL, Klippenstein J, Henderson A. Antichoice attitudes to abortion in women presenting for medical abortions. *J Obstet Gynaecol Can* 2005; **27**: 247–250.

37 DePuy C, Dovitch D. *The Healing Choice.* Simon & Schuster, New York, 1997.

38 Torre-Bueno A. *Peace After Abortion.* Pimpernel Press, San Diego, 1996.

39 Major B, Appelbaum M, Beckman L, Dutton MA, Russo NF, West C. Report of the APA task force on mental health and abortion [online]. Washington, DC: American Phychological Association, 2008 [cited 2008 Dec 29]. Available from: URL:http://www.apa.org/releases/abortion-report.pdf

6

CHAPTER 6

Clinical assessment and ultrasound in early pregnancy

Steven R. Goldstein, MD, and Matthew F. Reeves, MD, MPH

LEARNING POINTS

- Patient history alone is not sufficiently accurate to establish the diagnosis, duration, or status of pregnancy.
- Urine hCG testing is a simple and accurate way to diagnose pregnancy. Quantitative serum hCG is most useful when used serially to assess the status of a pregnancy.
- Ultrasound can reliably determine the gestational age of an intrauterine pregnancy by measurement of the mean sac diameter, crown-rump length, or biparietal diameter.
- Ultrasound can diagnose early pregnancy failures and assist in the diagnosis of ectopic pregnancy.

Introduction

When a woman requests an abortion, she presumes she is pregnant with a viable intrauterine gestation, and she usually has some idea of its duration. Because one or more of these assumptions may be incorrect, the preabortion evaluation includes confirming the diagnosis of pregnancy, evaluating its status and location, and estimating its gestational age. This information influences the options available to women and helps to prevent complications related to misdiagnosis of pregnancy and its gestational age (see Chapter 15).

In modern abortion practice, advances in pregnancy testing and imaging techniques have greatly enhanced safe and effective evacuation of the uterus. This chapter discusses the accuracy of clinical evaluation and assays for human chorionic gonadotropin (hCG) in diagnosing pregnancy. It also addresses the use of ultrasound in locating the pregnancy, determining gestational age, defining landmarks of normal and abnormal development, and interpreting ultrasound findings after medical or surgical abortion.

Clinical evaluation of early pregnancy

In contrast to embryologists who describe pregnancy events from the time of fertilization, clinicians typically date pregnancy from the first day of the last menstrual period (LMP). This calculation is based on an "ideal" menstrual cycle, with fertilization occurring on day 14 of the cycle. It is commonly referred to as "gestational age" and denoted as "days LMP" or "weeks LMP."

Patients commonly present for abortion services at or after the first missed menses, which in an "ideal" cycle corresponds to four or more weeks of gestational age [1,2]. They may or may not recall the date of their LMP, report symptoms related to the pregnancy, or have used a home pregnancy test to confirm their suspicion of pregnancy. Consequently, the clinical evaluation of a patient presenting for abortion must begin with a diagnosis of pregnancy and estimation of gestational age. This evaluation includes patient history, physical examination, biochemical testing and, when available or indicated, ultrasonography.

Symptoms of early pregnancy

Typical symptoms associated with early pregnancy include cessation of menses, nausea, vomiting, breast enlargement, breast tenderness, urinary disturbances, and fatigue [2]. Nausea occurs in 74% of pregnant women and may begin at 4 to 5 weeks LMP [3]. Abrupt onset of amenorrhea in a woman with previously regular menstrual cycles is the *sine qua non* of pregnancy, but this symptom can be misleading. Some women conceive without an identifiable prior menstruation. If sexual activity begins at a very early age, ovulation and conception can occur before menarche. If pregnancy rapidly follows delivery, and particularly if the woman is lactating, menses may not have resumed prior

Management of Unintended and Abnormal Pregnancy, 1st edition. By M Paul, ES Lichtenberg, L Borgatta, DA Grimes, PG Stubblefield, MD Creinin
 ISBN: 9781405176965.

to conception. Conversely, vaginal bleeding complicates 15 to 25% of all pregnancies [4]. Uterine bleeding sometimes occurs at the time of implantation or as the placenta expands (subchorionic bleeding) and may be misinterpreted as a menstrual period; other causes of irregular bleeding include use of hormonal contraception and abnormal pregnancy. Patient perception of first fetal movement, referred to as *quickening*, is a symptom that commonly occurs between 15 and 20 weeks of gestation. It is highly subjective and has poor reliability as a means of dating pregnancy.

A review of research examining the value of clinical assessment in diagnosing pregnancy concluded that clinicians should not depend solely on early pregnancy symptoms for this purpose, although a combination of symptoms is more predictive than amenorrhea alone [2]. "Morning sickness" had a sensitivity of 39% and a specificity of 86% in one study [5]. Reported sensitivities for amenorrhea were 63% in one study [5] and 68% in another [1]; specificities were 60 and 40%, respectively. The combination of amenorrhea, breast tenderness, and nausea (with or without vomiting) was most predictive of pregnancy, with a positive predictive value of 85% [5]. Clinical history alone also misclassifies many women who have abnormal pregnancies, including women with ectopic pregnancies or threatened spontaneous abortions [6,7].

Studies that have correlated patients' suspicion of pregnancy with the results of hCG assays show that women are better at ruling out pregnancy than ruling it in. In a pooled analysis of four studies carried out primarily in emergency department populations, pregnancy was confirmed in only 53% of 1,817 patients who suspected they were pregnant. Conversely, 84% of 1,692 women who did not think they were pregnant were correct [2]. These studies suggest that asking the question, "Is there any chance you could be pregnant now?" is more predictive than asking women if they believe they are pregnant [8]. Nonetheless, one study diagnosed pregnancy in 7% of women who reported regular, normal menses and who denied any chance of being pregnant [9].

Similarly, research indicates that women having early medical abortions are quite accurate in determining that they are no longer pregnant. In a large medical abortion study, women who had passed the pregnancy reported that they felt that they were no longer pregnant with a sensitivity of 97% and a positive predictive value of 99%. However, women's ability to predict accurately that expulsion had not occurred was limited [10].

Obstetrical research demonstrates that ultrasonography is superior to reported LMP for predicting the date of delivery, although these studies suffer from lack of a gold standard for determining true gestational age. Reassuring to abortion providers is the finding that LMP dating tends to overestimate the duration of pregnancy, probably because of delayed ovulation in some women [11,12]. A few studies have compared LMP with ultrasound dating in women seeking abortion care. In a study from a hospital-based clinic in the UK, McGalliard and Gaudoin [13] found that 237 (90%) of 262 women seeking pregnancy termination were sure of the date of onset of their LMP. In this group, the mean gestational age by ultrasound and LMP differed by only one day (61 days versus 62 days, respectively). However, the discrepancy between ultrasound and menstrual dates exceeded 7 days in 90 (38%) women, including 55 (23%) women whose LMP overestimated the gestational age by ultrasound and 35 (15%) women whose LMP underestimated it. Twenty-six (10%) women were more than 12 weeks' gestation by ultrasound, 18 (69%) of whom were less than 12 weeks by reported LMP.

Similar research has been conducted in women seeking early medical abortion. In US studies, transvaginal sonography using various dating formulas confirmed gestational age determined by LMP in only 40 to 60% of women receiving mifepristone or methotrexate regimens, although success rates were high regardless [14–16]. In a study of 673 women participating in a medical abortion feasibility study in South Africa, women's estimates of gestational age by LMP were within 1 week or 2 weeks of ultrasound estimates in 32 and 51% of cases, respectively; the LMP dating differed by more than three weeks in 35% [17]. In the absence of ultrasound, clinical assessment by the provider is superior to LMP alone in estimating gestational age [17,18]. In addition, only a small percentage of women underestimate their duration of pregnancy in a way that is inconsistent with safe use of mifepristone regimens for early medical abortion [17,18].

In summary, patient history provides an initial evaluation of the possibility of pregnancy and its duration. However, patient history is not sufficiently accurate to establish the diagnosis, duration, or status of pregnancy.

Physical examination in early pregnancy

Numerous physical signs occur with early pregnancy; they serve as markers of the presence of pregnancy and as a means to estimate gestational age [2,5]. These physical signs are found primarily on breast and pelvic examination. Appearance of these signs varies among individual gravidas, reducing the accuracy of physical diagnosis of early pregnancy [2].

Clinically apparent changes in the breasts are among the earliest signs of pregnancy [2,19]. These changes include increased visibility of the venous pattern, engorgement, and darkening and enlargement of the areolae [2,19]. Some combination of these signs occurs in about 40% of patients with early pregnancies, and they are evident as soon as 6 to 8 weeks' gestation. One study found that breast signs had a sensitivity of 56% and a specificity of 79% for the diagnosis of pregnancy [5].

Signs detectable on vaginal examination are quite specific (94%) but have low sensitivity (18%) [2,5]. The earliest signs detectable on pelvic examination are Hegar's sign, which is a softening of the cervical isthmus occurring at about 6 weeks' gestation [2,20], and a palpable uterine arterial pulse noted with the vaginal finger in the lateral fornix on bimanual examination [21]. Although a single study found uterine arterial pulsation a reliable indicator of early pregnancy, with a sensitivity of 76% and specificity of 93% [21], the diagnostic value of this sign requires confirmation. Chadwick's sign [22], a bluish discoloration of the cervix, vagina, and vulva because of venous congestion, can be noted by 8 to 12 weeks' gestation and is rarely present prior to 7 weeks.

Enlargement of the uterus begins shortly after implantation and initially results from hypertrophy of uterine smooth muscle. After approximately 4 weeks LMP, the size of the uterus increases by about 1 centimeter per week. In early gestation, prior to the emergence of the uterus from the pelvis, numerous clinicians utilize a system that relates the size of the uterus to the size of specific types of fruit [23]. For example, uterine size may be likened to the size of a small pear at 5 to 6 weeks' gestation, a medium orange at 8 weeks, and a grapefruit at 10 to 12 weeks.

Although clinical sizing of the uterus in the first trimester can provide a rough estimate of gestational age, it is imprecise. Incorrect estimation of gestational age by uterine sizing alone can occur even in the hands of experienced clinicians. In one study, for example, bimanual examination by obstetrics and gynecology faculty incorrectly assigned gestational age (as determined by ultrasound) by more than 2 weeks in 8% of women having first-trimester aspiration abortions; the corresponding proportion for first-year residents was 25% [24]. Nonetheless, research indicates that clinical assessment with only selective use of ultrasound suffices for safe and effective provision of early medical abortion. Fielding et al assessed the accuracy of medical history and bimanual examination in determining eligibility for medical abortion using mifepristone-misoprostol up to 63 days' gestation [25]. In this large study, clinicians correctly assigned gestational age as 63 days or less in 87% of women; in only 1% of cases did clinicians underestimate gestational age. Underestimation was associated with inexperience, but not with type of clinician (physician or advanced practice clinician). The clinicians were more likely to recommend sonography if LMP dating exceeded 49 days. Other studies have confirmed the safety of providing early medical abortion based on clinical assessment alone [17,18]. If gestational age estimates by LMP and physical exam are discordant, ultrasound should be considered [26].

After about 12 weeks' gestation, the uterus rises out of the pelvis and becomes an abdominal organ. It reaches the midpoint between the symphysis pubis and the umbilicus by 15 to 16 weeks' gestation and is at the level of the umbilicus by approximately 20 weeks. In obstetrical practice, fundal height is commonly used to approximate gestational age and assess fetal growth after 16 to 20 weeks by measuring the distance between the symphysis pubis and top of the fundus with a tape measure scored in centimeters. This measurement is not precise, however. Because accurate assessment of gestational age is critical for safe abortion in the second trimester, clinical practice guidelines of the National Abortion Federation require ultrasonographic assessment of gestational age before second-trimester abortion [26].

Human chorionic gonadotropin

Biochemistry of human chorionic gonadotropin in early pregnancy

Human chorionic gonadotropin (hCG) is a glycoprotein hormone produced by placental trophoblast cells during pregnancy. It consists of a dimer of two glycoprotein subunits designated alpha (α-hCG) and beta (β-hCG), which pair to form the complete hormone. The alpha subunit of hCG is morphologically and functionally identical to the alpha subunits of follicle-stimulating hormone, luteinizing hormone (LH), and thyroid-stimulating hormone. The beta subunit is 85% identical to the beta subunit of LH with the notable addition of a 24-amino-acid tail that acts to increase the serum half-life of hCG [27]. A single gene for the beta subunit appears to have evolved from a duplication of the LH beta subunit in the common ancestor to anthropoid primates [28,29]. Further duplication events have occurred in hominid evolution resulting in six genes for the hCG beta subunit in humans [29]. All six genes are homologous but, interestingly, they are not equally expressed [30]. Nonetheless, the beta subunits of the glycoprotein hormones are biochemically unique, accounting for their distinct biological characteristics.

Cytotrophoblasts within the blastocyst begin secreting hCG before implantation [31]. The blastocyst implants into the endometrium 6 to 12 days after ovulation [32] at which point the villous syncytiotrophoblasts assume production of hCG [33]. The appearance of detectable serum levels of hCG coincides with the timing of implantation [34], and hCG subsequently appears rapidly in maternal plasma and urine. Production of hCG during early pregnancy stimulates the corpus luteum to continue to produce progesterone, thereby providing hormonal support for the secretory endometrium [35], and forestalling menstruation.

The concentration of hCG rises exponentially in normal early pregnancy. Estimated doubling times range from 1.4 days to 2 days [36,37]; the minimum expected rise in 2 days is 53% [38] (see Chapter 18). The median serum concentration of hCG is approximately 100 mIU/ml (range 5–450 mIU/ml) at 4 weeks' gestation and approximately 60,000 mIU/ml (range 5,000–150,000 mIU/ml) at 10 weeks [39].

The wide individual variations in hCG concentrations make it impossible to use hCG levels as a means of determining gestational age [40]. After 10 weeks' gestation, hCG levels gradually decline, plateauing in the second and third trimesters [41,42].

During early pregnancy, serum and urine contain several different forms of hCG including intact hCG, free alpha and beta subunits, beta subunit core fragment (produced by degradation of the free beta subunit and present primarily in urine), and hyperglycosylated hCG (H-hCG) [43]. The latter variant has large oligosaccharide side-chains and is produced by early cytotrophoblasts; H-hCG is eventually replaced by regular intact hCG as the cells differentiate into syncytiotrophoblasts. During the first, second, and third weeks following implantation, H-hCG accounts for approximately 80%, 60%, and 50%, respectively, of the varying forms of hCG found in biological samples, after which it decreases rapidly [43].

As one of relatively few substances that are produced solely by trophoblast cells, hCG serves as a specific marker of pregnancy [40], although it is present as well in gestational trophoblastic disease and certain rare malignancies. In contrast to the long-held assertion that hCG concentrations in urine approximately equal those in serum, recent data indicate that urine levels are considerably lower than corresponding serum concentrations [43].

Testing for human chorionic gonadotropin

Types of assays

Assays for the presence of hCG in blood or urine are simple, inexpensive, and quite reliable methods of diagnosing or monitoring pregnancy. Immunoassays that quantify hCG in serum can detect levels as low as 2 to 10 mIU/ml, depending on the details of technique and calibration [40]. However, these assays have no advantages over currently available qualitative immunometric urine tests for the purpose of diagnosing pregnancy. Their use is usually confined to clinical management of abnormal pregnancies, such as suspected spontaneous abortions (Chapter 17), ectopic pregnancies (Chapter 18), or molar gestations (Chapter 19) or monitoring outcomes after early medical abortion (Chapter 9) when ultrasonography is not available.

Home pregnancy tests have been commercially available since the mid-1970s, and the results of a home pregnancy test are frequently part of the history given by a woman seeking an abortion [2,44]. In the past, home pregnancy tests used the agglutination-inhibition method of detecting hCG [44]. This immunoassay method employs reagents consisting of hCG-coated latex particles, or more commonly red cells, plus an antibody to hCG. When urine containing hCG is added, the hCG binds to the antibody and prevents agglutination of the particles [40]. Because these assays were not specific for the beta subunit of hCG, the threshold for detection of hCG was set at high levels (1,500–2,500 mIU/ml) to minimize cross-reactions with LH [40]. Therefore, the tests did not permit pregnancy diagnosis before about 6 weeks' gestation. These slide tests continue to have utility in abortion practice. For example, some facilities that do not offer very early abortions may use low sensitivity tests to assure that patients are at least 6 weeks' pregnant; if the results are negative, a positive high sensitivity test confirms the nascent pregnancy. In addition, tests with detection limits of 1,000 mIU/ml hCG or greater are usually negative 2 weeks following successful vacuum abortion [45]. A negative test provides reassurance of successful evacuation, whereas a positive test may signal failed attempted abortion, incomplete abortion, unsuspected ectopic gestation, or rarely, gestational trophoblastic disease. Unfortunately, neither low- nor high-sensitivity pregnancy assays have been found useful in determining medical abortion outcome because of frequent false-positive results 1 or 2 weeks following initiation of treatment [46].

Most modern pregnancy tests are "sandwich assays" that use two or more animal monoclonal antibodies raised against different sites on the hCG molecule. The "capture" antibody is in a solid phase and permanently anchored to a tube, bead, membrane, or plate; the labeled "tracer" antibody is in a liquid phase. When urine or blood containing hCG is added to the system, the hCG binds and links the capture and tracer antibodies. After the blood or urine and excess tracer is washed away, the amount of label bound to the solid phase is proportional to the amount of hCG [39]. These immunoassays are not subject to interference by medications or other factors.

The World Health Organization (WHO) distributes International Reference Preparations (IRPs) for the standardization of hCG immunoassays. Early IRPs were purified in 1972 and subsequent refinements were later adopted as the third and fourth International Standards for hCG and the first IRPs for its alpha and beta subunits [47]. All serum and urine pregnancy tests on the US market are calibrated against the WHO 3rd and 4th International Standards (IS). Recent research has led to the development of new reference preparations for hCG and its important variants, resulting in improved specificity and between-assay variability [47]. Further work in this field is particularly relevant to the monitoring of patients with abnormal pregnancies or those with cancer who can produce multiple or unusual forms of hCG [48].

Accuracy of hCG assays

Modern serum hCG assays rarely produce false-positive results, occurring in an estimated 1 in 1,000 to 1 in 10,000 tests [49]. The modest increase in pituitary secretion of hCG after menopause may account for this occurrence. Moreover, some individuals have serum antibodies directed against animal-derived antigens (heterophilic antibodies)

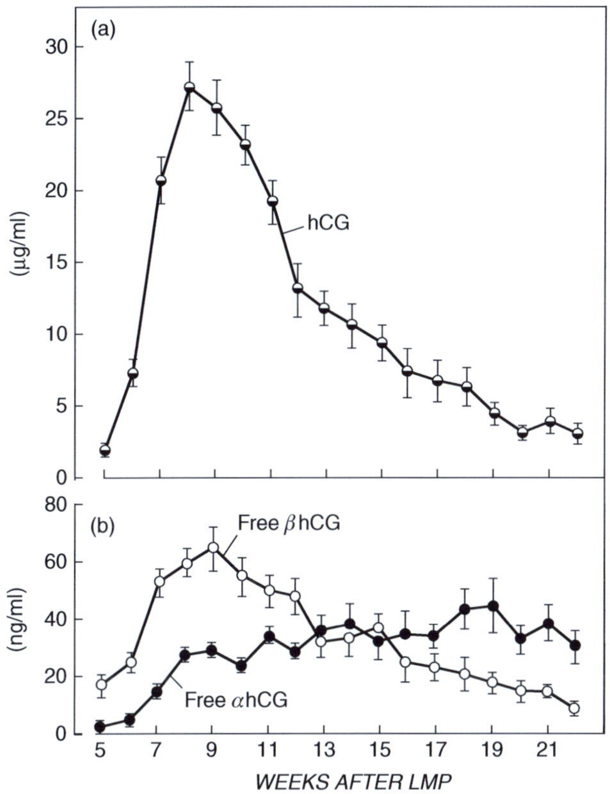

Figure 6.1 Mean levels (± standard error of the mean) of hCG, free hCG-α, and free hCG-β in maternal serum between 5 and 22 weeks after the last menstrual period (LMP) in normal pregnancies (Adapted with permission from Ozturk M, et al [41].)

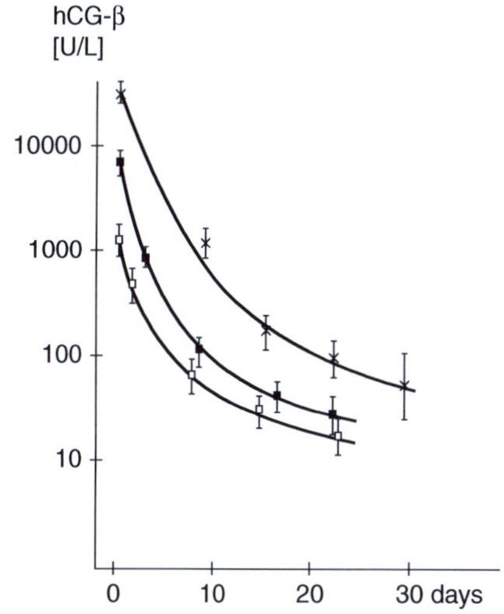

Figure 6.2 Disappearance curves of serum hCG in three groups of women. Top curve represents women ($n = 36$) who had elective vacuum aspiration abortions at 7–13 weeks LMP. Middle curve represents women ($n = 35$) with spontaneous abortions at 6–15 weeks LMP treated with uterine aspiration. Lower curve represents women ($n = 35$) with ectopic pregnancies diagnosed 2.5–11 weeks after LMP and removed surgically. In all three groups, the curves indicate an initial rapid drop in hCG followed by a gradual decline, and the elimination times correlate significantly with initial hCG levels. The differences in hCG concentrations between the groups with induced and spontaneous abortions are statistically significant ($p < 0.01$) both at the time of surgical aspiration and up to 4 weeks thereafter. The y-axis is in logarithmic scale. (Reprinted with permission from Steier JA, et al [51].)

that interfere with the antibodies used in immunoassays, causing false-positive results that have led to unwarranted intervention in some cases. Heterophilic antibodies are not excreted in urine. Therefore, a negative sensitive urine pregnancy test in the face of a serum assay persistently showing a low concentration of hCG (usually less than 1,000 mIU/ml) confirms interference [50].

An erroneous diagnosis of ongoing pregnancy can occur if sensitive assays are performed too soon after the termination of a pregnancy. Elimination of hCG is characterized by an initial rapid phase and a subsequent gradual decline (see Fig. 6.1). After first-trimester surgical abortion, it may take up to 60 days for hCG to fall to negligible levels from the high concentrations typically found at 7 to 10 weeks' gestation [51]. Disappearance of hCG is generally quicker after induced abortion earlier in the first trimester or in the second trimester, but low levels of hCG may still persist for a month or more [51,52]. Compared to first-trimester aspiration abortion, the disappearance time of hCG after surgical treatment for spontaneous abortion or ectopic pregnancy is significantly shorter (see Figs. 6.2 and 6.3).

False-negative results are a more common problem with hCG assays, particularly with home pregnancy tests. These problems are exacerbated by the large array of assays commercially available. Over 50 different quantitative hCG assays are sold in the USA [39]. Since their introduction in the mid-1970s, the number of home pregnancy test kits on the market has increased from 4 to more than 20 brands [53].

Numerous factors can contribute to false-negative results:

- Many women seek pregnancy testing around the time of a missed menses, and the package inserts of home pregnancy tests commonly advise testing around this time. However, even using reliable tests, up to 10% of women (95% CI 6, 16%) who will become pregnant will not test positive at the time of missed menses, due largely to delay in ovulation and implantation [54]. By one week after the missed menses, only 3% of pregnant women (95% CI 1, 6%) will have a negative test.
- Concentrations of hCG during early pregnancy vary widely among individuals, and concentrations in urine are only 50% or less of corresponding serum levels [43]. Some women will have levels of hCG below the detection limit of the assay if the test is performed during or before the week of the missed

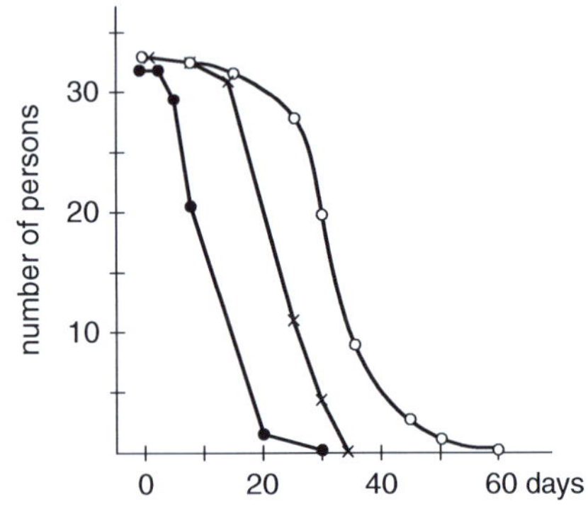

Figure 6.3 Numbers of patients with detectable levels of serum hCG (≥10 mIU/ml) after elective first trimester vacuum aspiration abortion (solid circles, left curve), uterine evacuation for spontaneous abortion (crosses, middle curve), or surgical removal of ectopic pregnancy (open circles, right curve) by time. These data are derived from the same patient population as Figure 6.2. Median time to disappearance of serum hCG was 30 days (range 16–60 days) in women with induced abortions, which was significantly longer than the median of 19 days (range 9–35 days) in the group receiving uterine aspiration for spontaneous abortion or 8.5 days (range 1–31 days) in the group treated surgically for ectopic pregnancy. (Reprinted with permission from Steier JA, et al [51].)

menses [43]. Using standardized concentrations of hCG to test home urine pregnancy assays, Cole et al [55] found that some brands became positive at an hCG concentration of 100 mIU/ml, whereas only one brand was consistently able to detect levels of 6 mIU/ml.

- Numerous forms of hCG are present in serum and urine during early pregnancy, including hyperglycosylated hCG, which predominates during the earliest weeks of gestation. An assay's detection limits for the various forms of hCG will affect its sensitivity. In a study of 15 brands of home pregnancy tests, Butler et al [56] found that the tests varied widely in their detection limits for regular hCG, and only six tests detected H-hCG as effectively as regular hCG.
- Although urine pregnancy tests are quite accurate in the hands of experienced laboratory technicians, sensitivity decreases when patients perform the tests [57]. Inaccurate results have been attributed to patient-related difficulty in understanding the instructions that accompany the kits, problems in interpreting the results of the test, and the absence of controls in some of the kits [58,59].

In summary, hCG assays are an essential tool in the armamentarium of abortion providers, but they have their limits. A negative urine assay at the time of the missed menses deserves repetition in one week or use of another diagnostic tool (e.g., ultrasound) to avoid missing an early diagnosis of pregnancy. Being knowledgeable about the assays used in facilities' reference laboratories will help providers know the strengths and limitations of the assays and facilitate their appropriate use.

Ultrasound evaluation of early pregnancy

Ultrasound plays a major role in pregnancy diagnosis. A thorough understanding of normal pregnancy and its growth milestones optimizes its utility. The milestones described in this section will consistently be imaged earlier with a vaginal, rather than abdominal, transducer.

Normal milestones in early pregnancy

With ultrasound, a gestational sac is the first definitive sign of pregnancy. It is characterized by a sonolucent center (chorionic cavity) that already contains the amnion, embryonic complex, and yolk sac, although these structures are still too small to be seen sonographically (see Fig. 6.4). The normal gestational sac has a symmetrical, thick echogenic rind (see Fig. 6.5) that results from symmetrical invasion of chorionic trophoblasts into the decidualized endometrium. When first seen, a healthy gestational sac should be round and located in the corpus of the uterus. As the sac implants into the endometrial wall, its position in the uterine cavity lateralizes. Using a basic two-dimensional static image, the gestational sac often appears centrally situated, but real-time or three-dimensional scanning reveals its true eccentric position.

The hCG level at which a given sac can first be seen is not as important clinically as the hCG concentration at which all normal sacs should be imaged (discriminatory level). The discriminatory level obtained transabdominally is approximately 3,600 mIU/ml [60,61]. When the sac is identified transvaginally, reported levels of hCG range from 935–2,388 mIU/ml [62–68]. Unfortunately, no clear-cut discriminatory level has yet been determined for transvaginal sonography, because visualization of the gestational sac by this route

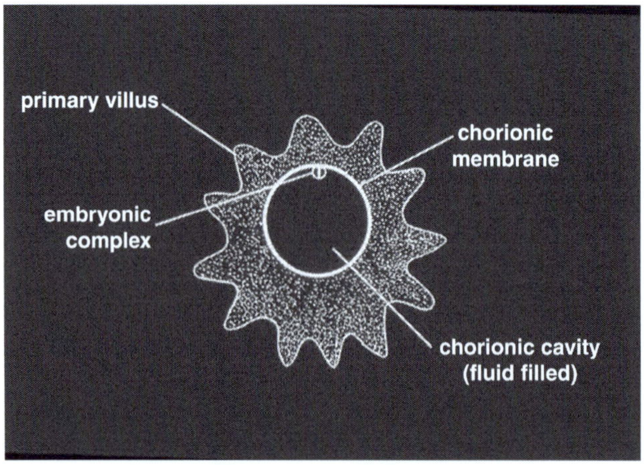

Figure 6.4 Schematic representation of a gestational sac. Note the fluid-filled chorionic cavity containing the embryonic complex consisting of yolk sac, trilaminar embryonic disc, and amnion. Projecting from the chorionic membrane are primary trophoblastic villi, which are round and symmetrical.

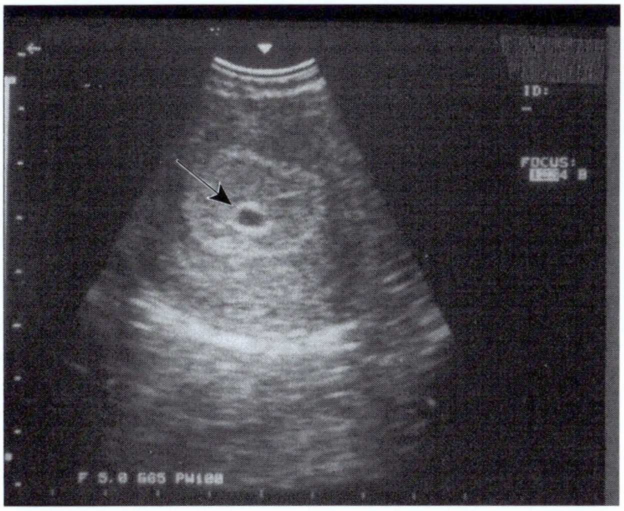

Figure 6.5 Ultrasonogram of a gestational sac depicted schematically in Figure 6.4. The echogenic ring (arrow) is the invasion of maternal decidua by primary trophoblastic villi. The sonolucent center is the fluid-filled chorionic cavity.

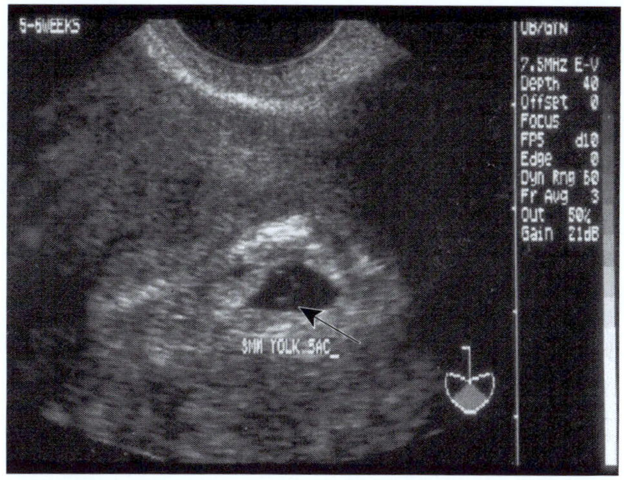

Figure 6.6 Endovaginal sonogram of an intrauterine pregnancy at 38 days LMP. A round symmetrical 3-mm yolk sac (arrow) is seen within the gestational sac.

is both operator and equipment dependent. Typically, discriminatory levels range from approximately 1,500–2,000 mIU/ml. Transvaginal sonographic visualization of the sac typically occurs 34.8 ± 2.2 days from onset of the LMP [64]. Delayed or failed visualization may occur because of the presence of fibroids, multiple gestation, a co-existing IUD, marked maternal obesity, uterine position, or previous uterine surgery [65,67].

The mean diameter of the sac grows approximately 1 mm per day during early pregnancy [69]. The yolk sac, and later the embryo, becomes progressively visible inside the chorionic cavity. The yolk sac is a perfectly round, symmetrical structure; when seen earliest in development, it may be only 2–3 mm in diameter (Fig. 6.6). Transvaginal visualization of the yolk sac is anticipated when the gestational sac has enlarged. The discriminatory level will depend on the type and frequency of the vaginal probe employed. With a 5-mHz transducer, a yolk sac should be seen by the time the mean sac diameter is 13 mm, a major discriminatory milestone [66,70]. In one small retrospective study using a more powerful 9-mHz transducer, the yolk sac could be visualized with a mean sac diameter as small as 5 mm [71].

Generally, the yolk sac can attain a maximum mean diameter of 6 mm [72]. As the amniotic cavity enlarges around the embryo, the yolk sac becomes recognizable as a distinct extra-amniotic entity. The embryo (also known as a somite) appears as a linear body (Fig. 6.7) until it attains 4 mm in length and develops a caudal and rostral neuropore [73]. At 49 days LMP when its greatest length is 7 mm, it appears C-shaped and tadpole-like, complete with tail. By 59 menstrual days, regression of the tail and extension of the head allow for identification of a true crown and rump, enabling measurement of the sitting height of the embryo (crown-rump length) (Fig. 6.8).

Gestational age assessment

Gestational sac size, expressed as a mean sac diameter, is used to measure menstrual age before visualization of an embryo. Typically, measurements are taken from the inner margins of the sac in three dimensions, with length and depth measured in the longitudinal axis and width measured in the transverse plane. These three measurements are then averaged to obtain the mean sac diameter. Conversion tables correlating sac diameter with menstrual age routinely assume that the sac being measured is a perfect sphere. Formulas have been devised by a number of investigators

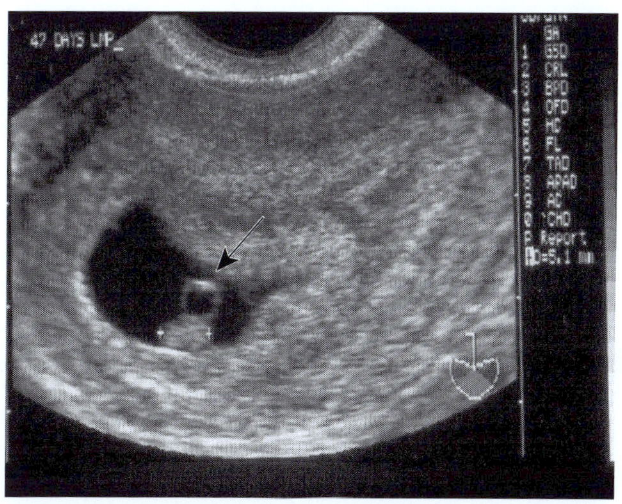

Figure 6.7 Endovaginal sonogram of an intrauterine gestation at 47 days LMP. A linear embryonic structure with cardiac activity is clearly seen (calipers) adjacent to the yolk sac (arrow). It measures 5.1 mm.

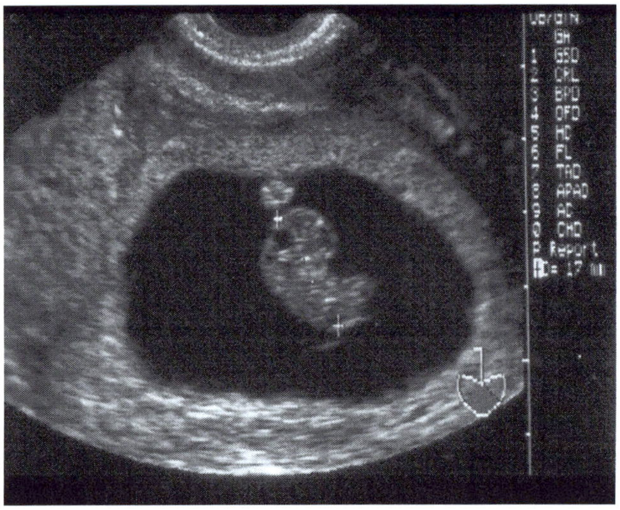

Figure 6.8 Endovaginal sonogram depicts crown-rump length (CRL) of 17 mm (calipers) at 8 weeks, 3 days LMP seen adjacent to the extra-amniotic yolk sac.

to describe this relationship [63,74,75]. One or more such conversion tables are generally installed in the software of commercially available ultrasounds. The equation in Box A provides a useful rule of thumb for conversion of mean sac diameter to gestational age [76]; the accuracy of this estimate is ±3 days.

Embryonic crown-rump length (Fig. 6.8) has been considered the most accurate method of dating a pregnancy sonographically. The original work of Robinson [77] performed with static arm scanners in 1975 remains the most widely used. However, its extrapolation may underestimate the true gestational age in very early pregnancy [78–80]; prior to 18–20 mm in length, the embryo has no true crown or rump and is measured by the ultrasound image that captures the greatest length of its long axis (Fig. 6.7). Correlation of embryo length and gestational age is conveniently expressed by the formula in Box B [80]. This method produces an estimate accurate to within three days (correlation coefficient = 0.87; confidence interval = 95%) (Table 6.1). By the time the embryo achieves a length of 25 mm (~9 weeks and 4 days LMP), the standard crown-rump length charts become the most reliable method of sonographic age determination through 12 gestational weeks [79] (Table 6.2).

After 12 weeks LMP, the fetus has grown sufficiently that a number of structures can be identified and measured using high-resolution, real-time ultrasound equipment. For the purpose of age assessment in abortion, biparietal diameter

Box A Calculation of Gestational Age from Mean Sac Diameter [76]

Gestational Age (±3 days) = Mean Sac Diameter (mm) + 30

Box B Calculation of Gestational Age from Embryo Length [80]

Gestational Age (±3 days) = Embryonic Size (mm) + 42

(BPD) is the easiest and most reproducible measurement. The BPD is measured transabdominally by imaging the fetal head in a transverse axial section. To achieve the most accurate determination, intracranial landmarks should include the falx cerebri anteriorly and posteriorly, the cavum septum pellucidum anteriorly in the midline, and if possible, the choroid plexus in the atrium of each lateral ventricle. The BPD is measured from the outer surface of the calvarium nearest the transducer to the inner margin of the opposite calvarium (often referred to as the "outer to inner") (Figure 6.9). Gestational age is then determined using a standard reference table (Table 6.3) [81,82]. Most equipment has software that calculates a result automatically. Depending on the formula used, the error in the BPD or any second-trimester fetal measurement may be up to two weeks.

Femur length is the second most convenient fetal measurement for assessment of gestational age. Femur length may be helpful in corroborating dating obtained with the BPD or in estimating gestational age when obtaining a BPD is technically difficult (e.g., fetal positioning, multiple gestation, maternal obesity) or impossible (e.g., anencephaly, hydrocephaly). The femur length measurement is made with the abdominal transducer aligned along the long axis of the bone, ideally with the beam exactly perpendicular to the shaft (Figure 6.10). For maximum accuracy, the measured ends of the bones should be blunt rather than pointed,

Table 6.1 Predicted gestational age (days) from embryonic size measurements in millimeters. The formula used to generate the gestational age is shown in Box B. The 95% confidence interval around the estimates is 3 days (Adapted with permission from Goldstein and Wolfson [80].)

Embryonic size (mm)	Gestational age (days)	Embryonic size (mm)	Gestational age (days)
1	43	14	56
2	44	15	57
3	45	16	58
4	46	17	59
5	47	18	60
6	48	19	61
7	49	20	62
8	50	21	63
9	51	22	64
10	52	23	65
11	53	24	66
12	54	25	67
13	55	26	68

Table 6.2 Predicted gestational age (GA) based on crown-rump length (CRL) in centimeters. The formula used to generate the gestational age is: GA (weeks) = exp (1.684969 + 0.315646 × CRL – 0.049306 × CRL^2 + 0.004057 × CRL^3 – 0.000120456 × CRL^4). The gestational age in days is 7 × (GA in weeks, unrounded). The same GA for two different CRL values is the result of rounding of the regression formula. The 95% confidence interval around the estimates is 8% of the predicted GA. Thus for GA of 75 days, the confidence interval would be 6 days [79].

CRL (cm)	GA (wk)	GA (days)	CRL (cm)	GA (wk)	GA (days)	CRL (cm)	GA (wk)	GA (days)
0.2	5.7	40	2.5	9.2	65	4.8	11.6	81
0.3	5.9	41	2.6	9.4	66	4.9	11.7	82
0.4	6.1	43	2.7	9.5	66	5.0	11.7	82
0.5	6.2	44	2.8	9.6	67	5.1	11.8	83
0.6	6.4	45	2.9	9.7	68	5.2	11.9	83
0.7	6.6	46	3.0	9.9	69	5.3	12.0	84
0.8	6.7	47	3.1	10.0	70	5.4	12.0	84
0.9	6.9	48	3.2	10.1	71	5.5	12.1	85
1.0	7.1	49	3.3	10.2	71	5.6	12.2	85
1.1	7.2	51	3.4	10.3	72	5.7	12.3	86
1.2	7.4	52	3.5	10.4	73	5.8	12.3	86
1.3	7.5	53	3.6	10.5	73	5.9	12.4	87
1.4	7.7	54	3.7	10.6	74	6.0	12.5	87
1.5	7.9	55	3.8	10.7	75	6.1	12.6	88
1.6	8.0	56	3.9	10.8	76	6.2	12.6	88
1.7	8.1	57	4.0	10.9	76	6.3	12.7	89
1.8	8.3	58	4.1	11.0	77	6.4	12.8	89
1.9	8.4	59	4.2	11.1	77	6.5	12.8	90
2.0	8.6	60	4.3	11.2	78	6.6	12.9	90
2.1	8.7	61	4.4	11.2	79	6.7	13.0	91
2.2	8.9	62	4.5	11.3	79	6.8	13.1	91
2.3	9.0	63	4.6	11.4	80	6.9	13.1	92
2.4	9.1	64	4.7	11.5	80	7.0	13.2	92

indicating that the entire femoral metaphysis has been captured on the image. Once again, these indices are compared to a standard reference table.

Computer-assisted estimations of fetal age demonstrate that the solitary BPD determination is, in practical terms,

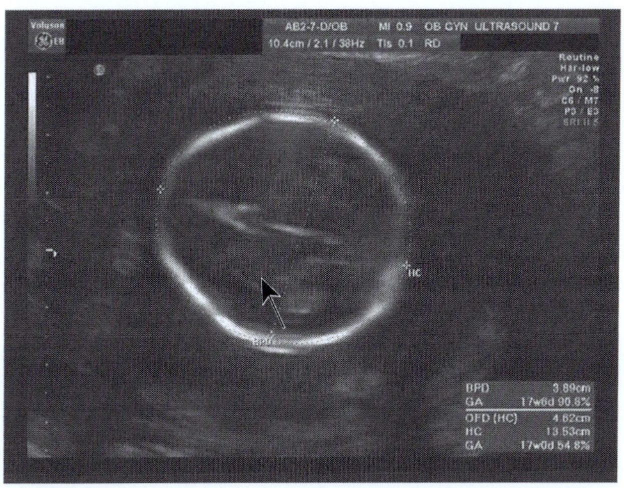

Figure 6.9 Ultrasonogram of a biparietal diameter (BPD) of 3.89 cm, corresponding to 17 weeks, 6 days LMP. Note that it is measured from outer skull table to inner skull table (referred to as "outer to inner").

Table 6.3 Predicted gestational age for biparietal diameter measurements. The confidence intervals around the estimates (± 2 standard deviations) are 1.2 at 12–18 weeks and 1.7 at 18–24 weeks (Adapted with permission from Hadlock et al [81], Hadlock et al [82].)

BPD (cm)	Gestational age (wk)	BPD (cm)	Gestational age (wk)
2.6	13.9	4.3	18.9
2.7	14.2	4.4	19.2
2.8	14.5	4.5	19.5
2.9	14.7	4.6	19.9
3.0	15.0	4.7	20.2
3.1	15.3	4.8	20.5
3.2	15.6	4.9	20.8
3.3	15.9	5.0	21.2
3.4	16.2	5.1	21.5
3.5	16.5	5.2	21.8
3.6	16.8	5.3	22.2
3.7	17.1	5.4	22.5
3.8	17.4	5.5	22.8
3.9	17.7	5.6	23.2
4.0	18.0	5.7	23.5
4.1	18.3	5.8	23.9
4.2	18.6	5.9	24.2

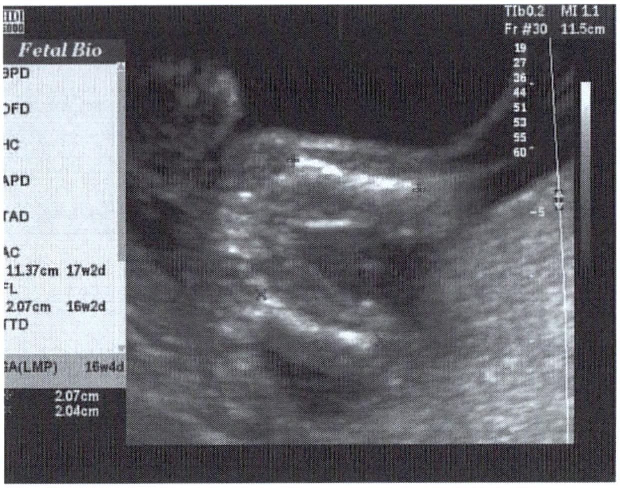

Figure 6.10 Femur length measurement of 2.07 cm (calipers), corresponding to 16 weeks, 2 days LMP. The abdominal transducer is aligned along the long axis of the femur.

virtually as accurate as any other single or combined set of fetal anatomic parameters in calculating gestational age [82].

Embryonic cardiac activity

The S-shaped endothelial heart tube folds upon itself and begins to beat by 21 days postconception (5 weeks' LMP) [73], which predates the ability to image it. For clinical purposes, the critical endpoint is defining the stage in gestation when the absence of cardiac activity is a definitive sign of pregnancy failure. The best approach is to relate presence or absence of cardiac activity to embryonic size. Discovery of cardiac activity will depend on the type and frequency of equipment employed, the degree of magnification available, the visual acuity of the operator, and any confounding anatomic variables (e.g., maternal obesity, coexisting myomas). By any criteria, however, cardiac motion is always present in normal pregnancy when the embryo reaches 5 mm in length [83–86], and its absence at this point signifies pregnancy failure. In more recent work employing an 8-mHz vaginal probe, absence of cardiac activity in an embryo measuring greater then 3.5 mm in its longest axis had 100% positive predictive value for embryonic demise [86].

Some investigators have attempted to correlate cardiac activity with hCG levels. These attempts yield a wide range of results from 6,636–26,356 mIU/ml [60,65,66,68]. Such an approach should be abandoned. As a criterion for diagnosing embryonic demise, the presence of cardiac activity should be correlated only with embryonic size.

Abnormal pregnancy

In addition to providing valuable help in diagnosing pregnancy and determining gestational age, ultrasonography can provide early diagnostic information about problematic pregnancies. A number of these conditions are relevant to the clinician providing gynecological, obstetrical, and abortion services. They include ectopic pregnancy (Chapter 18), early pregnancy failure (Chapter 17), and hydatidiform mole (Chapter 19).

Ectopic pregnancy

From a sonographic perspective, the presence of a definitive intrauterine pregnancy (IUP) virtually excludes ectopic pregnancy. A simultaneous intra- and extrauterine pregnancy has been reported to occur in 1 in 30,000 spontaneous pregnancies based on data from the 1940s [87], but modern-day estimates are closer to 1 in 6,500. Frequency is higher in women undergoing assisted reproductive technologies (Chapter 18).

The ability to diagnose an IUP definitively will rely on the aforementioned milestones. When no intrauterine gestation is seen on transvaginal ultrasound in a patient with a positive pregnancy test who is over 4 weeks LMP, the differential diagnosis should include incorrect dating, complete spontaneous abortion, failing IUP, or an extrauterine pregnancy. Obtaining a serum quantitative hCG measurement to determine if the level is above or below the discriminatory cutoff is the next step in making the diagnosis. In a retrospective cohort study by Barnhart et al [88] of clinically stable pregnant women with nondiagnostic transvaginal ultrasounds and an initial hCG level above the discriminatory zone (2,000 mIU/ml), 46% were ultimately diagnosed with ectopic pregnancies and 54% with failing IUPs. In a prospective observational study of pregnant women with no gestational sac on transvaginal ultrasound, the sensitivity and positive predictive value of a hCG level above 2,000 mIU/ml to detect ectopic pregnancy was 11 and 18%, respectively; the corresponding values for an hCG concentration above 1,500 mIU/ml was 15 and 18% [89]. Women with nondiagnostic transvaginal ultrasounds and hCG levels below the discriminatory level are more likely to have ectopic pregnancies than those with hCG concentrations above this cutoff [88].

If no intrauterine pregnancy is visualized above the discriminatory cutoff or if serial hCG monitoring demonstrates a subnormal rate of change, uterine aspiration is helpful in establishing the diagnosis (Chapter 18). Tissue examination that reveals the presence of chorionic villi proves an intrauterine gestation, except in the rare exception of cornual/interstitial ectopic pregnancy. The presence of only decidual tissue raises the index of suspicion for ectopic pregnancy, although complete abortion, especially when combined with prior bleeding, can account for such findings as well.

Some intrauterine fluid collections can look like a gestational sac (pseudosac). Visualization of a yolk sac within a gestational sac eliminates the possibility of misdiagnosis. If any doubt exists about the presence or normalcy of an

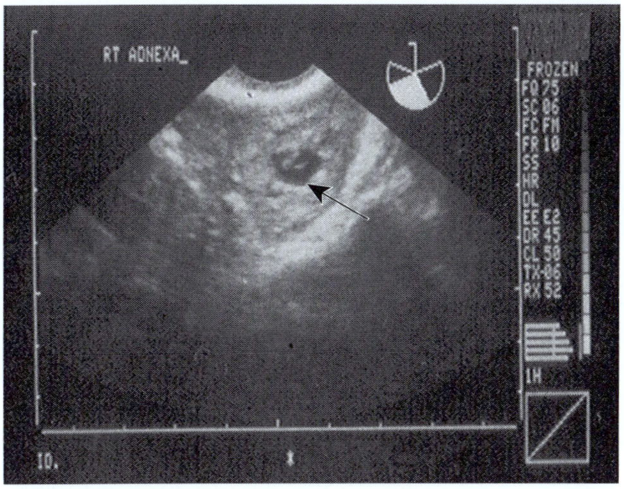

Figure 6.11 Endovaginal sonogram of right adnexa depicting a tubal ectopic pregnancy. Gestational sac (arrow) is seen containing yolk sac and attached embryonic structure. No intrauterine gestation was visible in the uterus in a separate scanning plane.

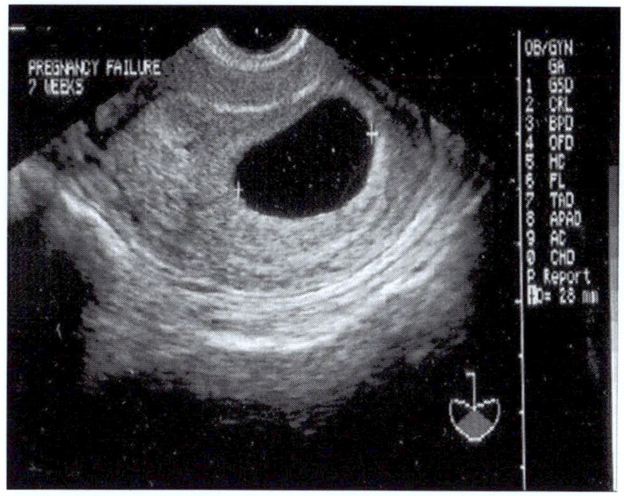

Figure 6.12 Endovaginal sonogram of an intrauterine gestation at 7 weeks LMP. The gestational sac measures 28 mm and lacks any yolk sac or embryonic structure. This is an example of early pregnancy failure (anembryonic pregnancy).

empty gestational sac, consultation with a more experienced sonographer or a follow-up ultrasound scan is warranted. Distinguishing eccentric (true sac) from central (pseudosac) location of the sonolucency is a key diagnostic maneuver (Fig. 6.5 and Fig. 18.3).

Extrauterine findings on ultrasound mirror those seen in the operating suite. Thirteen per cent to 28% of tubal ectopics will develop to the point that a yolk sac and/or cardiac activity are seen ultrasonographically [90–92] (Figure 6.11). Such pregnancies often follow normal doubling times of hCG until the tissue substrate (tubal implantation site) begins to break down because of placental hypoxia in an underperfused endosalpinx. Visualization of the gestational sac within the tube is facilitated by the contrast in density of surrounding tissues, particularly if embryonic cardiac activity is present. However, not all sonolucent or complex adnexal structures are extrauterine gestations. The ovaries should be identified on the side in question to aid in defining an ovarian corpus luteum site or a corpus luteum cyst that can be mistaken for an ectopic gestation. Finally, free fluid in the cul-de-sac may be helpful but is not pathognomonic. It is present in 41 to 83% of extrauterine pregnancies [90,91] but may be present physiologically or when adnexal cysts leak or rupture.

Early pregnancy failure

Clinicians routinely encounter patients with a failed pregnancy. These women are often asymptomatic, but they may present with bleeding or a size-dates discrepancy. Making a timely diagnosis allows patients to choose from a variety of management options (Chapter 17).

Ultrasound diagnosis of this condition is based on failure to achieve appropriate embryonic growth and the various landmarks described earlier. Sonographic findings diagnostic of early pregnancy failure include either an embryo 5 millimeters or greater in length without cardiac activity, or a gestational sac 13 millimeters or greater in mean diameter with absent yolk sac using a 5-mHz transducer (Figure 6.12). Importantly, a recent report using 5–6-mHz transducers found that 100% specificity was not attained until a mean sac diameter of 16 mm was applied as the cutoff for absent yolk sac [93]. Occasionally embryonic demise with resorption will cause a sac to appear to be empty, leading to the diagnosis of anembryonic pregnancy (Fig. 6.12).

An incomplete spontaneous abortion may show variable sonographic appearances within the uterine cavity. A true gestational sac is not seen, but echogenic material representing choriodecidua and blood is often present. In contrast, a complete spontaneous abortion usually has a thinner linear endometrial cavity echo. If tissue is available for inspection in this circumstance, identification of villi confirms the diagnosis. Otherwise, the clinician must consider the possibility of an ectopic pregnancy, because only a decidual cast may have passed. Of 152 women diagnosed with a completed abortion by transvaginal ultrasound, regardless of amount of bleeding by history, 6 ultimately proved to have ectopic pregnancy [94]. Thus, a diagnosis of complete abortion based solely on history plus scan findings is unreliable. These women warrant further evaluation, such as documentation that serum hCG has returned to nonpregnant levels.

During pharmacological management of early pregnancy failure, endometrial thickness is not predictive of the need for suction curettage [95,96]. Similarly, data suggest that endometrial thickness and volume of intracavitary content

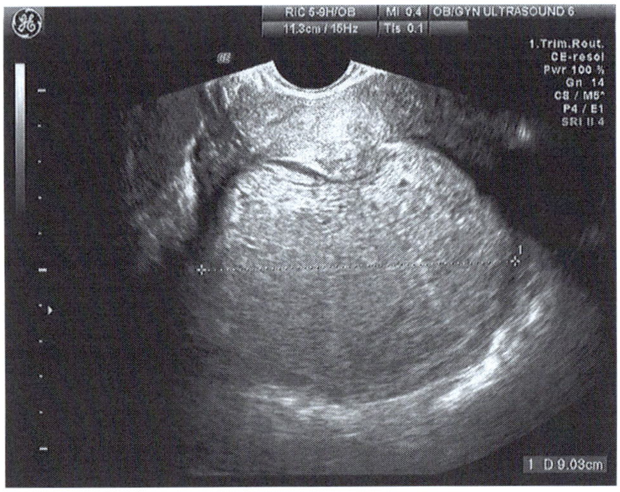

Figure 6.13 Endovaginal sonogram of molar pregnancy, showing blizzard-like pattern.

are not clinically useful endpoints in diagnosing failure of a medical abortion [97,98].

Hydatidiform mole

The appearance of hydatidiform mole on ultrasound has classically been called grape-like, corresponding to the edematous changes in the trophoblast (hydropic vesicles). Such a pattern on ultrasound is often not seen until 10 menstrual weeks or more. In a patient with vaginal bleeding early in pregnancy, ultrasound may simply show signs of IUP failure. In this case, instead of the classic ultrasound molar appearance ("blizzard" or "snowstorm" pattern, Figure 6.13), the cavity is expanded with inchoate homogeneous or mixed density echoes, resembling an incomplete abortion (Chapter 19).

In the USA and other developed countries, the widespread practice of early prenatal ultrasound screening of asymptomatic pregnancies has resulted in the early detection of most molar gestations, thereby dramatically reducing the number of moles seen clinically after 12 to 14 weeks LMP. Many early moles may not be suspected as other than failed intrauterine gestations. The detection of hydropic villi on fresh tissue examination after abortion warrants microscopic pathologic study to make a definitive diagnosis of molar pregnancy, although these changes are often lacking in early moles (Chapter 19). Early diagnosis of molar pregnancy enables counseling about risk of recurrence in future pregnancies and surveillance to detect the rare cases of gestational trophoblastic tumor or choriocarcinoma requiring chemotherapy.

Conclusion

Pregnancy diagnosis and accurate estimation of gestational age are integral aspects of abortion care. Although the initial clinical assessment provides important clues, no detail of the patient's history, reported symptoms, or physical signs allows the practitioner to make the diagnosis of early pregnancy with certainty. Fortunately, advances in pregnancy testing and imaging techniques now enable the clinician to identify pregnancy shortly after implantation and to assess the duration, location, and development of the pregnancy. These techniques have made it possible for providers to offer new options to women seeking abortion, including very early pregnancy termination by medical or surgical methods. Their judicious use also helps to minimize abortion-related complications and assists in the diagnosis and management of abnormal pregnancies.

In many cases, providers can safely proceed with first-trimester surgical abortion if clinical sizing of the uterus correlates with reliable menstrual dating. The use of ultrasound to confirm gestational age in the USA is increasingly common, however. A 2002 survey of National Abortion Federation member clinics revealed that 91% use ultrasound to confirm gestational age before first-trimester aspiration abortion, and virtually all do so before second-trimester abortion [99,100]. This practice allows for adequate preparation of the cervix before surgery and prevents complications related to incorrect estimation of gestational age (Chapter 15). In addition, a number of preexisting conditions such as leiomyomata, multiple gestation, and obesity may severely limit the accuracy of gestational age assessment by physical examination alone, recommending preprocedure assessment by ultrasound in these circumstances.

References

1 Zabin LM, Emerson MR, Ringers PA, Sedivy V. Adolescents with negative pregnancy test results: an accessible at-risk group. *JAMA* 1996; **275**: 113–117.

2 Bastian LA, Piscitelli JT. Is this patient pregnant? Can you reliably rule in or rule out early pregnancy by clinical examination? *JAMA* 1997; **278**: 586–591.

3 Lacroix R, Eason E, Melzack R. Nausea and vomiting during pregnancy: a prospective study of its frequency, intensity, and patterns of change. *Am J Obstet Gynecol* 2000; **182**: 931–937.

4 Wittels KA, Pelletier AJ, Brown DF, Camargo CA Jr. United States emergency department visits for vaginal bleeding during early pregnancy, 1993–2003. *Am J Obstet Gynecol* 2008; **198**: 523.e1-6.

5 Robinson ET, Barber JH. Early diagnosis of pregnancy in general practice. *J R Coll Gen Pract* 1977; **27**: 335–338.

6 Yip S K, Sahota D, Cheung LP, Lam P, Haines CJ, Chung TK. Accuracy of clinical diagnostic methods of threatened abortion. *Gynecol Obstet Invest* 2003; **56**: 38–42.

7 Chung TK, Sahota DS, Lau TK, Mongelli JM, Spencer JA, Haines CJ. Threatened abortion: prediction of viability based on signs and symptoms. *Aust N Z J Obstet Gynaecol* 1999; **39**: 443–447.

8 Stengel CL, Seaberg DC, MacLeod BA. Pregnancy in the emergency department: risk factors and prevalence among all women. *Ann Emerg Med* 1994; **24**: 697–700.

9 Ramoska EA, Sacchetti AD, Nepp M. Reliability of patient history in determining the possibility of pregnancy. *Ann Emerg Med* 1989; **18**: 48–50.

10 Rossi B, Creinin MD, Meyn LA. Ability of the clinician and patient to predict the outcome of mifepristone and misoprostol medical abortion. *Contraception* 2004; **70**: 313–317.

11 Savitz DA, Terry JW Jr, Dole N, Thorp JM, Siega-Riz AM, Herring AH. Comparison of pregnancy dating by last menstrual period, ultrasound scanning, and their combination. *Am J Obstet Gynecol* 2002; **187**: 1660–1666.

12 Mongelli M, Wilcox M, Gardosi J. Estimating the date of confinement: ultrasonographic biometry versus certain menstrual dates. *Am J Obstet Gynecol* 1996; **174**: 278–281.

13 McGalliard C, Gaudoin M. Routine ultrasound for pregnancy termination requests increases women's choice and reduces inappropriate treatments. *BJOG* 2004; **111**: 79–82.

14 Creinin MD, Jerald H. Success rates and estimation of gestational age for medical abortion vary with transvaginal ultrasonographic criteria. *Am J Obstet Gynecol* 1999; **180**: 35–41.

15 Creinin MD, Spitz IM. Use of various ultrasound criteria to evaluate the efficacy of mifepristone and misoprostol for medical abortion. *Am J Obstet Gynecol* 1999; **181**: 1419–1424.

16 Creinin MD, Fox MC, Teal S, Chen A, Schaff EA, Meyn LA. A randomized comparison of misoprostol 6 to 8 hours versus 24 hours after mifepristone for abortion. *Obstet Gynecol* 2004; **103**: 851–859.

17 Blanchard K, Cooper D, Dickson K et al. A comparison of women's, provider's and ultrasound assessments of pregnancy duration among termination of pregnancy clients in South Africa. *BJOG* 2007; **114**: 569–575.

18 Ellertson C, Elul B, Ambardekar S, Wood L, Carroll J, Coyaji K. Accuracy of assessment of pregnancy duration by women seeking early abortions. *Lancet* 2000; **355**: 877–881.

19 Hibbard BM. Pregnancy diagnosis. *Br Med J* 1971; **1**: 593–595.

20 MacDonald E. The diagnosis of early pregnancy, with report of one hundred cases and special reference to the sign of flexibility of the isthmus of the uterus. *Am J Obstet Dis Women Child* 1908; **57**: 323–346.

21 Meeks GR, Cesare CD, Bates GW. Palpable uterine artery pulsation as a clinical indicator of early pregnancy. *J Reprod Med* 1995; **40**: 194–196.

22 Chadwick JR. Value of the bluish discoloration of the vaginal entrance as a sign of pregnancy. *Trans Am Gynecol Soc* 1887; **11**: 399–418.

23 Margulies R, Miller L. Fruit size as a model for teaching first trimester uterine sizing in bimanual examination. *Obstet Gynecol* 2001; **98**: 341–344.

24 Nichols M, Morgan E, Jensen JT. Comparing bimanual pelvic examination to ultrasound measurement for assessment of gestational age in the first trimester of pregnancy. *J Reprod Med* 2002; **47**: 825–828.

25 Fielding SL, Schaff EA, Nam NY. Clinicians' perception of sonogram indication for mifepristone abortion up to 63 days. *Contraception* 2002; **66**: 27–31.

26 National Abortion Federation [Online]. Washington, DC: National Abortion Federation; c2008. Clinical policy guidelines; 2008 [cited 2008 Jun 5]. Available from: URL:http://www.prochoice.org/pubs_research/publications/downloads/professional_education/CPG2008.pdf

27 Fares FA, Suganuma N, Nishimori K, LaPolt PS, Hsueh AJ, Boime I. Design of a long-acting follitropin agonist by fusing the C-terminal sequence of the human chorionic gonadotropin beta subunit to the follitropin beta subunit. *Proc Natl Acad Sci USA* 1992; **89**: 4304–4308.

28 Jameson JL, Hollenberg AN. Regulation of human chorionic gonadotropin gene expression. *Endocr Rev* 1993; **14**: 203–221.

29 Maston GA, Ruvolo M. Chorionic gonadotropin has a recent origin within primates and an evolutionary history of selection. *Mol Biol Evol* 2002; **19**: 320–335.

30 Bo M, Boime I. Identification of the transcriptionally active genes of the human chorionic gonadotropin beta gene cluster in vivo. *J Biol Chem* 1992; **267**: 3179–3184.

31 Fishel SB, Edwards RG, Evans CJ. Human chorionic gonadotropin secreted by preimplantation embryos cultured in vitro. *Science* 1984; **223**: 816–818.

32 Wilcox AJ, Baird DD, Weinberg CR. Time of implantation of the conceptus and loss of pregnancy. *N Engl J Med* 1999; **340**: 1796–1799.

33 Sasagawa M, Yamazaki T, Endo M, Kanazawa K, Takeuchi S. Immunohistochemical localization of HLA antigens and placental proteins (αhCG, βhCG CTP, hPL and SP1) in villous and extravillous trophoblast in normal human pregnancy: a distinctive pathway of differentiation of extravillous trophoblast. *Placenta* 1987; **8**: 515–528.

34 Muyan M, Boime I. Secretion of human chorionic gonadotropin from human trophoblasts. *Placenta* 1997; **18**: 237–241.

35 Zeleznik AJ. In vivo responses of the primate corpus luteum to luteinizing hormone and human chorionic gonadotropin. *Proc Natl Acad Sci USA* 1998; **95**: 11002–11007.

36 Pittaway D, Reish R, Wentz AC. Doubling times of human chorionic gonadotropin increase in early viable intrauterine pregnancies. *Am J Obstet Gynecol* 1985; **152**: 299–302.

37 Kadar N, Freedman M, Zacher M. Further observations on the doubling time of human chorionic gonadotropin early asymptomatic pregnancies. *Fertil Steril* 1990; **54**: 783–787.

38 Barnhart KT, Sammel MD, Rinaundo PF, Zhou L, Hummel AC, Guo W. Symptomatic patients with an early viable intrauterine pregnancy. HCG curves redefined. *Obstet Gynecol* 2004; **104**: 50–55.

39 USA hCG Reference Service. hCG levels during pregnancy [Online]. Albuquerque: University of New Mexico Department of Obstetrics and Gynecology [cited 2008 July 5]. Available from: URL:http://www.hcglab.com

40 Chard T. Pregnancy tests: A review. *Hum Reprod* 1992; **7**: 701–710.

41 Ozturk M, Bellet D, Manil L, Hennen G, Frydman R, Wands J. Physiological studies of human chorionic gonadotropin (hCG), alpha hCG, and beta hCG as measured by specific monoclonal immunoradiometric assays. *Endocrinology* 1987; **120**: 549–558.

42 Nagy AM, Glinoer D Picelli G. Total amounts of circulating human chorionic gonadotrophin alpha and beta subunits can be assessed throughout human pregnancy using immunoradiometric assays calibrated with the unaltered and thermally dissociated heterodimer. *J Endocrinol* 1994; **140**: 513–520.

43 Davies S, Byrn F, Cole LA. Human chorionic gonadotropin testing for early pregnancy viability and complications. *Clin Lab Med* 2003; **23**: 257–264, vii.

44 Doshi ML. Accuracy of consumer performed in-home tests for early pregnancy detection. *Am J Public Health* 1986; **76**: 512–514.

45 van der Lugt B, Drogendijk AC. The disappearance of human chorionic gonadotropin from plasma and urine following induced abortion. Disappearance of HCG after induced abortion. *Acta Obstet Gynecol Scand* 1985; **64**: 547–552.

46 Godfrey EM, Anderson A, Fielding SL, Meyn L, Creinin MD. Clinical utility of urine pregnancy assays to determine medical abortion outcome is limited. *Contraception* 2007; **75**: 378–382.

47 Bristow A, Berger P, Bidart JM et al. Establishment, value assignment, and characterization of new WHO reference reagents for six molecular forms of human chorionic gonadotropin. *Clin Chem* 2005; **51**: 177–182.

48 Stenman UH. Standardization of assays for human chorionic gonadotropin. *Clin Chem* 2004; **50**: 798–800.

49 Braunstein GD. False-positive serum human chorionic gonadotropin results: causes, characteristics, and recognition. *Am J Obstet Gynecol* 2002; **187**: 217–224.

50 American College of Obstetricians and Gynecologists. Avoiding inappropriate clinical decisions based on false-positive human chorionic gonadotropin test results. *Obstet Gynecol* 2002; **100**: 1057–1059.

51 Steier JA, Bergsjø R, Myking OL. Human chorionic gonadotropin in maternal plasma after induced abortion, spontaneous abortion, and removed ectopic pregnancy. *Obstet Gynecol* 1984; **64**: 391–394.

52 Marrs RP, Kletzky OA, Howard WF, Mischell DR Jr. Disappearance of human chorionic gonadotropin and resumption of ovulation following abortion. *Am J Obstet Gynecol* 1979; **135**: 731–736.

53 Cole LA, Khanlian SA, Sutton JM, Davies S, Rayburn WF. Accuracy of home pregnancy tests at the time of missed menses. *Am J Obstet Gynecol* 2004; **190**: 100–105.

54 Wilcox AJ, Baird DD, Dunson D, McChesney R, Weinberg CR. Natural limits of pregnancy testing in relation to the expected menstrual period. *JAMA* 2001; **286**: 1759–1761.

55 Cole LA, Sutton-Riley JM, Khanlian SA, Borkovskaya M, Rayburn BB, Rayburn WF. Sensitivity of over-the-counter pregnancy tests: comparison of utility and marketing messages. *J Am Pharm Assoc* 2005; **45**: 608–615.

56 Butler SA, Khanlian SA, Cole LA. Detection of early pregnancy forms of human chorionic gonadotropin by home pregnancy test devices. *Clin Chem* 2001; **47**: 2131–2136.

57 Bastian LA, Nanda K, Hasselblad V, Simel DL. Diagnostic efficiency of home pregnancy test kits: a meta-analysis. *Arch Fam Med* 1998; **7**: 465–469.

58 Daviaud J, Fournet D, Ballonque C. Reliability and feasibility of pregnancy home-use tests: laboratory validation and diagnostic evaluation by 638 volunteers. *Clin Chem* 1993; **39**: 53– 59.

59 Hicks JM. Home testing: to do or not to do? *Clin Chem* 1993; **39**: 7–8.

60 Nyberg DA, Filly RA, Mahony BS, Monroe S, Laing FC, Jeffrey RB Jr. Early gestation: correlation of HCG levels and sonographic identification. *AJR Am J Roentgenol* 1985; **144**: 951–954.

61 Dashefsky SM, Lyons EA, Lindsay DJ. Suspected ectopic pregnancy: Endovaginal and transvesical US. *Radiology* 1988; **169**: 181–184.

62 Nyberg DA, Filly RA, Laing FC, Mack LA, Zarutskie PW. Ectopic pregnancy. Diagnosis by sonography correlated with quantitative HCG levels. *J Ultrasound Med* 1987; **6**: 145–150.

63 Bernaschek G, Rudelstorfer R, Csaicsich P. Vaginal sonography versus serum human chorionic gonadotropinin in early detection of pregnancy. *Am J Obstet Gynecol* 1988; **158**: 608–612.

64 Fossum GT, Davajan V, Kletzky OA. Early detection of pregnancy with transvaginal ultrasound. *Fertil Steril* 1988; **49**: 788–791.

65 Goldstein SR, Snyder JR, Watson C, Danon M. Very early pregnancy detection with endovaginal ultrasound. *Obstet Gynecol* 1988; **72**: 200–204.

66 Bree R, Edwards M, Böhm-Vélez M Beyler, S Roberts, J Mendelson, FB. Transvaginal sonography in the evaluation of normal early pregnancy: correlation with HCG level. *AJR Am J Roentgenol* 1989; **153**: 75–79.

67 Bateman B, Nunley WC Jr, Kolp LA, Kitchin JD III, Felder R. Vaginal sonography findings and hCG dynamics of early intrauterine and tubal pregnancies. *Obstet Gynecol* 1990; **75**: 421–427.

68 Cacciatore B, Tiitinen A, Stenman UH, Ylöstalo P. Normal early pregnancy: serum hCG levels and vaginal ultrasonography findings. *Br J Obstet Gynaecol* 1990; **97**: 899–903.

69 Nyberg DA, Mack LA, Laing FC, Patten RM. Distinguishing normal from abnormal gestational sac growth in early pregnancy. *J Ultrasound Med* 1987; **6**: 23–27.

70 Tongsong T, Wanapirak C, Srisomboon J, Sirichotiyakul S, Polsrisuthikul T, Pongsatha S. Transvaginal ultrasound in threatened abortions with empty gestational sacs. *Int J Gynaecol Obstet* 1994; **46**: 297–301.

71 Rowling S, Langer J, Coleman BG, Nisenbaum HL, Horii SC, Arger PH. Sonography during early pregnancy: dependence of threshold and discriminatory values on transvaginal transducer frequency. *AJR Am J Roentgenol* 1999; **172**: 983–988.

72 Lindsay DJ, Lovett IS, Lyons EA et al. Yolk sac diameter and shape at endovaginal US: predictors of pregnancy outcome in the first trimester. *Radiology* 1992; **183**: 115–118.

73 Moore KL, Persaud TVN. *The Developing Human: Clinically Oriented Embryology*. Saunders/Elsevier, Philadelphia, 2008.

74 Hellman LF, Kobayashi M, Fillisti L, Lavenhar M, Cromb E. Growth and development of the human fetus prior to the twentieth week of gestation. *Am J Obstet Gynecol* 1969; **103**: 784–800.

75 Daya S, Woods S, Ward S, Lappalainen R, Caco C. Early pregnancy assessment with transvaginal ultrasound scanning. *CMAJ* 1991; **144**: 441–446.

76 Rossavik IK, Torjusen GO, Gibbons WE. Conceptual age and ultrasound measurements of gestational sac and crown-rump length in in vitro fertilization pregnancies. *Fertil Steril* 1988; **49**: 1012–1017.

77 Robinson HP, Fleming JE. A critical evaluation of sonar "crown-rump length" measurements. *Br J Obstet Gynaecol* 1975; **82**: 702–710.

78 MacGregor SN, Tamura RK, Sabbagha RE, Minoque JP, Gibson ME, Hoffman DI. Underestimation of gestational age by conventional crown-rump length dating curves. *Obstet Gynecol* 1987; **70**: 344–348.

79 Hadlock FP, Shah YP, Kanon DJ, Lindsey JV. Fetal crown-rump length: Reevaluation of relation to menstrual age (5–18 weeks) with high-resolution real-time US. *Radiology* 1992; **182**: 501–505.

80 Goldstein SR, Wolfson R. Endovaginal ultrasonographic measurement of early embryonic size as a means of assessing gestational age. *J Ultrasound Med* 1994; **13**: 27–31.

81 Hadlock FP, Deter RL, Harrist RB, Park SK. Fetal biparietal diameter: a critical re-evaluation of the relation to menstrual age by means of real-time ultrasound. *J Ultrasound Med* 1982; **1**: 97–104.

82 Hadlock FP, Deter RL, Harrist RB, Park SK. Estimating fetal age: computer-assisted analysis of multiple fetal growth parameters. *Radiology* 1984; **152**: 497–501.

83 Brown DL, Emerson DS, Felker RE, Cartier MS, Smith WC. Diagnosis of early embryonic demise by endovaginal sonography. *J Ultrasound Med* 1990; **9**: 631–636.

84 Levi CS, Lyons EA, Zheng XH, Lindsay DJ, Holt SC. Endovaginal US: Demonstration of cardiac activity in embryos of less than 5.0 mm in crown-rump length. *Radiology* 1990; **176**: 71–74.

85 Goldstein SR. Significance of cardiac activity on endovaginal ultrasound in very early embryos. *Obstet Gynecol* 1992; **80**: 670–672.

86 Abaid L, As-Sanie S, Wolfe HM. Relationship between crown-rump length and early detection of cardiac activity. *J Reprod Med* 2007; **52**: 375–378.

87 DeVoe RW, Pratt JH. Simultaneous intrauterine and extrauterine pregnancy. *Am J Obstet Gynecol* 1948; **56**: 1119–1126.

88 Barnhart KT, Katz I, Hummel A, Gracia CR. Presumed diagnosis of ectopic pregnancy. *Obstet Gynecol* 2002; **100**: 505–510.

89 Condous G, Kirk E, Lu C et al. Diagnostic accuracy of varying discriminatory zones for the prediction of ectopic pregnancy in women with a pregnancy of unknown location. *Ultrasound Obstet Gynecol* 2005; **26**: 770–775.

90 Stiller RJ, Haynes de Regt R, Blair E. Transvaginal ultrasonography in patients at risk for ectopic pregnancy. *Am J Obstet Gynecol* 1989; **161**: 903–930.

91 Fleischer AC, Pennell RG, McKee MS et al. Ectopic pregnancy: features at transvaginal sonography. *Radiology* 1990; **174**: 375–378.

92 Condous G, Okaro E, Khalid A et al. The accuracy of transvaginal ultrasonography for the diagnosis of ectopic pregnancy prior to surgery. *Hum Reprod* 2005; **20**: 1404–1409.

93 Schouwink MH, Fong BF, Mol BW, van der Veen F. Ultrasonographic criteria for nonviability of first trimester intrauterine pregnancy. *Early Pregnancy* 2000; **4**: 203–213.

94 Condous G, Okaro E, Khalid A, Bourne T. Do we need to follow up complete miscarriage with serum human chorionic gonadotrophin levels? *BJOG* 2005; **112**: 827–829.

95 Reynolds A, Ayres-de-Campos D, Costa MA, Montenegro N. How should success be defined when attempting medical resolution of first-trimester missed abortion? *Eur J Obstet Gynecol Reprod Biol* 2005; **118**: 71–76.

96 Reeves MF, Lohr PA, Harwood BJ, Creinin MD. Ultrasonographic endometrial thickness after medical and surgical management of early pregnancy failure. *Obstet Gynecol* 2008; **111**: 106–112.

97 Reeves MF, Fox MC, Creinin M. Ability of endometrial thickness following medical abortion to predict subsequent surgical intervention [abstract]. *Contraception* 2007; **76**: 162.

98 Cowett AA, Cohen LS, Lichtenberg ES, Stika CS. Ultrasound evaluation of the endometrium after medical termination of pregnancy. *Obstet Gynecol* 2004; **103**: 871–875.

99 O'Connell K, Jones HE, Lichtenberg ES, Paul M. Second trimester surgical abortion practices: a survey of National Abortion Federation members. *Contraception* 2008; **78**: 492–499.

100 O'Connell K, Jones HE, Simon M, Saporta V, Paul M, Lichtenberg ES. First-trimester surgical abortion practices: a survey of National Abortion Federation members. *Contraception*, in press.

7

CHAPTER 7

Medical evaluation and management

Anne Davis, MD, MPH and Thomas Easterling, MD

LEARNING POINTS

- For healthy women, the evaluation before induced abortion is quick and simple.
- For women with chronic illness, the preoperative evaluation guides how or where the abortion is provided rather than whether it can be performed.
- Women with important medical conditions, such as a personal history of thrombosis or cardiac valvular disease, may benefit from care coordinated with their regular physician or another physician with appropriate expertise.
- Cervical infection with *C. trachomatis* or *N. gonorrhoeae* (or mucopurulent cervicitis) is a risk factor for post-abortal endometritis. No studies have compared outcomes after immediate preprocedure treatment versus delaying the abortion for a week to complete treatment.
- Women with chronic medical conditions should be encouraged to continue their regular medications around the time of the abortion with occasional modifications as needed (e.g., insulin in the fasting patient).

Introduction

For most healthy women choosing to have an abortion, care is straightforward. Other women decide to have an abortion in the context of a serious medical or psychiatric illness. Hence, abortion providers encounter women with a variety of medical and psychiatric problems. Determining the optimal setting for abortion is important. Safe, prompt abortion care is especially critical when maternal risks increase as the pregnancy advances. However, for most conditions, delays of a week or two are offset by achieving appropriate diagnosis, management, and referral to the safest environment.

Most women choose abortion for reasons other than threat to maternal health. One large, recent survey found that only 12% of women included a physical problem with their health among reasons for having an abortion [1]. Hospital-based abortion providers who receive referrals care for more women with medical problems than do providers in freestanding clinics.

This chapter reviews the preabortion assessment relevant to the care of healthy women as well as those with medical problems. For all women, appropriate assessment will include a targeted history, physical examination, and limited laboratory testing. We present additional relevant preabortion and management considerations for selected acute and chronic medical problems. We focus primarily on women having surgical abortions; few midtrimester abortions in the USA currently involve labor induction. Other chapters provide more information about management in the context of medical methods of abortion (Chapters 9 and 12), anesthesia (Chapter 8), and contraceptive care (Chapter 14).

This chapter also aims to assist providers in choosing the setting for the abortion. In some cases, women with serious illness benefit from additional testing prior to the abortion, referral to a hospital-based ambulatory care setting, or rarely, hospital admission. Unnecessary referrals, however, burden women with delays as well as increase the cost and complexity of care. Additionally, some hospitals lack an experienced abortion provider or may offer only labor-induction abortion in the second trimester. If acceptable for the patient, a discussion with her regular health care provider may clarify which, if any, special considerations require modification of routine abortion care.

Preabortion screening

History

A medical history should precede the abortion; in most cases, this evaluation will be brief. Providers may use a checklist to be self-administered in the waiting area or a standard interview. For women with chronic medical conditions (e.g., severe asthma with a current respiratory infection), a

Management of Unintended and Abnormal Pregnancy, 1st edition. By M Paul, ES Lichtenberg, L Borgatta, DA Grimes, PG Stubblefield, MD Creinin

discussion with the regular health care provider may help determine what, if any, modifications to care warrant consideration, such as the need for antibiotics or alteration in steroid therapy. Providers must obtain the woman's permission prior to such contact. The medical history should include an open-ended question about any medical problems as well as specific questions about common medical conditions affecting women of reproductive age: cardiac (murmurs, valvular disease, arrhythmias), pulmonary (asthma, respiratory infection), hematologic (bleeding or clotting disorders), endocrine (diabetes, thyroid), renal, and hepatic (kidney and liver impairment affect drug clearance and metabolism). Other elements of the history include but are not limited to the following:

- Obstetric history
- Gynecologic history
- Social history
- Family history
- Medications
- Allergies

Obstetric history

Clarify the type of previous abortion or early pregnancy failure management, mode of delivery for births, and any pregnancy or procedure-related complications. Some important risk factors include a history of failed attempted abortion or perforation with a prior surgical abortion (suggestive of a uterine anomaly, such as a bicorruate uterus) or multiple cesarean deliveries. The rate of initial and repeat cesarean delivery has increased in the USA and many other countries. For example, in 2006, 31% of US births were accomplished by cesarean delivery [2], whereas in some private hospitals in Brazil, the proportion is more than 80% [3]. The risk of abnormal placentation (previa, accreta, increta, percreta) increases progressively with the number of previous cesarean deliveries [4]. Additionally, the small risk of uterine rupture must be considered for women having labor-induction abortion after previous cesarean delivery (Chapter 12).

Gynecologic history

Determine the history of sexually transmitted infections (STI), including human immunodeficiency virus (HIV), and other risk factors that may indicate the need for STI screening, such as symptoms of infection, adolescent age, or recent change in sexual partner. A history of treatment for dysplasia, such as a loop electrosurgical excision procedure (LEEP) or cold-knife conization, may result in cervical stenosis requiring additional cervical preparation.

Social history

Determine recent and chronic use of tobacco, alcohol, and drugs that may influence administration of anesthesia or the ease of intravenous access. Some providers inquire about a history of sexual abuse, which if present, may affect the woman's tolerance of examinations and surgical procedures (Chapter 5).

Family history

A family history of venous thromboembolism (suggestive of an inherited thrombophilia) or problems with anesthesia (such as malignant hyperthermia) may be relevant.

Medications

The provider should query the patient about the name(s) of medication(s), drug regimens, and reasons for use. In most cases, women should continue their regular medications before and after the abortion and be asked to bring their medications with them to the abortion visit. Some medications, such as insulin, may need a regimen adjustment around the time of the abortion. Several online and print resources are available for providers to obtain information about unfamiliar medications [5] (such as www.Epocrates.com).

Allergies

Identify allergies to medications, latex, iodine, and eggs (for those who are to receive the anesthesia agent propofol, because of rare allergic reactions). Many reported "allergies" are normal side effects, such as nausea with narcotics or ampicillin-related rash, which does not represent true penicillin allergy.

Physical examination

A brief, focused physical examination will usually provide all needed information before an abortion. Providers vary in what they include, but may include the following:

- Height and weight
- Vital signs
- Pulmonary and cardiac examinations
- Abdominal examination
- Pelvic examination

Height and weight

Determining height and weight enables calculation of body mass index (BMI). Weight may affect the choice of procedure, setting, or anesthesia. The current epidemic of obesity in the USA is summarized in thirds: one-third of the US population is of normal weight, one-third is overweight, and one-third is obese (BMI $\geq$30) [6]. Obesity is associated with greater technical difficulty, longer operating times, and greater blood loss during surgical abortion [7,8]. Morbid obesity may make surgical abortion risky or impractical; a medical method of abortion may be the better approach for eligible patients.

Vital signs

If the blood pressure (BP) measurement is elevated, repeating the measurement after the patient has been sitting stationary for several minutes usually gives a lower, more accurate reading. Women with a large arm circumference may need a wider cuff. The correct measurement of BP is important when providers consider referral to a hospital-based setting at a certain threshold. Although tachycardia because of anxiety is common, it may also reflect active thyroid disease or serious anemia.

Pulmonary and cardiac examinations

Pulmonary auscultation is indicated for women with a history of asthma or current respiratory infection. Mild wheezes often respond to inhaled bronchodilators administered a few minutes before the abortion procedure. Local or regional anesthesia may be preferable in the setting of acute or chronic respiratory disease. Most murmurs in asymptomatic women are physiologic and require no change in usual care. A cardiac examination may be helpful in the setting of symptoms such as shortness of breath or exercise intolerance. Radiation of the murmur to the carotid artery may indicate a pathologic murmur.

Abdominal examination

An abdominal examination may reveal factors that increase operative difficulty: cesarean delivery limiting mobility of the uterus because of adhesions, leiomyomas (suggested by size-date discrepancy or an enlarged, irregular uterus), or central obesity.

Pelvic examination

A bimanual examination provides an estimate of gestational age (especially in the absence of ultrasound), uterine and cervical position, mobility of the uterus, cervical consistency, and the possible presence and location of leiomyomas.

Laboratory testing

Current recommendations for women undergoing abortion in the USA include determination of Rh(D) antigen status [9]. Because the earliest gestational age at which sensitization is possible is unknown, both the American College of Obstetricians and Gynecologists [10] and the Royal College of Obstetricians and Gynaecologists [11] recommend immunoprophylaxis in nonsensitized D negative women having abortions at any gestational age. An exception occurs if the father of the pregnancy is known to be D negative.

Many providers determine the hemoglobin or hematocrit. Although no evidence exists regarding the need for this practice before abortion [11], it provides a baseline in the event of hemorrhage and alerts providers to anemia requiring treatment afterwards. In rare cases, very low hemoglobin prompts preparation for transfusion. However, in most cases, women with anemia may safely undergo surgical or medical abortion, given the modest blood loss involved. Blood loss is greater during second-trimester abortion but is usually well tolerated; the need for transfusion is rare even at advanced gestational ages.

Thrombocytopenia rarely poses a problem. Unfortunately, no published data specific to abortion can guide practice. Provided the platelet count exceeds 100,000 per microliter, management for first or second-trimester abortion can be routine. First-trimester surgical abortions with counts less than 100,000 are probably safe as well; more caution is prudent in the midtrimester when greater blood loss is expected. When lower counts occur as part of a disease process (e.g., immunological thrombocytopenic purpura), platelet function as well as the platelet count should be considered. Severe thrombocytopenia (e.g., less than 20,000 per microliter) may require platelet transfusion, especially in the second trimester. When concerns arise about increased bleeding because of platelet dysfunction or thrombocytopenia, a hospital setting is preferable so that platelets and other blood products are available if needed.

Many providers screen for chlamydial infection or gonorrhea at the time of abortion, whereas others provide universal treatment regimens without screening. The latter strategy has been found to be more cost effective, at least in European countries with national health services, but it lacks the advantage of partner tracing and treatment [12]. Screening can be accomplished with a vaginal swab, cervical sample, or urine test. The prevalence of chlamydial infection is related to the number of sexual partners and inversely related to age, years of education, and household income [13]. One representative survey in the USA found that 6% of sexually experienced adolescents screened positive for *C. trachomatis* [13]. The Centers for Disease Control and Prevention (CDC) and the US Preventive Services Task Force (USPSTF) recommend universal screening of all sexually active women aged 25 years or younger and screening of older women with risk factors (e.g., those who have a new sex partner or multiple sex partners) [14]. Positive results must be communicated to the patient with a plan for treatment for her and her partner(s).

HIV counseling and testing should be offered as appropriate. Recommendations regarding screening are inconsistent: starting in 2006, the CDC advised screening all persons between 13 and 64 years of age [15]. Prompted by this policy change, the USPSTF reviewed the available evidence and confirmed its assessment that insufficient evidence exists to argue for or against screening those not at increased risk [16]. The USPSTF guidelines regarding screening of pregnant women are not germane for abortion practice, however, because they implicitly assume that all pregnant women choose to continue their pregnancies.

Physiological changes of pregnancy

The physiological changes of pregnancy are generally well tolerated by healthy women and most of those with medical conditions. Some women with more severe and complex medical problems may require special attention. By mid-pregnancy many of the changes are complete, such that treatment of some conditions at 22 to 24 weeks' gestation may be as potentially complicated as those in late pregnancy. More detailed information can be obtained from textbooks of obstetrics [17,18].

Cardiovascular

During pregnancy, cardiac output increases by approximately 40% because of volume expansion, increased stroke volume, and increased heart rate. Vascular resistance falls beginning early in the first trimester. The net effect is decreased BP in the first trimester. However, women with chronic hypertension may have an exacerbation of hypertension in the first trimester.

Serum albumin levels fall in pregnancy resulting in decreased serum oncotic pressure and increased leakage of fluid from capillaries into interstitial spaces. Endothelial integrity is also compromised in some pregnancies, again increasing the flux of fluid into interstitial spaces. Therefore, pregnant woman are more susceptible to cardiogenic or non-cardiogenic pulmonary edema.

These hemodynamic changes resolve rapidly after pregnancy ends. Immediately after uterine evacuation, blood is returned from the uterus to the central circulation; at term, this volume may reach 500 mL. Edema fluid is mobilized more gradually. These volume challenges to the cardiovascular system pose increased risks in women with mitral stenosis, dilated cardiomyopathy, or hypertrophic cardiomyopathy.

Renal

Because of augmented renal blood flow, the glomerular filtration rate (GFR) increases by approximately 40% very early in the first trimester, which manifests as a fall in serum creatinine from 0.9 to 0.6 mg/dL on average. Simultaneously, more avid sodium retention expands blood volume. The rise in GFR is associated with a proportionate increase in renal clearance of some drugs. Because of progesterone-mediated smooth muscle relaxation, the renal collecting system and ureters dilate, which increases urinary dead space and the risk for urinary tract infection.

Pulmonary

Progesterone induces a rise in minute ventilation so that pCO_2 falls from a normal value of 40 mmHg to approximately 30 mmHg. Renal compensation to the progesterone-induced hyperventilation results in a decline in bicarbonate (HCO_3) to approximately 22mEq/L. Oxygen consumption increases early in pregnancy because of the metabolic demand of cardiovascular and renal changes. Late in pregnancy, the fetus contributes to an increase in oxygen demand. The rise in cardiac output more than compensates for the increased demand for oxygen delivery, resulting in higher mixed venous pO_2 concentrations during pregnancy. The reduced HCO_3 in pregnancy can be mistakenly attributed to metabolic acidosis rather than to renal compensation to respiratory alkalosis.

Hematologic

The pregnant woman's blood volume expands more rapidly than her capacity to produce red blood cells, resulting in a physiologic anemia. Iron deficiency will exacerbate the anemia. During pregnancy a dramatic increase in the risk of deep venous thrombosis and pulmonary embolism occurs that peaks in the immediate postpartum period [19]. Women with hereditary or acquired thrombophilia may require prophylaxis.

Metabolic

Pregnancy increases insulin resistance and hyperglycemia. In the second trimester, women may develop gestational diabetes or an increased need for treatment with insulin or oral hypoglycemics. During the first trimester, prior to the development of insulin resistance, type I diabetes may become more brittle.

Management of selected medical conditions

Providers must ensure that they have sufficient medical expertise, supplies, and equipment to provide the necessary care. If not, referral is indicated.

In general, women should be encouraged to continue their regular medications (such as antihypertensive agents) unless specifically advised not to (such as discontinuing anticoagulants). Women may mistakenly fear that taking medications while pregnant is harmful; for example, a woman may arrive for abortion with hypertension out of control because she decided to stop her angiotensin-converting enzyme (ACE) inhibitor upon discovery of the pregnancy. With the patient's consent, a plan should be coordinated with the woman's regular health care provider whenever possible.

Vaginitis

Women with vaginitis can usually have the abortion proceed as planned. Candidiasis can be treated with either oral fluconazole 150 mg as a single dose or a topical nitroimidazole; oral therapy may be preferred, because uterine bleeding can dilute or wash out vaginal medication. Occasionally, a patient's vulva and vagina are so tender that she may require treatment before a procedure using only local anesthesia. Trichomoniasis likewise can be treated with metronidazole as usual. The CDC suggests either metronidazole 2.0 g or tinidazole 2.0 g orally in a single dose, with the same treatment for the male partner [14]. Metronidazole gel is less effective than oral metronidazole. Although many clinicians advise against any medication in the vagina in the days after an abortion, no evidence supports this recommendation.

Chlamydial and gonococcal cervicitis

Infection of the cervix with either of these pathogens increases several-fold the risk of endometritis after abortion. Hence, treatment and partner management should be initiated promptly. Some providers delay the abortion to complete treatment, whereas others initiate treatment on the day of cervical preparation or the abortion procedure; no randomized trials have compared outcomes. A single dose of oral azithromycin 1.0 g is the preferred treatment for chlamydial infection, although a 7-day course of oral doxycycline 100 mg twice daily is an alternative [14]. Because of the emergence of fluoroquinolone-resistant strains of gonorrhea, the CDC now recommends intramuscular ceftriaxone 125 mg or oral suspension of cefixime 400 mg for uncomplicated gonorrhea [14].

Bacterial vaginosis

Bacterial vaginosis is a common cause of vaginal discharge. Based on laboratory criteria and not symptoms, more than a quarter of abortion patients may have this condition [20,21]. Whether screening and treatment of asymptomatic bacterial vaginosis reduce post-abortal infection remains unclear. Randomized controlled trials have compared treatment with metronidazole versus placebo or metronidazole and doxycycline versus doxycycline alone [20–22]. Losses to follow up after randomization in these trials were so large that the validity of the results is suspect [23]. Hence, the evidence is insufficient to make a recommendation.

Women presenting for abortion with symptomatic bacterial vaginosis can receive usual therapy without delay. The CDC suggests metronidazole 500 mg by mouth twice daily for 7 days, which may be preferable to the vaginal medications metronidazole gel or clindamycin cream [14].

Human immunodeficiency virus infection

The advent of highly active antiretroviral therapy (HAART) has reduced the abortion ratio among HIV-infected women. Before HAART, seropositive women who became pregnant disproportionately chose induced abortion compared with seronegative women [24]. Since the introduction of HAART, higher proportions of infected women are electing to continue their pregnancies [25,26]. Nevertheless, underuse of highly effective contraceptives leaves many infected women at risk of unintended pregnancy [27].

Little is known about the potential interactions between HIV infection and abortion. One small cohort study found no increase in the risk of infectious morbidity after curettage abortion among HIV-infected women compared to those uninfected. The overall complication rate was higher among the infected women, but these events included retained placenta and anesthesia problems unlikely to be related to HIV [28]. Women taking antiretroviral drugs should continue them without interruption. Those with profound immunosuppression or overt acquired immune deficiency syndrome (AIDS) may need their abortion care to be coordinated with their patient's regular treating physician.

Cardiovascular disease

Hypertension

Hypertension is common among young women, often clinically silent and undertreated. In the absence of a history of hypertension, providers should confirm excessively high measurements before delaying the abortion for treatment or referring the woman to a hospital-based setting. Outpatient procedures are appropriate for women with mild to moderate hypertension. Poorly controlled hypertension (systolic BP >160 mmHg; diastolic BP >105 mmHg) probably warrants treatment before the procedure. Treatment is usually easily accomplished with a combination of drugs such as a beta-blocker and a vasodilator. Providers should probably avoid ergot drugs in women with hypertension; oxytocin or misoprostol is an acceptable uterotonic agent for such patients.

Heart disease

Most women presenting for an abortion with serious cardiac disease will be aware of their condition. Some may not know their specific diagnosis, however, particularly if the problem was identified and treated during childhood. Medical records represent an important source of information if they are obtainable. The woman's parents or guardian may also be helpful, provided the patient gives permission to contact them.

Impaired functional status [29,30] may suggest undiagnosed heart disease. Questions such as: "Can you walk up a flight of stairs?", "Do you wake up at night short of breath?", "Does your heart race from time to time?", "Do you have chest pain or discomfort with exercise?" may be helpful. New flow murmurs commonly occur during pregnancy because of increased cardiac output. A harsh murmur radiating to the carotid suggests aortic stenosis and is usually pathological. Low oxygen saturation also suggests underlying cardiac or pulmonary disease.

When a provider identifies the presence of congenital heart disease by history or the presence of a surgical scar, a review of medical records or an echocardiogram may clarify the nature of the condition. In general, the absence of cyanosis, nondilated left and right ventricles with normal contractility, and a normal functional status are reassuring. Congenital cardiac conditions such as ventricular septal defects, atrial septal defects, and surgically corrected tetralogy of Fallot will usually not pose a problem during abortion. Some women with congenital heart disease experience exacerbation of tachyarrhythmia in pregnancy that may require cardiac rate control. Women with uncorrected left-to-right shunts may have dramatically increased pulmonary blood flow resulting in shortness of breath and impaired functional status.

Valvular heart disease may be acquired or congenital. Acquired disease usually results from rheumatic fever and occurs more commonly in immigrant and disadvantaged populations. Rheumatic mitral stenosis should be considered if shortness of breath and oxygen desaturation develop within 2 weeks of an abortion (particularly a second-trimester abortion). Women with moderate mitral stenosis (valve area <1.5 cm^2) and moderate aortic stenosis (peak gradient >60 mmHg) usually tolerate an abortion procedure without difficulty. Similarly, mitral and aortic regurgitation without evidence of left ventricular dilation should not complicate an abortion.

Women with prosthetic valves usually are fit for abortion. The need for anticoagulation depends on the type of valve and location, the patient's history, and the gestational age of the pregnancy at the time of abortion. Anticoagulation seldom increases bleeding from an uncomplicated first-trimester procedure, because hemostasis occurs primarily through uterine contraction. The effect on bleeding may be more important, however, in the second trimester or in the rare event of a complication such as uterine perforation. When the risk of thrombosis is small, providers may choose to stop warfarin 2 to 3 days before the procedure and restart it immediately afterward. Higher risks of thrombosis warrant transitioning from warfarin to heparin, which can be briefly stopped around the time of the abortion.

Myocardial infarction (MI) is rare in women of reproductive age. Those with a history of MI will usually require management in a hospital environment with attention to cardiac rate control with a beta-blocker and pain management. Ergot drugs should be avoided; aspirin should be continued. Surgery after a recent MI poses extra risks. Data regarding the risk of an abortion shortly after MI are lacking; nevertheless, the potential risk of cardiac death, particularly in the context of advanced gestational age or a complicated procedure, warrants consideration.

Cardiomyopathy with a dilated or compromised left ventricle may lead to hemodynamic decompensation and arrhythmia. Women with a history of cardiomyopathy and a normal echocardiogram should tolerate an abortion procedure, but they may worsen afterwards. Management includes cardiac rate control, diuretics, and afterload reduction. Hypertrophic cardiomyopathy is an autosomal-dominant condition. Patients are at risk for malignant arrhythmia and sudden death; many will have a defibrillator in place. Diastolic dysfunction and a stiff ventricle will decrease tolerance to volume loading, whereas advanced disease with left ventricular outflow obstruction because of septal hypertrophy will lead to poor tolerance of hemorrhage with hypovolemia. Cardiac rate control, usually with a beta-blocker, and volume management are critical.

The American Heart Association [31] no longer recommends antibiotic prophylaxis with genitourinary operations to prevent infective endocarditis. No credible evidence supports a link between procedures on the genitourinary tract and infective endocarditis or establishes that prophylactic antibiotics in this setting lower the remote risk of endocarditis [32]. The revised guidelines emphasize that susceptible individuals with high-risk cardiac conditions are more likely to develop endocarditis from bacteremia associated with daily activities than from any dental procedure [31]. Regarding abortion, the incidence of bacteremia is unknown but probably related to gestational age; the presence of bacteremia at term delivery is well established. Performing first-trimester surgical abortion without antibiotics in women with low-risk conditions, such as mitral valve prolapse, is certainly reasonable. In the absence of clear guidelines related to abortion, providers may differ in their approach to women with high-risk conditions, such as prosthetic valves, where the consequences of infective endocarditis are dramatic. Consultation with cardiologists in the community regarding local practice for prophylaxis may be helpful.

Endocrine disorders

Diabetes

The epidemic of diabetes is growing in parallel with the epidemic of obesity. In 2005, 7% of the US population (21 million persons) had diabetes [33]; of these, about 6 million persons were undiagnosed. The prevalence of diabetes increases progressively with age to reach 21% of individuals aged 60 years and older. The disease occurs more commonly among Native American and Black people than among Hispanic American or non-Hispanic White people.

In general, pregnancy increases medication requirements for adequate glucose control in the second and third trimesters. Women with type I diabetes may become more brittle in the first trimester and therefore prone to hypoglycemia. In addition, hyperemesis may complicate oral intake for diabetic pregnant women. Management of diabetic women having surgical abortions depends in part on plans for pain management. No changes in diet or medication are required for those having abortions under local anesthesia. When deeper sedation requires preprocedure fasting, a common approach is to have the patient inject half her usual long-acting insulin dose the evening before and skip the morning dose. Ideally, a woman with diabetes is scheduled to have one of the first procedures of the day, so that she can eat and take her usual dose of morning insulin afterwards; morning NPH will be active in the afternoon. Glucose is monitored frequently by finger stick before, during, and after the procedure, with insulin given as needed until the patient resumes eating. Although sliding scales of insulin doses related to blood glucose levels have been used in hospitals for decades, little evidence supports this approach [34].

When advising women regarding medications and diet, providers should keep in mind that modest hyperglycemia poses no acute risk to women undergoing an abortion. "Loose" control of diabetes around the time of the procedure is preferred to "tight" control. For example, a transient blood glucose concentration of 180 to 200 mg/dL during an abortion is not worrisome, whereas a blood glucose level of 30 mg/dL is. Hence, providers should have food, intravenous glucose solutions, or glucagon available. After the procedure, the patient's medication requirements may decrease substantially. Coordination of care with her medical provider is recommended, especially during this transitional time.

Thyroid disease

Hyperthyroidism in pregnancy may present with tachycardia, vomiting, tremulousness, and wide pulse pressure (Box A). Rarely, women with hydatidiform mole present with clinical hyperthyroidism related to high human chorionic gonadotropin production [35]. Women with mild hyperthyroidism can undergo abortion as usual, but uncontrolled hyperthyroidism can lead to thyroid storm. Hence, treatment should begin promptly and the abortion should proceed after the disease is stabilized by medication. Consultation with an anesthesiologist is advisable if the patient is to receive deep sedation or general anesthesia.

Pulmonary disease

Asthma

Asthma is another common illness among women seeking abortion: in 2005, an estimated 8% of the US population (about 22 million persons) currently had asthma [36]. Women have a 40% higher prevalence of asthma than do men. In 2005, approximately 4% of the population had at least one asthma episode in the previous year.

Women with a history of childhood asthma without current symptoms may undergo usual care. If a woman reports current well-controlled asthma, she should be encouraged to use her usual medications and to bring an inhaler with her for her visit. Even if her lungs are clear on auscultation, prophylactic use of an inhaler with nebulized albuterol or metaproterenol before the procedure may be prudent. Additionally, the facility should be equipped to manage the rare acute asthma exacerbation. Concurrent respiratory infection or inadequately controlled asthma may require delaying the abortion until treatment achieves better control. The prostaglandin carboprost tromethamine is not recommended for women with asthma, because it may cause bronchoconstriction; misoprostol is not contraindicated.

The use of inhaled corticosteroids does not require "stress dose" steroids at the time of surgery. However, if the woman has received repeated oral glucocorticoid therapy for asthma control (doses equivalent to at least 20 mg of prednisone daily for 5 or more days) [37,38], stress dose(s) of hydrocortisone may be used to prevent adrenal insufficiency. The dose should be individualized; for example, not all patients need hydrocortisone 100 mg given intravenously at intervals.

Severe asthma with bronchospasm constitutes a medical emergency requiring intensive medical intervention. Indeed, the asthma mortality rate for women is 45% higher than that for men [36]. Women with a history of recent emergency department visits for asthma or intubation also may benefit from a hospital-based setting for the abortion. Management may include premedication with steroids and the availability of a team of pulmonary specialists. Local or regional anesthesia may be preferable if severe, uncontrolled asthma is present in order to avoid bronchospasm during deep sedation or intubation.

Box A

A woman presented at 23 weeks LMP with a history of thyroid disease of unknown etiology. She was clinically hyperthyroid with exophthalmia, tachycardia, and tremor. Her case was managed in consultation with the anesthesia service, which recommended beta-blockade prior to the procedure and a brief hospitalization afterward with telemetry to monitor for thyroid storm.

Restrictive lung disease

Pregnancy is usually well tolerated in women with restrictive lung disease if the vital capacity exceeds 50%. Increased oxygen demand may result in desaturation at rest or with exercise. Postprocedure volume shifts that complicate respiratory function can be managed with diuresis. Women with complicated cystic fibrosis may require hospital-based care because of altered pulmonary physiology. When functional status is normal, first-trimester abortion in an outpatient setting is acceptable.

Pulmonary hypertension

Pulmonary hypertension because of increased pulmonary vascular resistance is life-threatening in pregnancy, with maternal mortality as high as 50%. Systolic pulmonary artery pressures exceeding 60 mmHg, particularly in the context of a dilated right ventricle, are very concerning. Echocardiography can be used to evaluate pulmonary pressures. Women with pulmonary hypertension require hospital-based care, including providers experienced in treating the condition. Clinicians can use specific pulmonary vasodilators to lower pulmonary vascular resistance and improve right heart function and forward flow. In the context of a failing right heart, management of volume loading in the second trimester usually requires invasive hemodynamic monitoring. Even modest volume shifts may result in right heart decompensation. Aggressive but appropriate diuresis is critical postprocedure.

Renal disease

Asymptomatic bacteruria does not complicate abortion; hence, screening for it is not required. Women who have symptomatic cystitis usually are infected with *E. coli*, adequately treated by a 3-day course of antibiotics, such as fluoroquinolones or beta-lactams [39]. Longer courses, such as 5 to 10 days of therapy, yield higher bacteriological cure rates but have significantly more side effects. No evidence indicates an important interaction between abortion and pyelonephritis, although many providers would hesitate to perform an elective abortion on a febrile patient.

In the context of adequately controlled hypertension, renal disease should not complicate an abortion procedure. Postabortion volume shifts may complicate the control of hypertension and require more aggressive diuresis. Dialysis after an abortion may require additional hyperfiltration. Adjustments of chronic medications for dialysis patients can be made in consultation with a pharmacist.

Box B SELECTED RISK FACTORS FOR THROMBOEMBOLISM (Adapted from ACOG) [40].)

Hereditary
- Factor V Leiden deficiency (5–6% of Caucasian population; 1% of African American population)
- Prothrombin gene mutation (2–4% of general population)
- Antithrombin III deficiency (0.02–0.2% of general population)
- Protein C deficiency (0.2–0.5% of general population)
- Protein S deficiency (0.08% of general population)
- Hyperhomocysteinemia (1–11% of general population)

Other
- Prior venous thromboembolism
- Mechanical heart valve
- Atrial fibrillation
- Trauma
- Major operation
- Prolonged immobilization
- Antiphospholipid syndrome

Organ transplant recipients

Management of a woman with a solid organ transplant will depend on the allograft organ's function. Cyclosporine and tacrolimus must be adjusted during and after pregnancy. Many other medications, (e.g., erythromycin) given concurrently with cyclosporine and tacrolimus can increase drug levels into a toxic range.

Thrombophilia

Pregnancy increases the risk of venous thromboembolism (VTE), with the risk greatest in the postpartum interval. Women with thrombophilia have even greater risks of VTE during and after pregnancy. Identification of women at increased risk of VTE related to pregnancy can allow prophylactic measures to reduce the risk around the time of abortion. Recognized risk factors for VTE may be inherited or acquired (Box B [40]).

The most common inherited thrombophilias are Factor V Leiden deficiency and prothrombin gene mutation (e.g., G20210A) (Box C). Other genetic predispositions to VTE are less prevalent. If a woman requesting abortion is already receiving VTE prophylaxis, coordinating her abortion care with her treating physician is helpful. For patients identified as being at increased risk and not on prophylaxis, consultation with a hematologist is useful. How long to continue anticoagulants after an abortion remains unclear; little evidence exists to guide therapy [41]. Women at high risk for thromboembolism may require lifelong anticoagulation and deserve special consideration in contraceptive choice (Chapter 14).

For women at increased risk who are undergoing labor induction abortion, several approaches help to reduce the risk of VTE. Graduated compression stockings reduce the risk of calf-vein clots, but they must be properly fitted to avoid an inadvertent tourniquet effect. Pneumatic compression devices can be used if the woman is confined to bed. Low-dose unfractionated heparin, such as 5,000 units subcutaneously every 8 hours, has been shown to protect women having cancer operations from developing a VTE. Low-molecular-weight heparin is more convenient (enoxaparin 40 mg subcutaneously daily as a single injection) but incurs higher cost. Combinations of these strategies can be used, depending on the perceived risk. Women receiving anticoagulants should avoid spinal or epidural anesthesia because of the risk of spinal hematomas.

Neurologic disorders

Because pregnancy increases the metabolism of many antiepileptic medications, women with seizure disorders may require medication adjustment during pregnancy. Women with well-controlled epilepsy may undergo routine care. Hospital-based care should be considered for those with recent onset or uncontrolled seizures. For any woman with epilepsy, a seizure may occur at any time. If a seizure occurs during abortion in an awake patient, appropriate measures include maintaining patient safety (safe positioning with support) and interrupting the abortion procedure if possible until the seizure has ended. Most seizures resolve

Box C

A woman seeking abortion in the first trimester of pregnancy has a personal history of venous thromboembolism and is known to be heterozygous for Factor V Leiden deficiency. She may benefit from prophylactic anticoagulation at the time of the abortion and for a period of time afterwards. This can be accomplished appropriately with heparin (unfractionated or low molecular weight) or warfarin.

Box D INTRAVENOUS LOADING DOSE OF ANTIEPILEPTIC DRUGS USED IN STATUS EPILEPTICUS (From Sivven and Waterhouse [42].)

Diazepam 10–20 mg
Lorazepam 4 mg
Midazolam 0.2 mg per kg
Propofol 2 mg per kg

spontaneously and do not require intravenous anticonvulsants. Protecting the patient from falling is usually all that is required.

Fortunately, status epilepticus is rare. Stopping the prolonged or repetitive tonic-clonic seizures quickly is crucial to avoid neurologic and systemic injury [42]. This requires prompt administration of intravenous antiepileptic drugs; several of these benzodiazepines, such as midazolam, are commonly available in abortion settings (Box D [42]). Ancillary measures include airway maintenance, administration of oxygen and intravenous fluids, and monitoring of vital signs. Hospitalization for further evaluation and care should be prompt.

Contraceptive counseling in women with seizure disorders must include a careful review of antiepileptic drugs. Some, but not all, antiepileptic drugs induce the hepatic cytochrome p450 system that metabolizes oral contraceptive steroid hormones [43]. For instance, carbamazepine and phenobarbital decrease levels of contraceptive steroids but valproic acid does not. The decreases in serum levels of contraceptive steroids may lead to breakthrough bleeding and decreased efficacy; intrauterine contraception is often an easier and more effective approach.

Gastrointestinal disorders

A history of mild past or current liver disease does not affect usual care (e.g., hepatitis with mildly elevated transaminases). Coagulopathy may complicate cases of severe liver disease; an appropriate laboratory evaluation should precede the abortion. Women with portal hypertension warrant referral for hospital care.

Psychiatric conditions and substance abuse

Issues for women with psychiatric conditions seeking abortion include ensuring appropriate informed consent and identifying social support during and after the abortion. Some women seeking abortion are in a personal crisis; the request for abortion may reflect threats to the woman, such as an abusive partner, abandonment, or coerced sex. The current social situation and risk of suicide must be addressed (Chapter 5).

Women with a history of substance abuse may have a tolerance to narcotics and other drugs and thus require larger doses of medications (Chapter 8). With appropriate monitoring, larger than customary doses of narcotics and benzodiazepines can be administered safely in an outpatient setting. Establishing venous access in intravenous drug abusers can be challenging. Hence, clinicians should consider starting an intravenous line and securing it well with tape before the procedure begins.

Referral for abortion services

Abortion is a safe medical procedure. For a small number of women, a freestanding clinic or office may not offer the optimal conditions for care. Gestational age is important. Medical conditions easily managed at 8 weeks' gestation may be more complicated at 18 weeks. Similarly, the potential for uncommon but serious complications is greater in the second trimester than in the first.

Available medical services vary by site. Hospitals have more resources to manage complex problems (e.g., a full range of blood products, more anesthesia options, intensive care). Hospitals with perinatal services will have more resources than some community hospitals. Unfortunately, abortion expertise, particularly with dilation and evacuation at more advanced gestational ages, may be limited in hospitals. Although referral for hospital-based care can provide more sophisticated medical resources, it may limit the abortion options available to women.

The facility's resources to manage uncommon but potentially serious complications, such as hemorrhage or perforation, should be considered. A woman with moderate cardiac disease may easily tolerate a routine abortion but not one with complications. Is a hospital nearby, or would referral require transport of some distance?

Ideally, every freestanding clinic or office would have an established relationship with a Level III perinatal center where a patient with complications could receive appropriate counseling, medical management, and a safe abortion. Unfortunately, this scenario may be the exception rather than the rule in the USA. In some circumstances, referral to a hospital may be appropriate (Table 7.1). In other cases, consultation and coordination of care may permit a safe clinic-based procedure.

Conclusion

Although most women seeking abortion care are healthy, abortion providers also encounter women with a broad spectrum of medical and psychiatric illnesses. A focused history and physical examination, review of pertinent records, selective use of laboratory tests, and careful planning with treating physicians will enable safe outpatient care for many women with acute and chronic illness. Others will benefit from hospital-based or inpatient care. The overriding concern in deciding the optimal site for abortion care is patient safety. Although convenience and cost may have to be compromised, patient care must not be.

Table 7.1 Potential indications for referral to a hospital-based provider.

Here are some conditions seen in young women that may require intensive medical management around the time of an abortion. The list is not meant to be exhaustive or proscriptive. The decision about the optimal site of care depends on many factors such as gestational age, the severity of the medical condition, the capacity of the abortion facility to manage medical problems, and the availability or proximity of local referral resources.

Central nervous system
- Vascular – Arteriovenous malformation, untreated aneurysm
- Space-occupying lesions

Renal
- Impaired renal function (serum creatinine >2.5 mg/dL)

Hypertension
- Uncontrolled BP (systolic BP >160 or diastolic BP >105)

Endocrine
- Uncontrolled hyperthyroidism or diabetes
- Pheochromocytoma

Cardiac
- Congenital (cyanotic disease, right or left ventricular dilation, uncontrolled tachyarrhythmia)
- Coronary artery disease – (prior MI, angina)
- Cardiomyopathy – (current or history of pregnancy-related cardiomyopathy)

Pulmonary
- Uncontrolled asthma
- Restrictive lung disease (FVC <50%)
- Pulmonary hypertension (sPAP ≥50 mmHg)

Rheumatologic
- Lupus flare
- Lupus requiring anticoagulation

Gastrointestinal
- Hepatic disease with elevated prothrombin time
- Esophageal varices with history of bleeding
- Uncontrolled inflammatory bowel disease

Hematologic
- Severe anemia
- Sickle cell disease (current or recent crisis, history of thrombosis)
- Thrombophilia requiring anticoagulation

Oncology
- Counseling (timing of abortion relative to chemotherapy or radiation)
- Gynecologic cancers restricting access to the uterus

Transplant
- Impaired renal function (creatinine >2.5 mg/dL)
- Recent organ rejection
- Poorly functioning transplanted organ

Psychiatric
- Current suicidal ideation

References

1 Finer LB, Frohwirth LF, Dauphinee LA, Singh S, Moore AM. Reasons U.S. women have abortions: quantitative and qualitative perspectives. *Perspect Sex Reprod Health* 2005; **37**: 110–118.

2 Hamilton BE, Martin JA, Ventura SJ. Births: preliminary data for 2006. *National Vital Statistics Reports* 2007; **56**: Number 7.

3 Hopkins K. Are Brazilian women really choosing to deliver by cesarean? *Soc Sci Med* 2000; **51**: 725–740.

4 Silver RM, Landon MB, Rouse DJ et al. Maternal morbidity associated with multiple repeat cesarean deliveries. *Obstet Gynecol* 2006; **107**: 1226–1232.

5 Lacy CF, Armstrong LL, Goldman MP, Lance LL. *Drug Information Handbook: A Comprehensive Resource for All Clinicians and Healthcare Professionals*, 15th edn. Lexi-Comp, Hudson, OH, 2007.

6 Grimes DA, Shields WC. Family planning for obese women: challenges and opportunities. *Contraception* 2005; **72**: 1–4.

7 Dark AC, Miller L, Kothenbeutel RL, Mandel L. Obesity and second-trimester abortion by dilation and evacuation. *J Reprod Med* 2002; **47**: 226–230.

8 Marchiano DA, Thomas AG, Lapinski R, Balwan K, Patel J. Intraoperative blood loss and gestational age at pregnancy termination. *Prim Care Update Ob Gyns* 1998; **5**: 204–205.

9 National Abortion Federation. *National Abortion Federation Clinical Policy Guidelines 2008.* National Abortion Federation, Washington, DC, 2008.

10 American College of Obstetricians and Gynecologists. Prevention of Rh D alloimmunization. *ACOG Practice Bulletin* 1999; Number 4.

11 Royal College of Obstetricians and Gynaecologists. The care of women requesting induced abortion. *Evidence-Based Clinical Guideline* 2004; Number 7.

12 Cameron ST, Sutherland S. Universal prophylaxis compared with screen-and-treat for chlamydia trachomatis prior to termination of pregnancy. *BJOG* 2002; **109**: 606–609.

13 Datta SD, Sternberg M, Johnson RE et al. Gonorrhea and chlamydia in the United States among persons 14 to 39 years of age, 1999 to 2002. *Ann Intern Med* 2007; **147**: 89–96.

14 Centers for Disease Control and Prevention. Sexually transmitted diseases treatment guidelines, 2006. *MMWR Morbid Mortal Weekly Rep* 2006; **55**: No. RR-11.

15 Centers for Disease Control and Prevention. Revised recommendations for HIV testing of adults, adolescents, and pregnant women in health-care settings. *Morbid Mortal Weekly Rep* 2006; **55**: No. RR-14.

16 Agency for Healthcare Research Quality [Online]. Rockville, MD: U.S. Department of Health and Human Services. Screening for human immunodeficiency virus infection; 2005 Jul [cited 2008 Aug 8]. Available from: URL:http://www.ahrq.gov/clinic/uspstf/uspshivi.htm

17 Creasy RK, Resnik R, Iams JD, Lockwood CJ, Moore TR, eds. *Creasy & Resnik's Maternal-Fetal Medicine: Principles and Practice*, 6th edn. Saunders, Philadelphia, 2009.

18 Dildy GA, Belfort MA, Saade GR, Phelan JP, Hankins GDV, Clark SL, eds. *Critical Care Obstetrics*, 4th edn. Wiley-Blackwell, New York, 2003.

19 Heit JA, Kobbervig CE, James AH, Petterson TM, Bailey KR, Melton LJ III. Trends in the incidence of venous thromboembolism during pregnancy or postpartum: a 30-year population-based study. *Ann Intern Med* 2005; **143**: 697–706.

20 Crowley T, Low N, Turner A, Harvey I, Bidgood K, Horner P. Antibiotic prophylaxis to prevent post-abortal upper genital tract infection in women with bacterial vaginosis: randomised controlled trial. *BJOG* 2001; **108**: 396–402.

21 Miller L, Thomas K, Hughes JP, Holmes KK, Stout S, Eschenbach DA. Randomised treatment trial of bacterial vaginosis to prevent post-abortion complication. *BJOG* 2004; **111**: 982–988.

22 Larsson PG, Platz-Christensen JJ, Thejils H, Forsum U, Pahlson C. Incidence of pelvic inflammatory disease after first-trimester legal abortion in women with bacterial vaginosis after treatment with metronidazole: a double-blind, randomized study. *Am J Obstet Gynecol* 1992; **166**: 100–103.

23 Schulz KF, Grimes DA. Sample size slippages in randomised trials: exclusions and the lost and wayward. *Lancet* 2002; **359**: 781–785.

24 Sunderland A, Minkoff HL, Handte J, Moroso G, Landesman S. The impact of human immunodeficiency virus serostatus on reproductive decisions in women. *Obstet Gynecol* 1992; **79**: 1027–1031.

25 Massad LS, Springer G, Jacobson L et al. Pregnancy rates and predictors of conception, miscarriage, and abortion in U.S. women with HIV. *AIDS* 2004; **18**: 281–286.

26 Sharma A, Feldman JG, Golub ET et al. Live birth patterns among human immunodeficiency virus-infected women before and after the availability of highly active antiretroviral therapy. *Am J Obstet Gynecol* 2007; **196**: 541 e1-e6.

27 Massad LS, Evans CT, Wilson TE et al. Contraceptive use among U.S. women with HIV. *J Womens Health (Larchmt)* 2007; **16**: 657–666.

28 Stuart GS, Sheffield JS, Hill JB, McIntire DD, McElwee B, Wendel GD Jr. Morbidity that is associated with curettage for the management of spontaneous and induced abortion in women who are infected with HIV. *Am J Obstet Gynecol* 2004; **191**: 993–997.

29 Arena R, Myers J, Williams MA et al. Assessment of functional capacity in clinical and research settings: a scientific statement from the American Heart Association Committee on Exercise, Rehabilitation, and Prevention of the Council on Clinical Cardiology and the Council on Cardiovascular Nursing. *Circulation* 2007; **116**: 329–343.

30 American Heart Association [Online]. Dallas: American Heart Association; 2008. 1994 Revisions to classification of functional capacity and objective assessment of patients with diseases of the heart; 1994 [cited 2008 Aug 7]. Available from: URL:http://www.americanheart.org/presenter.jhtml?identifier=1712

31 Wilson W, Taubert KA, Gewitz M et al. Prevention of infective endocarditis: guidelines from the American Heart Association: a guideline from the American Heart Association Rheumatic Fever, Endocarditis, and Kawasaki Disease Committee, Council on Cardiovascular Disease in the Young, and the Council on Clinical Cardiology, Council on Cardiovascular Surgery and Anesthesia, and the Quality of Care and Outcomes Research Interdisciplinary Working Group. *Circulation* 2007; **116**: 1736–1754.

32 Strom BL, Abrutyn E, Berlin JA et al. Risk factors for infective endocarditis: oral hygiene and nondental exposures. *Circulation* 2000; **102**: 2842–2848.

33 Centers for Disease Control and Prevention. National diabetes fact sheet: general information and national estimates on diabetes in the United States, 2005 [Online]. Atlanta, GA: U.S. Department of Health and Human Services, Centers for Disease Control and Prevention; 2005 [cited 2008 Aug 7]. Retrieved June 26, 2008. Available from: URL:http://apps.nccd.cdc.gov/DDTSTRS/template/ndfs_2005.pdf

34 Umpierrez GE, Palacio A, Smiley D. Sliding scale insulin use: myth or insanity? *Am J Med* 2007; **120**: 563–567.

35 Erturk E, Bostan H, Geze S, Saracoglu S, Erciyes N, Eroglu A. Total intravenous anesthesia for evacuation of a hydatidiform mole and termination of pregnancy in a patient with thyrotoxicosis. *Int J Obstet Anesth* 2007; **16**: 363–366.

36 Akinbami L. Asthma prevalence, health care use, and mortality [Online]. Hyattsville, MD: National Center for Health Statistics; 2003–2005 [cited 2008 Aug 7]. Available from: URL:http://www.cdc.gov/nchs/products/pubs/pubd/hestats/ashtma03-05/asthma03-05.htm

37 Axelrod L. Perioperative management of patients treated with glucocorticoids. *Endocrinol Metab Clin North Am* 2003; **32**: 367–383.

38 Johnson BE, Porter L. Preoperative evaluation of the gynecologic patient: considerations for improved outcomes. *Obstet Gynecol* 2008; **111**: 1183–1194.

39 Milo G, Katchman EA, Paul M, Christiaens T, Baerheim A, Leibovici L. Duration of antibacterial treatment for uncomplicated urinary tract infection in women. *Cochrane Database Syst Rev* 2005; **2**: Art. No. CD004682.

40 American College of Obstetricians and Gynecologists. Thromboembolism in pregnancy. *ACOG Practice Bulletin* 2000; Number 19.

41 American College of Obstetricians and Gynecologists. ACOG Practice Bulletin No. 84: prevention of deep vein thrombosis and pulmonary embolism. *Obstet Gynecol* 2007; **110**: 429–440.

42 Sirven JI, Waterhouse E. Management of status epilepticus. *Am Fam Physician* 2003; **68**: 469–476.

43 Epilepsy Foundation of America [Online]. Landover, MD: Epilepsy Foundation of America. Contraception for women with epilepsy [cited 2008 July 2]. Available from: URL:http://www.epilepsyfoundation.org/answerplace/Life/adults/women/Professional/contraception.cfm

8

CHAPTER 8
Pain management

Mark Nichols MD, Glenna Halvorson-Boyd PhD, RN, Robert Goldstein MD, Clifford Gevirtz MD, MPH and David Healow MD

LEARNING POINTS

- Proper selection of medications and nonpharmacological interventions reduces pain and anxiety and enhances patient satisfaction.
- Several effective techniques exist for administration of local cervical anesthesia. Limited data support use of deep injections and adjunctive premedication with nonsteroidal antiinflammatory drugs.
- The most common conscious sedation regimen used by North American abortion providers is a combination of fentanyl and midazolam.
- Deep sedation and general anesthesia carry important benefits for certain patients, but they require specialized personnel and equipment.

Introduction

Managing pain associated with abortion procedures is an essential goal in the care of patients requesting pregnancy termination. Effective methods range from local cervical anesthesia, with or without supplemental oral or intravenous (IV) medications, to general anesthesia (GA). A number of factors influence the options available to patients, including local regulations, safety considerations, facility infrastructure and resources, cost, and insurance coverage. In the USA, where most abortions occur in freestanding clinics, cervical anesthesia with or without IV conscious sedation represents the most common method used [1]. On the other hand, in countries where abortions occur primarily in hospital operating rooms, general anesthesia predominates.

This chapter explores pain management for surgical abortion including the anatomy and physiology of pain; the use of local anesthesia, IV sedation, and GA; and challenging pain management cases. The chapter also investigates the relationship of psychosocial and emotional issues to abortion-related pain and describes nonpharmacological techniques to address them.

Management of Unintended and Abnormal Pregnancy, 1st edition. By M Paul, ES Lichtenberg, L Borgatta, DA Grimes, PG Stubblefield, MD Creinin
 ISBN: 9781405176965.

Pain associated with abortion

Pain management remains an important challenge in abortion practice, although studies suggest that progress in pain control has been achieved over time in the USA. In a survey in the late 1970s, 2,299 women having abortions with cervical anesthesia were asked to rate their pain as "mild, moderate, or severe." Forty-six per cent called the pain moderate, and 32% called it severe. [2] A survey conducted two decades later of more than 2,000 patients at 12 abortion facilities in the USA found that 30% of patients felt no pain, 25% mild pain, 29% moderate pain, and 14% severe pain. About 80% of patients said the pain was less than or similar to what they expected. [3]

Components of pain

Abortion-related pain requires stimulation of sensory fibers that innervate the uterus, the transmission of those impulses via afferent pathways to the spinal column and brain, and finally, interpretation of the signals as unpleasant by the higher cortical centers. The cervix and lower uterine segment are innervated by parasympathetic fibers from S2 to S4, which form a ganglia lateral to the cervix and enter along with the uterine blood vessels at about 3 o'clock and 9 o'clock (Fig. 8.1). The fundus is innervated by sympathetic fibers from T10 and L1 via the inferior hypogastric nerve, which enters the uterus at the uterosacral ligaments, as well as via the ovarian plexuses that enter at the cornua. By anesthetizing the nerve plexuses adjacent to the cervix along the

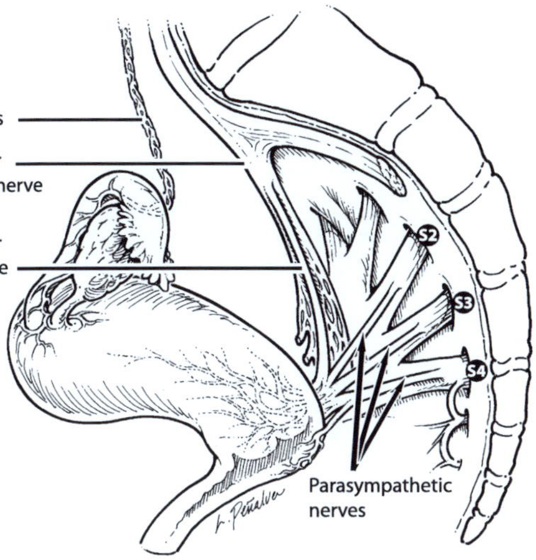

Figure 8.1 Innervation of the uterus. Paracervical anesthesia reaches the nerve plexuses that lie adjacent to the cervix, but not the nerves that accompany the ovarian vessels at the level of the uterine fundus.

lateral aspects at 3 and 9 o'clock as well as the uterosacral ligaments, paracervical anesthesia reduces pain from cervical manipulation, dilation, and to varying degrees, uterine aspiration. Because the anesthetic agent does not reach nerves that accompany the ovarian vessels at the fundus, it may have less effect on the cramping associated with uterine emptying. [4]

Factors influencing pain

Numerous patient-related variables are known to influence pain perception (Table 8.1). Factors associated with increased pain include younger age of the patient [2], fewer prior pregnancies [2], history of dysmenorrhea [5], preprocedure anxiety [5], and depression [4]. History of prior pelvic examination and gestational age of the pregnancy are not related to an increase in pain [2]. Regarding the procedure itself, both shorter procedure time [2] and provider experience [6] correlate with less pain; the amount of cervical dilation and cannula size are not associated with an increase in pain [2].

As these numerous factors suggest, perception of pain is a complex and multidimensional phenomenon. Recognized components of pain include physical (sensory), psychological (affective, motivational, and interpretive), and social (context and support) features and their constant interplay. As Melzack noted, "The quality of pain experiences must not be confused with the physical event."[7]

Choice of pain control methods

Patient preparation for abortion includes providing relevant information for an informed decision about pain management. This information includes a description of the procedure, the range of possible pain experiences, the available options for treatment, and the benefits and risks of each alternative. If the patient expresses a strong preference for a pain management method that the facility does not offer, then staff should provide her with appropriate referral resources.

Some women prefer local anesthesia for first-trimester aspiration abortion because they want to avoid the consciousness-altering effects of sedation and remain alert during the procedure, thereby quickening their recovery for discharge home. In addition, morbid obesity or certain medical conditions may preclude safe administration of IV sedation or GA in a nonhospital-based setting. Deeper levels of sedation, on the other hand, carry benefits for patients who are having second-trimester abortions, desire to be more relaxed or "asleep" during the experience, or whose elevated anxiety may affect their ability to remain still during the procedure. Deeper levels of sedation require more resources, including appropriately trained staff and monitoring equipment. Local, state, or provincial regulations may specify the facility design, equipment, and personnel necessary to offer IV sedation or GA.

Local anesthesia

Most first-trimester aspiration abortions in the USA and Canada take place at facilities that use local cervical anesthesia with or without IV sedation. A 2002 survey of National Abortion Federation (NAF) provider facilities ($n =$

Table 8.1 Factors that influence abortion-related pain.

Increased Pain	No Effect on Pain	Decreased Pain
Younger patient age [2]	Prior pelvic examinations [2]	Older patient age [2]
Fewer prior pregnancies [2]	Gestational age [2]	More prior pregnancies [2]
History of dysmenorrhea [5]	Amount of cervical dilation [2]	Shorter operative time [2]
Preprocedure anxiety [5]	Cannula size [2]	Increased provider experience [6]
Depression [4]		

Table 8.2 Selected properties of local anesthetic agents. (Adapted with permission from Bonica [9].).

Agent	Relative Lipid Solubility	Protein Binding (%)	pK_a	Relative Potency	Comments
AMINO ESTERS					More allergic reactions; more expensive
Procaine (Novocaine®)	1	5	8.9	1	
2-Chloroprocaine (Nesacaine®)	1	0	9.1	1	Low pH; more painful to inject
Tetracaine (Pontocaine®)	80	85	8.6	8	
AMINO AMIDES					Fewer allergic reactions
Lidocaine (Xylocaine®)	4	65	7.9	2	Least expensive
Bupivacaine (Marcaine®)	30	95	8.1	8	Long-acting
Mepivacaine (Carbocaine®)	1	75	7.6	2	
Prilocaine (Citanest®)	1.5	55	7.7	2	

364) examined anesthesia preferences for each facility by determining the method employed for 40 to 100% of first-trimester abortions. Of the 110 respondents that expressed a preference, 46% used cervical anesthesia with or without oral medications and 33% combined cervical anesthesia with IV conscious sedation; the remaining 21% offered deep sedation or GA. In general, smaller-volume providers tended to offer milder forms of anesthesia [1]. A 2007 survey of Planned Parenthood affiliates in the USA found that virtually all respondents provided local anesthesia during surgical abortion, and 85% of affiliates reported offering ibuprofen preoperatively. Two-thirds of the affiliates reported offering patients the option of IV sedation for pain management (Fjerstadt M, 2008, personal communication).

Types of local anesthetic agents

There are two classes of local anesthetics: amides and esters (Table 8.2). The metabolism of these drug groups differs. The esters are metabolized by acetyl cholinesterase in the plasma while the amides are metabolized in the liver. Amides have largely replaced esters in surgical abortion care because of their stability, affordability, and lower likelihood to cause an allergic reaction [8,9].

Safety, side effects, and allergies

Local anesthetic agents have a long history of safe use in abortion care. From 1988 to 1997 in the USA, complications of all forms of anesthesia accounted for 16% of total legal induced abortion mortality, a substantial decrease from the 29% figure reported for 1983 to 1987 [10]. Abortion-related deaths and notable adverse events with local anesthesia are rare. They may be related to the specific agent, excessive doses, or inadvertent IV injection. The maximum dose of lidocaine without epinephrine should not exceed 4.5 mg/kg; for paracervical anesthesia during pregnancy, the drug label recommends a total maximum dose of 200 mg per 90-minute period [11]. Lidocaine has less potential for cardiac toxicity than bupivacaine at similar serum levels.

In general, current commonly employed cervical anesthesia techniques that involve injections at multiple sites using standard dose ranges of procaine-analog agents, including bupivacaine, have not been associated with significant side effects [12] or toxic serum levels [13]. However in the 1970s, Grimes and Cates [14] reported a series of deaths from paracervical anesthesia that included overdoses, inadvertent bolus intravascular injections, and hypersensitivity reactions to preservatives. Serum levels of anesthetic agents correlate with toxicity and side effects. At low serum concentrations of lidocaine, patients may experience tinnitus, numbness of the lips or tongue, or a metallic taste in the mouth (see Question #1 in the Challenging Clinical Scenarios section). At higher levels, direct central nervous system (CNS) effects, including confusion or seizures, or cardiac effects of arrhythmia and collapse may occur [15] (Fig. 8.2).

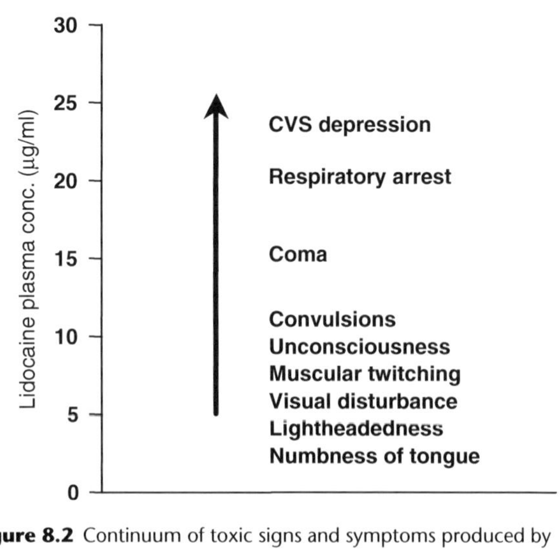

Figure 8.2 Continuum of toxic signs and symptoms produced by increasing plasma concentration of lidocaine. CVS = cardiovascular system (Reprinted with permission from Carpenter and Mackey [15].).

Adding vasoconstrictors, such as vasopressin or epinephrine, to procaine-analog anesthetics produces lower serum levels because of less vascular uptake of the anesthetic. Vasoconstrictors also produce longer lasting anesthesia because they cause slow reabsorption of the procaine analog.

True allergy to local anesthetic agents is extremely rare. The antioxidant preservative sodium metabisulfate present in vials of lidocaine with epinephrine may cause allergic reactions, particularly bronchospasm in some asthmatic patients. Vials of plain lidocaine do not contain this preservative [11].

Box A Sample Recipe for Preparation of the Anesthetic Solution (Adapted from Glick [21].).

1 Take a 50-ml vial of 1% or 0.5% lidocaine and draw off 5 ml (save or discard).
2 Add 5 ml of 8.4% sodium bicarbonate to buffer the solution.
3 Add 4-10 units (0.2-0.5 ml) of vasopressin (particularly useful in second-trimester procedures).
4 Use approximately 20 ml per patient.

Effectiveness

The mechanism of action in paracervical anesthesia is presumed to involve a direct anesthetic effect on the parasympathetic nerves near the cervix. One randomized clinical trial found no difference in pain between patients who received paracervical injections of 1% lidocaine or bacteriostatic saline [16], suggesting that mechanical distension of tissues with the anesthetic solution may contribute to the effect. However, the sterile saline solution contained benzyl alcohol as a preservative, which is a more effective analgesic than saline alone [17]. Based on these findings, bacteriostatic saline may prove useful in treating patients allergic to amino amides in medical settings where no amino ester procaine analogs are available (see Question #4 in the Challenging Clinical Scenarios section).

Efforts to improve effectiveness of paracervical anesthesia have included varying the type, concentration, and volume of anesthetic agents; injecting into different areas of the cervix; varying the waiting time; and supplementing with adjunctive medications and nonpharmacological techniques.

Anesthetic agents

Lidocaine is the most common local anesthetic agent used by North American abortion providers [1]. Abortion pain is similar in patients treated with either 1% lidocaine or 0.25% bupivacaine paracervical anesthesia according to a double-blind prospectively randomized trial; the 0.50% concentration of bupivacaine was not tested [18]. Another prospective randomized double-blinded study suggested that decreasing the concentration of lidocaine from 1.0 to 0.5% for paracervical anesthesia produced equivalent pain reduction during the procedure; however, the authors did not mention whether equivalent volumes of anesthetic were employed [19].

Wait time

A prospective randomized study found that delaying the abortion procedure 3 minutes compared to beginning cervical dilation immediately after deep paracervical injections of 1% buffered lidocaine at 4 o'clock and 8 o'clock did not affect pain scores during cervical dilation or aspiration of the uterus [20]. Evidence indicates that injecting buffered lidocaine slowly (over 60 seconds compared to 30 seconds) decreases the pain of the injection [18].

Additives

Preparation of the cervical anesthesia medication varies among providers and includes adding buffers, vasoconstrictors, uterotonics, narcotics, and/or atropine [21] (Box A). In 2001, 36% of NAF providers buffered the local anesthetic solution, and 41% added a vasoconstrictor to the solution [1]. Buffering the local anesthetic solution by adding sodium bicarbonate has been shown to make the injections less painful [18]. Low-dose vasopressin added to lidocaine solution reduces blood loss in second-trimester abortion [22] and softens the cervix in the nonpregnant patient, an effect that may decrease the force needed to dilate the cervix [23]. In 2001, 13% of NAF providers in North America added atropine to the paracervical anesthetic solution to prevent vasovagal reactions [1]. No published data have established the effectiveness or optimum dose of this treatment.

One randomized trial compared cervical and IV injection of fentanyl 100 μg in patients having first-trimester aspiration abortions. In the cervical injection group, the fentanyl was added to the lidocaine solution and injected intracervically or paracervically. Intravenous fentanyl was associated with significantly less pain. Mean pain scores were 4.7 and 3.8 during dilation and suctioning, respectively, in the IV fentanyl group compared to 5.7 and 5.6 for the cervical injection group. Women receiving IV fentanyl voiced more requests for antiemetic medication [24].

Technique

Several authors have advocated specific techniques for the injection, but only limited data have compared the effectiveness of these techniques. Most providers inject local anesthetic into the lip of the cervix before applying a tenaculum to position and stabilize the cervix for cervical anesthesia. Some providers advocate injecting the anesthetic agent directly into the stroma of the cervix, whereas others recommend injecting into the adventitial tissue paracervically where the nerve plexuses reside (Fig. 8.3). The clinician will encounter resistance to injection when administering

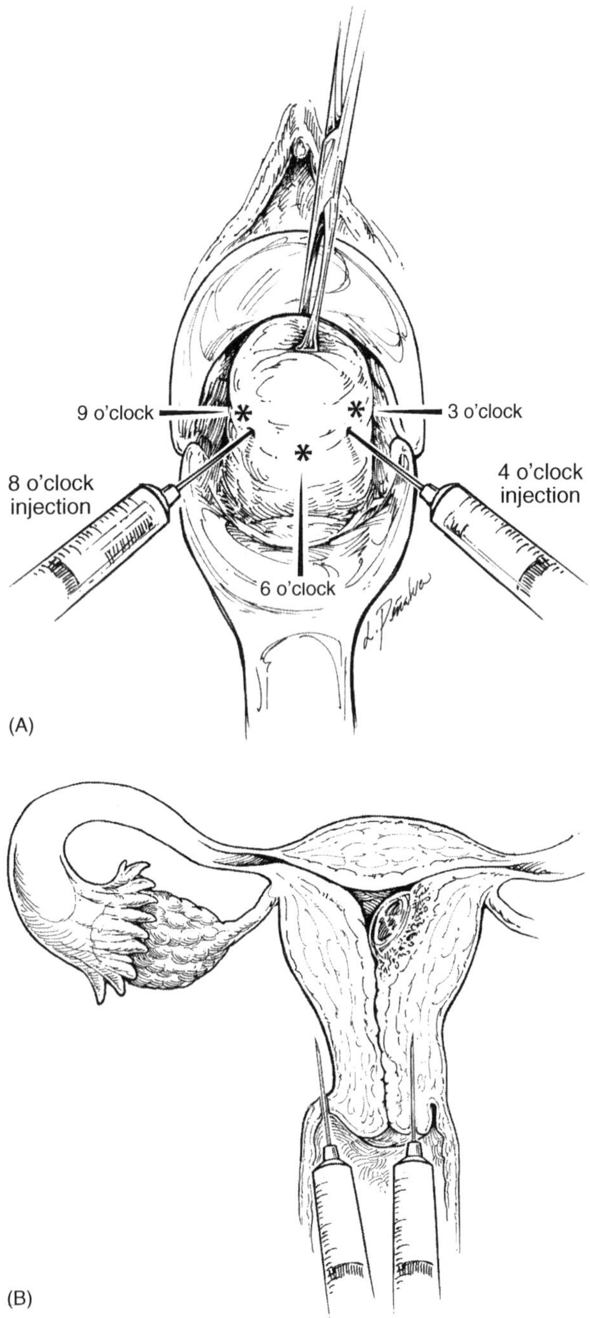

Figure 8.3 (A) Paracervical anesthesia injection at 4 o'clock and 8 o'clock positions, 1 cm under mucosa where vagina reflects off cervix. (Adapted with permission from Mann WJ, Stovall TG. eds. Gynecologic Surgery. Churchill Livingstone (Elsevier), New York, 1996, **799**). (B) Depiction of paracervical (left) and intracervical (right) deep injections.

anesthetic directly into the cervix and little or no resistance when injecting into the tissue lateral to the cervix.

The number and depth of injections also vary among providers. The most common paracervical anesthesia technique used by North American providers is a 4-point injection (2 o'clock, 4 o'clock, 8 o'clock, and 10 o'clock) to a depth of less than 3 cm using a maximum of 20 ml of total anesthetic volume (O'Connell K, unpublished observations, 2002). Techniques employing deeper injections appear to be more effective in reducing pain than superficial injections (Fig. 8.3). One study using 20 ml of 1% lidocaine at four paracervical locations demonstrated greater pain reduction with 3 cm deep injections compared to more superficial (1.5 cm) injections. The respective mean pain scores (on an 11-point scale) for the deep and superficial injections were 3.3 versus 4.0 during dilation and 3.0 versus 3.9 during aspiration [25]. Another randomized trial comparing 1% chloroprocaine injected superficially at 3 o'clock, 5 o'clock, 7 o'clock, and 9 o'clock (5 ml, 2 ml, 2 ml, and 5 ml, respectively) with injections at 4 o'clock and 8 o'clock (7 ml and 7 ml) found no difference between groups in pain following aspiration. The study was powered to detect a difference of 2.0 on an 11-point scale [26]. One study assumed patients would have less pain during cervical dilation on the side of the cervix where more anesthetic solution (6 ml vs. 2 ml) was injected [27]. The authors did not report the depth of injection, but did state that the injections were placed in the cervicovaginal junction. The majority of patients could not indicate which side was more painful, suggesting that cervical collateral circulation is abundant during pregnancy.

A recent small, randomized study ($n = 134$) investigated whether paracervical anesthesia had any appreciable effect during first-trimester vacuum abortion when patients also received IV conscious sedation and preoperative cervical priming with misoprostol. The investigators compared injecting or not injecting 5 ml of 1% lidocaine (total dose, 50 mg). The study groups, whose mean body weight was 51 kg (≈ 115 lbs), did not differ in patient-reported pain during cervical dilation or uterine aspiration [28].

Alternative techniques

Alternatives to paracervical injection of anesthetics have been investigated in several randomized trials. Application of lignocaine (lidocaine) gel to the cervix 1 minute before dilation resulted in pain reduction at the end of the suction procedure, but not during cervical dilation. The pain reduction occurred only among parous women. Both populations in this study had received 400 μg of vaginal misoprostol prior to the procedure [29]. Because of the effectiveness of intrauterine infusion of lidocaine for endometrial biopsies and hysteroscopies, some investigators have evaluated this approach for first-trimester abortion. A small ($n = 80$) randomized, blinded clinical trial found a mean reduction in pain scores with both cervical dilation ($p < 0.01$) and uterine suctioning ($p < 0.01$) when 5 ml of 4% lidocaine were infused transcervically immediately prior to vacuum abortion [30]. However no significant differences were found in a similar study design ($n = 80$) by the same investigators when patients received 10 ml of infused 1% lidocaine or an equal volume of infused saline in the same setting [12].

Taken together, these studies might suggest that a dose of at least 200 mg is needed for significant analgesic effect when a procaine-analog agent is infused. Infusion may be particularly useful for patients with an extreme aversion to receiving injections.

Pre-Procedure Medications

Providers commonly offer preoperative medications to decrease pain during abortion. Although pre-procedure anxiety correlates with abortion-related pain [5], available studies using preoperative oral anxiolytics have not demonstrated a salutary effect on pain. One study found that 1.0 mg of lorazepam given orally approximately 1 hour prior to first-trimester vacuum abortion did not reduce procedure-related pain compared to paracervical anesthesia alone [31]. In a prospective observational trial, 330 women having first-trimester abortions with cervical anesthesia and preoperative ibuprofen self-selected (1) no additional medication (local-only group); (2) sublingual lorazepam, 0.5 mg or 1.0 mg adjusted for body weight and administered 20 minutes preoperatively; or (3) intravenous conscious sedation using fentanyl 50–125 μg plus midazolam 1–2 mg. After controlling for several factors including gestational age, preoperative anxiety, depression, expected pain, and volume of cervical anesthesia, the investigators found that IV sedation reduced mean pain scores by 0.86 (95% CI 0.25, 1.46) on an 11-point verbal pain scale. Pain scores for the lorazepam group and the local-only group did not differ significantly [32].

Several studies suggest that pretreatment with nonsteroidal antiinflammatory drugs (NSAIDs) reduces the pain of abortion procedures, although accumulated evidence is conflicting. One nonrandomized study found that 550 mg of naproxen sodium taken orally 1 to 2 hours before surgical abortion reduced peak pain scores of the abortion and the pain at 15 to 30 minutes postoperatively [33]. Preoperative treatment with IV baclofen given immediately before the procedure decreased pain compared to placebo in a double-blinded trial; a dose of 0.6 mg/kg was more effective than a dose of 0.3 mg/kg [34]. In contrast, ibuprofen 600 mg taken orally 1 hour before the abortion had no effect on intraoperative pain, but it did decrease postoperative pain [18]. Also, diclofenac sodium 50 mg taken orally 4 hours before the procedure did not reduce the pain of the abortion in a randomized and blinded study of a population that also received preoperative misoprostol to ripen the cervix. None of the patients received IV sedation or paracervical anesthesia [35].

A blinded randomized trial compared the oral nonnarcotic analgesic agents, tramadol and ibuprofen, in women having first-trimester vacuum abortions. After ingesting either 50 mg of tramadol or 800 mg of ibuprofen, all 158 enrollees received cervical anesthesia using 20 ml 1% lidocaine with epinephrine and the option of nitrous oxide inhalation. Mean pain scores on an 11-point verbal rating scale were identical immediately after aspiration and significantly favored ibuprofen at 30 minutes, suggesting it has more durable effect [36].

Cervical ripening to reduce abortion-related pain

Ripening of the cervix with prostaglandins, laminaria, or nitric oxide-releasing agents has been found to ease dilation. Whether cervical ripening reduces the pain of dilation is less certain. One nonrandomized study found no pain reduction with use of laminaria; however, only 10% of the population received laminaria [6]. Misoprostol lessened the pain of surgical abortion compared to placebo in one study [37], but not in another [38]. Misoprostol causes more preoperative abdominal pain or cramping compared to placebo [39]. The effect of nitric oxide-releasing agents (e.g., nitroglycerin or amyl nitrite) on procedure pain has not been studied.

Summary: Local Anesthesia

A large body of literature describes multiple techniques for administration of paracervical anesthesia. No clearly superior approach can be extracted from this information, leaving several options available to the provider. The best evidence suggests that more effective anesthesia is obtained with deep injections and pretreatment with NSAID medications. No benefit appears to derive from imposing any waiting time between administering the cervical anesthesia and beginning a vacuum abortion, as long as deep injections are used.

Intravenous sedation and general anesthesia for abortion

Definitions

Because the drugs used for IV sedation produce dose-dependent CNS depression, the American Society of Anesthesiologists (ASA) approved in 1999 (and amended in 2004) a widely accepted and comprehensive definition of anesthesia described in the *Continuum of Depth of Sedation* [40]. This continuum consists of four discrete categories of anesthesia (Table 8.3):

- minimal sedation;
- moderate/conscious sedation;
- deep sedation; and
- general anesthesia.

The distinction among these categories derives from the observation of four key clinical parameters (Table 8.3):

- patient responsiveness;
- airway status/intervention;
- presence or absence of spontaneous ventilation; and
- overall cardiovascular function.

Occasionally, given doses of medications may induce greater sedative effects than anticipated. In the interest of

Table 8.3 Continuum of depth of sedation. Definition of general anesthesia and levels of sedation. (Approved by American Society of Anesthesiologists House of Delegates on October 13, 1999, and amended on October 27, 2004) (From ASA [40].).

	Minimal Sedation Anxiolysis	Moderate Sedation Analgesia ("Conscious Sedation")	Deep Sedation Analgesia	General Anesthesia
Responsiveness	Normal response to verbal stimulation	Purposeful response to verbal or tactile stimulation	Purposeful response following repeated or painful stimulation	Unarousable even with painful stimulus
Airway	Unaffected	No intervention required	Intervention may be required	Intervention often required
Spontaneous Ventilation	Unaffected	Adequate	May be inadequate	Frequently inadequate
Cardiovascular Function	Unaffected	Usually maintained	Usually maintained	May be impaired

patient safety, the ASA recommends that anesthesia providers be appropriately trained to "rescue" or manage a patient who progresses one level of anesthesia deeper along the continuum than was planned or intended [41]. For example, a provider attending to a woman scheduled for conscious sedation should be capable of managing her care if the sedative effects unintentionally result in a state of deep sedation [42]. This consideration is critical when facility managers are making decisions about the anesthesia needs of their patient population and who can best provide them.

Expense

The expense of anesthesia services for abortion will vary depending on the type of anesthesia offered. The majority of first-trimester abortion providers in North America use paracervical anesthesia alone or with IV conscious sedation [1,43]. For this level of anesthesia care, the cost of medications, staff, and equipment can be minimal. The demand for effective yet more costly deeper sedation or GA varies according to community expectations or standards, gestational age limits of abortion facilities, clinician and patient preferences, the availability of qualified anesthesia providers, economic considerations, and commonly, a combination of these factors. In North America, larger facilities [1] and those offering second-trimester abortions [44] are more likely to offer deeper levels of sedation or GA.

Many factors contribute to the costs of deep sedation and GA services. Administration of these methods requires licensed airway managers (anesthesiologist(s), certified registered nurse anesthetist(s) [CRNA], or both). In addition to the added expense of having such highly trained professionals, a facility must budget for additional monitoring devices, medications, anesthesia delivery machines, and emergency equipment and supplies (see chapter Appendix). These services also require more extensive anesthesia-specific policies and procedures, as well as more highly trained personnel for the preoperative and recovery areas.

Benefits

Patient satisfaction is an important benefit of IV sedation for the abortion patient. Several studies have evaluated patient satisfaction with abortion procedures. In general, three measures comprise patient satisfaction perioperatively: pain, nausea and vomiting, and anxiety/recall of the experience. A sleeping patient avoids any memory of the physical discomfort of the procedure, as well as the environmental noise of surgical equipment and staff. In one study, women receiving paracervical anesthesia and conscious sedation for abortion had improved pain control and better overall satisfaction than those receiving only paracervical anesthesia [32]. In another study, women who had GA voiced fewer perioperative complaints than those who received paracervical anesthesia with conscious sedation [45]. In another setting, patients receiving GA also had less postoperative nausea and vomiting and a faster recovery time [46]. Women who receive IV sedation or GA for abortion generally require less postoperative analgesia in the recovery room. Resumption of daily activities and full recovery are hastened when pain is not a significant factor [8,47]. Overall, the addition of some form of IV sedation has been shown to improve patient satisfaction with the abortion experience [48].

Increasing evidence suggests that monitoring and treating pain effectively confer substantial physiological benefits to patients [8]. In addition, general anesthesia or IV sedation may improve operative conditions for the surgeon by facilitating muscle relaxation and visualization. This benefit is especially important in a teaching setting or when the provider anticipates difficulties because of patient anxiety, history of prior emotionally or physically traumatic experiences, uterine anomalies, obesity, or serious medical conditions.

Morbidity and mortality

According to the Centers for Disease Control and Prevention (CDC), the US case-fatality rate associated with reported legal induced abortion decreased remarkably in the 1970s and has remained at less than 1 death per 100,000 abortions since 1980 [49]. In 1972, the CDC recorded 24 deaths from all causes known to be associated with legal induced abortions (notably, infection, hemorrhage, embolism, and anesthesia complications). By 1990, this figure had fallen to nine deaths and has varied little since [49]. The most recent CDC tabulation of abortion-related deaths for the period 1988 to 1997, using voluntary reports by state health departments, medical examiners, review committees, and the media, found that anesthesia complications were responsible for 16% of deaths [10].

The leading cause of anesthesia-related abortion mortality in the early CDC surveillance data was hypoventilation and/or loss of airway resulting in hypoxia, implying inadequate perioperative patient monitoring [50,51]. Facilities can minimize the risk of these occurrences by developing policies and procedures that require surveillance appropriate to the type of anesthesia they provide. Since the late 1970s, advances in monitoring equipment have dramatically decreased anesthesia-related morbidity and mortality for all surgical procedures. According to the ASA, the chance of a healthy patient dying under anesthesia is now 1 in 200,000 cases.

Studies from a large Planned Parenthood affiliate illustrate the safety of deep sedation in modern settings using appropriately trained personnel. This affiliate introduced a fully equipped anesthesia service with modern monitoring equipment in 1979. Of the 170,000 women who had abortions at the affiliate from 1971 to 1987, approximately 51,000 received IV methohexital and the rest had local cervical anesthesia. A retrospective chart review of these cases revealed no deaths and comparable complication rates for local anesthesia and deep sedation [47]. The authors concluded that deep sedation is a safe alternative when administered with appropriate equipment to properly selected patients by well-trained personnel. More recently, researchers at this same Planned Parenthood affiliate reviewed the medical records of more than 61,000 consecutive abortion patients who received primarily propofol for deep sedation anesthesia without endotracheal intubation during the period 2001 to 2007. The cohort included more than 10,000 women who had D&E abortions up to 24 weeks' gestation. No patient developed pulmonary aspiration or required transfer to the hospital for airway or ventilatory compromise (Dean G., unpublished observations, 2007).

A study of over 54,000 first-trimester abortions performed in US hospitals and nonhospital facilities from 1971 through 1975 found comparable major surgical complication rates for local or general anesthesia [52]. However, a different spectrum of complications occurred with each type of anesthesia. Whereas general anesthesia was associated with higher rates of hemorrhage and uterine trauma, local anesthesia carried more febrile and convulsive morbidity. Another early study of second-trimester D&E abortions found a major complication rate of 0.72 per 100 abortions for general anesthesia and 0.32 per 100 abortions for local anesthesia [53]. Rates of uterine perforation and cervical trauma were not significantly different. General anesthesia carried higher risks of hemorrhage or sustained fever, but lower risks of retained products, excessive postoperative bleeding, and repeat curettage. The majority of anesthesia-related complications occurs with abortions after 8 weeks' gestation [10].

Patient preparation

The licensed airway manager should perform and document a targeted history and physical examination of the patient. Important consideration should be given to the past medical history and review of systems including:

- *Pulmonary*: In general, risk of hypoxia is higher in pregnancy because of a decrease in functional residual capacity and an increase in oxygen consumption. Patients with chronic or acute pulmonary conditions, including asthma or upper respiratory infection, may be especially vulnerable.
- *Airway*: Swelling of the oral and nasal airway occurs during pregnancy because of capillary engorgement. This factor can increase the risk of bleeding during airway manipulation while also making intubation difficult (if necessary electively or in an emergency).
- *Gastrointestinal*: Symptoms of heartburn may indicate reduced tone of the lower esophageal sphincter, posing added risk of reflux.
- *Cardiac*: Cardiac output and heart rate are increased during pregnancy. Patients with a history of cardiac conditions or complaints should be thoroughly evaluated prior to their procedure.

Other important features of the patient history include the following:

- Current medications, particularly those that may interact with the medications planned for sedation;
- History of smoking, alcohol, or illicit substance abuse: acute or chronic overuse of drugs or alcohol has implications for the type and amount of anesthesia as well as the overriding decision regarding whether to proceed at all (see Question #6 in the Challenging Clinical Scenarios);
- Previous experiences with sedation and anesthesia, including untoward events in the patient or family members. This line of questioning may elicit a history of malignant hyperthermia or prolonged mechanical ventilation following surgery (consistent with pseudocholinesterase deficiency), both very serious risk factors for the patient;
- Allergies to medications.
- NPO (*nil per os*, or nothing by mouth) status: To minimize the risk of aspiration, the ASA standards suggest that clear liquids (water, clear juice, black coffee) may be consumed up to 2 hours prior to surgery while at least 6 hours must pass after a meal [41]. Chewing gum,

lozenges, or breath mints stimulate gastric secretions; therefore, many anesthesiologists prefer to wait and treat these infractions as if they involved a clear liquid.

All available laboratory studies should be reviewed. Patients with a concerning history of diabetes may require blood glucose monitoring (via an on-site glucometer). Targeted physical examination includes auscultation of the heart and lungs as well as an evaluation of the airway and extremities.

After completion of the history and physical examination, patients are classified according to the ASA physical status classification as follows:

- ASA Class 1 – healthy;
- ASA Class 2 – mild systemic disease;
- ASA Class 3 – severe systemic disease that limits activity but is not incapacitating; and
- ASA Class 4 – severe systemic disease that is a constant threat to life.

In general, ASA 1 and 2 patients are good candidates for an outpatient abortion under deep sedation or GA. With appropriate personnel and monitoring, some if not most ASA 3 patients can undergo outpatient abortion under deep sedation or GA. ASA 4 patients are not appropriate candidates for an outpatient procedure using deep sedation or GA.

A retrospective chart review of over 1,500 consecutive women having first-trimester vacuum abortions at a Planned Parenthood affiliate for the period April 1 to December 31, 2006, examined outcomes of IV conscious sedation without NPO restrictions or routine use of an indwelling IV catheter. The maximum allowable dosages were 100 µg of fentanyl plus 2 mg of midazolam. Most patients received a 1-mg dose of midazolam and 100 µg of fentanyl via a single syringe and given by the surgeon. Oral ibuprofen 800 mg administered 30 minutes before the procedure and paracervical anesthesia with 20 ml of 0.25% bupivacaine rounded out the anesthetic. Complications were rare, mild, and treated without hospital transport [54].

Facility preparation

Anesthesia personnel

Licensed airway managers must have requisite skills including experience and training giving brief anesthetics, efficiency, diligence, personal rapport, and if applicable, comfort performing in an outpatient facility without other comparably trained colleagues on-site. In many US communities, the pool of licensed airway managers willing to provide outpatient abortion anesthesia is thin or nonexistent. An anesthesiologist assumes the full risk, responsibility, and liability for the care he or she provides. As of 2008, in 14 US states, a CRNA can practice independently and similarly assume responsibility and liability. In the other 36 states, the CRNA must be supervised or directed by a physician who shares in the risks, responsibility, and obligations of the anesthesia care.

Recovery/preoperative personnel

The recovery area for the postanesthesia patient requires qualified personnel with a specific skill set. A registered nurse (RN) with experience in this realm of care should monitor the acute recovery area. Unlicensed medical assistants and licensed practical or vocational nurses play an important role as physician- and RN-extenders in perioperative care. Regardless of licensure or training, personnel having contact with patients acutely recovering from consciousness-altering levels of anesthesia should be trained in basic life support.

Equipment

Prior to administering deep sedation or GA, the anesthesia provider should re-confirm the presence and adequacy of equipment and supplies in the procedure or operating room (OR) (see chapter Appendix). A common mnemonic can be used as a reminder before each case: ***POSE MD.***

Positive pressure ventilation. The OR must have either a bag-valve mask (Ambu bag) or an anesthesia machine/ventilator with an anesthesia circuit and mask.

Oxygen source. The OR must have a consistent and available source of oxygen. Clean nasal cannulas and nonrebreather masks should be readily available to administer oxygen.

Suction. A mechanism for active suctioning of the airway must be available.

Equipment. Readily available equipment should include airway devices (assorted sizes of working laryngoscope handles and blades, laryngeal mask airways, oral and nasal airways, and endotracheal tubes), Ambu bags and masks, and IV supplies (IV catheters, tubing).

Monitors and Machines. In facilities offering GA, anesthesia machines require regular maintenance by a certified technician. The OR should have individual or multiparameter monitors that record noninvasive blood pressure, electrocardiogram (ECG), and pulse oximetry. The anesthesia provider should document these parameters on an anesthesia record at intervals no less than every 5 minutes. Ideally, most of these parameters are monitored even when administering conscious sedation. End-tidal carbon dioxide detection, capnography, is a standard of care if a patient is intubated. Means of recording a patient's temperature should be easily obtainable.

Drugs. The OR should be stocked with appropriate medications (along with syringes and needles) to induce anesthesia, maintain anesthesia, and reverse the anesthetic agent (if an antidote exists). Muscle relaxants to facilitate intubation are kept in most ORs, as are their reversing agents. Additionally, medications should be available to manage changes in blood pressure and heart rate and to treat allergic reactions. Commonly, medications for treating pain, nausea, and vomiting are also supplied. A separate emergency cart must be at hand in case of cardiac arrest.

Medications

The ideal outpatient anesthetic has a rapid onset, a short duration of action, is easily modulated, eliminates pain, induces amnesia, and causes limited nausea and vomiting. Recovery space is often small, and many patients bypass the acute recovery area altogether. Thus, the chosen anesthetic should compress the induction time and the return to wakefulness to the fullest extent [55]. For IV conscious sedation, the combination of fentanyl and midazolam works very well. For deep sedation and GA, bolus IV methohexital or propofol meet these specifications with high patient satisfaction in an outpatient setting [56].

Medications used for conscious sedation

Fentanyl and midazolam are the most common medications used in combination for IV conscious sedation by North American members of the National Abortion Federation (O'Connell, K., unpublished observations, 2002).

Midazolam (Versed)

Midazolam (Versed) is a benzodiazepine. Benzodiazepines are sedatives and anxiolytics. They confer anterograde amnesia but do not diminish a patient's stored information (retrograde amnesia). In addition, they have minimal impact on the cardiovascular and pulmonary systems. Midazolam provides an optimum level of amnesia while leaving the patient responsive and coherent [57]. Importantly, benzodiazepines, including midazolam, can be reversed by an antagonist, flumazenil (Romazicon®). When administered in 0.2-mg increments intravenously over 30 seconds, flumazenil reverses benzodiazepines, arousing the patient from the hypnotic effects while often preserving the amnesia [58]. Flumazenil has a short half-life of action and re-sedation may recur if the patient received large doses of the agonist drug. The elimination half-life of midazolam is 1 to 4 minutes but may vary among pregnant women. Other benzodiazepines, such as diazepam or lorazepam, are longer-acting than midazolam and have the potential to delay discharge from the facility.

Fentanyl

Fentanyl is a narcotic. Narcotics provide potent analgesia and a mild euphoria. Narcotics produce significant respiratory depression that can occur quickly and is dose-related. They have little impact on the cardiovascular system even at higher doses. Fentanyl has a very rapid onset and short duration of action, but it is as much as 100 times more potent than morphine (the narcotic to which all others are compared). Narcotics can be reversed using the antagonist naloxone (Narcan®). Naloxone efficiently reverses fentanyl if titrated intravenously in 0.04-mg increments; the respiratory depression can be reversed without compromising the analgesic effect [59]. Naloxone's duration of action is about 30 minutes, so additional dosing may be necessary. High doses of naloxone can awaken a patient quickly and amplify pain as well as sympathetic nervous system responses. The elimination half-life of fentanyl is 185 to 219 minutes but may vary among pregnant women.

The combination of midazolam and fentanyl can be given IV push in the same syringe to produce safe and effective sedation [54]. The key to administering these medications is the concept of titration. No dose is ideal for every patient; the most common regimen used by North American members of the National Abortion Federation is 1 to 3 mg of midazolam and 50 to 100 μg of fentanyl (O'Connell, K., unpublished observations, 2002). Initial and cumulative doses can be increased safely in obese or anxious patients or during protracted cases.

Older narcotics, such as morphine or meperidine (Demerol), have distinct disadvantages compared to fentanyl. In the case of meperidine [60], the drawbacks include less potency, a longer elimination half-life, and occurrence of more nausea and vomiting. Morphine carries the potential for histamine-induced hypotension and peripheral vasodilation [61].

Ketamine

Ketamine, a phenylcyclidine derivative, is a powerful dissociative anesthetic. Induction doses can result in patients becoming cataleptic with eyes open and nystagmus present. In smaller doses, however, ketamine can be a potent analgesic and bronchodilator. These smaller doses, as an adjunct to other agents [62], can be useful in abortion care when a patient requires re-suctioning for retained tissue but is no longer NPO. The concomitant administration of anticholinergics and benzodiazepines is highly recommended to offset the undesirable side effects of ketamine that include increased airway secretions and the potential for emergence delirium. One desirable effect of ketamine is a decrease in airway resistance that results from stimulation of the sympathetic nervous system. This property makes ketamine a good choice for asthmatic patients [63].

Medications used for deep sedation and general anesthesia

In 2001, 21 and 36% of North American NAF member facilities provided at least 40% of their patients with deep sedation/GA during first- and second-trimester surgical abortions, respectively [1,44]. These deeper levels of anesthesia may require interventions to assure airway patency and cardiovascular stability. GA is sometimes described in terms of a progression through four stages from awake to fully anesthetized:

Stage 1: Amnesia (memory loss with continued perception of pain)

Stage 2: Delirium (irregular respirations, divergent gaze, dilated pupils, excitation)
Stage 3: Surgical anesthesia (constricted pupils, regular respirations, no response to painful stimuli)
Stage 4: Overdosage (shallow respirations, dilated pupils, hypotension)

Patients passing through stage 2 during induction or reemergence from anesthesia are at risk of airway compromise, including laryngospasm. Intubation or extubation should be avoided during this time.

Propofol (Diprivan®)

Propofol (Diprivan®) is the most common drug used by North American provider members of the National Abortion Federation for deep sedation and GA, as of 2001 (O'Connell, K., unpublished observations, 2002). It has the attractive qualities of rapid onset (unconsciousness in less than 30 seconds with induction dosing) and offset (awakening in 4 to 8 minutes after induction) with minimal residual side effects. In addition to these properties, propofol has been shown to decrease the frequency of postoperative nausea and vomiting compared to methohexital [56]. As with any total IV anesthetic, incremental dosing may be necessary to maintain the desired depth of anesthesia. Combining propofol with other medications, such as fentanyl, enhances analgesia during and after surgery but increases the potential for respiratory depression. The only major weakness of propofol is the lack of a specific reversal agent. For this reason, the manufacturer strictly limits the use of this drug to clinicians trained in the administration of GA. Propofol can be painful on injection (an effect moderated by aiding a procaine-analog agent during infusion), has the potential for degradation during storage, can lead to allergic reactions in some susceptible patients (depending on the manufacturer, those with egg allergy or sulfite allergy), and should be avoided in patients with known seizure disorders [64].

Other common agents that have been found to have less safety, less utility, or both, in the abortion setting include:

- Etomidate is expensive, can activate seizure foci, induce nausea and vomiting, and depress the adrenal cortex. It has greatest utility in unstable cardiac patients who are unlikely candidates for outpatient settings [65].
- Droperidol has a black box warning on the drug label for potentiating unwanted extrapyramidal side effects as well as hypotension [66].
- Methohexital (Brevital®), previously the most commonly used induction agent in abortion facilities, is no longer available in the USA, having been superseded by the superior performance and generic pricing of propofol.
- Potent halogenated inhalation agents (isoflurane, sevoflurane, desflurane) have a limited role in deep sedation and GA for abortion because of their uterine relaxation properties at all doses, particularly above 1% concentration. Uterine relaxation can result in rapid, clinically significant blood loss. In addition, along with succinylcholine, these potent agents are triggers for malignant hyperthermia (MH). MH is extremely rare but results in a life-threatening emergency.

Nitrous oxide

Nitrous oxide is not an MH trigger and is not a potent inhalation agent. Nitrous oxide is an inorganic gas with great utility because it dissipates very rapidly. It can be administered only by anesthesia providers or licensed professionals skilled in its use. Nitrous oxide must be used in combination with at least 30% oxygen to prevent hypoxia. An oxygen analyzer should be used to ensure an appropriate mixture of nitrous oxide and oxygen. When given by mask at dosages between 25 and 50%, nitrous oxide can provide analgesia and, importantly, has no uterine relaxant effects. Potent inhalation agents as well as nitrous oxide require a scavenging system to assure removal of waste gases from the facility, thereby limiting exposure of the staff to these agents.

Neuromuscular-blocking agents

Neuromuscular-blocking agents (NMBAs) are indicated if intubation is planned. Short procedures like abortions rarely require intubation, but it may be indicated in some cases. NMBAs should be administered only by appropriate anesthesia providers trained in the delivery of GA, because they cause paralysis of skeletal muscle including muscles of respiration. Once a patient receives NMBAs, the anesthesia provider must assume control of her airway and breathing.

Recovery and discharge

Following surgery, patients who received GA or deep IV sedation are observed in a recovery area or postanesthesia care unit (PACU) with established rules of operation and conduct. The physicians, CRNAs, and nurses that supervise the PACU share responsibility for admitting and releasing patients postoperatively.

PACU nurses will receive a patient and often assign a numerical value to her condition on entry, graded in much the same fashion as Apgar scores for newborns. Criteria include reflex activity, respiration, circulation, state of consciousness, and color. Pertinent vital signs, including pulse rate, blood pressure, respiratory rate, and oxygen saturation via pulse oximetry should be assessed at frequent intervals (at least every 15 minutes). For patients receiving GA or deep IV sedation, monitoring is continued until the patient is awake and has no need for supplemental oxygen. At no time should the recovery area be left unattended, no matter how alert patients may appear, because recovering from anesthesia may involve lapses in consciousness or sudden vomiting. Some patients require antiemetics and additional pain medication.

Various scoring systems (e.g., the Aldrete system) have been developed to assess discharge readiness, but only good judgment can ultimately determine when a patient should be discharged. Common objective criteria include that the patient is oriented and ambulatory with stable vital signs and minimal pain, nausea/vomiting, and bleeding [42]. The PACU chart becomes part of the permanent clinical record and provides a summary of the postoperative period. Personnel should document pertinent observations and physical findings and note all therapeutic measures in the order administered. When a patient has received IV sedation or GA, documenting that she has an escort and her mode of transportation is important. She also should be advised not to operate a motor vehicle or heavy equipment until the following day. All patients must receive instructions outlining the signs and symptoms of postoperative complications and emergency contact information [42].

Summary: IV Sedation and General Anesthesia

Safe administration of IV sedation and general anesthesia in the outpatient abortion setting requires appropriately trained personnel, adequate equipment and supplies, and established protocols for patient eligibility and routine and emergency care. Fentanyl (50-100 μg) and midazolam (1-3 mg) comprise the most common drug regimen for IV moderate ("conscious") sedation among US abortion providers. For deep sedation and general anesthesia, propofol permits rapid onset and awakening with minimal side effects, making it the currently favored agent in US abortion practice.

Nonpharmacological aspects of pain management

Optimum pain management enables the patient, in the short term, to cope with the pain associated with medical or surgical abortion and, ultimately, to integrate the abortion psychologically as a positive life experience. These goals can be achieved consistently when clinicians employ nonpharmacological strategies as adjuncts to effective sedative, analgesic, and anesthetic agents. Although nonpharmacological methods may seem most applicable to patients having abortions with local anesthesia or light sedation, they also assist the more deeply sedated patient in coping with the abortion experience and in managing any later pain.

Successful pain management strategies must fit the needs and abilities of the individual patient. This fit can be achieved only through collaboration between the abortion provider and the patient. The provider should make an initial assessment of the woman's motivation and potential coping skills, have experience with and flexibility in the use of a variety of pain management interventions, and remain open to feedback from the patient about their effectiveness.

Although formal training in counseling and the use of hypnotic techniques is helpful, any motivated staff member working in a setting committed to the success of nonpharmacological pain management can acquire adequate skills on the job. Abortion providers may feel reluctant to make this commitment because of perceived time and cost restraints. Once the skills are mastered, however, research indicates that relaxation and hypnotic techniques result in shorter procedure times [67,68] and less medication use [69], thus saving both time and money. In a small unblinded randomized trial ($n = 30$) examining the effects of preoperative hypnosis, patients undergoing first-trimester aspiration abortion received optional nitrous oxide supplementation in addition to cervical anesthesia using 12 ml of 0.5% lidocaine. Only 36% of hypnotized patients versus 87% of those not hypnotized requested nitrous oxide supplementation [70].

Preparation prior to the abortion

Most patients will benefit from actively participating in their own pain management. They will experience increased control over their own life situation and feel better equipped to face future challenges. In preparation for the abortion, the clinician and counselor can facilitate this process by: (1) affirming the patient's existing point of view whenever possible; (2) providing medical education in manageable doses; (3) avoiding the temptation to offer glib reassurances; (4) advising the patient that her fears are widely shared; and (5) helping the patient to distinguish between emotional pain and physical pain.

During the intake interview, the provider or counselor should explore with the patient her pain history and expectations of pain with this abortion, her existing ways of coping with pain, the source and intensity of any fears she may have about the abortion, and her sense of control of the present situation. These elements overlap and blend in the inner world of the patient's experience, and disentangling them unobtrusively is of benefit. This phase of the interview also reinforces the patient's positive expectations and coping skills.

Providing information in the context of the patient's own worries enhances the likelihood that the information will be heard. For example, if the patient expresses fear about pain during the procedure, the clinician might respond: "Most patients are worried about pain, and they are often surprised when it is easier then they had expected. As we proceed, let us know how you are feeling so that we can make adjustments. We want this to go well for you." Such statements blend compassion, medical fact, and positive suggestion. Explaining that fear intensifies pain and teaching a relaxation response that can diminish pain are far more effective than attempts to downplay a patient's anxieties. Exploring any negative feelings about having an abortion is important for successful pain management. Although the decision may be difficult, what most patients feel badly about is less the abortion per se than the life situation that makes abortion their best choice.

The general rule that guides all interventions is to accept and respect the patient's feelings, thoughts, and associations rather than trying to take them away. After carefully listening and empathizing, the clinician and counselor can help the patient distinguish any emotional pain that may underlie her decision to abort from the physical sensations of the abortion. Because the words "feel," "hurt," and "pain" apply to both emotions and sensations, the patient's use of these words provides opportunities to point out the difference. The physical sensations of the abortion and postprocedure period become far more manageable when they are separated from the whirl of emotions and fears that some patients bring to the abortion.

Selected techniques

The nonpharmacological pain management techniques discussed in this section are known to be effective in reducing pain associated with medical and surgical procedures [71,72]. Clinical applications of these methods are adapted to the provision of abortion services.

Positive suggestion

Positive suggestion is a simple method that involves providing information to the patient in ways that emphasize the positive meaning of routine medical events and presume effective coping [73]. Examples of positive suggestions that providers can use during and after surgical abortion are presented in Table 8.4.

Relaxation

The technique of relaxation is notably effective in reducing pain [67]. In addition, several investigators report that hypnotic induction of relaxation decreases the incidence of vasovagal events [67,74]. This technique can be explained to the patient as follows:

> "A natural reaction to pain, or even the fear of pain, is to tense our muscles. I'll teach you a way to let your muscles relax. Focus your attention on your pelvis and buttocks. Tighten those muscles...hold them tight. Now let them go loose. Feel the difference. Practice that several more times, paying special attention to just how limp your muscles can go when you let them. Whenever you feel strange sensations during the abortion, you will know that you can control those muscles. By letting them go very loose, you can help to make your abortion easier and safer, and it will actually go more quickly."

Another relaxation technique can be used as the patient is lying on the examining table waiting for the abortion to begin. The following script is an example:

> "Begin by letting your mind focus on my voice. Follow along with me, and you can become very...deeply... relaxed. Take one...or two...deep, slow breaths...and allow the relaxation to begin to flow...deeply, pleasantly...throughout your body. You might think about how it feels to be calm...to be peaceful...and completely at ease. Imagine that feeling...of tranquility...peacefulness...spreading deeply...throughout your entire body. At the same time let all of your muscles relax. Begin with your feet...and your legs...and let those muscles go loose and limp. Feel the relaxation flow into your thighs and hips...as all the tension flows out. Let your mind relax along with your body. Feeling calm...at ease...it feels so good to be relaxed and at ease. Everything is going just the way it should..."

Guided imagery

Guided imagery (visualizing sensory images) is an effective technique in a wide range of acute and chronic pain states [75]. Some studies have shown that guided imagery can decrease anxiety, analgesic requirements, and length of stay

Table 8.4 Examples of positive suggestions for use during and after surgical abortion.

Medical Event	Positive Suggestion
Administration of IV medication	I am giving you a powerful pain medicine to make you much more comfortable throughout your procedure. You may begin to notice its effect... as your body feels lighter and you feel more dreamlike. If you need to be any more comfortable later, you can just let me know.
Patient feels pain with cervical anesthesia	That is the medicine numbing your cervix. You may feel heat or cold, pressure or stinging for a moment. You may be surprised how quickly the sensation passes as the numbness spreads... making everything else we will be doing much easier for you.
Patient feels pain with mechanical dilation	That sensation is your cervix gently opening so that the pregnancy can be safely and easily removed... Yes, it is opening more... just as it should...
Sound of the vacuum aspirating machine/device	That sound means that your abortion is proceeding just as it should. Each time you hear that sound, you can know that we are closer and closer to completing your abortion.
Patient has cramping following evacuation	That cramping sensation means that your procedure is almost over.
Patient reports cramping postoperatively	That cramping sensation means that your uterus is shrinking back to its normal size. Your body is healthy... It is naturally doing just what it needs to do to prevent you from bleeding more than normal.

for surgical patients [76]. This technique is especially effective when used in conjunction with pharmacological agents. The patient's imagination is harnessed to focus attention on pleasant sensory experiences. Prior to the abortion, the patient is invited to describe a favorite place or activity. This exercise is then reenacted during the procedure by recalling the cues that prompted the original imagery, as the following example illustrates:

> "When you are ready, you can see yourself in the meadow. Look around and notice what you see... hear... feel... Reach out and touch the grass... or a flower. What color is it? And notice the path leading to the hill nearby. When you're ready, you can follow the path and begin climbing the hill... What is happening now? As you near the top of the hill, you'll see the house... What is it like? And you can open the door and go in... look around... What do you see? And you'll enter your favorite room... noticing your favorite things... What do you see? You can touch... and the smell... is so familiar... What is it?" And so forth.

Challenging clinical scenarios

In this section, challenging situations that may occur during abortion procedures are presented as "Frequently Asked Questions."

1. What should I do if my patient experiences circumoral numbness and ringing in her ears during or soon after an injection with a procaine-analog drug, such as lidocaine?

Local anesthetic toxicity can result from inadvertent intravascular injection, which raises blood levels of the drug. Injections in more vascular areas also result in higher uptake and the potential for toxicity. Initial symptoms of toxicity often include circumoral numbness, tinnitus, restlessness, and even blurred vision (Fig. 8.2). These symptoms can be frightening to some patients, but they usually resolve within a minute or two. No specific interventions are needed. Generally, informing patients that their symptoms will pass shortly suffices to reassure them. If the patient is not overly distressed, the abortion procedure can continue. Techniques to minimize the risk of intravascular injection of anesthetic agents include aspirating before injecting or, for deep injections, injecting the solution *while moving the needle* into or out of the paracervical tissue.

For plain lidocaine the maximum allowable dose is 3–5 mg/kg, although the drug label advises a 200-mg total dose limit over a 90-minute period for paracervical anesthesia during pregnancy [11]. Epinephrine-containing anesthetics permit somewhat higher doses because the vasoconstrictive effect of epinephrine decreases vascular uptake. The dosage is easy to calculate by using the following formula:

$$\text{Total dose (mg)} = \text{Concentration (mg/ml)} \times \text{Volume (ml)}$$

To convert per cent concentration to mg/ml, simply move the decimal point one place to the right, for example, 1% is 10 mg/ml, 0.5% is 5 mg/ml, and so forth. Using this formula, 20 ml of 1% lidocaine contains 200 mg of lidocaine (10 mg/ml × 20 ml).

2. What do I need to consider in selecting and administering a safe anesthetic for an obese patient?

Obesity is best defined using body mass index (BMI). A person with a BMI of 30 or greater is considered obese. Morbid obesity is defined as a BMI of 40 or greater. Almost one-half of US women of childbearing age are overweight (BMI between 25 and 30). The prevalence of overweight status continues to rise, particularly among children and teenagers [77].

Obese patients are at increased risk for many medical problems, several of which may impact their anesthesia care. Obstructive sleep apnea [78,79], diminished lung capacity, pulmonary hypertension, hypercholesterolemia, hypertension, ischemic heart disease, cardiomegaly, diabetes, hypothyroidism, hiatal hernia, and arthritis are all more prevalent in obese patients. Specific considerations in the care of obese patients include the following:

- *Dosing of medication:* The dose of medication appropriate for an obese patient varies because of several factors. Obese patients may have increased blood volume, which in turn decreases plasma concentration of a drug and can result in underdosing. Conversely, obese patients also have a large amount of adipose tissue that is poorly perfused; greater amounts of an administered medication may distribute to highly perfused tissues and result in overdosing. Initial dosing based on the patient's ideal body weight (rather than actual weight) is logical in order to observe the response, with subsequent administration of the medications gauged accordingly. Recovery from muscle relaxants can be prolonged in obese patients for unknown reasons.
- *Airway/Pulmonary:* Obese patients have excess adipose tissue throughout their body. When sedation or anesthesia is administered, excessive soft tissue around the airway can relax and result in airway obstruction and, eventually, in difficulty with ventilation or intubation. Decreased functional residual capacity in the obese patient leads to rapid drops in oxygenation during periods of hypoventilation or apnea. Therefore, maximizing oxygenation via mask or nasal oxygen prior to sedation is important. Higher ventilatory pressure and the prevalence of gastroesophageal reflux disease raise the risk of aspiration. Measures to minimize this risk include strict adherence to NPO guidelines and possibly prophylaxis with metoclopramide (Reglan) or a histamine (H_2) blocker preoperatively. Once a patient is extubated, airway obstruction may make ventilation difficult. Desaturation is likely to occur quickly in the face of hypoventilation, and aspiration remains a risk.

- *Cardiac:* A proper preoperative history and comprehensive review of systems, as well as a thorough cardiac physical examination, should reveal most problems. When taking blood pressures, appropriately sized cuffs are important.
- *Recovery:* In addition to heightened patient vigilance, a sitting position may improve the mechanics of ventilation and minimize hypoxemia. Supplemental oxygen is usual. Early ambulation, regardless of the duration of the surgical procedure, will improve oxygenation and decrease the risk of deep vein thrombosis.

3. What do I need to consider in selecting and administering safe pain control options for an asthmatic patient?

Asthma of any severity is present in 8% of the US population [80]; 25% of these patients wheeze after anesthetic induction, and 1.7% experience a severe respiratory outcome postoperatively. Patients with asthma who merit special concern during presurgical screening are those with: (1) symptoms requiring continuous antiinflammatory or steroid therapy; (2) frequent exacerbations or nocturnal dyspnea (more than one to two episodes per week); (3) a recent attack requiring medical therapy; or (4) acute symptoms on presentation. Therapeutic medications commonly used by asthmatics include beta-adrenergic agonists (e.g., albuterol), theophyllines, systemic or inhaled corticosteroids, and leukotriene antagonists (e.g., montelukast [Singulair®]).

When a patient with asthma calls for her appointment, instruct her to continue her current treatment regimen until the time of her procedure and to bring her medications with her to the clinic. Significant signs observed on-site, such as wheezing on auscultation, increased respiratory effort, use of accessory muscles, and complaints of dyspnea, may warrant delay of the abortion procedure. Patients with mild scattered wheezes on auscultation, or even those whose lungs are clear, may benefit from use of an inhaler before the abortion procedure (Chapter 7).

The commonly used sedatives midazolam and fentanyl usually reduce the risk of bronchospasm, most likely because of anxiolysis and slowed respiratory rate. If GA involving intubation is planned, precipitation of bronchospasm is an important consideration. Ketamine is a possible choice because it is a sympathomimetic and dilates bronchial smooth muscle. Side effects of ketamine (see previous section) may outweigh its benefits, but low adjunctive doses are usually well tolerated. Other anesthetic drugs such as halogenated gases (does not include nitrous oxide) are efficient bronchodilators but they decrease uterine tone, which can result in greater surgical blood loss.

4. My patient told me that she had an allergic reaction to the numbing medicine at the dentist's office. What should I do?

Allergic reactions to local anesthetics are estimated to account for less than 1% of problematic reactions to these agents. A good history can be extremely helpful in determining what to do for this patient. Often patients describe symptoms consistent with local anesthesia toxicity (see Question #1) rather than true allergy. A true allergic reaction is a histamine-mediated event. Signs of true allergy comprise a continuum that may include erythematous raised rash, bronchoconstriction (wheezing and dyspnea), hypotension, and laryngeal edema.

True allergic reactions occur more commonly with esters (e.g., 2-chloroprocaine, [Nesacaine®]; procaine [Novocaine®] Table 8.2). Ester local anesthetics that produce metabolites like para-amino benzoic acid (PABA) are more likely to evoke allergic reactions. PABA is also found in sunscreen, so patients allergic to sunscreen may not be candidates for ester local anesthetics. Amides (e.g., lidocaine [Xylocaine®], mepivacaine [Carbocaine®], bupivacaine [Marcaine®]) are not metabolized to PABA.

The classes of local anesthetics have no cross-sensitivity to true allergy. Therefore a patient allergic to an ester can receive an amide, and vice versa. Occasionally, a patient will be allergic to the preservative found in some local anesthetic preparations (e.g., the antioxidant sodium metabisulfite used with epinephrine-containing procaine-analog agents). Preservative-free local anesthetics are readily available. Other alternatives include use of bacteriostatic saline [16] or IV sedation.

5. My patient had an uncomplicated vacuum aspiration procedure at 8 weeks' gestation using deep sedation with propofol. She needs resuctioning for a large hematometra that she developed 30 minutes postop. She is in so much pain that she wants to go to sleep again, but she ate a saltine cracker and some apple juice in the recovery room. What are her options?

Because the patient ate a "meal" consisting of clear liquids and solid food, she no longer qualifies as NPO and is at some risk for aspiration of gastric contents. Medications such as nonparticulate antacids (sodium citrate [Bicitra®]), gastropropulsive agents (metoclopramide [Reglan®]), H_2 blockers (cimetidine [Tagamet®]), or proton pump inhibitors (omeprazole [Prilosec®]) will not resolve the patient's non-NPO status, although prior to induction the anesthetist may use one or more of these medications prophylactically to reduce the chance of vomiting and the acidity of gastric contents. If the patient's procedure cannot be delayed or the provider feels the case cannot wait, then the safest and best option is to reaspirate the uterine cavity using local anesthesia only or local anesthesia with conscious sedation.

6. My patient is addicted to heroin. Should I give her less fentanyl and midazolam for conscious sedation? Chronic abusers of illicit drugs and/or alcohol are often extremely anxious and fearful. They commonly distrust the medical system and thereby fail to reveal their substance abuse. They may even anticipate decreased tolerance of pain, often a self-fulfilling prophecy that may have a chemical basis. Moreover, they may be under the influence of drugs at the time of their visit, potentially prolonging or antagonizing the effect of anesthetic agents and altering their tolerance to medications.

Chronic use of narcotics stimulates hepatic cytochrome P-450 enzymes causing more rapid metabolism of medications and drugs. Chronic use also depletes endogenous endorphin reserves, thereby compromising the normal release of endorphins during painful stimuli. Because of these factors, these patients may need larger doses of IV narcotics than nonabusers to achieve similar levels of sedation. Acutely intoxicated patients (drugs or alcohol) should have their procedure postponed. However, sometimes the anesthesia provider may unwittingly encounter a patient already under the influence of a drug or a medication that may alter her state of consciousness. This situation warrants judicious administration of IV sedation, because these patients may require less medication to achieve the desired level of sedation.

Although standard protocols require patients to abstain from drugs for some time prior to the abortion, patients frequently are unable or unwilling to comply. A policy of nonjudgmental discussion of prescription and street drug use may result in more complete disclosure of the patient's drug abuse history, especially when framed in the context of avoiding risks, including the risk of death. This approach will help the abortion provider to individualize the types and doses of pain medications and anesthetics for these patients. Assessing the impaired patient's ability to give informed consent to the abortion is also critical (Chapter 5).

7. How do I treat a seizure that occurs during administration of anesthesia, surgery, or postoperatively?

Causes of seizures during administration of anesthesia, surgery, or postoperatively include a history of seizure disorder, systemic toxicity from intravascular injection of local anesthetics (Fig. 8.2), hypoxia or hypercarbia because of airway obstruction, or an acute CNS event. Patients with a history of seizures may exhibit them because of the physical and emotional stress of the surgery itself. Seizures resulting from hypoxia or hypercarbia may occur while administering deep sedation or GA or during recovery because of airway obstruction or hypoventilation. Seizures predicated on any of these circumstances may occur subsequent to or in the absence of earlier signs of CNS toxicity such as light-headedness, dizziness, visual blurring, metallic taste, and tinnitus. Other sedative or excitatory symptoms and signs may also occur such as disorientation, drowsiness, shivering, twitching, and tremors, both in the face and distal extremities.

Ideally patients known to be at high risk for seizure activity will have a primary practitioner or specialist who oversees their care. If a patient does not present with a clearance note, a simple call to her doctor may lend valuable information. Patients who are compliant with their antiseizure medications based on past history or current signs may require no special preoperative preparation. Noncompliance may warrant postponement of the procedure in order to evaluate and adjust the patient's medication as needed. Premedicating a patient with an antiepileptic agent may be appropriate in some cases. Common intravenous regimens include 100 mg of phenytoin (Dilantin®) or 5–10 mg of diazepam (Valium®) just prior to administration of anesthesia.

In the case of a seizure associated with cervical anesthesia, treatment is based on supporting the patient until the high CNS levels of the procaine-analog agent are reduced by distribution to other tissues. *In most cases, resolution occurs with simple supportive measures including protecting against head trauma and assuring an adequate airway.* However, respiratory depression, hypercarbia, and the ensuing combined acidosis associated with major motor seizure will exacerbate and prolong the seizure by lowering the seizure threshold and amplifying drug toxicity.

Distinguishing the normal twitching and tremors of an earlier excitatory stage from a partial motor seizure can prove challenging, so clinicians may want to consider ventilatory support any time a seizure seems imminent or questionable. Providing such support requires the availability of supplemental oxygen and, in some circumstances, positive pressure ventilation equipment including an Ambu bag or mechanical ventilator, such as an anesthesia machine.

Maneuvers of jaw lift, head extension with neck flexion (the sniffing position), or jaw thrust may be needed to keep the upper airway open and maintain air exchange. Inability to keep the airway open with appropriate support warrants use of an oral airway, nasal airway, or a laryngeal mask airway. The airway device should be removed as soon as the patient starts to object to it in the form of posturing or gagging. The onset of apnea requires positive pressure ventilation support. Use of the currently employed bag-valve mask device can require two persons to achieve adequate mask seal, upper airway support, and positive pressure simultaneously. Endotracheal intubation is rarely necessary if the appropriate intermediate steps are utilized. *Because endotracheal intubation requires prolonged paralysis and has potential complications even in experienced hands, continuing airway support (even if inadequate) until emergency assistance arrives may be the most appropriate course of action.* Case analysis of lawsuits that have been decided (closed case analysis) reveals that a stable nasal or oral airway plus ventilation, even if not fully adequate in restoring saturation to normal levels, is preferable to a difficult, prolonged endotracheal intubation [81].

Supporting the Airway, Breathing, and Circulation (ABC) is important. Drugs (D) may also be necessary if a true ongoing seizure is occurring. Benzodiazepines, such as midazolam (Versed®), are effective and frequently available in the outpatient abortion setting. Thiopental (Penthothal®)

or propofol also is useful but less widely available. Use of these agents will likely prolong the duration required for ventilatory support. Medications known to potentiate or induce seizures, including ketamine, etomidate, and meperidine (Demerol®), should be avoided.

Treatment can end when the patient assumes independent respiratory status and achieves a clear sensorium. Further neurological evaluation is not indicated based solely on the occurrence of a procaine analog-induced or other seizure in a patient with no prior history suggestive of a neurological disorder.

8. One of the providers in the facility elicits more pain during procedures than the other providers. What can staff do to support patients and the provider?

Pain management is an acquired skill like any other, and can be learned. The provider's supervisor can refer the provider to resources (such as this chapter) that describe the sources of pain associated with abortion provision and offer a variety of pain control techniques. Any practitioner is apt to do a better job with pain management when he or she recognizes the multifaceted nature of pain that can occur during induced and spontaneous abortion, does not feel blamed or criticized, and has the benefit of nurturing instruction. Relating to an understanding and patient colleague with strong pain management skills who can act as a model and mentor may be immensely salutary.

Reducing patients' anxiety is particularly important in this context, because anxiety is known to increase perception of pain. Support staff must remember that patients are naïve to the situation. Therefore, staff members can modulate the messages, both verbal and nonverbal, that they send patients about what to expect from the provider. They should emphasize the provider's strengths, whether it is low complication rates, speed of surgery, genuine commitment to women's reproductive rights, or a caring demeanor. A patient who is primed to respect and appreciate the provider will be more easily reassured that everything is going well despite any transitory painful sensations. Additionally, staff members typically know which part of the procedure is apt to be most painful with any given provider. They can talk the patient through that event using the nonpharmacological techniques illustrated in this chapter.

Conclusion

Pain management is a critical aspect of abortion care. Effective control of pain and anxiety confers substantial physiologic and psychological benefits and results in greater patient satisfaction. Safety and patient preference should direct the choice of anesthetic medications and techniques. Newer medications and advances in anesthetic techniques and monitoring allow providers to offer a range of safe pain management options from local anesthesia to IV sedation or GA. Nonpharmacological approaches serve as important adjuncts to pharmacological treatments. By attending to the psychosocial and affective factors that influence pain perception, providers can improve the overall quality of the abortion experience.

Appendix

Procedure or operating room setup requirements

The following equipment, supplies, and medications are required for anesthesia setup of a procedure or operating room at an abortion center providing general anesthesia.

1 Anesthesia gas machine, including ventilator with pipelined supply of oxygen and nitrous oxide meeting or exceeding ASA and state requirements
2 Vaporizers for anesthesia machine: sevoflurane and isoflurane
3 Vital sign monitor to monitor the following:
  Blood pressure
  Continuous EKG
  Oxygen saturation
  Gases
  End-tidal CO_2
4 Syringe infusion pump, time- and volume-controlled (optional)
5 Suction machine with minimum capacity of 25 cm H_2O
6 Nerve stimulator
7 Anesthesia cart
8 Laryngoscope set
  Handle, medium: two each
  Handle, stubby: one
  Blades MAC 1, 2, 3: one each
  Blades MILLER 2, 3: one each
9 Magill forceps and scissors
10 Laryngeal mask airway: sizes 3, 4, 5
11 Emergency cart (see chart)
12 Difficult airway cart (optional)
13 Malignant hyperthermia cart (only if using triggered agents)
14 Fluid warmer (optional)
15 Patient warmer (Bair Hugger) (optional)
16 Defibrillator (synchronization preferred)
17 IV stand
18 Double-door, double-lock narcotic cabinet meeting or exceeding US federal DEA (Drug Enforcement Agency) and state requirements
19 Patient monitor in recovery area to monitor blood pressure, continuous EKG, oxygen saturation
20 Suction apparatus for acute recovery area

Emergency cart contents and setup

Cart must be unlocked and checked at least once per week and after each use.

Drawer #1 Medication Tray	Qty
Albuterol inhaler	1
Cordarone	5
Adenosine 3 mg/ml	3
Aminophylline 25mg/ml	4
Atropine sulphate 1mg/syringe	4
Calcium chloride 10 ml	2
D50	1
Dopamine 400 mg	2
Dobutamine 250 mg/vial	2
Epinephrine 1 mg/syringe	4
Epinephrine ampules	4
Ephedrine ampules	4
Furosemide ampules	4
Phenytoin	4
Isuprel	2
Phenylephrine	4
2% lidocaine syringe	3
Magnesium sulfate	4
Lanoxin	2
Levophed	4
Procainamide	1
Sodium bicarbonate	4
Naloxone	4
Sodium nitroprusside	1
Drawer #2	
Suction catheter	3
Yankauer suction tips	3
Electrodes EKG	
Laryngoscope handle	1
Assorted blades	1
Scissor	1
Endotracheal tube (ETT) 7.5	1
Endotracheal tube (ETT) 8.0	1
Endotracheal tube (ETT) 8.5	1
Adult oral airway	3
Drawer #3	
18G needles	5
IV catheter 20G/18G	3
IV catheter 16G	3
IV catheter 14G	3
Silk tape	1
Pink tape	1
Alcohol wipes	
Ethilon suture	1
16G central venous catheter	1
Syringes all sizes	5
Mini drip set	2
Drawer #4	
1000cc NS	2
500cc D_5W	2
100cc D_5W	2
Loose IV labels	10
Drawer #5	
Box gloves	
Betadine solution	
Sterile gloves	
4 × 4 gauze sponges	
Tracheostomy set	
Adult oxygen mask	

Estimated costs of equipment for procedure or operating room setup (US dollars, 2008)

Monitor	$4,000–$5,000
Defibrillator	$1,000–$1,500
O_2 concentrator	$800
Oxygen tank	$200
Tank holder	$35
Suction machine	$275
Cart	$180
Banyan kit	$550
Anesthesia machine and all required components (if necessary)	$7,000 and up

References

1 O'Connell K, Jones HE, Simon M, Saporta V, Paul M, Lichtenberg ES. First-trimester abortion practices: a survey of National Abortion Federation members. *Contraception*, in press.

2 Smith GM, Stubblefield PG, Chirchirillo L, McCarthy MJ. Pain of first-trimester abortion: its quantification and relations with other variables. *Am J Obstet Gynecol* 1979; **133**: 489–498.

3 Henry J. Kaiser Family Foundation, The Picker Institute. *From the Patient's Perspective: Quality of Abortion Care.* Kaiser Family Foundation and The Picker Institute, Menlo Park, CA, 1999.

4 Stubblefield PG. Control of pain for women undergoing abortion. *Suppl Int J Gynecol Obstet* 1989; **3**: 131–140.

5 Pud D, Amit A. Anxiety as a predictor of pain magnitude following termination of first-trimester pregnancy. *Pain Med* 2005; **6**: 143–148.

6 Borgatta L, Nickinovich D. Pain during early abortion. *J Reprod Med* 1997; **42**: 287–293.

7 Melzack R. Toward a new concept of pain. In: Waldman SD & Winnie AP, eds. *Interventional Pain Management.* W.B. Saunders Company, Philadelphia, 1996: 1–9.

8 Wiklund RA, Rosenbaum SH. Anesthesiology. Second of two parts. *N Engl J Med* 1997; **337**: 1215–1219.

9 Bonica JJ. *Principles and Practice of Obstetric Analgesia and Anesthesia*. FA Davis, Philadelphia, 1967, 476.

10 Bartlett LA, Berg CJ, Shulman HB et al. Risk factors for legal induced abortion-related mortality in the United States. *Obstet Gyencol* 2004; **103**: 729–737.

11 *Physician's Desk Reference*, 62nd edn. Medical Economics, Montvale, 2008.

12 Edelman A, Nichols MD, Leclair C, Astley S, Shy K, Jensen JT. Intrauterine lidocaine infusion for pain management in first-trimester abortions. *Obstet Gynecol* 2004; **103**: 1267–1272.

13 Blanco LJ, Reid PR, King TM. Plasma lidocaine levels following paracervical infiltration for aspiration abortion. *Obstet Gyencol* 1982; **60**: 506–508.

14 Grimes DA, Cates W Jr. Deaths from paracervical anesthesia used for first-trimester abortion, 1972–1975. *N Engl J Med* 1976; **295**: 1397–1399.

15 Carpenter RL, Mackey DC. Local anesthetics. In: Barash PG, Cullen BF, & Stoelting RK, eds. *Clinical Anesthesia*, 3rd edn. Lippincott-Raven, Philadephia, 1997.

16 Miller L, Jensen MP, Stenchever MA. A double-blind randomized comparison of lidocaine and saline for cervical anesthesia. *Obstet Gynecol* 1996; **87**: 600–604.

17 Grekin RC, Auletta MJ. Local anesthesia in dermatologic surgery. *J Am Acad Dermatol* 1988; **19**: 599–614.

18 Wiebe ER, Rawling M. Pain control in abortion. *Int J Gynaecol Obstet* 1995; **50**: 41–46.

19 Wiebe ER, Rawling M, Janssen P. Comparison of 0.5% and 1.0% lidocaine for abortions. *Int J Gynaecol Obstet* 1996; **55**: 71–72.

20 Phair N, Jensen JT, Nichols MD. Paracervical block and elective abortion: the effect on pain of waiting between injection and procedure. *Am J Obstet Gynecol* 2002; **186**: 1304–1307.

21 Glick E. *Surgical Abortion*. West-End Women's Medical Group, Reno, NV, 1998.

22 Schulz KF, Grimes DA, Christensen DD. Vasopressin reduces blood loss from second-trimester dilatation and evacuation abortion. *Lancet* 1985; **2**: 353–356.

23 Phillips DR, Nathanson HG, Milim SJ, Haselkorn JS. The effect of dilute vasopressin solution on the force needed for cervical dilatation: a randomized controlled trial. *Obstet Gynecol* 1997; **89**: 507–511.

24 Wiebe ER, Trouton KJ, Savoy E. Intra-cervical versus IV fentanyl for abortion. *Hum Reprod* 2005; **20**: 2025–2028.

25 Cetin A, Cetin M. Effect of deep injections of local anesthetics and basal dilatation of cervix in management of pain during legal abortions. A randomized, controlled study. *Contraception* 1997; **56**: 85–87.

26 Glantz JC, Shomento S. Comparison of paracervical block techniques during first-trimester pregnancy termination. *Int J Gynaecol Obstet* 2001; **72**: 171–178.

27 Grossman RA. Women cannot discriminate between different paracervical block techniques applied to opposite sides of the cervix. *Am J Obstet Gynecol* 1995; **173**: 935–936.

28 Kan AS, Ng EH, Ho PC. The role and comparison of two techniques of paracervical block for pain relief during suction evacuation for first-trimester pregnancy termination. *Contraception* 2004; **70**: 159–163.

29 Li HW, Wong CY, Lo SS, Fan SY. Effect of local lignocaine gel application for pain relief during suction termination of first-trimester pregnancy: a randomized controlled trial. *Hum Reprod* 2006; **21**: 1461–1466.

30 Edelman A, Nichols MD, Leclair C, Jensen JT. Four percent intrauterine lidocaine infusion for pain management in first-trimester abortions. *Obstet Gynecol* 2006; **107**: 269–275.

31 Wiebe E, Podhradsky L, Dijak V. The effect of lorazepam on pain and anxiety in abortion. *Contraception* 2003; **67**: 219–221.

32 Allen RH, Kumar D, Fitzmaurice G, Lillford KL, Goldberg AB. Pain management of first-trimester surgical abortion: effects of selection of local anesthesia with and without lorazepam or intravenous sedation. *Contraception* 2006; **74**: 407–413.

33 Suprapto K, Reed S. Naproxen sodium for pain relief in first-trimester abortion. *Am J Obstet Gynecol* 1984; **150**: 1000–1001.

34 Corli O, Roma G, Bacchini M et al. Double-blind placebo-controlled trial of baclofen, alone and in combination, in patients undergoing voluntary abortion. *Clin Ther* 1984; **6**: 800–807.

35 Li CF, Wong CY, Chan CP, Ho PC. A study of co-treatment of nonsteroidal anti-inflammatory drugs (NSAIDs) with misoprostol for cervical priming before suction termination of first-trimester pregnancy. *Contraception* 2003; **67**:101–105.

36 Romero I, Turok D, Gilliam M. A randomized trial of tramadol versus ibuprofen as an adjunct to pain control during vacuum aspiration abortion. *Contraception* 2008; **77**: 56–59.

37 Saxena P, Salhan S, Sarda N. Sublingual versus vaginal route of misoprostol for cervical ripening prior to surgical termination of first-trimester abortions. *Eur J Obstet Gynecol Reprod Biol* 2006; **125**: 109–113.

38 Okanlomo KA, Ngotho D, Moodey J. Effect of misoprostol for cervical ripening prior to pregnancy interruption before twelve weeks of gestation. *East Afr Med J* 1999; **76**: 552–555.

39 Li CF, Chan CW, Ho PC. A comparison of isosorbide mononitrate and misoprostol cervical ripening before suction evacuation. *Obstet Gyencol* 2003; **102**: 538–583.

40 American Society of Anesthesiologists. Continuum of depth of sedation: definition of general anesthesia and levels of sedation/analgesia [Online]. Washington, DC: American Society of Anesthesiologists; 2004 [cited 2008 Aug 19]. Available from: URL:http://www.asahq.org/publicationsAndServices/standards/20.pdf

41 American Society of Anesthesiologists. Standards for basic anesthetic monitoring [Online]. Washington, DC: American Society of Anesthesiologists; 2005 [cited 2008 Aug 19]. Available from:

URL:http://www.asahq.org/publicationsAndServices/standards/02.pdf

42 National Abortion Federation [Online]. Washington, DC: National Abortion Federation; 2008. Clinical policy guidelines; 2008 [cited 2008 Aug 19]. Available from: URL:http://www.prochoice.org/pubs_research/publications/downloads/professional_education/CPG2008.pdf

43 Grimes DA, Creinin MD. Induced abortion: an overview for internists. *Ann Intern Med* 2004; **140**: 620–626.

44 O'Connell K, Jones HE, Lichtenberg ES, Paul M. Second-trimester surgical abortion practices: a survey of National Abortion Federation members. *Contraception*, 2008; **78**: 492–499.

45 Raeder JC. Propofol anaesthesia versus paracervical blockade with alfentanil and midazolam sedation for outpatient abortion. *Acta Anaesthesiol Scand* 1992; **36**: 31–37.

46 Tablov V, Tsafarov M, Tablov B, Popov I, Partenov P. Diprivan versus midazolam in combined anaesthesia with ketamine for minor gynecological surgery. *Akush Ginekol (Sofia)* 2007; **46**: 41–43.

47 Hakim-Elahi E, Tovell HM, Burnhill MS. Complications of first-trimester abortion: a report of 170,000 cases. *Obstet Gynecol* 1990; **76**: 129–135.

48 Keder LM. Best practices in surgical abortion. *Am J Obstet Gynecol* 2003; **189**: 418–422.

49 Strauss LT, Gamble SB, Parker WY, Cook DA, Zane SB, Hamdan S. Abortion Surveillance-United States, 2004. *MMWR Surveill Summ* 2007; **56**: 1–33.

50 Peterson HB, Grimes DA, Cates W Jr, Rubin GL. Comparative risk of death from induced abortion at less than or equal to 12 weeks' gestation performed with local versus general anesthesia. *Am J Obstet Gynecol* 1981; **141**: 738–763.

51 Atrash HK, Cheek TG, Hogue CJ. Legal abortion mortality and general anesthesia. *Am J Obstet Gynecol* 1988; **158**: 420–424.

52 Grimes DA, Schulz KF, Cates W Jr, Tyler CW Jr. Local versus general anesthesia: which is safer for performing suction curettage abortions? *Am J Obstet Gynecol* 1979; **135**: 1030–1035.

53 MacKay HT, Schulz KF, Grimes DA. Safety of local versus general anesthesia for second-trimester dilatation and evacuation abortion. *Obstet Gynecol* 1985; **66**: 661–665.

54 Wilson L, Chen BA, Creinin MD. Low-dose fentanyl and midazolam in outpatient surgical abortion up to 18 weeks of gestation. Contraception, in press.

55 Apfelbaum JL, Grasela TH, Walawander CA. Bypassing the PACU–a new paradigm in ambulatory surgery. *Anesthesiology* 1997; **87**: A32.

56 Lichtenberg ES, Hill LJ, Howe M, Heber W, Peipert JF. A randomized comparison of propofol and methohexital as general anesthetics for vacuum abortion. *Contraception* 2003; **68**: 211–217.

57 Reves JG. Valium–Fentanyl interaction. In: Reves JG & Hall KD, eds. *Common Problems in Cardiac Anesthesia*. Year Book Medical Publishers, Chicago, 1987: 357.

58 Brogden RN, Goa KL. Flumazenil. A reappraisal of its pharmacological properties and therapeutic efficacy as a benzodiazepine antagonist. *Drugs* 1991; **42**: 1061–1089.

59 Bailey PL, Clark NJ, Pace NL et al. Antagonism of postoperative opioid-induced respiratory depression: nalbuphine versus naloxone. *Anesth Analg* 1987; **66**: 1109–1114.

60 Estafanous FG, ed. *Opioids in Anesthesia*. Butterworth, Boston, 1984, 38.

61 Rosow CE, Moss J, Philbin DM, Savarese JJ. Histamine release during morphine and fentanyl anesthesia. *Anesthesiology* 1982; **56**: 93–96.

62 Friedberg BL. Propofol-ketamine technique. *Aesthetic Plast Surg* 1993; **17**: 297–300.

63 Stoelting RK, Miller RD. *Basics of Anesthesia*, 5th edn. Churchill Livingstone (Elsevier), Philadelphia, 2007.

64 Finley GA, MacManus B, Sampson SE, Fernandez CV, Retallick R. Delayed seizures following sedation with propofol. *Can J Anaesth* 1993; **40**: 863–865.

65 Famewo CE, Odugbesan CO. Further experience with etomidate. *Can Anaesth Soc J* 1978; **25**: 130–132.

66 Wooltorton E. Droperidol: cardiovascular toxicity and deaths. *CMAJ* 2002; **166**: 932.

67 Lang EV, Benotsch EG, Fick LJ et al. Adjunctive nonpharmacological analgesia for invasive medical procedures: a randomised trial. *Lancet* 2000; **355**: 1486–1490.

68 Schupp CJ, Berbaum K, Berbaum M, Lang EV. Pain and anxiety during interventional radiologic procedures: effect of patients' state of anxiety at baseline and modulation by nonpharmacologic analgesia adjuncts. *J Vasc Interv Radiol* 2005; **16**: 1585–1592.

69 Faymonville ME, Mambourg PH, Joris J et al. Psychological approaches during conscious sedation. Hypnosis versus stress reducing strategies: a prospective randomized study. *Pain* 1997; **73**: 361–367.

70 Marc I, Rainville P, Verreault R, Vaillancourt L, Masse B, Dodin S. The use of hypnosis to improve pain management during voluntary interruption of pregnancy: an open randomized preliminary study. *Contraception* 2007; **75**: 52–58.

71 Mobily PR, Herr KA, Kelley LS. Cognitive-behavioral techniques to reduce pain: a validation study. *Int J Nurs Stud* 1993; **30**: 537–548.

72 Rowbotham MC. Chronic pain: from theory to practical management. *Neurology* 1995; **45**: S5–S10; discussion S35–S36.

73 Bejenke CJ. Painful medical procedures. In: Barber J, ed. *Hypnosis and Suggestion in the Treatment of Pain: A Clinical Guide*. W.W. Norton, New York, 1996: 209–266.

74 Elkins G, White J, Patel P, Marcus J, Perfect MM, Montgomery GH. Hypnosis to manage anxiety and pain associated with colonoscopy for colorectal cancer screening: case studies and possible benefits. *Int J Clin Exp Hypn* 2006; **54**: 416–431.

75 Syrjala KL, Donaldson GW, Davis MW, Kippes ME, Carr JE. Relaxation and imagery and cognitive-behavioral training reduce pain during cancer treatment: a controlled clinical trial. *Pain* 1995; **63**: 189–198.

76 Tusek DL, Church JM, Strong SA, Grass JA, Fazio VW. Guided imagery: a significant advance in the care of patients undergoing elective colorectal surgery. *Dis Colon Rectum* 1997; **40**: 172–178.

77 Centers for Disease Control and Prevention [Online]. Atlanta: Center for Disease Control and Prevention. US obesity trends 1985–2007; 2008 [cited 2008 Aug 19]. Available from: URL:http://www.cdc.gov/nccdphp/dnpa/obesity/trend/maps/

78 Strollo PJ Jr, Rogers RM. Obstructive sleep apnea. *N Engl J Med* 1996; **334**: 99–104.

79 American Society of Anesthesiologists Task Force on Perioperative Management of Patients with Obstructive Sleep Apnea. Practice guidelines for the perioperative management of patients with obstructive sleep apnea. *Anesthesiology* 2006; **104**: 1081–1093.

80 Akinbami L. Asthma prevalence, health care use, and mortality: United States, 2003–2005 [Online]. Washington, DC: Centers for Disease Control and Prevention; 2006 Nov. [cited 2008 Aug 19]. Available from: URL:http://www.cdc.gov/nchs/products/pubs/pubd/hestats/asthma03-05/asthma03-05.htm

81 Bhananker SM, Posner KL, Cheney FW, Caplan RA, Lee LA. Injury and liability associated with monitored anesthesia care: a closed claims analysis. *Anesthesiology* 2006; **104**: 228–234.

CHAPTER 9

Medical abortion in early pregnancy

Mitchell D. Creinin MD, and Kristina Gemzell Danielsson MD, PhD

LEARNING POINTS

- The standard or classic regimen of mifepristone 600 mg followed 36 to 48 hours later by a prostaglandin analog, typically misoprostol 400 μg orally, is highly effective for abortion up to 49 days' gestation.
- Mifepristone can be used at a dose of 200 mg, instead of 600 mg, with equal efficacy and lower cost.
- When the misoprostol is used vaginally, the gestational age limit can be extended to 63 days and the medications can be administered as little as 6 to 8 hours apart or even simultaneously.
- Buccal and sublingual misoprostol also are effective when used at 24- to 48-hour intervals after mifepristone. These alternative routes appear to have more side effects than vaginal administration.
- Ultrasound examination 1 week after administering the medications is highly predictive of long-term success of the medical abortion procedure.
- Methotrexate and misoprostol can be used as an alternative regimen in women up to 49 days' gestation. The methotrexate does not appear to have immediate effect in the abortion process; rather, by rendering the pregnancy nonviable, methotrexate may serve as a backup for women who do not abort shortly after misoprostol administration.
- Misoprostol alone, in repeated doses, can be used for abortion where mifepristone is too expensive or unavailable. The recommended regimen for pregnancies up to 63 days' gestation is 800 μg administered vaginally every 3 to 24 hours for a maximum of three doses.

Introduction

The phrase *medical abortion* commonly refers to use of medications up to 63 days' gestation to effect abortion, although some regimens are effective beyond 63 days. Medical abortion allows a woman to have a safe, effective abortion without a surgical procedure. Since the early 1990s, millions of women in Europe, China, and North America have used mifepristone in combination with a prostaglandin analog for early abortion. However, in many regions of the world mifepristone is not available, prompting use of alternative regimens, including methotrexate in combination with misoprostol and misoprostol alone. This chapter reviews accumulated research on these medical methods of abortion and presents guidelines for their use in clinical practice.

Management of Unintended and Abnormal Pregnancy, 1st edition. By M Paul, ES Lichtenberg, L Borgatta, DA Grimes, PG Stubblefield, MD Creinin

History of medical abortion

Early agents

Although using medications to induce abortion dates back centuries, effective medical regimens have emerged only in the last 50 years. In the early 1950s, Thiersch and colleagues [1] experimented with the folic acid antagonist, 4-aminopteroylglutamic acid (aminopterin) in mice, rats, and humans. Aminopterin was noted to induce embryonic demise and resorption in mice and rats during the first week of gestation. Oral aminopterin was then used to induce medically indicated abortions in women less than 3 months' gestation. Ten of 12 women aborted.

In the 1970s, natural prostaglandins such as PGE_2 and $PGF_{2\alpha}$ were found to induce early abortion effectively [2,3]. However, regimens that resulted in high efficacy also caused intolerable side effects, including nausea, vomiting, diarrhea, fever, and pain. Prostaglandin analogs developed in the mid-1970s acted more selectively on the myometrium, allowing use of lower doses to effect abortion, but their instability limited long-term use. By 1980, more stable analogs proved efficacious, including the vaginal suppository, gemeprost (16, 16-dimethyl-*trans*-Δ^2-PGE_1 methyl ester) [4–6], and the injectable analog, sulprostone (16-phenoxy-tetranor PGE_2

sulfonylamide) [7]. Gastrointestinal side effects were less severe with the analogs than with natural prostaglandins, but they still occurred commonly, thus limiting their clinical utility [4,8].

Modern era of medical abortion: Mifepristone

While investigating compounds that would block glucocorticoid receptors, a research team led by Dr. Etienne-Emile Baulieu recognized that some compounds also bound strongly to the similarly shaped progesterone receptor and blocked the action of progesterone. Further refinement led to the production of mifepristone, and clinical testing began in 1982. Initially, clinical investigators administered mifepristone alone for early abortion. For gestations up to 49 days, complete abortion occurred in approximately 60 to 80%, incomplete abortion in 6 to 30%, and continuing pregnancies in 7 to 40% [9–12]. Outcomes were not improved by varying the dose from 50 to 400 mg daily or by using single or divided doses over multiple days. At best, 80% of women treated with mifepristone alone in early pregnancy completely aborted within a few days. Adding small doses of a prostaglandin analog increased the complete abortion rate to almost 100% [10,13].

In 1988, France and China licensed mifepristone in combination with a prostaglandin analog for abortion up to 49 days' gestation. Subsequently, the United Kingdom and Sweden approved mifepristone for use up to 63 days' gestation. Beginning in late 1998 many other European countries approved mifepristone for sale and use, followed in 2001 by the USA.

Since the introduction of mifepristone in combination with a prostaglandin analog for medical abortion, research has continued with the goals of finding cost-effective regimens that maximize access and acceptability. Initial regimens used a single 600-mg oral dose of mifepristone followed by a prostaglandin analog. This dose of mifepristone is still used in many parts of the world, and it is the only dose included in the USA's Food and Drug Administration (FDA) labeling for mifepristone. Prostaglandin analogs used initially with mifepristone included gemeprost 1 mg vaginally or sulprostone 0.25 to 0.50 mg intramuscularly. Abortion occurred in 95 to 96% of women with pregnancies up to 49 days' gestation [14,15].

The single largest medical abortion trial included women through 49 days' gestation who received mifepristone with varying doses of gemeprost or sulprostone [15]. Three hundred centers enrolled 16,369 patients, and 15,709 women were included in the final analysis. Overall efficacy was 95.3% (95% CI 95.0, 95.6%), with no difference in treatment success rates by dose or type of prostaglandin analog. A small percentage (2.8%) of patients aborted after receiving mifepristone and before prostaglandin administration. Abortion occurred within 4 and 24 hours after the prostaglandin in 57 and 87% of subjects, respectively. Failures included continuing pregnancies (1.2%), incomplete abortions (2.8%), and curettage because of heavy vaginal bleeding (0.7%). Four serious cardiovascular complications (one myocardial infarction and three cases of severe hypotension) occurred with sulprostone injection. As a result of these and other reported cardiovascular events, use of sulprostone in medical abortion regimens ceased.

Effective regimens using mifepristone 600 mg and gemeprost 1 mg vaginally still resulted in considerable rates of vomiting (reported rates of 13 to 26%) [16–18] and diarrhea (reported rates of 10 to 13%) [16,17]. Using a lower (0.5 mg) dose of gemeprost approximately 48 hours after 600 mg of mifepristone resulted in similar efficacy and side effect rates [19]. In 391 women up to 63 days' gestation 97% (95% CI 95, 99%) aborted, with no difference by gestational age. Although gemeprost is the prostaglandin analog approved for use with mifepristone for medical abortion up to 63 days' gestation in the United Kingdom, Sweden, and Norway, it has several disadvantages compared to misoprostol. Gemeprost is more expensive and requires refrigeration, important drawbacks in developing countries. Moreover, clinical trials have suggested that mifepristone followed by vaginal misoprostol demonstrates superior efficacy, lower rates of continuing pregnancy, and similar side effects as compared to mifepristone with gemeprost [20]. These aspects have led to the gradual substitution of misoprostol for gemeprost over the last few years; today, misoprostol is the most commonly used prostaglandin analog in regimens for medical abortion.

Although mifepristone is approved in more than 30 countries worldwide, most women live in countries where mifepristone is not available or not widely affordable or where access to legal abortion is lacking [21]. Even where mifepristone is approved for medical abortion, usage patterns may vary among countries or within different regions of the same country. As of 2000, for example, more than half of abortions within approved gestational limits were accomplished using a mifepristone regimen in France (56%), Scotland (61%), and Sweden (51%) compared to only 18% in England and Wales [22]. In various regions of Sweden, use of mifepristone for abortion ranges from 10 to 60% of eligible abortions [23]. Similar variations exist throughout the USA, where medical abortion use by state varies from 0 to 32% of all abortions [24]. In 2005 medical abortion accounted for 13% of all abortions and 22% of abortions before 9 weeks' gestation [25] (Chapter 3). Danco Laboratories, LLC, the company that supplies mifepristone in the USA, estimates that more than 1 million women in the USA used the product for abortion by the end of 2008 (Danco Laboratories, LLC, personal communication).

Further research has revealed other medical uses for mifepristone. In Europe, subsequently approved indications include labor-induction abortion, labor induction for fetal demise, and cervical ripening. Additionally, mifepristone is used in China for emergency contraception. Other potential uses include treatment of symptomatic leiomyomata uteri, endometriosis, Cushing's syndrome, contraception, depression, breast cancer, and glaucoma.

Modern era of medical abortion: Nonmifepristone regimens

Because mifepristone was not available in most countries, investigators searched for alternative means to provide a medical abortion. With the publication of studies demonstrating the effectiveness of low-dose methotrexate for treatment of extrauterine pregnancy [26], this agent emerged as a potential candidate. In January 1993, researchers in the USA started clinical trials using low-dose methotrexate and misoprostol for early abortion [27], leading to the clinical protocols in use today. However, in many developing countries, even access to methotrexate is limited.

Whereas past studies evaluating prostaglandins and prostaglandin analogs alone for medical abortion did not result in clinically useful regimens, the emergence of misoprostol as an inexpensive agent that was stable at room temperature reignited interest in such regimens. Misoprostol was initially evaluated as a single agent for use in the management of early pregnancy failure and abortion beyond 11 weeks' gestation. Subsequent research indicated that vaginal administration of misoprostol 800 μg repeated up to three times at intervals ranging from 3 to 24 hours effected complete abortion in 85 to 90% of women up to 9 weeks' gestation. Sublingual administration at 3-hour intervals had similar efficacy but with more frequent side effects. As expected, oral administration is less effective [28].

Although not as effective as combined regimens, misoprostol alone, with repeated doses if necessary, does provide an important medical abortion option for women in many countries. In countries where mifepristone is not available, misoprostol-alone regimens are now widely used and have been shown to reduce mortality and morbidity associated with illegal unsafe abortion [29,30] (Chapters 2 and 22).

Agents

Mifepristone

Overview

Progesterone, as its names suggests ("pro-gestation"), is fundamentally important for sustaining an early pregnancy. Withdrawal of progesterone support during early human pregnancy results in uterine contractions with expulsion of the embryo by a prostaglandin-mediated mechanism [31]. Inhibition of progesterone effects is accomplished by preventing its synthesis or blocking its action at the receptor. Mifepristone (Figure 9.1), a derivative of norethindrone, binds to the progesterone receptor with an affinity greater

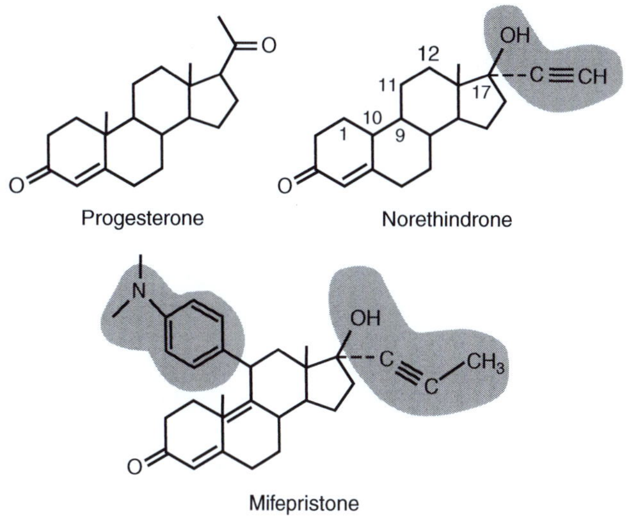

Figure 9.1 Structural formulas of mifepristone, norethindrone, and progesterone. To create mifepristone from norethindrone, a long side-chain is added at the 17-carbon position, which makes it bind very tightly to the progesterone receptor, and a bulky side-chain is added at the 11-carbon position, rendering it inactive.

than progesterone itself without activating the receptor, thereby acting as an "antiprogestin"[32].

Mifepristone has several effects on the uterus and cervix during early pregnancy:

- Mifepristone induces uterine contractility directly by reversing progesterone-induced inhibition in gap junction formation [33]. In addition, contractility is indirectly affected by a resultant increase in myometrial sensitivity to prostaglandins [34].
- Mifepristone alters the endometrium directly by affecting the capillary endothelial cells of the decidua; it has no direct effect on the trophoblast [35,36]. Decidual necrosis results in separation of the trophoblast from the decidua, causing bleeding and a decrease in human chorionic gonadotropin (hCG) secretion into the maternal system. The decidual action also increases prostaglandin release [37].
- Mifepristone softens the cervix to allow expulsion.

Notably, mifepristone is not effective as a primary treatment for extrauterine pregnancy [38], most likely because of a lack of progesterone receptor expression in fallopian tubes containing an ectopic pregnancy [39].

Human studies have suggested that uterine contractility does not increase until 24 to 36 hours after mifepristone administration but is preceded by an increase in myometrial sensitivity to prostaglandins [34]. At this point, the myometrium is five times more sensitive to the stimulatory effects of exogenous prostaglandins. However, recent studies have shown high efficacy when vaginal misoprostol is administered less than 15 minutes after mifepristone [40]. The effectiveness of such a regimen cannot be attributed to the actions of the misoprostol, as misoprostol alone has a much lower efficacy. Accordingly, these studies suggest that some or all of these actions occur sooner or that the effects of mifepristone that are important and necessary for its abortifacient activity remain incompletely understood.

Pharmacokinetics

When administered orally, mifepristone is easily absorbed, reaching peak serum concentrations in pregnant and non-pregnant women within 2 hours regardless of dose [41]. The pharmacokinetics of mifepristone differ for daily doses less than 100 mg than for higher doses; at doses of 100 mg or more, serum levels are similar [42–44]. Comparable peak serum concentrations of 2.0 to 2.5 μg/ml occur in women given 100 mg, 400 mg, 600 mg, or 800 mg of mifepristone [45]. The nonlinear pharmacokinetics may be due to saturation of a specific transport protein for mifepristone, serum alpha-1-acid glycoprotein; this protein is saturated at doses of 100 mg or more [46]. These data indicate that single doses as low as 100 mg are likely to be as effective as 600 mg. The half-life of mifepristone is approximately 24 to 29 hours [44,45]. Because mifepristone without a prostaglandin failed to induce abortion consistently, researchers sought to determine if failure was related to serum concentrations of mifepristone and its metabolites. In women receiving a single 600-mg dose of mifepristone, serum levels of mifepristone or its metabolites did not differ between those who did and did not abort [47]. Therefore, increasing the dose to more than 600 mg is unlikely to result in a better outcome.

Methotrexate

Overview

Methotrexate blocks the enzyme dihydrofolate reductase, thereby inhibiting the production of reduced folates required for DNA synthesis. Methotrexate primarily affects rapidly dividing cells. Medical conditions in which rapid cell division occurs include cancers, autoimmune diseases, and pregnancy. More than 50 years ago, the US FDA approved methotrexate to treat certain neoplastic diseases, rheumatoid arthritis, and psoriasis. Since 1982, multiple investigators have used various multidose regimens of methotrexate off-label to treat ectopic pregnancy, with efficacy rates in the 90 to 95% range (Chapter 18). Because methotrexate should have similar effects on both extrauterine and intrauterine trophoblast, its potential for abortion was obvious.

In contrast to the high-dose regimens required to treat cancer, low doses of methotrexate suffice for other medical conditions, including early abortion and treatment of unruptured ectopic pregnancy. This distinction is important, because toxicity is dose-dependent. High-dose versus low-dose, though, is not actually a comparison of absolute quantity administered at one time, but the total dose administered over a given period of time (area under the curve). Thus, a patient given a single 85-mg injection of methotrexate is receiving low-dose therapy compared to a person who receives a 50-mg injection 5 days in a row.

High-dose methotrexate can affect the lining of the gastrointestinal tract, bone marrow, and pulmonary interstitium; with very high doses, renal toxicity and alopecia also can occur. However, with the low doses used for ectopic pregnancy or abortion, side effects are usually limited to mild gastrointestinal problems like nausea, vomiting, or diarrhea. Women treated with methotrexate for gestational trophoblastic tumors have normal future reproductive function [48]. After low-dose methotrexate treatment for ectopic pregnancy, menses return normally and pregnancy rates are similar to those achieved by traditional surgical treatment [26]. Thus, methotrexate has no effect on future fertility and does not increase the risk of anomalies in subsequent pregnancies.

Pharmacokinetics

Very limited pharmacokinetic information is available for methotrexate in pregnant women. In 10 women up to 49 days' gestation who received methotrexate 50 mg/m^2 intramuscularly to induce abortion, serum levels peaked within 1 to 2 hours, which is similar to results in nonpregnant subjects [49]. The mean peak serum concentration was 4.4 ± 0.9 μmol/l and did not exceed 5.0 μmol/l at 24 hours in any patient. Serum levels were nondetectable within 48 hours. The renal clearance rate was the same as that for men and nonpregnant women receiving methotrexate in lower doses for rheumatoid arthritis or asthma.

Misoprostol

Overview

Misoprostol (11α, 13E, 16-dihydroxy-16-methyl-9-oxoprost-13-en-1-oic acid methyl ester) is a synthetic prostaglandin E_1 analog developed in 1973 for the treatment and prevention of gastric ulcers. Misoprostol tablets are produced primarily for oral use in doses of 100 μg and 200 μg. Treatment and prevention of gastric ulcer is still the only licensed indication for misoprostol, with the exception of Gymiso® in France (200 μg tablets for abortion) and a 25 μg vaginal suppository approved in Brazil and Egypt for induction of labor. Despite the lack of an approved indication for use alone in medical abortion, misoprostol is specifically mentioned as the prostaglandin analog of choice in the marketing authorization for mifepristone in the USA and European countries and, together with gemeprost, in the United Kingdom, Sweden, and Norway.

Misoprostol has become an important drug in obstetrics and gynecology because of its uterotonic and cervical priming actions. Misoprostol has several advantages over other prostaglandins on the market: it is inexpensive, has no effect on the bronchi or blood vessels, and can be stored at room temperature for many years; moreover, the tablets for oral use are also effective when used vaginally, sublingually, or rectally. Because mifepristone is more costly and less available, the use of misoprostol alone for medical abortion has become common through both medical and informal routes of provision [50]. However, the misoprostol-alone regimens are less effective, require higher doses of misoprostol, and thus result in more side effects.

Pharmacokinetics

Misoprostol is rapidly and extensively absorbed from the gastrointestinal tract and undergoes rapid first-pass metabolism (de-esterification) to form the free acid, which is responsible for its clinical activity. Unlike the parent compound, misoprostol acid is detectable in plasma [51,52]. Taking misoprostol orally with food diminishes maximum plasma concentrations of misoprostol acid and concomitant use of antacid reduces its total availability [53].

The pharmacokinetics of misoprostol differ by route of administration. Following a single dose of 400 μg oral misoprostol, the plasma misoprostol level increases rapidly and peaks at about 30 minutes; the plasma level then declines rapidly by 120 minutes [54–57]. After vaginal administration, the plasma concentration rises gradually, reaching a maximum after 70 to 80 minutes; it then slowly declines, with levels detectable up to 6 hours after administration. Compared to the oral route, the peak plasma concentration following vaginal administration is lower (Figure 9.2) but the "area under the curve" (AUC), or total bioavailability, is significantly greater [54,55,58]. Whereas initial findings of tablet remnants hours after vaginal administration led clinicians to assume that absorption is variable and incomplete, the remnants likely reflect the lack of complete breakdown of the tablet fillers with vaginal administration rather than any variance in absorption. Attempts have been made to improve the absorption of vaginal misoprostol. Athough the addition of water to the misoprostol tablets is a common practice, it does not significantly improve the bioavailability of vaginal misoprostol [55].

Buccal and sublingual routes of misoprostol administration have also been investigated for medical abortion. With both routes, the tablets are usually swallowed after 30 minutes, so a small amount of gastric absorption may occur as well. Systemic bioavailability as measured by the AUC is highest following sublingual use [55,59]. With buccal use, the shape of the absorption curve is similar to that of the vaginal route; however, the plasma drug levels attained are lower, and the AUC is only half that observed after vaginal administration [57]. The AUC for sublingual misoprostol is four times that seen after buccal administration [60]. However, measures of uterine contractility comparing buccal or sublingual administration to the vaginal route are quite similar [61].

Medical abortion regimens

Mifepristone regimens

Standard ("classic") regimen

The standard or "classic" regimen derives from early studies of mifepristone and a prostaglandin analog adapted for the use of misoprostol in place of earlier analogs. The

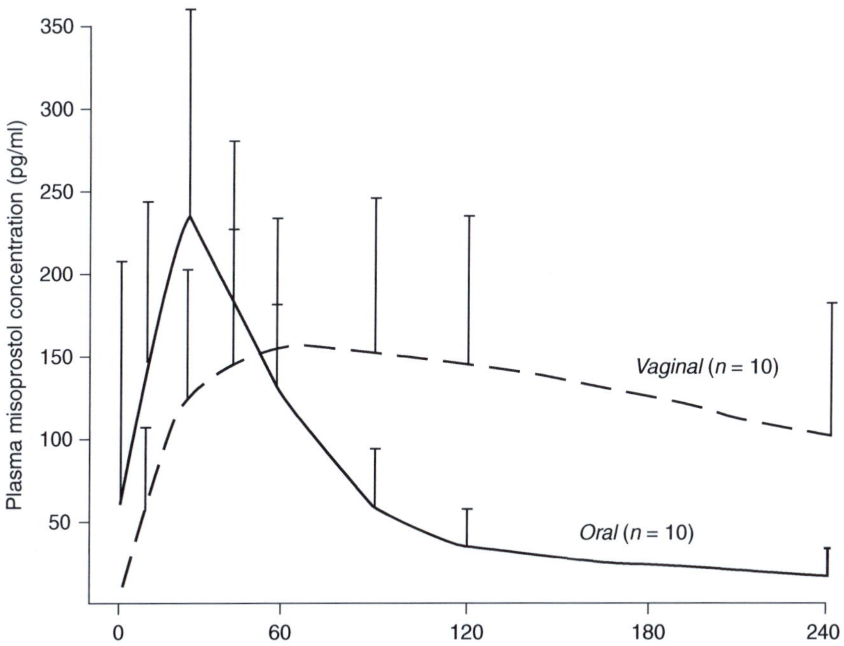

Figure 9.2 Mean plasma concentrations of misoprostol acid over time with oral (solid line) and vaginal (dotted line) administration. Arrow bars represent one standard deviation [54]. (Reprinted with permission from the American College of Obstetricians and Gynecologists.)

first large-scale study using the mifepristone/misoprostol combination involved 873 women up to 49 days' gestation [62]. Peyron and colleagues described two consecutive studies in which all women received mifepristone 600 mg orally followed 48 hours later by a single oral dose of misoprostol 400 μg. Women in the second study were also eligible to receive an additional 200 μg of misoprostol orally if abortion had not occurred within 4 hours. Overall 4% of women aborted solely from the mifepristone. Complete abortion occurred in 96.9% (95% CI 94.1, 97.7%) of the 488 women treated in the first study and in 98.7% (95% CI 96.8, 99.5%) of the 385 subjects in the second study, a nonsignificant difference. The abortion rates in the first 4 hours after misoprostol administration were 61 and 69% in the two studies, respectively, implying that the difference in overall efficacy was not necessarily a factor of the second dose. One woman (in group 1) required a transfusion. Nausea, vomiting, and diarrhea occurred after the misoprostol in approximately 40%, 15%, and 10% of women, respectively.

The use of mifepristone and oral misoprostol is approved in France, the USA, and other countries through 49 days' gestation. The efficacy of this regimen falls significantly thereafter, as well demonstrated by the first large-scale US clinical trial, which was performed by the Population Council in women up to 63 days' gestation [63]. Women at 17 clinical sites received mifepristone 600 mg orally and returned 2 days later to receive misoprostol 400 μg orally. The women stayed in the clinic for a minimum of 4 hours of observation then returned 12 days later for a final visit, at which time a physical or ultrasound examination was performed to confirm complete expulsion.

For the 2,005 women included in the final analysis of efficacy, failure rates at 49 days' or less, 50 to 56 days', and 57 to 63 days' gestation were 7.9%, 17.0%, and 22.5%, respectively. In pregnancies up to 49 days' gestation, the rate of ongoing pregnancy was comparable to previously published trials (approximately 1%); however, the rates at 50 to 56 days' and 57 to 63 days' gestation were higher than European studies (3.7 and 9.0%, respectively).

The time of expulsion was known for 1,468 subjects; 49% aborted within 4 hours and 75% within 24 hours after misoprostol administration. The median duration of bleeding was 13 days in the group up to 49 days' gestation and 15 days in women with more advanced gestations; 9% of women had bleeding that lasted more than 30 days. Four women received blood transfusions including one subject at 49 days' gestation or less, one at 57 to 63 days' gestation, and two subjects at 50 to 60 days' gestation.

The practical clinical application of this standard regimen requires three visits. The first visit involves patient education and consent, gestational age determination, and treatment. In some regions, specific counseling or consent must take place well in advance of treatment as mandated by law. Gestational age is determined in different ways depending on local standards and resources. Some practitioners use the woman's menstrual history and pelvic examination primarily, with sonography reserved only for questionable cases; others, especially in the USA, use sonography routinely for all patients. Similarly, some providers obtain hemoglobin or hematocrit measurements only in women at risk for anemia because of poor health, poor nutrition, or a history of bleeding, and others obtain such measurements in all women. Treatment with mifepristone is 600 mg (three 200-mg pills) taken orally in front of the provider.

The second visit occurs 2 days later, approximately 36 to 48 hours after the mifepristone. If the woman gives a history compatible with abortion, she typically is examined to see if she has expelled the pregnancy, which occurs in less than 5% of women. Women who are still pregnant receive misoprostol 400 μg (two 200-μg tablets) orally and stay at the center for a maximum of 4 hours. Women receive pain medication as needed and may leave after expulsion of the pregnancy is confirmed clinically. If 4 hours pass without apparent expulsion, an examination is performed before women leave because sometimes the expelled gestational sac is in the vagina. The third visit occurs approximately 2 weeks later. Women without confirmed expulsion undergo sonographic examination. Women with a persistent gestational sac, whether or not gestational cardiac activity is present, are typically offered vacuum aspiration.

Slight variations of the standard regimen include not requiring that women stay in the clinic following misoprostol treatment and administering additional doses of misoprostol at the clinic. The former adaptation followed agency approval in the USA, with the US FDA not mandating a 4-hour observation period. Additional misoprostol doses have been studied systematically without evidence of benefit. In addition to the work of Peyron and Aubeny et al [62] discussed previously, Aubeny and Peyron et al. [64] performed a multicenter trial that included 1,108 women up to 63 days' gestation who were treated with this regimen but were also offered an additional 200 μg of misoprostol orally. Complete abortion rates were highest at lower gestational age: 97.6% up to 42 days' gestation, 94.8% from 42 to 49 days' gestation, 93.4% from 50 to 56 days' gestation, and 86.8% from 57 to 63 days' gestation. Similarly, continuing pregnancy rates increased with advancing gestational age: 0.8%, 1.4%, 1.6%, and 5.1%, respectively. Overall, 61.6% of women had not expelled the pregnancy within 3 hours of misoprostol administration and received a second dose. The group of women through 49 days' gestation was compared with a historical cohort of women who received only a single dose of misoprostol with no significant improvement in the expulsion rate using the repeat dose. A randomized, blinded study in India evaluated a routine second dose of misoprostol 3 hours later as compared to placebo [65] in women up to 56 days' gestation. The study was significantly underpowered so an apparent trend toward a benefit did not show statistical significance. Treatment success rates in the single-dose and multiple-dose groups were 86 and 92%, respectively ($p = 0.11$). Continuing pregnancy rates, though, were significantly different (7% vs. 1%, $p = 0.005$). The gestational ages of the continuing pregnancies were not described. This study, in combination with those mentioned previously, fails to support any benefit of the routine use of a second misoprostol dose in women up to 49 days' gestation using the standard mifepristone-misoprostol regimen.

Alternative evidence-based regimens

Despite the early acceptance in France and most other countries of the standard regimen in women up to 49 days' gestation [38], alternative regimens using these agents were sought that would cause fewer side effects, be less expensive, or be more acceptable to providers and patients. Studies have led to lower doses of mifepristone, non-oral dosing of misoprostol, home administration of the misoprostol, earlier follow-up, and altering the timing of the misoprostol dose following mifepristone.

Lower doses of mifepristone

As expected based on the pharmacokinetics of mifepristone, lower doses of mifepristone are equally as effective as the 600-mg dose when combined with either gemeprost or misoprostol [18,66,67]. Because mifepristone is the more expensive of the medications, lower-dose regimens are more economical. In 1992, Thong and Baird [68] first reported using mifepristone 200 mg followed 48 hours later by misoprostol 600 μg orally in 100 women up to 56 days' gestation. Overall, the regimen was 92% effective, with 79% of women aborting within 4 hours of misoprostol administration. A randomized trial performed by the World Health Organization (WHO) [67] included women up to 63 days' gestation who received either mifepristone 200 mg ($n = 792$) or 600 mg ($n = 797$) followed 48 hours later by misoprostol 400 μg orally. Complete abortion rates were similar for both groups (89 and 88%, respectively) and were gestational age dependent: 92% up to 42 days, 89% at 43 to 49 days, 87% at 50 to 56 days, and 80% after 56 days. Rates of side effects were comparable in the groups. Subsequent to these trials, most large studies and commonly used clinical protocols have employed 200 mg of mifepristone for medical abortion. Efficacy is still maintained when mifepristone 200 mg is used with misoprostol 400 μg orally through 49 days' gestation [69]. Additionally, in 2007 the 200-mg mifepristone dose, when used with a vaginal prostaglandin analog, received regulatory approval by the European Medicines Agency, affecting the entire European Union.

Alternate routes for misoprostol

Administering misoprostol vaginally, as compared to the standard oral route, allows the effective use of mifepristone regimens after 49 days' gestation (Table 9.1). In general, efficacy rates are approximately 95 to 98% up to 49 days' gestation, 93 to 98% from 50 to 56 days, and 92 to 98% from 57 to 63 days. Despite the success with vaginal dosing, studies suggest that women prefer an oral route [70]. Both buccal and sublingual regimens have been investigated with success, although the magnitude of the literature is much smaller than that for vaginal misoprostol. Additionally, use after 63 days' gestation has been investigated.

Use of buccal misoprostol appears equivalent to vaginal misoprostol. Middleton and colleagues [71] randomized 442 women with gestations of 56 days or less to 200 mg mifepristone orally followed 1 to 2 days later by 800 μg misoprostol given by the vaginal or buccal route. Buccal administration consisted of allowing the tablets to dissolve for 30 minutes after which the remaining fragments were swallowed. The complete abortion rate was 95% in the buccal group and 93% in the vaginal group ($p = 0.51$). With the exception of diarrhea, which occurred more frequently in the buccal group (36% vs. 24%, $p = 0.006$), the side effect profiles were similar. Overall satisfaction rates were high in both groups (92% buccal vs. 95% vaginal, $p = 0.18$). When women were queried regarding their preferences for the route of administration, 16% of women in the buccal group would have preferred vaginal administration compared with 11% in the vaginal group who would have preferred buccal. A recent study confirmed this high efficacy with use of mifepristone and buccal misoprostol through 63 days' gestation [72].

Three studies have been published that combine mifepristone and sublingual misoprostol. Hamoda and colleagues [73] randomized 340 women up to 13 weeks' gestation to receive mifepristone 200 mg followed by misoprostol 600 μg sublingually ($n = 171$) or 800 μg vaginally ($n = 169$) 36 to 48 hours later. Most (62%) subjects were beyond 63 days' gestation. Subjects were admitted for observation during misoprostol treatment. In women up to 9 weeks' gestation, an additional dose of misoprostol 400 μg was administered by the same route 3 hours later. Women over 9 weeks' gestation received additional misoprostol 400 μg if the pregnancy had not passed within 3 more hours. Overall efficacy in both groups was the same (97 to 98%); however, women who received sublingual misoprostol experienced significantly more diarrhea (71% vs. 52%), shivering (84% vs. 64%), and unpleasant taste (71% vs. 32%).

Singh and colleagues [74] reported a pilot study of 40 women up to 8 weeks' gestation who received mifepristone 200 mg followed 24 hours later by three doses of misoprostol 200 μg sublingually administered 6 hours apart. All of the women had complete abortions. Another recent report from Taiwan included 356 women up to 49 days' gestation treated with mifepristone 200 mg followed 48 hours later by misoprostol 600 μg sublingually [75]. This study also demonstrated high efficacy, with complete abortion in 98% of participants.

Table 9.1 Outcome of treatment with mifepristone 200 mg followed by misoprostol 800 μg vaginally by gestational age.

		≤49 Days			50–56 Days			57–63 Days		
Primary Author	Interval between Mifepristone and Misoprostol	Number	Complete Abortion (%)	Continuing Pregnancy (%)	Number	Complete Abortion (%)	Continuing Pregnancy (%)	Number	Complete Abortion (%)	Continuing Pregnancy (%)
Ashok (1998) [106]	36–48 hours	928	98.5	0.2	1,072[a]	96.7[a]	0.8[a]			
Schaff (1999) [79]	48 hours	660	97.4	0.3	273	96.3	1.1			
Schaff (2000) [80]	48 hours	578	97.7	0.2	251	96.8	0.4	308	96.0	1.0
Bartley (2001) [20]	48 hours	232	99.6	0	164	98.2	0	55	96.5	1.8
Schaff (2002) [122]	36–48 hours	349	98.2	0.6	113	98.2	0	60	93.3	0
Tang (2003) [147]	48 hours	26	96.2	0	86	93.1	2.7			
von Hertzen (2003) [148]	36–48 hours	223	95.1	–	242	93.4	0.4[b]	268	92.2	0
	36–48 hours[c]	240	94.6	–	246	93.1	0.2[b]	254	96.5	0
Creinin (2004) [88]	6–8 hours	245	97.1	0	154	94.2	0	126	95.2	0.8
	23–25 hours	258	98.4	0	157	97.5	0.6	116	98.3	0
Shannon (2006) [149][d]	24–48 hours	240	95.4	0	59	90.8	0			
Creinin (2007) [40]	<15 minutes	266	95.5	0.4	159	94.3	1.3	129	95.3	0.8
	23–25 hours	229	98.3	0.4	172	95.3	0	145	96.6	0

[a] Women 50–63 days' gestation.
[b] Continuing pregnancy rate for combined groups up to 56 days' gestation.
[c] Received misoprostol 400 μg orally twice daily for 1 week after vaginal misoprostol.
[d] Subjects could self-administer a second dose after 24 hours if they had little bleeding.

One of the primary advantages of non-oral misoprostol dosing is the continued efficacy of these regimens to 63 days' gestation and beyond. Limited trials have demonstrated continued efficacy of mifepristone and misoprostol between 9 and 13 weeks' gestation. In addition to the experience with vaginal and sublingual misoprostol previously described [73], multiple studies and case series have reported the successful use of mifepristone and vaginal misoprostol after 63 days' gestation. Regimens typically include additional doses of misoprostol 400 μg orally, vaginally, or sublingually every 3 hours as deemed necessary by the treating clinician. Unlike regimens up to 9 weeks' gestation, all of these studies have kept women in the office or hospital for observation during treatment. Vacuum aspiration is reported in approximately 5 to 10% of women overall, with higher rates with advancing gestation [76–78].

Home administration of misoprostol

Although initial protocols for use of mifepristone and a prostaglandin analog included in-office observation, home use of the prostaglandin analog with self-administration has become the standard of care in much of the world. Most trials using mifepristone and misoprostol in North America include home administration, and even the regulatory labeling for mifepristone in the USA does not require that the patient remain under observation after using the prostaglandin analog. Two large studies specifically evaluated adverse events in the hours after misoprostol during home use; only four (0.1%) women were noted to have emergencies [79,80]. Two of these women presented for an emergent aspiration for heavy bleeding; neither required a blood transfusion. One patient had a vasovagal reaction, and one woman had a syncopal episode while bleeding and fell and broke her nose. Only the latter occurrence (1 out of approximately 4,500 women) would potentially have been avoided with in-office observation. A recent pilot investigation of home use of misoprostol from Sweden and France demonstrated that women in those countries also manage well without being observed in the clinic. Of the 130 women using oral misoprostol at home, 98% reported no trouble with the regimen and 98% would use it at home again for a next abortion [81,82]. In 2004, Sweden changed its regulatory guidelines to allow medical abortion with mifepristone and home use of misoprostol up to 63 days' gestation.

Earlier follow-up

Women receiving the standard regimen are scheduled for follow-up approximately 2 weeks after initiating treatment. By this time, a woman who has successfully aborted will likely have light to no bleeding, a lack of pregnancy symptoms, and a small uterus on examination. Sonography is commonly reserved for situations where the outcome cannot be determined by a simple history and physical examination.

Multiple clinical trials have included earlier follow-up with the use of routine sonography. Although routine use of sonography could potentially increase cost, it does allow for earlier determination of success with high predictability. Studies using sonography have included follow-up as early as 24 hours posttreatment. To determine success, most investigators simply look for the absence of a gestational sac whereas others also use endometrial thickness. Although endometrial thickness can be slightly greater in women who ultimately need a uterine evacuation procedure, studies of women receiving medical treatment for abortion or early pregnancy failure have shown that the measurement has poor positive predictive value and no clinical utility [83–87].

Only a few recent studies have included routine follow-up beyond 2 weeks [40,88–90]. In two studies by Creinin and colleagues, the investigators evaluated women 1 week after treatment using transvaginal sonography and continued to follow the subjects for a total of 5 weeks. In these studies, 78% [88] and 88% [40] of subjects who had not already had a vacuum aspiration were contacted 5 weeks after initiating treatment. A total of 14 (1.7%) and 13 (1.3%) women required an aspiration procedure during the prolonged follow-up. Thus, women in these trials were very unlikely to need further intervention, demonstrating the high predictability of sonography at 1 week.

Time interval between mifepristone and misoprostol

In the past decade much research has focused on the time interval between mifepristone and misoprostol administration. Acceptability is higher with shorter time intervals [91]. The combination of mifepristone with oral misoprostol at an interval of less than 36 to 48 hours is not effective. Creinin et al [92] randomized 86 women taking the standard regimen to use the misoprostol 24 or 48 hours after the mifepristone. Expulsion at 24 hours was evaluated for potential efficacy of this new regimen, with complete abortion rates of 50% and 91%, respectively (RR = 0.55 [95% CI 0.42, 0.73]).

Regimens with non-oral misoprostol routes, however, allow for high efficacy with a shorter interval. Schaff et al [91] reported a multicenter randomized trial in 2,295 women up to 56 days' gestation who self-administered misoprostol 800 μg vaginally 24, 48, or 72 hours after taking mifepristone 200 mg orally. The misoprostol dose was repeated at a 1-week follow-up visit if vaginal ultrasound examination did not confirm expulsion. Complete medical abortion occurred in 98% (95% CI 97, 99%), 98% (95% CI 97, 99%), and 96% (95% CI 95, 97%), respectively. The time waiting for expulsion was acceptable in 86%, 79%, and 76%, respectively ($p = 0.001$). In a later trial, the same investigative team showed continued high efficacy of the combination of mifepristone and misoprostol 800 μg vaginally 24 hours later up to 63 days' gestation [70].

A stepwise progression of studies has demonstrated that vaginal misoprostol can be used simultaneously with the mifepristone. First, Creinin et al [88] performed a multicenter, randomized trial of 1,080 women up to 63 days' gestation who received the misoprostol either 6 to 8 hours ($n = 540$) or 23 to 25 hours ($n = 540$) following the mifepristone. Complete abortion rates were equivalent (96 and 98%, respectively). Continuing pregnancy rates were 0.4 and 0.1%, respectively. Surprisingly, side effects after mifepristone administration were significantly more common in the women who received misoprostol 23 to 25 hours later. Additionally, nausea, vomiting, and heavy bleeding were significantly greater after misoprostol treatment in this group. Pain and subject acceptability were similar between groups.

Investigators in the UK attempted a similar comparative multicenter trial, randomizing 450 women up to 63 days' gestation to receive the misoprostol either 6 hours ($n = 225$) or 36 to 48 hours ($n = 225$) following the mifepristone [90]. Women in the 6-hour group returned for the misoprostol and then went home. Women in the 36- to 48-hour group returned for the misoprostol and stayed in the clinic for 4 to 6 hours. Complete abortion rates were 89 and 96%, respectively (RR = 0.92 [95% CI 0.84, 0.98]). The results of this smaller study are quite discrepant from those of the US trial. More women were considered to have incomplete abortions in the UK trial (4% vs. 2%), and more women had vacuum aspirations for persistent gestational sacs (4% vs. 0.6%). Most likely, the differences in protocol led to higher use of aspiration in the UK: specifically, conducting the follow-up sooner, requiring women to stay in the clinic longer if they wanted a repeat dose (which encouraged choice of a quicker aspiration procedure), and using incorrect ultrasound criteria to define incomplete abortion.

Additional work from the USA indicates that the timing can be decreased further when using misoprostol vaginally. Creinin et al [40] performed a multicenter, randomized trial of 1,128 women up to 63 days' gestation who received the misoprostol either within 15 minutes of the mifepristone administration ($n = 567$) or 23 to 25 hours ($n = 561$) following the mifepristone. Complete abortion rates were statistically equivalent (95 and 97%, respectively). Continuing pregnancy rates were 0.7% and 0.2%, respectively. Women who used simultaneous dosing had a lower likelihood of expulsion with a single dose of misoprostol as compared to the 23- to 25-hour interval (91 vs. 94% $p = 0.10$ for noninferiority). However, simultaneous use of misoprostol has a practical advantage in that the misoprostol cannot be improperly placed or lost.

Studies using buccal and sublingual misoprostol similarly have demonstrated that a 24-hour interval can be used with high success [74,78]. However, unlike with vaginal misoprostol, the combination of mifepristone and buccal misoprostol is not effective when the two are used simultaneously [89].

Methotrexate regimens

Initial clinical trials of methotrexate and misoprostol for early abortion began in 1993, 11 years after the start of human testing on mifepristone [27]. The encouraging results led to larger trials that have investigated a longer interval between methotrexate and misoprostol administration, the effects of moistening the misoprostol, and use of oral methotrexate (Table 9.2).

In general, it appears that the methotrexate has little effect as an abortifacient, as abortion rates in the short term are similar to those of misoprostol alone. Rather the methotrexate acts to create a nonviable gestation should the misoprostol not work. A randomized trial in women up to 7 weeks' gestation supports this point. Wiebe and colleagues [93] reported in brief about a randomized comparison of the combined regimen of methotrexate 50 mg/m^2 intramuscularly followed 72 hours later by misoprostol 800 μg vaginally ($n = 149$) and a misoprostol-only regimen that combined misoprostol 400 μg sublingually and 400 μg vaginally ($n = 149$). Efficacy in both groups following one treatment was about 60%. A recent review counters this finding. Aldrich [94] reported a large study of sequential cohorts, using first misoprostol alone and subsequently methotrexate and vaginal or buccal misoprostol. Success rates were 77% for misoprostol alone and 82 to 84% for methotrexate regimens. The nature of the review, however, limits its utility.

As with mifepristone regimens, recent studies have evaluated methotrexate combined with nonvaginal misoprostol. Wiebe and Trouton [95] compared buccal and vaginal misoprostol used after intramuscular methotrexate 50 mg/m^2. Women with gestations up to 49 days were randomized to 600 μg of misoprostol administered vaginally or buccally 3 to 6 days after receiving methotrexate. Women in the buccal group were instructed to allow the tablets to dissolve for 1 hour and then to spit out any remaining fragments. The overall complete abortion rate 8 days after misoprostol administration was statistically higher in the vaginal misoprostol group (67.5% vs. 53.5%, $p = 0.01$); the acceptability was similar in both groups, as was the eventual need for surgical abortion, likely reflecting the efficacy of methotrexate. The efficacy rate in this study is lower than that previously reported for methotrexate used with 800 μg of vaginal misoprostol (Table 9.2), suggesting that the lower dose of misoprostol rather than the route of administration may have contributed to the findings. In addition, expelling the remaining fragments of misoprostol after 1 hour may have lowered the overall dose of misoprostol in the buccal group, although serum concentrations were not determined.

Comparison to mifepristone regimens

A randomized trial in Canada compared the efficacy and side effects of mifepristone 600 mg followed 36 to 48 hours later by misoprostol 400 μg orally ($n = 518$) and methotrexate 50 mg/m^2 intramuscularly followed 4 to 6 days later

Table 9.2 Selected studies of medical abortion using methotrexate (MTX) and vaginal misoprostol (MIS).

Primary Author	N	Gestational Age (Days)	MTX Dose, Route of Administration	MIS Dose[a]	Interval between MTX and MIS (days)	Repeat Dose of MIS (days after MIS dose)[b]	Follow-up Period (days after MTX)	Overall Success (%)
Hausknecht (1995) [150]	178	≤63	50 mg/m^2 IM	800 μg	5 to 7	7	14	96.1
Creinin (1995) [151]	46	≤56	50 mg/m^2 IM	800 μg	3	4	56	82.6
	40				7	1		97.5
Creinin (1996) [115]	300	≤56	50 mg/m^2 IM	800 μg	7	7	14/35	69.7/91.7
Creinin (1997) [152]	100	≤49	75 mg IM	800 μg	5 to 6	7	14/44	77.8/94.9
Creinin (1997) [116]	299	≤49	50 mg PO	800 μg	5 to 6	7	14/44	80.6/91.3
Carbonell (1997) [153]	93	≤63	50 mg/m^2 IM	800 μg[c,d]	3	2 and 2	14	92.5
	98				4			91.8
	96				5			92.7
Wiebe (1999) [154]	45	<49	50 mg/ m^2 IM	600 μg[d]	5 to 7	1 and 7	28	88.9
	55		50 mg/m2 PO	800 μg[d]				94.5
	37		50 mg/m2 IM					97.3
	50		50 mg/m2 PO					90.0
Creinin (1999) [155]	126	≤49	50 mg/ m^2 IM	800 μg[d]	5 to 6	7	14/42	87.3/95.2
	122			800 μg			14/42	81.1/91.8
Carbonell Esteve (1999) [156]	148	≤56	25 mg PO	800 μg[c,d]	7	2 and 2	14	91.2
	154		50 mg PO					90.3
Borgatta (2001) [157]	1987	≤49	50 mg/ m^2 IM	800 μg	4 to 6	1 to 2	43	84.1
Wiebe (2002) [96]	518	≤49	50 mg/ m^2 IM	800 μg[d]	4 to 6	1 and 3	35	94.5

PO = orally
IM = intramuscularly
[a] Self-administered as dry tablets unless otherwise indicated.
[b] Repeated if gestational sac was still present.
[c] Regimen included additional misoprostol 400–1200 μg over a 24-hour period after expulsion confirmed.
[d] Moistened misoprostol.

by misoprostol 800 μg vaginally ($n = 524$) in women up to 49 days' gestation [96]. Women self-administered the misoprostol and repeated the dose 24 hours later if bleeding was less than typical menstrual flow. Subjects returned 7 days after the initiation of treatment for vaginal ultrasonography; those with a persistent gestational sac received misoprostol 800 μg vaginally. A vacuum aspiration was performed if a viable gestation persisted at a second follow-up visit 2 weeks after initiation of treatment or if the gestational sac had not expelled by 5 weeks after initiation of treatment. The abortion rate by the 1-week follow-up examination was 75% in the methotrexate group and 90% in the mifepristone group ($p < 0.001$). Aspiration rates were 4% in both groups. Side effects were similar between the mifepristone/misoprostol and methotrexate/misoprostol regimens with statistically significant differences in the incidence of headache after the mifepristone or methotrexate (19.1% vs. 11.3%, $p = 0.001$), diarrhea after the misoprostol (15.9% vs. 27.0%, respectively, $p < 0.001$), fever after the misoprostol (11.5% vs. 21.7%, respectively, $p < 0.001$), chills after the misoprostol (23.2% vs. 49.3%, respectively, $p < 0.001$), and headache after the misoprostol (28.6% vs. 17.0%, respectively, $p < 0.001$). The mean number of bleeding days was slightly greater with the mifepristone regimen (14.6 vs. 13.3 days, $p = 0.032$), whereas the mean pain score using an 11-point scale was significantly greater with the methotrexate regimen (6.3 vs. 5.8, $p = 0.003$). Overall, this study shows a similar overall efficacy for the two regimens in women up to 49 days' gestation; however, women who use the methotrexate regimen are more likely to expel the pregnancy beyond the first week of treatment.

Misoprostol-alone regimens

Where mifepristone is not accessible, various misoprostol-only regimens are being used. Brazil is the only country that has granted regulatory approval for a medical abortion regimen using only misoprostol. However, its widespread use in countries with restricted abortion laws appears to be associated with reduction in maternal morbidity and mortality [29,30].

Reported regimens differ with respect to several factors, including the intervals between doses (3 to 48 hours), the time point for assessing the outcome (a few days to several weeks), and the gestational age (Table 9.3). These multiple variables make it difficult to determine the most effective regimen. When misoprostol is used alone, the oral route is less effective than the vaginal route [97]. Vaginal doses of 800-μg misoprostol are usually repeated several times at intervals from 3 to 48 hours if abortion has not occurred. Typical success rates range from 85 to 95%, with continuing pregnancies occurring in about 4 to 10% of women. A recent review concluded that the evidence supported a recommendation of using misoprostol 800 μg vaginally every 6, 12, or 24 hours for a maximum of three doses [28].

Although the interval for vaginal administration, ranging in studies from 3 to 24 hours, may not be critical, a recent

Table 9.3 Selected studies with misoprostol 800 μg vaginally without mifepristone or methotrexate for medical abortion.

Primary Author	Number	Gestation (weeks)	Moistened with Saline	# Doses	Interval	Observation Time (days)	Complete Abortion (%)	Continuing Pregnancy (%)
Carbonell (1999) [99]	720	5–9	Yes	3[a]	24h	21	89	6.5
Jain (1999) [158]	100	≤8	Yes	2	24h	1	73	12.0
						15	88	8.0
Ngai (2000) [159]	40	≤9	Yes	3	48h	42	85	2.5
	40	≤9	No	3	48h	42	65	10.0
Bugalho (2000) [160]	103	≤6	Yes	2	7d	1	72	NR
						8	92	NR
Jain (2001) [161]	100	≤8	Yes	3	24h	3	93	5.0
Jain (2002) [102]	125	≤8	Yes	3	24h	1	72	NR
						15	88	4.8
Zikopoulos (2002) [162]	80	≤6	Yes	3[a]	24h	3	96	1.3
	80	6–8	Yes	3[a]	24h	3	86	2.5
Carbonell (2003) [163]	452	5–9	Yes	3[a]	8h	21	91	4.2
Singh (2003) [164]	150	8	Yes	3[b]	3h	43	96	4.0
Von Hertzen (2007) [98]	513	≤9	Yes	3	3h	14	85	3.9
	512	≤9	Yes	3	12h	14	83	4.9

[a] Subjects treated with additional misoprostol once expulsion confirmed.
[b] Repeat doses were 400 μg.
NR = Not reported.
Continuing pregnancy = Viable pregnancy.

WHO trial showed that the interval did matter for sublingual administration, with 3 hours being more effective than 12 hours [98]. Investigators recorded complete abortion rates after 2 weeks of follow-up for 431 (84%) women in the sublingual group and 434 (85%) women in the vaginal group when misoprostol 800 μg was given at 3-hour intervals. However, complete abortion occurred in 399 (78%) and 425 (83%), respectively, when the dosing occurred at 12-hour intervals. The rate of continuing pregnancy also was significantly higher for the 12-hour interval as compared with the 3-hour interval when using sublingual misoprostol (difference 4% [95% CI 0.4, 6.8%], $p = 0.03$) but not for vaginal dosing (difference 1% [95% CI 1.5, 3.5%], $p = 0.44$). The sublingual route was associated with more frequent gastrointestinal side effects (such as nausea, vomiting, shivering, and hyperthermia) than vaginal administration. In this large study, the efficacy was noted to decrease with advancing gestation regardless of route of misoprostol. The risk of failure was twice as high for women at 8 to 9 weeks' gestation compared with those at 7 weeks' gestation or less. This finding is similar to previous studies using misoprostol-only regimens [99].

Misoprostol as a single agent has been used for higher gestational ages, with two studies reporting success rates of 84% to 89% using repeated vaginal doses of 800 μg for women with pregnancies from 9 to 13 weeks' gestation [100,101].

Comparison to mifepristone regimens

A single randomized trial has compared mifepristone and misoprostol to misoprostol alone [102]. This double-blind trial included women up to 56 days' gestation using mifepristone 200 mg ($n = 119$) or placebo ($n = 125$) followed 48 hours later by misoprostol 800 μg vaginally. Misoprostol was repeated every 24 hours up to three doses. Complete abortion rates were 95.7 and 88.0%, respectively ($p < 0.05$). The women who received mifepristone aborted much more quickly and required fewer doses of misoprostol compared to women who received misoprostol alone. Complete abortion by 24 hours after misoprostol treatment was 89.9 and 72.0%, respectively ($p < 0.001$). Women experienced slightly more side effects with the mifepristone regimen, which may be due to a higher rate of treatment success resulting in effects related to the abortion process.

Medical abortion practice

Patient eligibility

Although medical contraindications to abortion with mifepristone, methotrexate, or misoprostol alone are few, social or psychological considerations are more common. Women are not optimal candidates for medical abortion if they:

- wish to minimize participation in their abortion;
- are anxious to have the abortion over quickly;
- cannot return for follow-up visits; or
- cannot communicate easily with the provider because of language or comprehension barriers (phone interactions are more common with medical than with surgical abortion patients).

Due to the risk of teratogenicity in an ongoing pregnancy, women also must intend to have a surgical abortion should the medical method fail. Other nonmedical considerations include access to a telephone in case of an emergency and distance from emergency medical treatment (e.g., suction curettage for hemorrhage). A few reports have examined use of medical abortion by adolescents, with outcomes similar to older women [103,104].

Some medical issues are important regardless of the regimen being used. Most studies exclude anemic women with hemoglobin levels less than 9.5 or 10 g/dl; accordingly, the safety of medical abortion in anemic women is unknown. Transfusion rates with medical abortion are 0.1 to 0.4% in large trials [15,40,63,88,105,106]. Although these rates are low, they exceed that reported for surgical abortion in early pregnancy (0.01%) [107]. Women with a coagulopathy or actively using anticoagulants are excluded from medical abortion studies for similar reasons. Accordingly, providing a medical abortion for a woman with hemoglobin less than 9.5 g/dl or who is anticoagulated warrants caution.

Similarly, medical abortion side effects, although limited in nature, could be consequential in women with severe hyperemesis gravidarum or other conditions that cause nausea, vomiting, or diarrhea. Gynecologic contraindications include suspected ectopic pregnancy and an intrauterine device (IUD) *in situ* that will not be removed. The outcomes for multiple pregnancies do not appear to differ from those for singletons [108].

Misoprostol, the agent commonly used with all regimens, has no contraindications in principle. However, because a small number of female smokers over the age of 35 years experienced adverse cardiac events following sulprostone administration [15], the medical commission in France extended the same restriction to women using misoprostol or gemeprost. In the USA, clinical practice guidelines of the American College of Obstetricians and Gynecologists and the National Abortion Federation do not advise against misoprostol use in smokers [109,110]. In breastfeeding women, small amounts of misoprostol or its active metabolite may appear in breast milk [111]. Thus, breastfeeding or pumping milk for feeding should be avoided for at least 6 hours after misoprostol administration. Breastfeeding women who use methotrexate-misoprostol regimens should pump and discard the milk for 72 hours.

Contraindications to the use of mifepristone or methotrexate regimens include known allergy to any of the agents being used. Because of the antiglucocorticoid properties of mifepristone, women with chronic renal insufficiency and long-term corticosteroid use should not use mifepristone. Contraindications to the methotrexate regimens include active liver or renal disease. Asthma is not a contraindication for any regimen; both methotrexate and misoprostol are bronchodilators, and mifepristone has no effect on the respiratory system. However, severely asthmatic patients may require chronic corticosteroid therapy, and providers should ask about such medication use prior to administering mifepristone.

Patient education, informed consent, and preparation

As with all abortion methods, the informed consent process must assure that a woman is certain about her decision to have an abortion and that she understands the alternatives available and their risks and benefits (Chapter 5). Patient uncertainty warrants a delay, even if waiting means that she will be unable to choose an early medical option.

The process of medical abortion is quite similar regardless of the agent used, although the timing and efficacy may vary. Patient education (Table 9.4) [112] includes explaining the medical abortion process and ways in which it differs from surgical abortion (Chapter 10). Heavier bleeding and more severe cramping may occur as compared to surgical abortion; describing the bleeding and cramping as comparable to a miscarriage, rather than menses, helps to prepare some patients. Mean days of bleeding are higher with medical (14 days) than surgical abortion (9 days), but days of spotting (about 10) are similar [113]. Increasing gestational age predicts more bleeding or spotting days after medical, but not surgical, abortion.

In contrast to surgical abortion, patients experience passage of the products of conception firsthand, and women may wonder if they will identify the tissue. The pregnancy and the decidua may pass at the same time or separately. The decidualized endometrium commonly appears thick and solid as it passes either in fragments or as a complete decidual cast. The gestational sac and placenta frequently pass intact, often with adherent clot (Figure 9.3). The clots may be quite large and obscure the pregnancy tissue. However, some patients may see a tiny sac or conceptus, particularly if the pregnancy is more than 7 weeks' gestation. Using true-to-size illustrations that show early products of conception may help prepare the patient for this event.

Although complications occur infrequently, providers must provide patients with clear instructions for accessing emergency services in case of hemorrhage. Medical abortion patients with severe hemorrhage or ongoing viable pregnancies warrant uterine aspiration. Therefore, clinicians who are

Table 9.4 Patient education for early medical abortion.

1. Discuss the decision to have an abortion and confirm that it is certain and voluntary.
2. Discuss the treatment alternatives (medical abortion or aspiration) and the benefits and risks of each method.
3. Describe the medical regimens available and their approval status. For mifepristone-misoprostol abortion in the USA, explain the differences between the FDA-approved regimen and other evidence-based regimens. For methotrexate-misoprostol abortion, explain that the FDA has approved these drugs for other uses, but not for medical abortion.
4. Explain what to expect. Bleeding and cramping typically intensify during expulsion of the pregnancy (usually 2–4 hours) and then gradually subside. Passage of clots is common during expulsion; lighter bleeding or spotting typically lasts about 2 weeks, but may be longer.
5. Explain that the patient is unlikely to see products of conception unless she is beyond 7 to 8 weeks' gestation, in which case the embryo will be very small and often obscured by blood clots.
6. Discuss known side effects of the medical abortion regimen including mild gastrointestinal symptoms; short-term fever, warmth, or chills; or oral ulcers (methotrexate only).
7. Explain that the drugs used for medical abortion may increase the risk of birth defects in continuing pregnancies. Emphasize that aspiration is advised if the medical abortion fails.
8. Discuss possible complications including failed abortion, incomplete abortion, hemorrhage, or infection. Emphasize that atypical infections have occurred rarely after use of mifepristone combined with misoprostol (see text).
9. Provide how to insert the misoprostol vaginally (deep into the vagina after washing hands), buccally (tucked between cheek and gum), or sublingually (under the tongue) and how to use pain medications.
10. Explain the time commitment and expected number of visits.
11. Provide 24-hour emergency contact information and emphasize warning signs that may warrant evaluation, including:
    a. Prolonged or heavy bleeding (≥ two soaked maxi pads for 2 consecutive hours);
    b. Fever (≥ 38°C) lasting more than 4 hours or beginning in the days after misoprostol administration;
    c. Abdominal pain or discomfort or "feeling sick" (including weakness, nausea, vomiting, or diarrhea, with or without fever) more than 24 hours after using misoprostol.
12. Provide information about available contraceptive methods and when to initiate the chosen method, if any.
13. Address issues of confidentiality.
14. Review all required consent forms, which must be signed before administration of the medications.

Adapted with permission from Paul M, Stewart F. Abortion. In *Contraceptive Technology* 2008. [112]

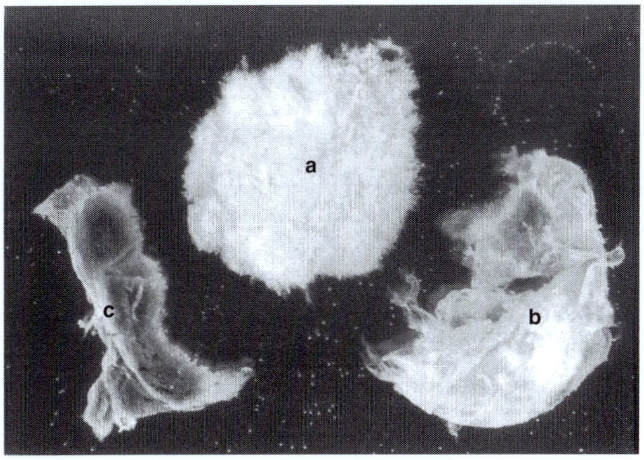

Figure 9.3 Tissue passed within several hours of taking misoprostol (mifepristone abortion). The gestational sac (a) and placenta measure about 3.0 cm. The decidual cast (b) and the blood clot (c) are approximately the same size. (Photographer Daniel Benevento, with permission).

not trained in suction curettage must have collaborative arrangements or referral mechanisms in place for patients who require this intervention.

Treatment

Mifepristone is manufactured in 200-mg tablets and use of doses exceeding 200 mg are of no benefit. In the USA, mifepristone is not available through pharmacies; rather, it is sold by the drug distributor directly to licensed physicians after they sign and return a Prescriber's Agreement. Prescribers agree to report adverse events and to give each patient a Medication Guide to read and a Patient Agreement to read and sign. Instructions for enrolling as a mifepristone provider are available at the distributor's website (http://www.earlyoptionpill.com). Because the distributor's forms pertain to the standard regimen, clinicians who offer an alternative regimen should have patients sign an additional consent or addendum that provides information about the alternative and its benefits and risks.

Due to the impressive accumulation of research on medical abortion, numerous regimens have emerged that are evidence-based, safe, and effective (Table 9.5). The regimen chosen will depend on the availability of medications, cost, patient preference, and other factors. When available, mifepristone regimens offer distinct advantages over other regimens in terms of efficacy, efficiency, and/or side effects.

Women can safely self-administer misoprostol at home. Regardless of route of administration, the same tablets are used as approved for oral dosing. Special suppositories of misoprostol described in some studies are not commercially available and are not necessary. Producing these suppositories and requiring an office visit for misoprostol administration increase cost and inconvenience. When dispensing the tablets, review with the patient how to place the tablets correctly in the vagina, under the tongue, or between the cheek and gums (Table 9.4). With vaginal use, patients need not remain at rest after misoprostol administration or use a tampon to hold the tablets in place.

When using methotrexate, women who are taking folate-containing medications (e.g., prenatal vitamins) should discontinue them for 1 week following methotrexate administration. Some clinicians also advise patients to avoid foods rich in folate, but no studies have evaluated the necessity of this practice.

All unsensitized Rh(D)-negative patients should receive anti-D immune globulin [109,110]. A dose of 50 μg suffices for gestations of 12 weeks or less. If the Rh status is unknown when mifepristone or methotrexate is administered, the patient can receive anti-D immune globulin anytime before or within 72 hours after she uses the misoprostol.

Patients are given appropriate instructions and prescribed oral narcotic analgesics to use if ibuprofen or acetaminophen provides inadequate pain relief. Providers may choose to use narcotics without acetaminophen (e.g., codeine, 30-mg tablets) to allow patients to self-medicate without concern for acetaminophen overdose. Nonsteroidal antiinflammatory drugs (NSAIDs) such as ibuprofen are not contraindicated and do not decrease the likelihood of successful medical abortion after misoprostol administration [114].

Although heavy bleeding is common, the patient needs to know how much bleeding is considered too much. Typical instructions include advising the patient to contact the provider if she soaks two sanitary pads per hour for 2 hours in a row. Clinicians who receive such calls can talk to the woman at 20-minute to 30-minute intervals until the bleeding slows, as long as the patient is feeling all right. Advise the patient to seek emergency care if the bleeding does not slow down; the urgency depends on how the patient is feeling, her baseline hemoglobin, and how far she is from emergency treatment.

Follow-up typically occurs 2 weeks after initiation of treatment if the provider is using clinical evaluation to determine outcome; it can be scheduled sooner if vaginal ultrasonography is used. Sonography should be used only as a means of determining the presence or absence of the gestational sac (Figure 9.4) and not for measurement of endometrial thickness when deciding if a medical abortion is successful. Most protocols with mifepristone or methotrexate include follow-up approximately 1 week after initiating treatment, whereas protocols using misoprostol alone follow women at frequent intervals to assess the need for repeat dosing. If the gestational sac remains, women have the option of a repeat dose of misoprostol (administered in the office or self-administered at home), expectant management (if the pregnancy is nonviable), or a vacuum aspiration should she want to complete the abortion without further delay. Approximately 20 to 30% of women using mifepristone or

Table 9.5 Comparison of medical abortion regimens.

	Standard Mifepristone-Regimen	Alternative Mifepristone- Misoprostol Misoprostol Regimens	Methotrexate-Misoprostol Regimens	Misoprostol-Only Regimens
Gestational Age Limit	49 days	63 days; efficacy continues throughout first trimester, but studies have included in-hospital observation	49 days	63 days
Mifepristone Dose	600 mg oral[a]	200 mg oral	N/A	N/A
Methotrexate Dose	N/A	N/A	50 mg/m^2 IM or 25–50 mg oral[b]	N/A
Misoprostol Dose	400 μg oral; administered during second office visit	800 μg vaginal, buccal, or sublingual; tablets supplied during first office visit and administered at home	800 μg vaginal; tablets supplied during first office visit and administered at home	800 μg vaginal; other routes can be used but are not well studied, have more side effects, or are not as effective
Misoprostol Timing	36–48 hours after mifepristone	24 hours after mifepristone for all routes; vaginal misoprostol may be used earlier, with studies supporting simultaneous administration of misoprostol and mifepristone up to 63 days' gestation	3–7 days after methotrexate	Every 6, 12, or 24 hours for a maximum of three doses
Advantages and Drawbacks	Some women prefer the oral route of misoprostol administration	Compared to regimens using oral misoprostol: extends gestational age eligibility, higher complete abortion rates, fewer side effects, more flexibility in timing of misoprostol	Useful in areas with limited access to mifepristone	Useful in areas with limited access to mifepristone, but not as effective as mifepristone-misoprostol regimens

[a] Mifepristone 200 mg oral followed by misoprostol 400 μg oral 36–48 hours later is also effective up to 49 days' gestation.
[b] Methotrexate tablets come in 2.5-mg doses, so packaging the tablets into gelatin capsules facilitates administration.

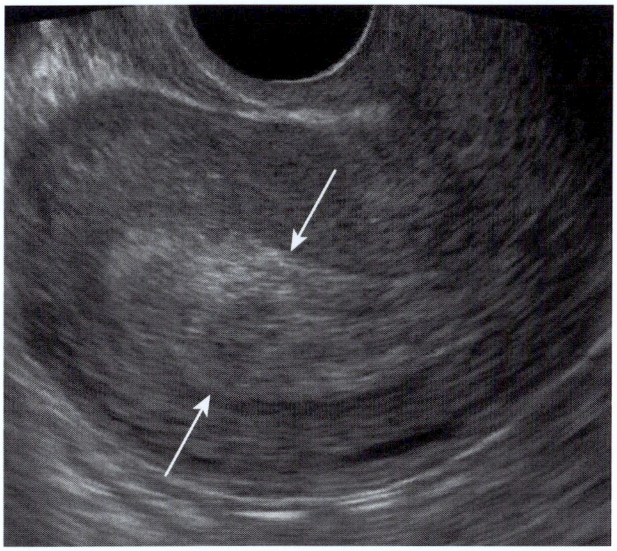

Figure 9.4 Vaginal ultrasound examination of uterine cavity 1 day after medical abortion. Heterogeneous intracavitary echoes are present (arrows) but no gestational sac is visible. These findings are consistent with successful abortion and do not require intervention.

methotrexate regimens will abort following a second dose of misoprostol [40,88,115,116]. Follow-up is scheduled for 1 week, although some methotrexate studies have delayed this second follow-up for 4 weeks if gestational cardiac activity is absent.

A few studies have attempted to investigate alternative methods of follow-up, including human chorionic gonadotropin (hCG) evaluation. Serum hCG is predictive of expulsion when values obtained before and 24 hours after misoprostol treatment are compared [117]. The average decline with successful treatment is 66% with a lower limit of 50% considered acceptable. Monitoring hCG values 1 week after treatment also can be used, with a decline of 80% indicating success [118,119]. Urine hCG testing 1 or 2 weeks after treatment is not clinically useful whether high or low sensitivity tests are used [120] (Chapter 6). An evaluation of nearly 1,000 women suggests that clinical history alone is as or more predictive than any of these objective measures [121].

Methotrexate regimens include the possibility that women who do not abort following misoprostol treatment will expel the pregnancy after a delay of a few days to a few weeks. On average, this event will happen approximately 3 to 3½ weeks after methotrexate administration. While waiting for the pregnancy to pass, the patient's bleeding and pregnancy symptoms will subside. Usually, she will have slight cramping or light bleeding a day or two before expulsion occurs. Of the women who have to wait for the pregnancy to pass, approximately 96% will abort completely within 35 days after the methotrexate injection [115]. Whereas mifepristone and misoprostol-only regimens commonly include a vacuum aspiration if expulsion has not occurred within 2 weeks, women with a nonviable pregnancy could be treated in the same way (expectant management) should they not desire surgical intervention.

Because medical abortion is not 100% effective, patients need access to surgical abortion services if the medical method fails or if significant hemorrhage occurs. Clinicians who offer medical abortion but not aspiration abortion must ensure the availability of 24-hour back-up coverage that includes competent surgical abortion services.

Side effects and complications

Bleeding

The mean duration of bleeding is 9 days, but the range is from 1 to 45 days; some women bleed until their next menstrual period. The average drop in hemoglobin is 0.7% [62]. The few women who present with excessive bleeding typically do so at least 10 days after misoprostol, and most have retained pregnancy tissue. Vacuum aspiration, which is rarely emergent, can be performed at this point.

Abdominal pain and cramping

The majority of women experience some cramping; for most women, it is like an intense menstrual period. Pain medication use varies significantly between countries. Narcotic pain medicine is used by 60% of women in the UK [20]. In a French study, when women were asked to rate their pain on a visual analog scale on the day of misoprostol use, the mean rating was 3.1 (0 = no pain at all, 10 = unbearable pain) [62]. Clinicians commonly advise women to use an NSAID or other non-narcotic pain medication initially and to add a narcotic medication if needed. Because the dose of acetaminophen must not exceed 4 grams in a 24-hour period to avoid liver toxicity, use of narcotics without acetaminophen (e.g., codeine or oxycodone) allows women to use as much as they need to ensure adequate pain control.

Gastrointestinal distress

Many women experience some nausea, vomiting, or diarrhea. However, these symptoms are generally self-limiting and usually resolve 2 to 6 hours after taking misoprostol. Diarrhea appears to be less frequent with vaginal administration of misoprostol and more common when women are exposed to higher serum levels of misoprostol, as with sublingual administration.

Infection

Endometritis is a rare complication of medical abortion, which typically involves no instrumentation of the cervix or uterine cavity. In large trials including 1,000 participants or more, infection rates typically vary from 0.1 to 0.9% [15,40,63,87,91,122]. A review of medical abortion studies suggests that the infection rate is approximately 0.9% [123].

Severe neutropenia has been described in two women who received methotrexate 50 mg/m^2 intramuscularly for the treatment of ectopic pregnancy [124]. A sustained fever exceeding 38°C following the use of methotrexate, especially if stomatitis is also present, requires a complete blood count for evaluation of neutropenia. In the very rare event of severe neutropenia following the use of methotrexate, the theoretical risk of secondary opportunistic infection warrants appropriate preventive measures.

Whereas some clinicians recommend the universal use of perioperative antibiotics for surgical abortion [125], no data currently exist to support such treatment with medical abortion. Rare fatal infections with *Clostridium sordellii* and *perfringens* have been reported in North America in women who received mifepristone and misoprostol [126,127]. Symptoms seen with such infections include weakness, nausea, vomiting, or diarrhea with or without abdominal pain that persists after expulsion of the pregnancy. Although patients typically lack a fever, they exhibit rapid pulse, low blood pressure, and very high red and white blood cell counts. The US Centers for Disease Control and Prevention have also reported deaths from the same organism after other reproductive outcomes (Chapter 15), including in two women who had spontaneous abortions without use of mifepristone or misoprostol [128]. On the basis of available information, serious infection and death from medical abortion seem most likely related to the physiologic process of abortion, whether spontaneous or induced, and not the medicines themselves.

Teratogenicity

The risk of congenital anomalies in pregnancies that continue after administration of medical abortifacients is a concern. Methotrexate is an antimetabolite that can damage a fetus; however, most reports of teratogenicity involve high doses used for chemotherapy or doses exceeding normal ranges [129,130]. A review of teratogenicity with low-dose oral methotrexate in early pregnancy found no effect [130]. No reports have linked any teratogenic effects to mifepristone.

Misoprostol, however, has been associated with multiple congenital anomalies whether used alone or with other agents, albeit the risk is low. Case reports suggesting its potential teratogenicity were first reported in 1991 from Brazil, where abortion is highly restricted and misoprostol was commonly used to induce abortion illegally [131]. Malformations most likely are due to disruption of the blood supply to the developing embryo during misoprostol-induced myometrial contractions. Central nervous system and limb defects are the most commonly reported anomalies, specifically Möbius syndrome, which is characterized by congenital facial paralysis with or without limb defects. A recent meta-analysis including 4,899 cases of congenital anomalies and 5,742 controls showed an increased risk for any congenital defect (OR = 3.56 [95% CI 0.98, 12.98]), Möbius sequence (OR = 25.31 [95% CI 11.11, 57.66]) and terminal transverse limb defects (OR = 11.86 [95% CI 4.86, 28.90]) [132].

Uterine rupture

Another concern about the use of medical abortion regimens using a prostaglandin analog is the risk of uterine rupture, especially in women with previous uterine scarring. Case reports of uterine rupture are rare in first-trimester medical abortion [133,134]. Four case series of women with prior uterine surgery (primarily cesarean sections) have been reported. These series include women who received mifepristone and oral misoprostol [135,136] and methotrexate and vaginal misoprostol [137] for medical abortion, and women who received vaginal misoprostol alone for treatment of early pregnancy failure [138]. They include a total of 392 women with no reported uterine rupture, giving a 95% confidence interval of 0 to 0.8%.

Acceptability

Early medical abortion is well accepted. Acceptability appears to be driven primarily by efficacy (i.e., when women are asked if a regimen is acceptable, they will view one with high efficacy positively) [139]. To no surprise, all studies that ask women if the experience was positive report a high percentage of favorable responses regardless of the regimen, typically with more than 80% of women finding the method acceptable [140–143].

Few studies have evaluated factors that affect acceptability. Findings are similar for all types of medical abortion regimens. Women who have had a prior surgical abortion are somewhat less likely to choose a medical method for a future abortion as compared to women who have never experienced a surgical abortion [142–144].

Although studies indicate that women prefer oral administration of misoprostol, this type of inquiry is questionable because it presumes that all else is equal (e.g., efficacy, side effects, risks). Accordingly, Lohr et al [89] attempted to evaluate factors beyond overall acceptability by asking women about their feelings regarding buccal administration of misoprostol. As expected, most women who used the mifepristone and buccal misoprostol regimen would choose the method again (91%), and almost all (97%) would recommend the option to a friend. With further open-ended questioning, however, 72% disliked the buccal route; only 6% said so because the regimen did not work. Forty-three per cent of women found the taste of buccal administration objectionable; 30% found buccal retention uncomfortable; and 10% experienced oral irritation, numbness, or oral ulcers.

Henshaw and colleagues [145] followed women who chose their method of abortion and those with no preference who were then randomized to the standard regimen of mifepristone and misoprostol or vacuum aspiration under general anesthesia. Although 95% of women who elected medical abortion would choose it again, only 74% of those randomized to medical abortion would choose that option again. A similar disparity was evident for women who had a surgical abortion; 90% of those who chose, and 87% of those who were randomized and received, a surgical abortion would choose that option again. The lower acceptability for women who were randomized to medical abortion only applied to those more than 49 days' gestation. This study suggests that women with no preference tend to be happy with either method early in pregnancy.

Interestingly, Creinin [146] randomized 50 women up to 49 days' gestation to medical or surgical abortion. The medical abortion regimen included methotrexate 50 mg/m^2 intramuscularly followed 5 to 6 days later by misoprostol 800 μg self-administered vaginally at home. The surgical abortion method involved manual vacuum aspiration with local anesthesia in the office. Of the women randomized to aspiration, 92% stated they would choose a surgical procedure for a next abortion, whereas only 63% of women randomized to a medical abortion would choose that option in the future ($p < 0.001$).

Conclusion

Mifepristone in combination with misoprostol or another prostaglandin analog is the most effective and efficient abortifacient combination. Acceptable gestational age limits for using mifepristone depend on the type and route of administration of the prostaglandin analog. Regimens using mifepristone with gemeprost are effective through 63 days' gestation. When mifepristone is combined with oral misoprostol 400 μg, complete abortion occurs in more than 90% of women through 49 days' gestation. Using misoprostol 800 μg vaginally results in high efficacy through 63 days' gestation or more. Although less studied, buccal or sublingual misoprostol administration appears to have similar efficacy to vaginal regimens, albeit with more side effects. Unlike vaginal administration, regimens with buccal misoprostol may not be effective with time intervals of less than 24 hours.

In some countries where mifepristone is not available, methotrexate and misoprostol can be effective for abortion up to 49 days'gestation when methotrexate is administered as either 50 mg/m^2 intramuscularly or 50 mg orally. As with mifepristone regimens, efficacy is highest under 42 days' gestation and appears to decrease after 49 days, but no sharp decline is evident at any particular gestational age. The overall efficacy of methotrexate regimens is achieved only with patience, as only about 60% to 75% of women expel the pregnancy during the week after misoprostol treatment.

The more commonly used alternative when mifepristone is not accessible is misoprostol alone. The recommended regimen up to 63 days' gestation is 800 μg vaginally every 3 to 24 hours for a maximum of three doses. As an alternative, sublingual misoprostol shows similar efficacy to the vaginal route when 800 μg is given at 3-hour, but not 12-hour, intervals. Side effects appear to occur more frequently following sublingual administration. When available, mifepristone regimens are preferable. Whereas the continuing pregnancy rate after mifepristone followed by a single vaginal dose of 800 μg misoprostol is less than 1% (Table 9.1) in pregnancies up to 9 weeks' gestation, it rises to 4 to 10% with misoprostol-alone regimens using vaginal or sublingual dosing (Table 9.3). Complete abortion rates are also about 10 to 15% higher with combination regimens.

Overall, medical abortion is effective, safe, and acceptable to women. Because most women find a regimen acceptable if it works, studies have begun to examine acceptability of misoprostol dosing methods in more depth. These studies suggest that buccal or sublingual dosing produces side effects that may make the regimens less acceptable than vaginal dosing. More research into what factors women feel are important other than efficacy will help us to provide the best medical abortion options for each patient.

References

1 Thiersch JB. Therapeutic abortions with a folic acid antagonist, 4-aminopteroyglutamic acid (4-amino P.G.A.) administered by the oral route. *Am J Obstet Gynecol* 1952; **63**: 1298–1304.

2 Karim SMM. Once-a-month vaginal administration of prostaglandins E2 and F2 alpha for fertility control. *Contraception* 1971; **3**: 173–183.

3 Mocsary P, Csapo AJ. Menstrual induction with PGF2 alpha and PGE2. *Prostaglandins* 1975; **10**: 545–547.

4 Smith SK, Baird DT. The use of 16-16 dimethyl trans delta 2 PGE1 methyl ester (ONO 802) vaginal suppositories for the termination of early pregnancy: a comparative study. *Br J Obstet Gynaecol* 1980; **87**: 712–717.

5 Bygdeman M, Christensen NJ, Gréen K, Zheng S, Lundström V. Termination of early pregnancy: future development. *Acta Obstet Gynecol Scand Suppl* 1983; **113**: 125–129.

6 Cameron IT, Baird DT. Early pregnancy termination: a comparison between vacuum aspiration and medical abortion using prostaglandin (16,16-dimethyl-trans-delta 2-PGE1 methyl ester) or the antiprogestogen RU 486. *Br J Obstet Gynaecol* 1988; **95**: 271–276.

7 Anonymous. Menstrual regulation by intramuscular injections of 16-phenoxy-tetranor PGE_2 methyl sulfonylamide or vacuum aspiration. A randomized multicentre study. World Health Organisation Task Force on Post-ovulatory Methods of Fertility Regulation. *Br J Obstet Gynaecol* 1987; **94**: 949–956.

8 Bygdeman M, Bremme K, Christensen N, Lundström V, Gréen K. A comparison of two stable prostaglandin E analogs for termination of early pregnancy and for cervical dilatation. *Contraception* 1980; **22**: 471–482.

9 Kovacs L, Sas M, Resch BA et al. Termination of very early pregnancy by RU 486: an antiprogestational compound. *Contraception* 1984; **29**: 399–410.

10 Bygdeman M, Swahn ML. Progesterone receptor blockage: effect on uterine contractility and early pregnancy. *Contraception* 1985; **32**: 45–51.

11 Shoupe D, Mishell DR Jr, Brenner PF, Spitz IM. Pregnancy termination with a high and medium dosage regimen of RU 486. *Contraception* 1986; **133**: 455–461.

12 Birgerson L, Odlind V. Early pregnancy termination with antiprogestins: a comparative clinical study of mifepristone given in two dose regimens and Epostane. *Fertil Steril* 1987; **48**: 565–570.

13 Swahn ML, Cekan S, Wang G, Lundstrom V, Bygdeman M. Pharmacokinetics and clinical studies of RU 486 for fertility regulation. In: Baulieu EE, Siegel S, eds. *The Antiprogestin Steroid RU 486 and Human Fertility Control.* Plenum, New York, 1985: 249–258.

14 Silvestre L, Dubois C, Renault M, Rezvani Y, Baulieu EE, Ulmann A. Voluntary interruption of pregnancy with mifepristone (RU 486) and a prostaglandin analogue: a large-scale French experience. *N Engl J Med* 1990; **322**: 645–648.

15 Ulmann A, Silvestre L, Chemama L et al. Medical termination of early pregnancy with mifepristone (RU 486) followed by a prostaglandin analogue: study in 16,369 women. *Acta Obstet Gynecol Scand* 1992; **71**: 278–283.

16 Hill NC, Ferguson J, MacKenzie IZ. The efficacy of oral mifepristone (RU 38,486) with a prostaglandin E1analog vaginal pessary for the termination of early pregnancy: complications and patient acceptability. *Am J Obstet Gynecol* 1990; **162**: 414–417.

17 Anonymous. The efficacy and tolerance of mifepristone and prostaglandin in first trimester termination of pregnancy. UK multicentre trial. *Br J Obstet Gynaecol* 1990; **97**: 480–486.

18 Anonymous. Termination of pregnancy with reduced doses of mifepristone. World Health Organisation Task Force on Post-ovulatory Methods of Fertility Regulation. *BMJ* 1993; **307**: 532–537.

19 Baird DT, Sukcharoen N, Thong KJ. Randomized trial of misoprostol and cervagem in combination with a reduced dose of mifepristone for induction of abortion. *Hum Reprod* 1995; **10**: 1521–1527.

20 Bartley J, Brown A, Elton R, Baird DT. Double-blind randomized trial of mifepristone in combination with vaginal gemeprost or misoprostol for induction of abortion up to 63 days' gestation. *Hum Reprod* 2001; **16**: 2098–2102.

21 World Health Organization. *Unsafe Abortion: Global and Regional Estimates of the Incidence of Unsafe Abortion and Associated Mortality in 2003.* 5th edn. World Health Organization, Geneva, 2007.

22 Jones RK, Henshaw SK. Mifepristone for early medical abortion: experiences in France, Great Britain, and Sweden. *Perspect Sex Reprod Health* 2002; **34**: 154–161.

23 Bygdeman M, Danielsson KG, Marions L. Medical termination of early pregnancy: the Swedish experience. *J Am Med Womens Assoc* 2000; **55** (Suppl.): 195–196.

24 Gamble SB, Strauss LT, Parker WY et al. Abortion surveillance–United States, 2005. *MMWR Surveill Summ* 2008; **57**: No. SS–13.

25 Jones RK, Zolna MR, Henshaw SK, Finer LB. Abortion in the United States: incidence and access to services, 2005. *Perspect Sex Reprod Health* 2008; **40**: 6–16.

26 Stovall TG, Ling FW, Buster JE. Reproductive performance after methotrexate treatment of ectopic pregnancy. *Am J Obstet Gynecol* 1990; **162**: 1620–1623.

27 Creinin MD, Darney PD. Methotrexate and misoprostol for early abortion. *Contraception* 1993; **48**: 339–348.

28 Faúndes A, Fiala C, Tang OS, Velasco A. Misoprostol for the termination of pregnancy up to 12 completed weeks of pregnancy. *Int J Gynaecol Obstet* 2007; **99** (Suppl.): S172–S177.

29 Faúndes A, Santos LC, Carvalho M, Gras C. Post-abortion complications after interruption of pregnancy with misoprostol. *Adv Contracep* 1996;**12**: 1–9.

30 Miller SE, Lehman T, Campbell M et al. Misoprostol and declining abortion-related morbidity in Santo Domingo, Dominican Republic: a temporal association. *BJOG* 2005; **112**: 1291–1296.

31 Csapo AI, Pulkkinen MO, Wiest WG. Effects of luteectomy and progesterone replacement therapy in early pregnant patients. *Am J Obstet Gynecol* 1973; **115**: 759–765.

32 Gravanis A, Schaison G, George M et al. Endometrial and pituitary responses to the steroidal antiprogestin RU 486 in postmenopausal women. *J Clin Endocrinol Metab* 1985; **60**: 156–163.

33 Garfield RE, Blennerhassett MG, Miller SM. Control of myometrial contractility: role and regulation of gap junctions. *Oxf Rev Reprod Biol* 1988; **10**: 436–490.

34 Swahn ML, Bygdeman M. The effect of the antiprogestin RU 486 on uterine contractility and sensitivity to prostaglandin and oxytocin. *Br J Obstet Gynaecol* 1988; **95**: 126–134.

35 Johannisson E, Oberholzer M, Swahn ML, Bygdeman M. Vascular changes in the human endometrium following the administration of the progesterone antagonist RU 486. *Contraception* 1989; **39**: 103–107.

36 Schindler AM, Zanon P, Obradovic D, Wyss R, Graff P, Herrmann WL. Early ultrastructural changes in RU-486-exposed decidua. *Gynecol Obstet Invest* 1985; **20**: 62–67.

37 Herrmann WL, Schindler AM, Wyss R, Bishof P. Effects of the antiprogesterone RU 486 in early pregnancy and during the menstrual cycle. In: Beaulieu EE, Siegel S, eds. *The Antiprogestin Steroid RU 486 and Human Fertility Control.* Plenum, New York, 1985: 259–262.

38 Avrech OM, Golan A, Weinraub Z, Bukovsky I, Caspi E. Mifepristone (RU486) alone or in combination with a prostaglandin analog for termination of early pregnancy: a review. *Fertil Steril* 1991; **56**: 385–393.

39 Land JA, Arends JW. Immunohistochemical analysis of estrogen and progesterone receptors in fallopian tubes during ectopic pregnancy. *Fertil Steril* 1992; **58**: 335–337.

40 Creinin MD, Schreiber CA, Bednarek P et al. Mifepristone and misoprostol administered simultaneously versus 24 hours apart

for abortion: a randomized controlled trial. *Obstet Gynecol* 2007; **109**: 885–894.

41 Shi YE, Ye ZH, He CH et al. Pharmacokinetic study of RU 486 and its metabolites after oral administration of single doses to pregnant and nonpregnant women. *Contraception* 1993; **48**: 133–149.

42 Lähteenmäki P, Heikinheimo O, Croxatto H et al. Pharmacokinetics and metabolism of RU 486. *J Steroid Biochem* 1987; **27**: 859–863.

43 Heikinheimo O, Lähteenmäki PL, Koivunen E et al. Metabolism and serum binding of RU 486 in women after various single doses. *Hum Reprod* 1987; **2**: 379–385.

44 Heikinheimo O. Pharmacokinetics of the antiprogesterone RU 486 in women during multiple dose administration. *J Steroid Biochem* 1989; **32**: 21–25.

45 Heikinheimo O, Tevilin M, Shoupe D, Croxatto H, Lähteenmäki P. Quantitation of RU 486 in human plasma by HPLC and RIA after column chromatography. *Contraception* 1986; **34**: 613–624.

46 Philibert D, Moguilewsky M, Bonnat C et al. (1986) Influence of human alpha-1-acid glycoprotein (AAG) on pharmacokinetics and biologic activity of RU 486. In: *Abstracts of the 68th Meeting of the Endocrine Society*. The Endocrine Society, Bethesda, MD, 1986: 282.

47 Heikinheimo O, Ylikorkala O, Turpeinen U, Lähteenmäki P. Pharmacokinetics of the antiprogesterone RU 486: no correlation to clinical performance of RU 486. *Acta Endocrinol* 1990; **123**: 298–304.

48 Walden PA, Bagshawe KD. Reproductive performance of women successfully treated for gestational trophoblastic tumors. *Am J Obstet Gynecol* 1976; **125**: 1108–1114.

49 Creinin MD, Krohn MA. Methotrexate pharmacokinetics and effects in women receiving methotrexate and misoprostol for early abortion. *Am J Obstet Gynecol* 1997; **177**: 1444–1449.

50 Lara D, Abuabara K, Grossman D, Díaz-Olavarrieta C. Pharmacy provision of medical abortifacients in a Latin American city. *Contraception* 2006; **74**: 394–399.

51 Schoenhard G, Oppermann J, Kohn FE. Metabolism and pharmacokinetic studies of misoprostol. *Dig Dis Sci* 1985; **30** (Suppl.): 126S–128S.

52 Karim A. Antiulcer prostaglandin misoprostol: single and multiple dose pharmacokinetic profile. *Prostaglandins* 1987; **33** (Suppl.): 40–50.

53 Karim A, Rozek LF, Smith ME, Kowalski KG. Effects of food and antacid on oral absorption of misoprostol, a synthetic prostaglandin E1 analog. *J Clin Pharmacol* 1989; **29**: 439–443.

54 Zieman M, Fong SK, Benowitz NL, Bankster D, Darney PD. Absorption kinetics of misoprostol with oral or vaginal administration. *Obstet Gynecol* 1997; **90**: 88–92.

55 Tang OS, Schweer H, Seyberth HW, Lee SW, Ho PC. Pharmacokinetics of different routes of administration of misoprostol. *Hum Reprod* 2002; **17**: 332–336.

56 Khan RU, El-Refaey H, Sharma S, Sooranna D, Stafford M. Oral, rectal, and vaginal pharmacokinetics of misoprostol. *Obstet Gynecol* 2004; **103**: 866–870.

57 Meckstroth KR, Whitaker AK, Bertisch S, Goldberg AB, Darney PD. Misoprostol administered by epithelial routes: drug absorption and uterine response. *Obstet Gynecol* 2006; **108**: 582–590.

58 Danielsson KG, Marions L, Rodriguez A, Spur BW, Wong PYK, Bygdeman M. Comparison between oral and vaginal administration of misoprostol on uterine contractility. *Obstet Gynecol* 1999; **93**: 275–280.

59 Aronsson A, Fiala C, Stephansson O et al. Pharmacokinetic profiles up to 12 h after administration of vaginal, sublingual, and slow-release oral misoprostol. *Hum Reprod* 2007; **22**: 1912–1918.

60 Schaff EA, DiCenzo R, Fielding SL. Comparison of misoprostol plasma concentrations following buccal and sublingual administration. *Contraception* 2005; **71**: 22–25.

61 Tang OS, Gemzell-Danielsson K, Ho PC. Pharmacokinetic profiles, effects on the uterus and side-effects. *Int J Gynaecol Obstet* 2007; **99** (Suppl.): S160–S167.

62 Peyron R, Aubény E, Targosz V et al. Early termination of pregnancy with mifepristone (RU 486) and the orally active prostaglandin misoprostol. *N Engl J Med* 1993; **328**: 1509–1513.

63 Spitz IM, Bardin CW, Benton L, Robbins A. Early pregnancy termination with mifepristone and misoprostol in the United States. *N Engl J Med* 1998; **338**: 1241–1247.

64 Aubény E, Peyron R, Turpin C et al. Termination of early pregnancy (up to and after 63 days of amenorrhea) with mifepristone and increasing doses of misoprostol. *Int J Fertil* 1995; **40** (Suppl.): 85–91.

65 Coyaji K, Krishna U, Amberdekar S et al. Are two doses of misoprostol after mifepristone for early abortion better than one? *BJOG* 2007; **114**: 271–278.

66 McKinley C, Thong KJ, Baird DT. The effect of dose of mifepristone and gestation on the efficacy of medical abortion with mifepristone and misoprostol. *Hum Reprod* 1993; **8**: 1502–1505.

67 Anonymous. Comparison of two doses of mifepristone in combination with misoprostol for early medical abortion. A randomised trial. World Health Organisation Task Force on Post-ovulatory Methods of Fertility Regulation. *BJOG* 2000; **107**: 524–530.

68 Thong KJ, Baird DT. Induction of abortion with mifepristone and misoprostol in early pregnancy. *Br J Obstet Gynaecol* 1992; **99**: 1004–1007.

69 Shannon CS, Winikoff B, Hausknecht R et al. Multicenter trial of a simplified mifepristone medical abortion regimen. *Obstet Gynecol* 2005; **105**: 345–351.

70 Schaff EA, Fielding SL, Westhoff C. Randomized trial of oral versus vaginal misoprostol at one day after mifepristone for early medical abortion. *Contraception* 2001; **64**: 81–85.

71 Middleton T, Schaff E, Fielding SL et al. Randomized trial of mifepristone and buccal or vaginal misoprostol for abortion through 56 days of the last menstrual period. *Contraception* 2005; **72**: 328–332.

72 Winikoff B, Dzuba IG, Creinin MD, et al. Two distinct oral routes of misoprostol in mifepristone medical abortion. A randomized controlled trial. *Obstet Gynecol* 2008; **112**: 1303–1310.

73 Hamoda H, Ashok PW, Flett GM, Templeton A. A randomised controlled trial of mifepristone in combination with misoprostol administered sublingually or vaginally for medical abortion up to 13 weeks of gestation. *BJOG* 2005; **112**: 1102–1108.

74 Singh KC, Ummat S, Rajaram S, Goel N. First trimester abortion with mifepristone and three doses of sublingual misoprostol: a pilot study. *Aust N Z J Obstet Gynaecol* 2005; **45**: 495–498.

75 Lin M, Li YT, Chen FM et al. Use of mifepristone and sublingual misoprostol for early medical abortion. *Taiwan J Obstet Gynecol* 2006; **45**: 321–324.

76 Hamoda H, Ashok PW, Flett GM, Templeton A. Medical abortion at 9–13 weeks' gestation: a review of 1,076 consecutive cases. *Contraception* 2005; **71**: 327–332.

77 Garbin O, Vayssiere C, Bettahar-Lebugle K, Nisand I. Consistency of medical abortion efficacy from 5 through 14 weeks' gestation. *Eur J Obstet Gynecol Reprod Biol* 2006; **129**: 36–40.

78 Bracken H, Ngoc NTN, Schaff E et al. Mifepristone followed in 24 hours to 48 hours by misoprostol for late first-trimester abortion. *Obstet Gynecol* 2007; **109**: 895–901.

79 Schaff EA, Eisinger SH, Stadalius LS, Franks P, Gore BZ, Poppema S. Low-dose mifepristone 200 mg and vaginal misoprostol for abortion. *Contraception* 1999; **59**: 1–6.

80 Schaff EA, Fielding SL, Eisinger SH, Stadalius LS, Fuller L. Low-dose mifepristone followed by vaginal misoprostol at 48 hours for abortion up to 63 days. *Contraception* 2000; **61**: 41–46.

81 Fiala C, Winikoff B, Helström L, Hellborg M, Gemzell-Danielsson K. Acceptability of home-use of misoprostol in medical abortion. *Contraception* 2004; **70**: 387–392.

82 Clark WH, Hassoun D, Gemzell-Danielsson K, Fiala C, Winikoff B. Home use of two doses of misoprostol after mifepristone for medical abortion: a pilot study in Sweden and France. *Eur J Contracept Reprod Health Care* 2005; **10**: 184–191.

83 Harwood B, Meckstroth KR, Mishell DR, Jain JK. Serum beta-human chorionic gonadotropin levels and endometrial thickness after medical abortion. *Contraception* 2001; **63**: 255–256.

84 Luise C, Jermy, K, Collons WP, Bourne TH. Expectant management of incomplete, spontaneous first-trimester miscarriage: outcome according to initial ultrasound criteria and value of follow-up visits. *Ultrasound Obstet Gynecol* 2002; **19**: 580–582.

85 Cowett AA, Cohen LS, Lichtenberg ES, Stika CS. Ultrasound evaluation of the endometrium after medical termination of pregnancy. *Obstet Gynecol* 2004; **103**: 871–875.

86 Reynolds A, Ayres-de-Campos D, Costa MA, Montenegro N. How should success be defined when attempting medical resolution of first-trimester missed abortion? *Eur J Obstet Gynecol Reprod Biol* 2005; **118**: 71–76.

87 Reeves MF, Lohr PA, Harwood BJ, Creinin MD. Ultrasonographic endometrial thickness after medical and surgical management of early pregnancy failure. *Obstet Gynecol* 2008; **111**: 106–112.

88 Creinin MD, Fox MC, Teal S et al. A randomized comparison of misoprostol 6 to 8 hours versus 24 hours after mifepristone for abortion. *Obstet Gynecol* 2004; **103**: 851–859.

89 Lohr PA, Reeves M, Hayes JL, Harwood B, Creinin MD. Oral mifepristone and buccal misoprostol administered simultaneously for abortion. *Contraception* 2007; **76**: 215–220.

90 Guest J, Chien PFW, Thomson MA, Kosseim ML. Randomised controlled trial comparing the efficacy of same-day administration of mifepristone and misoprostol for termination of pregnancy with the standard 36- to 48-hour protocol. *BJOG* 2007; **114**: 207–215.

91 Schaff EA, Fielding SL, Westhoff C et al. Vaginal misoprostol administered 1, 2, or 3 days after mifepristone for early medical abortion: a randomized trial. *JAMA* 2000b; **284**: 1948–1953.

92 Creinin MD, Schwartz JL, Pymar HC, Fink W. Efficacy of mifepristone followed on the same day by misoprostol for early termination of pregnancy: report of a randomised trial. *BJOG* 2001; **108**: 469–473.

93 Wiebe ER, Trouton KJ, Lima R. Misoprostol alone vs. methotrexate followed by misoprostol for early abortion. *Int J Gynaecol Obstet* 2006; **95**: 286–287.

94 Aldrich T, Winikoff B. Does methotrexate confer a significant advantage over misoprostol alone for early medical abortion? A retrospective analysis of 8,678 abortions. *BJOG* 2007; **114**: 555–562.

95 Wiebe ER, Trouton K. Comparing vaginal and buccal misoprostol when used after methotrexate for early abortion. *Contraception* 2004; **70**: 463–466.

96 Wiebe E, Dunn S, Guilbert E, Jacot F, Lugtig L. Comparison of abortions induced by methotrexate or mifepristone followed by misoprostol. *Obstet Gynecol* 2002; **99**: 813–819.

97 Blanchard K, Shochet T, Coyaji K, Thi Nhu Ngoc N, Winikoff B. Misoprostol alone for early abortion: an evaluation of seven potential regimens. *Contraception* 2005; **72**: 91–97.

98 von Hertzen H, Piaggio G, Huong NT et al. Efficacy of two intervals and two routes of administration of misoprostol for termination of early pregnancy: a randomised controlled equivalence trial. *Lancet* 2007; **369**: 1938–1946.

99 Carbonell JLL, Varela L, Velazco A, Tanda R, Cabezas E, Sánchez C. Early abortion with 800 μg of misoprostol by the vaginal route. *Contraception* 1999; **59**: 219–225.

100 Carbonell Esteve JL, Varela L, Velazco A, Cabezas E, Tanda R, Sánchez C. Vaginal misoprostol for late first trimester abortion. *Contraception* 1998; **57** : 329–333.

101 Carbonell JL, Velazco L, Varela L et al. Misoprostol for abortion at 9–12 weeks' gestation in adolescents. *Eur J Contracept Repro Health Care* 2001; **6**: 39–45.

102 Jain JK, Dutton C, Harwood B, Meckstroth KR, Mishell DR Jr. A prospective, randomized, double-blinded, placebo-controlled trial comparing mifepristone and vaginal misoprostol to vaginal misoprostol alone for elective termination of early pregnancy. *Hum Reprod* 2002; **17**: 1477–1482.

103 Creinin MD, Wiebe E, Gold M. Methotrexate and misoprostol for early abortion in adolescent women. *J Pediatr Adolesc Gynecol* 1999; **12**: 71–77.

104 Velazco A, Varela L Tanda, R et al. Misoprostol for abortion up to 9 weeks in adolescents. *Eur J Contracep Reprod Health Care* 2000; **5**: 227–233.

105 Winikoff B, Sivin I, Koyaji KJ et al. Safety, efficacy, and acceptability of medical abortion in China, Cuba, and India: a comparative trial of mifepristone-misoprostol versus surgical abortion. *Am J Obstet Gynecol* 1997; **176**: 431–437.

106 Ashok PW, Penney GC, Flett GM, Templeton A. An effective regimen for early medical abortion: a report of 2000 consecutive cases. *Hum Reprod* 1998; **13**: 2962–2965.

107 Hakim-Elahi E, Tovell HM, Burnhill MS. Complications of first-trimester abortion: a report of 170,000 cases. *Obstet Gynecol* 1990; **76**: 129–135.

108 Hayes JL, Achilles S, Reeves MF, Creinin MD. Outcomes of medical abortion through 63 days in women with twin gestations. *Contraception* 2008; **78**: 168–169.

109 American College of Obstetricians and Gynecologists. ACOG practice bulletin. Clinical management guidelines of obstetrician-gynecologists. Number 67, October 2005. Medical management of abortion. *Obstet Gynecol* 2005; **106**: 871–872.

110 National Abortion Federation. NAF protocol for mifepristone/misoprostol in early abortion [Online]. Washington, DC: National Abortion Federation; 2008 [cited 2008 Aug 15]. 6 p. Available from: URL:http://www.prochoice.org/pubs_research/publications/downloads/professional_education/medical_abortion/protocol_mife_miso.pdf

111 Abdel-Aleem H, Villar J, Gülmezoglu AM et al. The pharmacokinetics of the prostaglandin E1 analog misoprostol in plasma and colostrum after postpartum oral administration. *Eur J Obstet Gynecol Reprod Biol* 2003; **108**: 25–28.

112 Paul M, Stewart F. (2007) Abortion. In: Hatcher RA, Trussell J, Nelson AL, Cates W Jr., Stewart FH, Kowal D, eds. *Contraceptive Technology*, 19th ed. Ardent Media, New York, 2007.

113 Davis A, Westhoff C, De Nonno L. Bleeding patterns after early abortion with mifepristone and misoprostol or manual vacuum aspiration. *J Am Med Womens Assoc* 2000; **55** (Suppl.): 141–144.

114 Creinin MD, Shulman T. Effect of nonsteroidal antiinflammatory drugs on the action of misoprostol in a regimen for early abortion. *Contraception* 1997; **56**: 165–168.

115 Creinin MD, Vittinghoff E, Keder L, Darney PD, Tiller G. Methotrexate and misoprostol for early abortion: a multicenter trial. I. Safety and efficacy. *Contraception* 1996; **53**: 321–327.

116 Creinin MD, Vittinghoff E, Schaff E, Klaisle C, Darney PD, Dean C. Medical abortion with oral methotrexate and vaginal misoprostol. Obstet Gynecol 1997; **90**: 611–616.

117 Creinin MD. Change in serum beta-human chorionic gonadotropin after abortion with methotrexate and misoprostol. *Am J Obstet Gynecol* 1996; **174**: 776–778.

118 Clark W, Panton T, Hann L, Gold M. Medication abortion employing routine sequential measurements of serum hCG and sonography only when indicated. *Contraception* 2007; **75**: 131–135.

119 Fiala C, Safar P, Bygdeman M, Gemzell-Danielsson K. Verifying the effectiveness of medical abortion: ultrasound versus hCG testing. *Eur Obstet Gynecol Reprod Biol* 2003; **109**: 190–195.

120 Godfrey EM, Anderson A, Fielding SL, Meyn L, Creinin MD. Clinical utility of urine pregnancy assays to determine medical abortion outcome is limited. *Contraception* 2007; **75**: 378–382.

121 Rossi B, Creinin MD, Meyn LA. Ability of the clinician and patient to predict the outcome of mifepristone and misoprostol medical abortion. *Contraception* 2004; **70**: 313–317.

122 Schaff EA, Fielding SL, Westhoff C. Randomized trial of oral versus vaginal misoprostol 2 days after mifepristone 200 mg for abortion up to 63 days of pregnancy. *Contraception* 2002; **66**: 247–250.

123 Shannon C, Brothers P, Philip NM, Winikoff B. Infection after medical abortion: a review of the literature. *Contraception* 2004; **70**: 183–190.

124 Isaacs JD Jr, McGehee RP, Cowan BD. Life-threatening neutropenia following methotrexate treatment of ectopic pregnancy: a report of two cases. *Obstet Gynecol* 1996; **88**: 694–696.

125 Sawaya GF, Grady D, Kerlikowske K, Grimes DA. Antibiotics at the time of induced abortion: the case for universal prophylaxis based on a meta-analysis. *Obstet Gynecol* 1996; **87**: 884–890.

126 Fischer M, Bhatnagar J, Guarner J et al. Fatal toxic shock syndrome associated with Clostridium sordellii after medical abortion. *N Eng J Med* 2005; **353**: 2352–2360.

127 Cohen AL, Bhatnagar J, Reagan S et al. Toxic shock associated with *Clostridium sordellii* and *Clostridium perfringens* after medical and spontaneous abortion. *Obstet Gynecol* 2007; **110**: 1027–1033.

128 Zane SB, Berg CJ. Deaths from *Clostridium sordellii* after medical abortion. *New Engl J Med* 2006; **354**: 1645–1647.

129 Darab DJ, Minkoff R, Sciote J, Sulik KK. Pathogenesis of median facial clefts in mice treated with methotrexate. *Teratology* 1987; **36**: 77–86.

130 Kozlowski RD, Steinbrunner JV, MacKenzie AH, Clough JD, Wilke WS, Segal AM. Outcome of first-trimester exposure to low-dose methotrexate in eight patients with rheumatic disease. *Am J Med* 1990; **88**: 589–592.

131 Fonseca W, Alencar AJ, Mota FS, Coelho HL. Misoprostol and congenital malformations. *Lancet* 1991; **338**: 56.

132 da Silva Dal Pizzol T, Knop FP, Mengue SS. Prenatal exposure to misoprostol and congenital anomalies: systematic review and meta-analysis. *Reprod Toxicol* 2006; **22**: 666–671.

133 Kim JO, Han JY, Choi JS et al. Oral misoprostol and uterine rupture in the first trimester of pregnancy: a case report. *Reprod Toxicol* 2005; **20**: 575–577.

134 Jwarah E, Greenhalf JO. Rupture of the uterus after 800 micrograms misoprostol given vaginally for termination of pregnancy. *BJOG* 2000; **107**: 807.

135 Gao P, Wang P. Clinical observation on termination of early pregnancy of 213 cases after caesarian section with repeated

use of mifepristone and misoprostol. *Reprod Contracept* 1999; **10**: 227–233.

136 Xu J, Chen H, Ma T, Wu X. Termination of early pregnancy in the scarred uterus with mifepristone and misoprostol. *Int J Gynaecol Obstet* 2001; **72**: 245–251.

137 Gautam R, Agrawal V. Early medical termination pregnancy with methotrexate and misoprostol in lower segment cesarean section cases. *J Obstet Gynaecol Res* 2003; **29**: 251–256.

138 Chen BA, Reeves MF, Creinin MD et al. Misoprostol for treatment of early pregnancy failure in women with previous uterine surgery. *Am J Obstet Gynecol* 2008; **198**: 626.e1–5.

139 Lohr P, Reeves M, Creinin M. Eliciting women's preferences in medical abortion treatment using willingness to pay. *Contraception* 2007; **76**: 164.

140 Holmgren K. Women's evaluation of three early abortion methods. *Acta Obstet Gynecol Scand* 1992; **71**: 616–623.

141 Bachelot A, Cludy L, Spira A. Conditions for choosing between drug-induced and surgical abortions. *Contraception* 1992; **45**: 547–559.

142 Creinin MD, Park M. Acceptability of abortion with methotrexate and misoprostol. *Contraception* 1995; **52**: 41–44.

143 Creinin MD, Burke AE. Methotrexate and misoprostol for early abortion: a multicenter trial: acceptability. *Contraception* 1996; **54**: 19–22.

144 Tang GWK, Lau OW, Yip P. Further acceptability evaluation of RU486 and ONO 802 as abortifacient agents in a Chinese population. *Contraception* 1993; **48**: 267–276.

145 Henshaw RC, Naji SA, Russell IT, Templeton AA. Comparison of medical abortion with surgical vacuum aspiration: women's preferences and acceptability of treatment. *BMJ* 1993; **307**: 714–717.

146 Creinin MD. Randomized comparison of efficacy, acceptability, and cost of medical versus surgical abortion. *Contraception* 2000; **62**: 117–124.

147 Tang OS, Chan CC, Ng EH, Lee SW, Ho PC. A prospective, randomized, placebo-controlled trial on the use of mifepristone with sublingual or vaginal misoprostol for medical abortions of less than 9 weeks gestation. *Hum Reprod* 2003; **18**: 2315–2318.

148 von Hertzen H, Honkanen H, Piaggio G et al. WHO multinational study of three misoprostol regimens after mifepristone for early medical abortion. I: Efficacy. *BJOG* 2003; **110**: 808–818.

149 Shannon C, Wiebe E, Jacot F et al. Regimens of misoprostol with mifepristone for early medical abortion: a randomised trial. *BJOG* 2006; **113**: 621–628.

150 Hausknecht RU. Methotrexate and misoprostol to terminate early pregnancy. *New Engl J Med* 1995; **333**: 537–540.

151 Creinin MD, Vittinghoff E, Galbraith S, Klaisle C. A randomized trial comparing misoprostol three and seven days after methotrexate for early abortion. *Am J Obstet Gynecol* 1995; **173**: 1578–1584.

152 Creinin MD. Medical abortion with methotrexate 75 mg intramuscularly and vaginal misoprostol. *Contraception* 1997; **56**: 367–371.

153 Carbonell JL, Velazco A, Varela L, Cabezas E, Fernández C, Sánchez C. Misoprostol 3,4, or 5 days after methotrexate for early abortion. A randomized trial. *Contraception* 1997; **56**: 169–174.

154 Wiebe ER. Oral methotrexate compared with injected methotrexate when used with misoprostol for abortion. *Am J Obstet Gynecol* 1999; **181**: 149–152.

155 Creinin MD, Carbonell JL, Schwartz JL, Varela L, Tanda R. A randomized trial of the effect of moistening misoprostol before vaginal administration when used with methotrexate for abortion. *Contraception* 1999; **59**: 11–16.

156 Carbonell Esteve JL, Varela L, Velazco A, Tanda R, Sánchez C. 25 mg or 50 mg of oral methotrexate followed by vaginal misoprostol 7 days after for early abortion. *Gynecol Obstet Invest* 1999; **47**: 182–187.

157 Borgatta L, Burnhill MS, Tyson J, Leonhardt KK, Hausknecht RU, Haskell S. Early medical abortion with methotrexate and misoprostol. *Obstet Gynecol* 2001; **97**: 11–16.

158 Jain JK, Meckstroth KR, Mishell DR Jr. Early pregnancy termination with intravaginally administered sodium chloride solution-moistened misoprostol tablets: historical comparison with mifepristone and oral misoprostol. *Am J Obstet Gynecol* 1999; **181**: 1386–1391.

159 Ngai SW, Tang OS, Chan YM, Ho PC. Vaginal misoprostol alone for medical abortion up to 9 weeks of gestation: efficacy and acceptability. *Hum Reprod* 2000; **15**: 1159–1162.

160 Bugalho A, Mocumbi S, Faúndes A, David E. Termination of pregnancies of <6 weeks' gestation with a single dose of 800 microg of vaginal misoprostol. *Contraception* 2000; **61**: 47–50.

161 Jain JK, Harwood B, Meckstroth KR, Mishell DR Jr. Early pregnancy termination with vaginal misoprostol combined with loperamide and acetaminophen prophylaxis. *Contraception* 2001; **63**: 217–221.

162 Zikopoulos KA, Papanikolaou EG, Kalantaridou SN et al. Early pregnancy termination with vaginal misoprostol before and after 42 days gestation. *Hum Reprod* 2002; **17**: 3079–3083.

163 Carbonell JL, Rodriguez J, Velazco A et al. Oral and vaginal misoprostol 800 microg every 8 h for early abortion. *Contraception* 2003; **67**: 457–462.

164 Singh K, Fong YF, Dong F. A viable alternative to surgical vacuum aspiration: repeated doses of intravaginal misoprostol over 9 hours for medical termination of pregnancies up to eight weeks. *BJOG* 2003; **110**: 175–180.

10

CHAPTER 10 First-trimester aspiration abortion

Karen Meckstroth MD, MPH, and Maureen Paul MD, MPH

LEARNING POINTS

- When using misoprostol for preprocedure cervical preparation, 400 μg vaginally 3 to 4 hours prior to aspiration abortion is the optimum regimen.
- Clinicians may perform aspiration abortion very early in pregnancy, even before ultrasound reveals a gestational sac, if meticulous tissue examination and appropriate follow-up are employed to ensure complete evacuation of the pregnancy.
- The uterine aspirate must be examined to identify chorionic villi, gestational sac or membranes, and in the later first trimester, fetal parts.
- Perioperative antibiotics reduce infection with aspiration abortion, even in low-risk women.

Introduction

Approximately one in five pregnancies worldwide end in abortion. The likelihood that a woman will have an abortion is similar if she lives in a developed or developing area of the world. Western Europe has the lowest abortion rate in the world (12 per 1,000 women aged 15 to 44). The rate is 17 in Northern Europe and 21 in Northern America [1]. In 2005, approximately 1.2 million women obtained abortions in the USA, making abortion one of the most common medical procedures provided to women of reproductive age [2].

Approximately 90% of abortions in the USA occur during the first trimester. Advances in pregnancy testing, ultrasonography, and medical and surgical abortion techniques have accelerated the trend toward earlier abortion care, with the proportion of abortions obtained during the first 6 weeks of gestation doubling from 14% in 1992 to 29% in 2005 [3]. The remarkable safety and technical simplicity of early modern induced abortion place it well within the scope of practice of diverse types of clinicians. Although nonphysicians are often proscribed from providing abortions in the USA (Chapter 4), data from around the world indicate that appropriately trained clinicians can provide first-trimester aspiration or medical abortion with an impressive safety record [4–9].

Virtually all modern first-trimester surgical abortions are accomplished by vacuum aspiration [3], with dilation and sharp curettage (D&C) confined to some countries where abortion is illegal. Manual vacuum aspiration (MVA), once a technology more common in low-resource settings, is now widely used and often preferred by providers in developed countries [10].Even in developing countries with restrictive abortion laws, increasing use of MVA and medical abortion methods has reduced abortion-related mortality [11,12].

This chapter focuses on vacuum aspiration throughout the first trimester, which has been variably defined as ending at 12 or 13 completed weeks of gestation. The chapter addresses current practices, acceptable variations in technique, and approaches to uterine evacuation in very early pregnancy. Although we use the terminology *surgical abortion* at times, *aspiration abortion* more accurately reflects the procedure [13].

Historical perspective

Vacuum methods for uterine evacuation were first described in the latter half of the 19th century. In 1872, Sir James Young Simpson, the Scottish obstetrician to Queen Victoria, fashioned a "tube resembling in length and size a male catheter, with a large number of thickly-set small orifices stretching along for about two inches from its extremity." Attaching "an exhausting syringe" to this primitive cannula, Simpson used "a few strokes of the piston of the syringe" to perform the first reported endometrial aspiration [14]. More than 50 years passed before this method was applied to pregnancy interruption: in 1927, Bykov, a Russian physician, used a handheld syringe to induce menstruation [15].

Management of Unintended and Abnormal Pregnancy, 1st edition. By M Paul, ES Lichtenberg, L Borgatta, DA Grimes, PG Stubblefield, MD Creinin
 ISBN: 9781405176965.

In 1934, Hungarian Bela Lorinez added electric suction for sampling endometrium [16].

Greater dissemination of the vacuum aspiration technique began in the late 1950s. Shortly after China removed restrictions on abortion in 1957, two case series of induced abortion by electric vacuum aspiration appeared in *The Chinese Journal of Obstetrics and Gynecology* [17,18]. In the 1960s, clinicians from Eastern Europe and Great Britain reported favorable experiences as well. The Czechoslovakian physician Vojta [19] and the British tandem Kerslake and Casey [20] published their series in US journals; the latter are credited with introducing this technique in North America. In the early 1970s, California psychologist Harvey Karman introduced inexpensive, disposable, flexible plastic cannulae for aspiration abortion that were smaller and more pliable than their metal counterparts. Karman and Potts [21] reported their success using a manual aspiration method for early abortion in 1972.

Vacuum aspiration soon became the most common method of first-trimester abortion in the USA and other developed countries, proving superior to traditional D&C in speed, comfort, and safety [22–24]. During the past decade, several developing countries have introduced manual vacuum aspiration for abortion as well, in keeping with the World Health Organization's recommendation that suction methods replace sharp curettage as the safe standard for first-trimester surgical abortion [25].

Safety—morbidity and mortality

As a result of abortion surveillance efforts initiated in the USA by the Centers for Disease Control and Prevention (CDC) in the late 1960s, "We have come to know more about legally induced abortion than any other operation"[26]. The CDC collects data on abortion incidence and demographics from state health departments, and it ascertains abortion-related deaths using numerous sources. Reporting is voluntary, and depending on the year, three or four states (including California where more than 23% of US abortions occur) do not provide abortion data to the CDC [3]. Organizations such as the Guttmacher Institute perform additional surveillance, integrating surveys of all known abortion providers with CDC data.

Notwithstanding these limitations, CDC surveillance clearly demonstrates a dramatic drop in abortion-related mortality following nationwide legalization of abortion. The case-fatality rate for legal induced abortion decreased approximately 80% between 1972 and 1980, from 4.1 to 0.7 deaths per 100,000 abortions, and it has remained essentially stable since [3]. Today, the risk of death from legal induced abortion is less than that from an injection of penicillin [27] and substantially below the risk of carrying a pregnancy to term (Fig. 10.1). Infection and anesthesia complications comprise the most frequent causes of death from

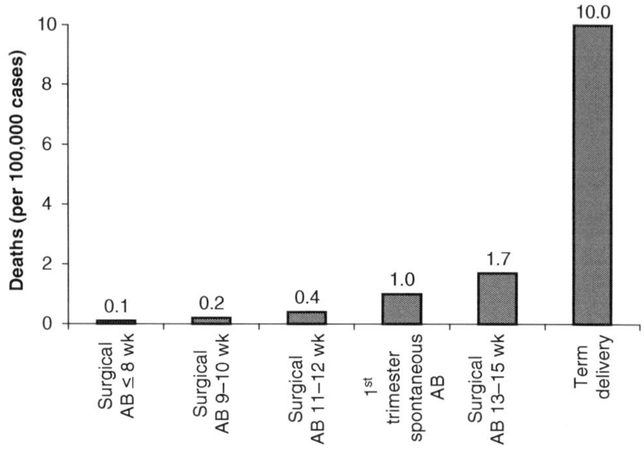

Figure 10.1 USA mortality rates (deaths per 100,000 induced abortions, spontaneous abortions, or deliveries). AB = abortions; wk = weeks. (Data from Bartlett et al [28], Saraiya et al [29], Christiansen and Collins [30], Grimes [31].).

first-trimester aspiration abortion in the USA (Fig. 10.2) [28]. When abortions take place under unsafe conditions, as they do for half of the abortions worldwide, deaths and serious complications are much more common (Chapter 2). The CDC discontinued its research on nonfatal complications of abortion in the early 1980s, after its numerous large prospective studies clearly documented the safety of legal induced abortion. Subsequent studies by various investigators that include newer surgical or medical approaches have confirmed that serious complications from early abortion are rare (Chapter 15). Of women having first-trimester surgical abortions, 97% report no complications; 2.5% have minor complications that can be handled at the medical office or abortion facility; and less than 0.5% have more serious complications that require some additional surgical procedure or hospitalization [32].

Data on long-term sequelae provide reassurance as well (Chapter 16). Accumulated research on first-trimester vacuum aspiration shows that it poses virtually no risk of infertility, ectopic pregnancy, spontaneous abortion, or preterm or low-birth-weight delivery [33–36]. Less extensive evidence suggests that repeat aspiration abortion poses no

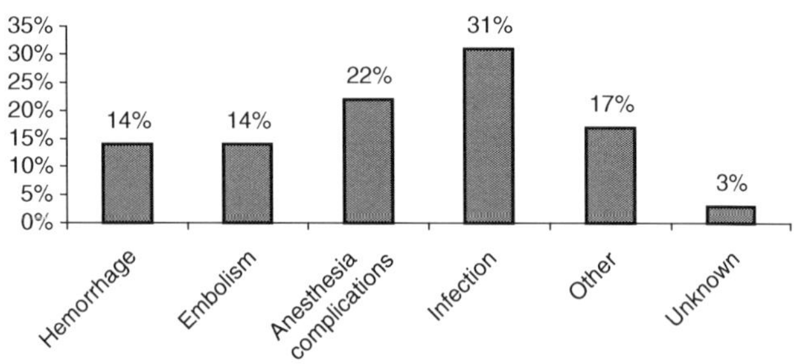

Figure 10.2 Causes of death for first-trimester aspiration abortion in the USA, 1988–1997. (Data from Bartlett et al [28].).

additional risk [37]. Exhaustive reviews by US and British government expert panels have found no association between abortion and breast cancer, and no data indicate that abortion is a risk factor for other types of cancer [37]. In repeated studies since the early 1980s, leading experts and organizations such as the American Psychiatric Association have concluded that abortion does not pose a hazard to women's mental health [38].

Service settings

Worldwide, laws often specify where abortions may take place and who may perform them. In Great Britain and India, for example, abortions must take place in government hospitals or authorized health care facilities. Most abortions in the USA are provided in freestanding clinics; in 2005, only 5% occurred in hospitals, down from 22% in 1980, and only 2% took place in physicians' offices [2]. First-trimester aspiration abortions performed in an office or clinic are as safe as those performed in hospitals [39] and considerably less expensive [2,40].

The freestanding clinic model holds some benefits for patients and clinicians including uniformly pro-choice staff, cost, efficiency, and a supportive, high-volume training environment [8]. This service model, however, marginalizes abortion from mainstream medical care and may make providers and patients more susceptible to antiabortion harassment and violence [8,41]. Integration of early abortion services into primary care practice settings mitigates these drawbacks and optimizes continuity of care. Hospitals offer a critical alternative for women who have serious medical conditions or require intensive anesthesia, and they serve as the primary venue for abortion care in many countries.

Aspiration abortion using local anesthesia with or without oral or moderate ("conscious") intravenous (IV) sedation can be provided safely and appropriately in outpatient settings with only modest changes, if any, in infrastructure and supplies. Although the National Abortion Federation (NAF) and the American College of Obstetricians and Gynecologists (ACOG) do not recommend specific appointment timelines, the British Royal College of Obstetricians and Gynaecologists (RCOG) advises that assessment appointments for abortions occur within 5 days of contact and maximally within 2 weeks. Ideally, abortion should be available within 7 days of the woman's decision to proceed [42].

The type and number of staff needed depends in part on the methods of abortion offered, available pain management options, and abortion volume. Clinics with higher patient volumes usually employ dedicated health educators or counselors who explore the abortion decision with patients and provide verbal and written information regarding the procedure, its alternatives, and the benefits and risks of each (Chapter 5). In smaller settings, medical assistants, nurses, or physicians may assume these responsibilities. In the USA, some states require that patients receive specific information before abortion and dictate the type of staff who can convey the information (Chapter 4).

The American Society for Anesthesiologists and NAF issue guidelines for IV sedation that delineate minimum personnel requirements, patient monitoring, and recovery requirements [43,44] (Chapter 8). The Joint Commission on Accreditation of Healthcare Organizations also provides requirements for sedation and anesthesia. Relaxation or pain medications that induce milder sedation, such as oral benzodiazepines and narcotics, entail less regulation because of their lower risk.

Numerous resources are available for providers who are considering starting abortion services (Appendix). The NAF website (www.prochoice.org) includes annually updated clinical guidelines, training modules, and patient education handouts, and the World Health Organization's *Safe Abortion: Technical and Policy Guidance for Health Systems* [25] is an excellent global resource. The Guttmacher Institute website (www.guttmacher.org) details requirements and laws governing abortion provision in the various states.

Aspiration versus medical abortion

Most women seeking abortion perceive a choice of methods as extremely important [45]. Women who are permitted to choose aspiration or medical abortion have high satisfaction rates with both methods [45,46]. In countries such as France, Scotland, and Sweden, where both options have been available for over a decade, 50 to 60% of eligible women elect medical abortion over aspiration abortion (Chapter 9). In the USA, aspiration abortion remains the most common method of early pregnancy termination, although use of medical abortion is increasing. In 2005, early medical abortions accounted for 14% of all US nonhospital abortions (compared with 6% in 2001) and 22% of nonhospital abortions at 9 weeks' gestation or less [2]. Fifty-seven per cent of US abortion providers offered medical abortion services in 2005, a 70% increase from 2001 [2].

Given that both early medical and aspiration methods are highly effective and safe, the decision usually turns on personal preferences. Some women opt for medical abortion because they like that it is noninvasive and offers more privacy and control. Others prefer aspiration because it is quick, predictable, and may be combined with sedation or anesthesia (Table 10.1). Although a few conditions render women ineligible for medical abortion (Chapter 9), aspiration abortion has no contraindications given the appropriate setting. Medical abortion, however, may be the best option in some situations such as very early pregnancy, marked obesity that limits visualization of the cervix [47], or obstructive uterine fibroids that make access to the pregnancy difficult or infeasible [48–50]. When efficacy is defined according to frequency of continuing pregnancies, early aspiration abortion

Table 10.1 Characteristics of early abortion methods.

Aspiration Abortion	Medical Abortion
Highly effective	Highly effective
Procedure brief	Abortion process takes one to several days to complete (sometimes longer)
Involves invasive procedure	Avoids invasive procedure (aspiration) if successful
Allows option of sedation or general anesthesia	Avoids anesthesia
Usually requires only one visit	May involve two visits or more
Lighter perceived bleeding	Heavier perceived bleeding
Requires clinical setting	May occur in privacy of home

and medical abortion using contemporary evidence-based regimens have similar efficacy [6,51]. Safety of medical versus aspiration abortion is difficult to compare because the causes of adverse events differ, but both methods have low rates of complications (Chapters 9 and 15).

Patient preparation

Before providing an abortion, the clinician must assure that the patient has considered her options, wants to have an abortion, and has given voluntary and informed consent for the procedure (Chapter 5). Each patient will need information about the abortion methods available at her gestational age, the risks and benefits of each method, and pain management options. Discussing contraceptive methods beforehand allows the patient to choose and consent to a method if she so desires; preprocedure consent for contraception is particularly important if the patient will receive sedation or desires insertion of an intrauterine system or transdermal implant immediately following the abortion (Chapter 14).

Depending on the setting, providers may use menstrual history and bimanual examination or ultrasonography to estimate gestational age (Chapter 6). Nearly all US members of the National Abortion Federation have ultrasound machines on-site, and 91% perform dating ultrasounds routinely before first-trimester aspiration abortion [52]. Although routine ultrasound is not required for provision of safe early suction abortion, its use is recommended in patients with uncertain menstrual dates, indeterminate pelvic examinations, size/dates discordance, and in cases of suspected ectopic pregnancy. When preprocedure ultrasound has not documented an intrauterine pregnancy, the provider must consider the possibility of ectopic pregnancy (Fig. 10.3).

The medical history may identify allergies to medications, latex, or antiseptic solutions used in abortion care as well as medical conditions that warrant preprocedure management. Laboratory evaluation typically includes confirmation of pregnancy (through urine pregnancy testing or sonography), determination of Rh(D) antigen status, and hematocrit or hemoglobin, at least in areas where anemia is prevalent. Patients with acute or chronic illnesses may require more extensive assessment (Chapter 7). Most providers defer bimanual examination to the time of the aspiration procedure, especially when they use routine ultrasonography. Confirming the size and flexion of the uterus helps the provider to direct instruments along the appropriate axis and anticipate conditions, such as large leiomyomata, that may present challenges (Chapter 13).

Cervical preparation

The degree of cervical dilation required to accomplish first-trimester suction abortion varies with gestational age. Most North American providers dilate the cervix mechanically using tapered Pratt or Denniston dilators, although in early gestation, a small cannula may pass without dilation. Some clinicians advocate routine use of osmotic dilators prior to first-trimester aspiration abortion based on early evidence that it may reduce the risk of cervical injury and possibly uterine perforation, at least for less experienced providers [53,54]. In a more recent case series of 170,000 first-trimester abortions performed by experienced physicians using Pratt dilators alone, cervical lacerations occurred in only 1 in 1,000 cases [55]. Cervical preparation with pharmacologic agents, such as prostaglandin analogs or progesterone antagonists, has also become increasingly common, especially in the later first trimester. No studies have been large enough to compare complication outcomes [56]. The low risk of cervical injury and perforation must be balanced against added cost, discomfort, and inconvenience for the patient.

Guidelines from professional organizations support use of cervical preparation before late first-trimester aspiration abortion; some advocate earlier use for nulliparous women or adolescents, because a higher rate of cervical injury has been reported in adolescents [56]. The WHO recommends cervical priming for all women younger than age 18 years, nulliparous women over 9 weeks' gestation, and all women over 12 weeks' gestation [25]. The RCOG advises cervical priming for women who are less than age 18 years or more than 10 weeks' gestation [42]. The Society of Family Planning Clinical Guidelines recommend cervical priming for all women at 12 to 14 weeks' gestation, with consideration of priming for all adolescents [56]. NAF does not recommend cervical priming after a particular week of gestation in the first trimester [44].

Pharmacologic preparation

Misoprostol, a prostaglandin E_1 analog, is commonly employed for cervical ripening. Other analogs, such as dinoprostone and gemeprost (not available in the USA), are more expensive yet no better than misoprostol for cervical ripening [57,58]. When providers in Europe, Scandinavia,

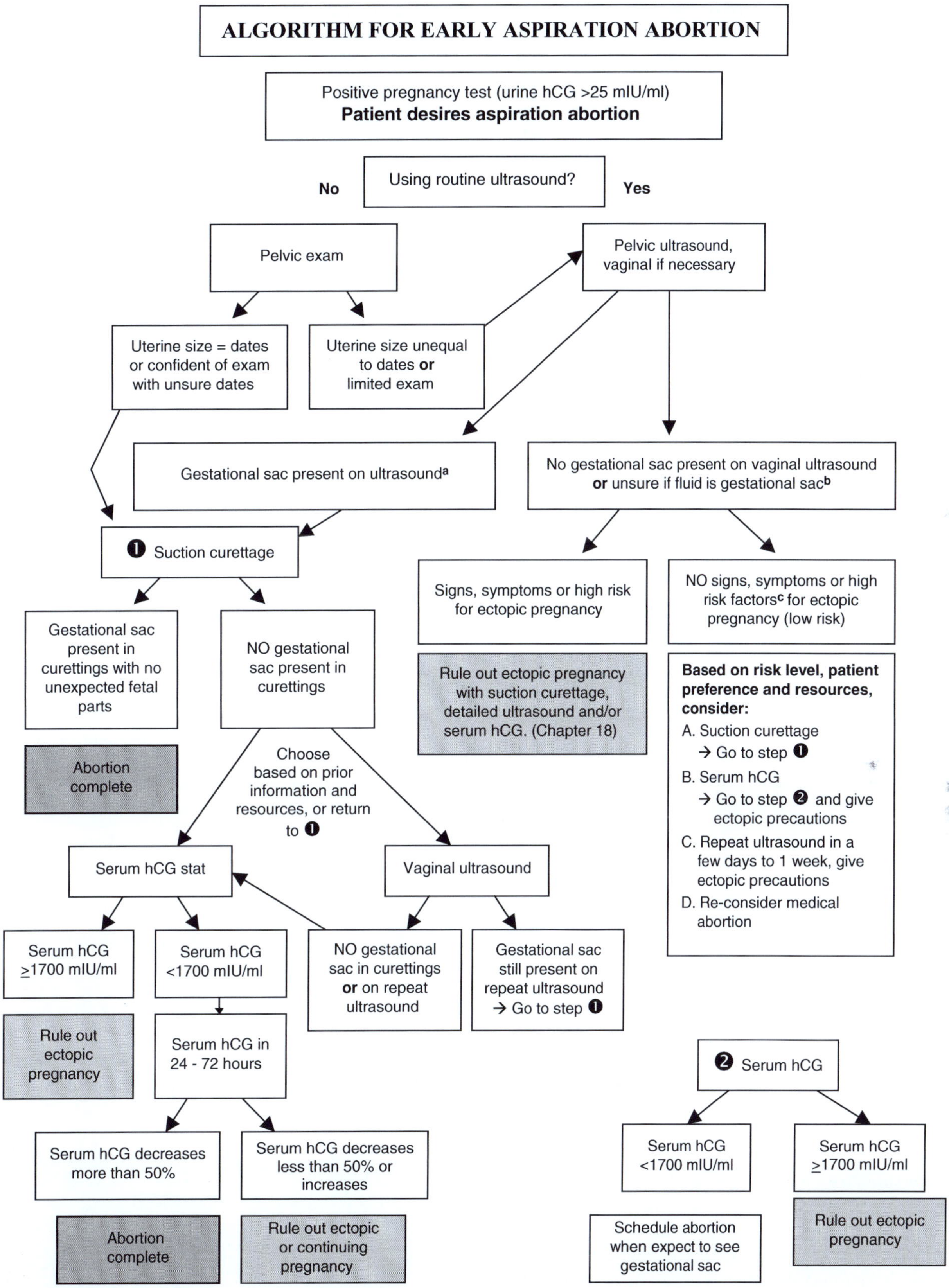

Figure 10.3 Algorithm for early aspiration abortion. [a]Gestational sac is confirmed when yolk sac is visualized. [b]When feasible, evaluate for adnexal masses and for presence of free peritoneal fluid. [c]May also choose to consider moderate or minor risk factors for ectopic pregnancy.

and other countries use gemeprost, a 1-mg vaginal suppository is placed vaginally for 3 to 12 hours prior to abortion. Mifepristone also effectively primes the cervix if used 36 to 48 hours prior to the procedure [59–61]. After 48 hours, mifepristone may cause more cervical dilation than misoprostol used for 2 to 4 hours [62]; however, its use for cervical priming is limited as a result of the long preparation time, high cost, and lack of availability in some settings.

Researchers have evaluated several routes of misoprostol administration. The appropriate route takes into account efficacy, side effects, and patient and staff preferences. The many studies of misoprostol for cervical priming define efficacy by a variety of outcome measures including baseline cervical dilation, need for mechanical dilation, force required for mechanical dilation, and duration of procedure. Studies that evaluate patient acceptance have found that women generally prefer 1-day procedures to 2-day and prefer misoprostol to laminaria [63,64]. Studies have not been large enough to detect a difference in complication rates.

When using vaginal misoprostol, the optimum regimen is 400 μg given 3 to 4 hours prior to the procedure. This conclusion derives from studies that demonstrate the following:

- Vaginal misoprostol is equally or more effective than oral administration and causes fewer side effects [63,65].
- Vaginal misoprostol 200 μg is inferior to 400 μg [66–69].
- Doses higher than 400 μg result in higher rates of side effects such as pain, bleeding, and fever [67,68].
- Vaginal misoprostol 600 μg for 2 hours is inferior to 400 μg for 3 hours [68,69].
- More than 4 hours of vaginal misoprostol does not improve dilation and causes increased bleeding and passage of products of conception prior to the procedure [63,70].

Misoprostol 400 μg is also effective when given orally 8 to 12 hours prior or sublingually 2 to 4 hours before the procedure [56]. However, sublingual dosing results in higher rates of nausea, vomiting, and diarrhea as compared to vaginal dosing [71]. Although buccal misoprostol is effective for cervical priming prior to second-trimester abortion [72,73], it has not been evaluated for cervical priming in the first trimester. Although the mechanism of action of misoprostol involves induction of endogenous prostaglandins, one study found that using nonsteroidal antiinflammatory drugs (NSAIDs) for pain relief did not alter the efficacy of misoprostol for cervical ripening [74].

Osmotic dilators

Osmotic dilators absorb water from the surrounding tissues and gradually increase in diameter to dilate the cervix (Appendix, Fig. A-13). All osmotic dilating devices induce endogenous prostaglandins and some additionally create radial force on the cervix [75,76]. A trained provider must place the dilators during a speculum exam. Women may experience pain with placement necessitating local cervical anesthesia, especially if multiple dilators are placed. More than one osmotic dilator is rarely needed, though, in the first trimester. Three types of osmotic dilators are used in abortion care: laminaria (*Laminaria digitata, Laminaria japonica*); Dilapan-S™ (GelMed International, Czech Republic), and Lamicel® (no longer available in the USA). Chapter 11 reviews osmotic dilators in detail.

Setup and equipment

First-trimester suction abortions are performed in operating rooms, outpatient surgical centers, clinics with procedure rooms, and regular office examination rooms.

Room setup

The room setup typically includes an examination or operating table, seating, focused lighting, a table or stand, and appropriate equipment and supplies. For women who are awake, a calm warm atmosphere may facilitate relaxation and comfort during the procedure.

The treatment table should provide comfortable support for the patient in lithotomy position. Tables equipped with knee stirrups allow the patient to relax her legs as the crutches hold them apart, although foot stirrups also function well in awake patients. Where resources permit, a hydraulic table affords the clinician a more comfortable posture and provides flexibility in patient positioning. Lighting concentrated in the provider's work area minimally disturbs the patient. Better lighting is occasionally necessary for patient monitoring, particularly when general anesthesia is administered. Supplies for postprocedure tissue examination may be located in the treatment room or at a station in a nearby room. Backlighting, such as an x-ray view box, and a clear dish in which to suspend the tissue facilitate visualization (Fig. 10.4).

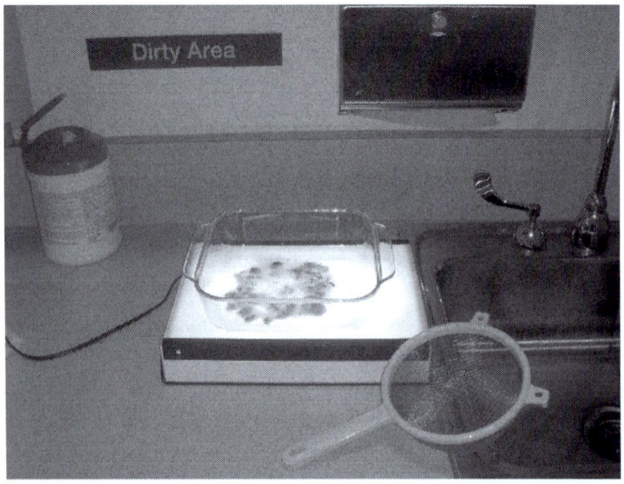

Figure 10.4 Tissue examination area with a backlight and glass dish.

Manual versus electric suction

Use of manual vacuum aspirators (MVA; also called manual uterine aspirators or Karman syringes), once associated with resource-poor settings, has become increasingly common in developed countries in the past decade. These small handheld devices create up to 60 mmHg of suction, and they are quiet, small, and easy to transport. About 50% of US abortion providers use MVAs, particularly during the earliest weeks of pregnancy [52]. There is no clear gestational age limit in the first trimester at which MVAs are no longer appropriate. After 9 weeks' gestation, the MVA must be emptied a few times, so some providers prefer to switch to the electric machine. Other providers routinely use the MVA up to 14 weeks' gestation. MVA involves lower costs and service delivery resources [77].

A recent systematic review of randomized trials comparing MVA with electric vacuum aspiration (EVA) found no differences in complete abortion rates or patient satisfaction. At less than 50 days' gestation, women having MVA procedures experienced less blood loss and reported less severe pain, whereas women undergoing EVA had shorter procedure times [78]. Several of the trials included in this review are in Chinese and have not yet been translated into English. US trials have not demonstrated a difference in immediate complications [79] or pain between the two methods [10,80]. In several comparative studies, women reported the absence of noise as an advantage of MVA [10,81,82]. In one study, women who had EVA reported that the noise associated with the electric pump increased their pain, although pain scores did not differ [82]. Some clinicians who use MVA have commented that women ask for "the quiet procedure," indicating their preference for this aspect of MVA [81].

MVA devices

The components of an MVA aspirator include a cylinder, plunger, and valves (Fig. 10.5). The aspirator accommodates various sizes of cannulae, although some aspirator-cannulae combinations require adapters. Aspirators are clean but not usually sterile when shipped, and they do not need to be sterile for use (although the cannula that enters the uterus must be sterile). The reusable models require high-level disinfection between each patient, and some models are designed to tolerate steam sterilization techniques. There are a number of MVA manufacturers worldwide including Ipas (Chapel Hill, NC) and MedGyn (Lombard, IL) that sell MVA instruments in the USA. In 2004, EngenderHealth published the *Practical Guide for Selection of MVA Instruments* [83], which details instrument handling, cleaning, and processing as well as compatibility with various cannulae. The package inserts for the devices also detail methods of disinfection and sterilization as well as assembly.

Use of MVA

With most manual vacuum aspirators, the provider closes the valves and pulls on the plunger to create a vacuum (Fig. 10.6). Some providers prefer to seat the cannula firmly into the aperture of the syringe before inserting it into the uterus, whereas others choose to insert the cannula into the uterus and then attach the prepared syringe. Once the cannula is situated inside the uterus, the clinician releases the valves and evacuates the uterine contents using the same movements as described in a later section for other first-trimester procedures. With other MVA syringes, the provider creates the vacuum after inserting the cannula into the uterus; these devices have a locking plunger that prevents loss of pressure during the procedure.

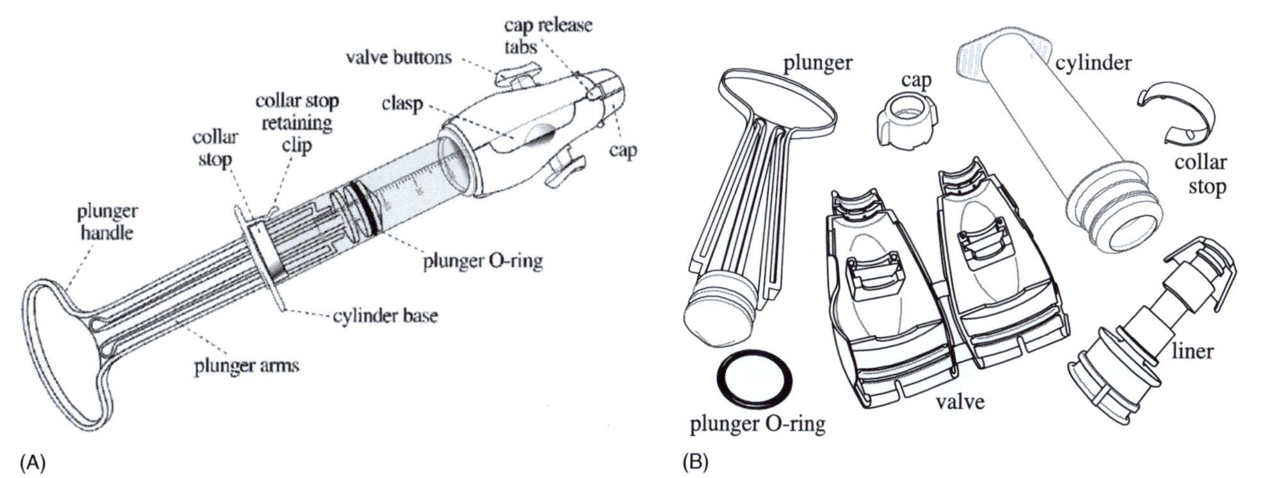

Figure 10.5 (A) Ipas manual vacuum aspirator (MVA Plus) consisting of a cylinder, plunger, and valves. This model and other aspirators accommodate flexible and rigid cannulae of various types and sizes. (B) The device comes apart for cleaning or sterilizing and must be reassembled. Used with permission from Ipas.

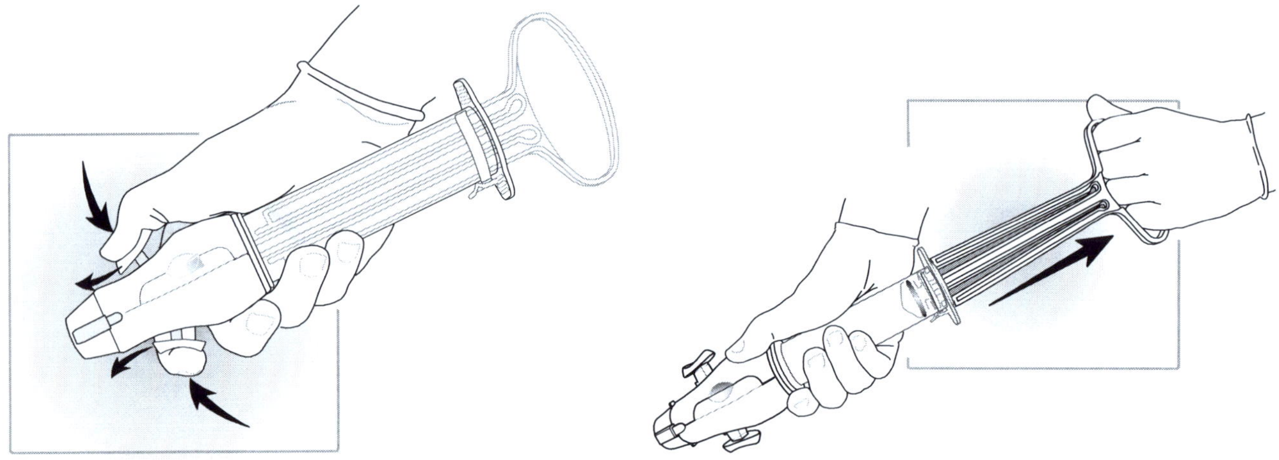

(A) (B)

Figure 10.6 Use of a manual vacuum aspirator: to create a vacuum, the provider closes the valves by pushing the buttons down and forward (A) and then pulls the plunger back until the plunger arms snap outward and catch on the wide sides of the cylinder base (B). Never grasp the aspirator by the plunger arms, and be sure that both plunger arms are secured over the edges of the cylinder to prevent them from slipping back inside the cylinder. A collar stop prevents the plunger from pulling out of the cylinder. Because the clear plastic cylinder pulls apart from the white plastic valve cap for cleaning and emptying, the provider should hold the cylinder to prevent separation while creating the vacuum. Used with permission from Ipas.

Electric aspiration machine

Electric aspiration machines have become quieter over the years, but they still create a low rumbling noise. One end of a plastic hose connects to a bottle on or in the aspiration machine, and the other end has a rotating handle that accommodates the sterile cannula. Single-use or reusable hoses are available. Reusable hoses require high-level disinfection. Some facilities use adjustable wall suction attached to collection bottles, which functions similarly to a portable electric machine.

Instruments and supplies

A standard surgical tray containing only a small number of instruments suffices for termination of most first-trimester pregnancies (Appendix, Fig. A-1). Selection of particular instruments depends largely on provider preference. Keep the tray as simple as possible, and place the instruments in a standard configuration so that they can be located quickly. This predictability increases efficiency, keeps noise from instrument handling to a minimum, and is especially helpful during difficult or emergent cases. Instruments commonly included on a first-trimester aspiration abortion tray include the following:

- Speculum
- Tenaculum, usually single-toothed or atraumatic
- Ring-type forceps
- Set of graduated cervical dilators, commonly Pratt sizes 13 to 39 French
- Gauze sponges or cotton balls
- Antiseptic solution in a small basin

Additionally, a syringe and needle will be needed for administration of cervical anesthesia. Instruments that are used occasionally can be sterilized and stored separately in or near the procedure room so that they are readily available when needed.

Specula

Commonly used specula include adult Graves and its modifications, juvenile, and Pederson models. The Weisman-Graves and Moore-Graves specula have shorter blades that permit the cervix to be drawn closer to the perineum. Narrow blade designs, like Pederson and juvenile specula, may be more comfortable and effective in cases of extreme patient guarding or a narrow introitus. Open-sided or tri-blade models are useful in special circumstances. Specula with a more obtuse angle between the blade and handle can be helpful for women with anterior cervices or large buttocks (Appendix, Figs. A-2 to A-4).

Tenacula

Providers commonly use single-toothed tenaculum for first-trimester vacuum abortion [52]. Some clinicians prefer designs with blunt teeth or grooves, such as Allis or Bierer vulsellum tenacula. They cause tears less often but may slip off the cervix more readily if strong traction is applied. Ring-type forceps function well on fleshy, parous cervices (Appendix, Fig. A-6).

Dilators

Most providers use graduated and finely taped dilators, including Pratt dilators (Appendix, Fig. A-1) and their plastic equivalents, the Denniston dilators [52]. The curved tips of these models are particularly helpful when the endocervical canal is angled or tortuous. Pratt dilators are sized by the French designation, which refers to the circumference of the dilator in millimeters, and they increase by 2-mm increments. Dividing by pi (approximately 3) provides the diameter of the dilator in millimeters. Denniston dilators are sized by the largest diameter in millimeters, and they increase by 1-mm increments. Blunter designs, like Hegar or Hanks dilators, are less favored because they require greater force to dilate the cervix [84,85].

Cannulae

Disposable plastic suction cannulae come in flexible (e.g., Karman) and curved or straight rigid models (Appendix, Fig. A-9). Rigid plastic cannulae increase in diameter by 1-mm increments from 6 to 16 mm; flexible cannulae increase in a similar fashion from 4 to 12 mm. Nondisposable metal cannulae rarely are used; they come in only five diameters ranging from 8 to 16 mm and require sterilization before reuse. Cannulae from various manufacturers are not always compatible with MVA devices; although most combinations maintain pressure, some lose pressure rapidly [83,86]. Adapters on flexible cannulae are usually removable, so switching the adaptor may alleviate loss of suction if it occurs.

Forceps

A ring-type forceps is useful for retraction, to hold gauze sponges, and to tamponade a bleeding cervical laceration or tenaculum site (Appendix, Fig. A-6). In some cases of late first-trimester evacuation, standard sponge forceps or their heavier modifications are used as an adjunct to suction. When cervical dilation is snug, placental tissue or, in later gestations, the calvarium may have difficulty passing through the cannula. In these cases, the clinician can use the forceps to bring the tissue to the cervical os and remove it. Both ring-type and polyp forceps require at least 12 mm of cervical dilation to introduce them through the cervix.

Box A Supplies for Initial Office Management of Hemorrhage

- Supplies to provide IV fluids
- Uterotonics (Methergine, prostaglandin F2α, and/or misoprostol)
- Vasopressin (for cervical injection if not used routinely)
- Foley catheter with 30-cc balloon; small diameter, large syringe; sterile water to fill balloon
- Vaginal packing gauze

Uterine curettes

Routine use of metal uterine curettes is decreasing in first-trimester abortion practice [52]. Metal curette sizes start at a few millimeters in width and gradually increase (Appendix, Fig. A-12). No studies have examined the benefits or risks of routine sharp curettage following suction aspiration.

Gauze

Surgeons are often familiar with sponge-sticks made by carefully wrapping a large gauze sponge around a ring forceps. Because awake patients may experience considerable discomfort from passing large gauze through the vagina, use of cotton balls or smaller gauze may be preferable.

Syringe and needle

A standard 10-cc syringe and small-gauge (e.g., 21- to 25-gauge), 1.5-inch needle typically suffice for cervical anesthesia injections. A larger syringe may compromise visibility and a shorter needle limits the depth of injections, although use of a spinal needle circumvents these limitations. Some practitioners prefer a "control" syringe with finger loops to accomplish injections comfortably using one hand.

Emergency supplies

In addition to the typical supplies found in medical settings for airway management and treatment of anaphylaxis, abortion providers need emergency supplies for management of hemorrhage (Box A). Additional supplies depend on the type of anesthesia (Chapter 8).

Ultrasound

Ultrasound machines with basic features generally suffice for abortion services. A sector transducer "abdominal probe" of 3- to 5-MHz permits documentation of an intrauterine pregnancy at 7 weeks' gestation and greater for many women. A 5- to 10-MHz vaginal probe improves visualization of earlier pregnancies or retroverted uteri, allows evaluation of the adnexae if necessary, and permits more detailed assessment of the endometrium when retained tissue is suspected.

Determining which personnel are allowed to perform ultrasound examinations remains a controversial issue within institutions and is sometimes specified by hospitals or insurance policies. Only persons who have had adequate didactic and supervised hands-on experience should perform ultrasound examinations. Ultrasound examinations require permanently recorded images.

Pain control

Anesthesia options reflect available resources, patient and provider preferences, and risk assessment (Chapter 8). Regardless of the method used, the objective is to provide comfort and relaxation sufficient for patient satisfaction and completion of the abortion safely. Pain perception and response are extremely complex, interwoven into the psychological and social context, and vary widely among individuals. One Indian study found that when women were permitted to choose between the two extremes of general and local anesthesia, 60% chose general and 40% chose local. General anesthesia patients reported that having no pain (95%) or anxiety (38%) were the best features, whereas those having local anesthesia liked being ambulatory (26%), avoiding side effects (26%), and feeling awake (21%) [87].

Although offering a range of pain management options is ideal, not all facilities are equipped to provide deeper levels of sedation. A 2002 survey of NAF member facilities examined first-trimester pain management preferences for each clinic by determining the method employed for 40 to 100% of procedures. Of those clinics that expressed a preference, 46% used local cervical anesthesia with or without oral premedication, 33% combined local anesthesia with IV moderate ("conscious") sedation, and 21% offered deep sedation or general anesthesia [52]. Chapter 8 reviews these methods in detail, and they are only briefly summarized here.

- *Local Cervical Anesthesia*: No one method of cervical anesthesia clearly stands out as most effective. Most North American providers use 1% lidocaine [52], and they show a modest preference for paracervical injection at four or more sites (Chapter 8). Studies that demonstrate improved pain control with larger volumes of medication [88] and deeper injections [89] suggest that deposition of sufficient medication at the nerve site is at least part of the mechanism of analgesia.
- *Oral Medications*: In the office setting, nonsteroidal anti-inflammatory drugs (NSAIDs), oral or sublingual benzodiazepines, or oral narcotics commonly are combined with local anesthesia. In randomized trials, preoperative naproxen sodium demonstrated decreased pain compared to placebo [90], and ibupofen proved superior to tramadol (Ultram™) in reducing postoperative pain [91]. Although a low-dose benzodiazepine (lorazepam 1 mg) does not appear to help with pain in women who desire relaxation [88,92], it does decrease periprocedure anxiety [92]. Higher doses of oral or sublingual benzodiazepines (i.e., 1 to 3 mg of lorazepam) are used in clinical office settings for abortion, but they have not been evaluated in controlled trials.
- *Moderate ("Conscious") Sedation*: Typical regimens for moderate sedation in the outpatient setting include parenteral fentanyl, 50 to 100 μg, and midazolam, 1 to 3 mg (Chapter 8). Studies differ as to whether moderate sedation improves pain with abortion compared to local anesthesia alone, although it does appear to improve satisfaction with the experience [93,94]. Moderate sedation has not been compared to oral pain and relaxation medications.
- *Deep Sedation or General Anesthesia*: When local cervical anesthesia with mild relaxation or sedation is not sufficient to prevent agitation and abrupt movements, injury can result. Therefore, deep sedation or general anesthesia may be beneficial for extremely anxious patients or in cases of technically challenging procedures.

Principles of surgical technique

Adherence to principles of sound surgical technique enhances the safety of abortion. These principles include techniques to reduce the risk of infection, meticulous and gentle instrumentation, and sufficient knowledge and skills to perform the surgery efficiently and safely.

Wearing sterile gloves does not assure asepsis, because contamination occurs as soon as the gloved hands contact the patient. In addition, eradicating the natural microflora of the vagina is impossible. Therefore, providers typically employ a "no-touch" technique in surgical abortion practice: whether wearing sterile or nonsterile gloves, the clinician avoids touching the parts of instruments that will enter the uterus. For example, holding dilators in their midportion avoids contaminating the tips that pass into the uterine cavity (Fig. 10.7). Establishing a separate area on the field for sterile instruments ensures that other items that have contacted the provider's hands or the patient do not touch the

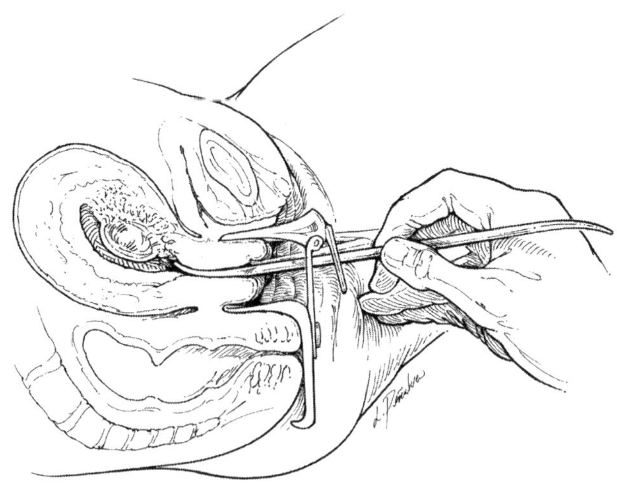

Figure 10.7 Dilation of the cervix with a Pratt dilator. Note that the provider holds the dilator in its midportion and avoids touching the tip of the dilator that enters the sterile uterine cavity ("no-touch" technique). The fourth and fifth fingers rest against the perineum and buttocks to prevent the dilator from thrusting forward as it passes through the internal os.

cannula or dilator tips. Taking care that instruments are inserted directly into the cervix without touching the vaginal sidewalls is also important.

Gentle manipulation of tissue helps to avoid trauma to the cervix or uterus. Forcible dilation of a noncompliant cervix can result in lacerations or perforations, and vigorous metallic curettage may produce intrauterine scarring, albeit rarely (Chapter 15). If the cervix is stenotic or rigid and a small-sized cannula will not complete the evacuation safely, delaying the procedure to effect cervical preparation with osmotic dilators or ripening agents is a better alternative than using excessive force.

The skill and experience of the provider are important determinants of the safety of abortion [54,95]. In most cases, first-trimester aspiration abortion is a simple procedure with low morbidity; even less experienced operators may perform several hundred cases before encountering a serious complication. Although abortion training opportunities for physicians have increased over the past decade in the USA, they still remain inadequate [96]. Providers must remain cognizant of their skill levels, experience, and limitations and know when to ask for help or to refer difficult cases.

Skills in abortion care also encompass the ability to communicate effectively with patients (Chapter 5). Confidence and comfort are enhanced when the provider acts professionally, conveys warmth and empathy, provides useful information, and addresses the patient's questions and concerns. During the abortion procedure, informing awake patients of what sensations to expect and reminding them to breathe deeply and rhythmically help prevent sudden movements that may jeopardize safety (Chapter 8).

Vacuum aspiration procedure

Providers use a variety of techniques to perform first-trimester abortions. This section provides a general description of first-trimester vacuum aspiration using cervical anesthesia, followed by a discussion of variations in technique used routinely or in particular situations. Administration of sedation or analgesia should occur about 30 to 90 minutes prior to the procedure for oral medications and immediately prior to the procedure for IV medications.

1. Align the patient's hips just beyond the edge of the table. For very heavy patients, the knee-chest position may facilitate visualization of the cervix. In the unusual case of an extremely anterior cervix that defies visualization, placing the patient in Trendelenburg position via an adjustable table may help.
2. Perform a gentle bimanual examination to assess the position, size, and contour of the uterus. Note the angle between the cervix and body of the uterus, which may approach 90 degrees in cases of extreme anteflexion or retroflexion. Substantial size/dates discrepancy or anatomic abnormalities warrant ultrasound if one was not already performed.
3. Insert a speculum gently into the vagina and open the blades to visualize the cervix. In very overweight women, the speculum handle will commonly sit between the cheeks of the buttocks unless a speculum with a wider angle is used.
4. Using a squeeze or spray bottle, cotton ball, or gauze swab, cleanse the cervix with antiseptic solution such as povidone-iodine or chlorhexidine.
5. Anesthetize the tenaculum site, either by injecting 2 to 5 cc of local anesthetic solution into the lip of the cervix or performing a complete block of the anterior lip (e.g., 5 cc each at 2 o'clock and 10 o'clock on the cervical face). Position the tenaculum either horizontally or vertically with the inferior tooth near the cervical canal, being sure to grasp the stroma of the cervix and not only the epithelium.
6. Applying gentle traction to the cervix, administer cervical anesthesia (Chapter 8).
7. Perform cervical dilation. Using a "no-touch" technique, grasp a small tapered dilator in its midportion and hold it much like a pencil (Fig. 10.7). Applying traction on the tenaculum to straighten the angle between the cervical canal and the uterine cavity, carefully insert the smaller end of the dilator to a depth just beyond the internal cervical os. Resting the fourth and fifth fingers against the perineum and buttocks during insertion prevents the dilator from thrusting forward as it overcomes the resistance of the internal os (Fig. 10.7). Some experienced providers prefer to rotate the dilator within the canal (Fig. 13.2) rather than inserting it directly. As the instrument traverses the endocervical canal, sense the smooth surface of the glandular mucosa. Deviation from this sensation, especially if accompanied by a subtle shearing sensation, suggests creation of a false channel (Fig. 13.6). Continuing to apply pressure in the wrong direction can result in perforation. Only when the direction of the canal is certain should dilation proceed using progressively larger dilators to achieve an opening sufficient to accommodate a plastic cannula of appropriate size.
8. Insert a rigid or flexible plastic cannula through the internal os, positioning it in the mid to upper fundus. As a general rule of thumb, use a cannula with a diameter in millimeters that approximates the gestational age in weeks (e.g., a 7-mm cannula for a 7-week gestation). If you are using Pratt dilators that are measured in circumference, multiply the cannula size by 3 (pi) to determine the largest Pratt dilator size necessary to achieve sufficient dilation (e.g., dilation to a size 21 or 23 Pratt will accommodate a 7-mm cannula). Avoid touching the end of the cannula that enters the uterus to anything except the cervical os. Attach the cannula to the suction machine tubing either before or after insertion.

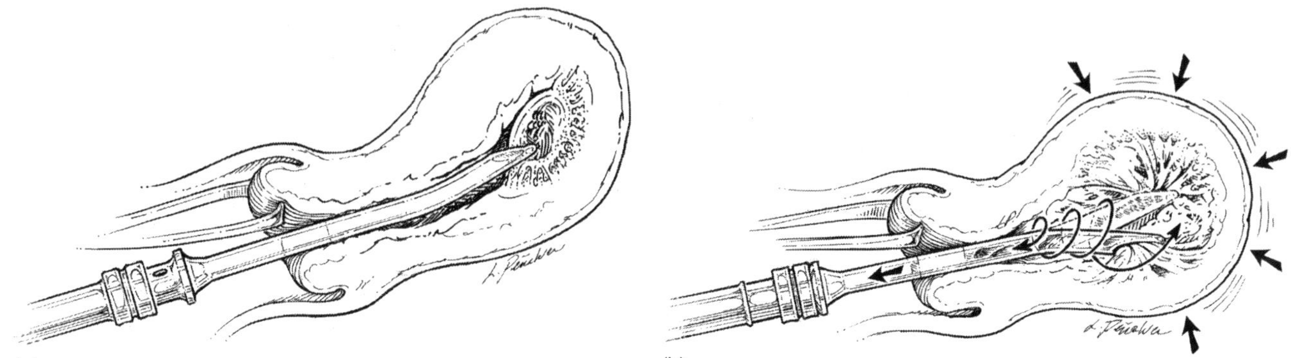

Figure 10.8 Technique of electric vacuum aspiration. (A) The cannula is placed in the mid to upper fundus before suction is created. (B) After closing the thumb valve to create suction, the provider rotates the cannula while gradually withdrawing it to the internal os. The motion is repeated until evacuation is complete.

9 Aspirate the uterine contents. If using electric vacuum, close the thumb valve on the hose and turn on the vacuum machine, assuring that it achieves a negative pressure of at least 55 to 60 mmHg. Evacuate the uterus by rotating the cannula while gradually and gently withdrawing it to the internal os (Fig. 10.8); advance the cannula and repeat this motion until flow of tissue through the cannula and hose ceases. Back-and-forth motions promote rapid evacuation, but they require the provider to remain cognizant of the depth of the fundus and create more movement that the patient may detect. Signs of complete evacuation include bubbles in the cannula and hose; contraction of the uterus around the cannula, making rotation increasingly difficult; and a "gritty" sensation when the cannula moves against the endometrial surface. At this point, withdraw the cannula from the cervix, releasing the pressure with the thumb valve as the tip of the cannula reaches the external os.

10 Remove the tenaculum and inspect the cervix for bleeding, then withdraw the speculum. Reassure the patient before you leave the room or before she moves to a recovery area.

11 Examine the fresh tissue aspirate as described in a later section.

Sometimes the flow through the cannula stops because the products are too large to pass. The provider can usually restore flow by releasing pressure with the thumb valve and quickly restoring it by closing the valve. If this technique fails, release and restore the vacuum while advancing the cannula a few centimeters into the cavity and then withdrawing it in a pumping motion. If the cannula still remains plugged, simply withdraw the cannula, releasing vacuum at the external os, and use a ring forceps to remove any material that is wedged in the end of the cannula or lodged at the external os. Final suctioning after the uterus has involuted may require a slightly smaller cannula to allow for unimpeded motion.

Failure to detect the gritty sensation that typically signals an empty uterine cavity may indicate retained products of conception, myomata, or uterine anomalies. If the curette reveals a slick area of uterine wall, repeat suctioning of the area often demonstrates retained placental fragments.

Variations in technique

Cleansing the cervix

Not all providers cleanse the cervix with dilute antiseptics prior to surgical abortion. Vaginal scrubbing does not notably decrease bacterial counts in the endocervix [97]. Two randomized studies of cervical cleaning with chlorhexidine did not demonstrate a difference in postabortal infection [98,99]. The infection rate in the 2005 study by Varli et al was 2.4% with cleaning and 2.1% without [99]. Prophylactic antibiotics were not used in either study.

Placement of tenaculum

When the uterus is retroflexed, some providers feel that placing the tenaculum on the posterior lip allows for more effective traction. Other providers feel that anterior placement is still preferable for a retroflexed uterus, as the tenaculum can be used to torque the uterus and allow easier access to the posterior wall. No studies have evaluated if any specific technique is more advantageous.

Uterine sounding

A small proportion of providers routinely uses a uterine sound to measure fundal depth prior to evacuation [52]. This practice, however, carries risk. In an early study of abortion complications in over 37,000 women, 23% of perforations were associated with uterine sounding, although the incidence of recognized perforations was low (0.16%)[100]. A 13-year retrospective review of patients who sustained perforations during first-trimester abortions found that the suction cannula represented the most common perforating instrument (25%), followed by the uterine sound (23%) and the dilator (20%) [101].

The uterine sound, however, has value as an adjunct in performing aspiration abortion. Because a metal sound is visualized easily with real-time ultrasound, it is a useful marker for locating elusive pregnancy sacs in abortions complicated by congenital or acquired anomalies. Some providers use a sound to identify and evaluate suspected uterine perforations, especially in conjunction with ultrasound. Documenting that a perforation does not exist or is small often permits experienced clinicians to complete uterine evacuation immediately and safely.

Choice of cannula

Providers' preferences vary for desired size and type of cannula. A 2002 survey of North American abortion providers found that, for first-trimester abortions after 7 weeks' gestation, 54% dilate to a diameter in millimeters corresponding to the number of gestational weeks, whereas 37% dilate 1 to 2 mm more [52]. A minority of clinicians prefers to dilate to 1 to 3 mm less than the gestation age to minimize discomfort in awake patients. A relatively larger cannula facilitates the ease and speed of uterine evacuation and may permit more intact tissue to facilitate gross examination. A smaller cannula may cause less discomfort and often slides without resistance (especially as the uterus involutes). Some products of conception may not fit through a smaller cannula, in which case pulling the cannula through the cervix with a small amount of suction often brings the tissue through the cervical os where the provider can remove it with ring forceps. No studies have compared rigid and flexible cannulae. Rigid cannulae have a slightly larger internal aperture and a larger single opening at the tip. Providers have varying opinions regarding which cannulae permit them to best feel the gritty texture of the empty uterus.

Mechanical dilation

A small Pratt dilator usually passes with no resistance, even in the early first trimester, and a larger dilator may pass initially with a soft or previously dilated cervix or a later gestation. Some providers prefer to attempt to pass a small cannula without dilation or pass successively larger cannulae instead of dilators. In most cases, providers dilate incrementally in order to expand the cervix gradually. When the internal os is compliant, however, clinicians can skip dilator sizes. A minority of abortion providers uses blunt dilators some or all of the time. Blunt dilators increase in size more rapidly than tapered dilators, requiring fewer instrument passes.

Some reports suggest that cervical resistance notably drops when mechanical dilation achieves a diameter of approximately 11 mm; whether this occurrence represents minor cervical injury or is of clinical import is unknown [102]. No controlled trials have compared outcomes after lesser versus greater mechanical dilation in first-trimester abortion; at the same time, no epidemiologic evidence supports an increased risk of cervical incompetence after first-trimester vacuum aspiration abortion (Chapter 16).

Providers use a variety of techniques when the internal os is difficult to locate (Chapter 13). These approaches include increased cervical traction, repeat pelvic examination to reassess the angle of the canal, and probing gently at varied angles to locate the os. In difficult cases, abdominal ultrasound usually provides a clear view of the cervix and dilator, allowing for safe dilation under direct vision (Chapter 13).

When the cervical canal or internal os is tight, providers may use special, thinner instruments including ultrathin dilators, plastic or metal sounds, IV catheter sheaths, lacrimal duct probes, or plastic os finders (Appendix, Fig. A-7). Applying sterile lubricant or a detergent antiseptic to the dilator helps reduce resistance. Once a dilating instrument successfully passes the internal os, allowing it to reside in the canal for a short time facilitates subsequent dilation. In some cases of difficult dilation, the provider can evacuate the uterus using a smaller cannula than is ordinarily employed. Failing these maneuvers, osmotic dilators or cervical ripening agents (e.g., misoprostol) are effective in softening and expanding the cervix; their use delays the abortion for only a few hours. In very rare cases of extremely difficult dilation in an early pregnancy, a 1- to 2-week wait will almost always result in a more compliant cervix. Medical abortion is also an alternative for women with early pregnancies.

Suction technique

Providers vary in positioning the cannula within the uterine cavity; some prefer placing it at the top of the fundus whereas others choose the midfundus. Outcomes have not been statistically compared. The same is true for differences in the rotary or back-and-forth motions employed during aspiration. Most providers apply a combination of the two motions. Some clinicians prefer a technique of serial side-by-side strokes with the cannula placed flush to the walls of the uterus.

Modulating control of suction pressure during aspiration is another variation in technique. By adjusting the sliding sleeve on the thumb valve or turning the dial on the aspiration machine, the clinician can modify vacuum pressure from zero, when the valve is open, to the usual upper range of 55 to 75 mmHg. Intermediate levels may allow for freer motion of the cannula as the uterine cavity begins to involute. Switching to a smaller cannula during uterine involution also achieves this objective. When using a manual suction device, pulling back the plunger part way prior to cocking the valves (or placing the cannula, depending on the device) reduces the level of suction. The amount of suction also decreases as the MVA chamber fills with the products of conception and blood.

Confirming a complete procedure

Although the cannula is the primary instrument of curettage, nearly 50% of North American providers determine completeness of evacuation by gentle sharp curettage followed by final suctioning [52]. In most cases meticulous suctioning suffices to empty the uterus. No data suggest that additional sharp curettage lessens the risk of retained products or failed attempted abortion, and sharp curettage causes more pain than suction curettage [103].

Perioperative ultrasound

Only 21% of North American specialists use intraoperative ultrasound routinely during first-trimester aspiration abortion, although most use it for difficult cases [52]. Ultrasound can help the practitioner determine the direction of the endocervical canal during dilation, locate intrauterine gestational sacs in uteri distorted by congenital or acquired anomalies, or assess complete evacuation. In addition, ultrasound may provide confirmation of suspected uterine perforation and enable experienced operators to complete evacuation in the face of such injuries. In the later first trimester or with multifetal pregnancies, intraoperative ultrasound may speed the procedure by identifying what tissue remains and when complete evacuation has occurred.

Few studies have assessed the value of perioperative ultrasound for first-trimester aspiration abortion. One randomized trial from a teaching hospital in the UK found a 4% rate of immediate complications in 108 women who had ultrasound-guided early aspirations versus 16% in 107 women who had their procedures without ultrasound [104]. Complications were ill defined in this study, and the reported rates were substantially higher than those found in most surgical abortion studies [55,105]. In a recent randomized trial from Israel, Debby et al [106] allocated 809 women who had aspiration abortions at 7 to 14 weeks' gestation to routine postprocedure ultrasound with immediate reaspiration for an endometrial thickness of 8 mm or more or no postoperative ultrasound. Women in the no ultrasound group were significantly more likely to undergo subsequent procedures for suspected retained tissue, although the indications for this intervention remain unclear. Other investigators have found endometrial thickness a poor predictor of retained products in the days following first-trimester aspiration abortion [107–109]. An Israeli group has developed a special speculum and device that permits real-time vaginal sonography during uterine procedures. One report of use during 45 first-trimester abortions noted no complications and favorable responses from the nine participating physicians [110]. The device may be especially helpful in cases of difficult dilation or a distorted endometrial cavity.

Prophylactic uterotonics and vasoconstrictors

Although uterotonic medications are useful in the emergent management of hemorrhage, few data support their routine use during first-trimester abortion. Two first-trimester abortion studies found that intraoperative administration of IV oxytocin only minimally decreased blood loss when used at or after 9 weeks' gestation [111,112]. A 1998 review found no evidence supporting the routine use of methylergometrine to reduce blood loss during first-trimester abortion [113]. The advantages of vasopressin therapy in controlling blood loss are greater in late first-trimester abortion and beyond [114]. However, intracervical administration of low-dose, dilute vasopressin at the time of first-trimester vacuum abortion may reduce the incidence of reaspiration for postoperative bleeding and cramping [115]. Moreover, in a randomized trial of women undergoing operative hysteroscopy, administration of dilute vasopressin decreased the force required for mechanical dilation [116]. One to six units of vasopressin are typically added to the local anesthetic solution. Sands et al [117] reported a reduced incidence of postabortal hematometra with routine administration of intramuscular ergonovine 0.1 mg immediately after first-trimester surgical abortion.

Very early abortion

Very early abortion became possible with the introduction of plastic cannulae that permitted diameters smaller than the 8-mm width feasible with metal. Advantages include early relief from the symptoms and anxiety of undesired pregnancy and more psychological comfort with terminating an early pregnancy. According to CDC data, the proportion of US abortions occurring during the earliest weeks of gestation has increased steadily since 1992 [3]. Surveys by the Guttmacher Institute indicate that the proportion of US providers offering abortion at 4 weeks' gestation rose from 7% in 1993 to 40% in 2005 [2]; the latter figure is similar to that found in a large survey of NAF member clinics conducted in 2002 [52].

With the use of modern technologies of pregnancy detection, meticulous technique, and appropriate follow-up, no gestational age may be too early to attempt aspiration abortion. One large case series of aspiration abortions performed at less than 6 weeks' gestation by a single practitioner using a uniform protocol found a continuing pregnancy rate of only 0.1%, although the rate of follow-up was not reported [118,119]. A later observational study with rigorous follow-up of patients having abortions before 6 weeks' gestation by multiple providers at Planned Parenthood clinics found a continuing pregnancy rate of 2%[120]. These rates compare favorably with those reported after early medical abortion, and they are lower than early surgical reports showing failed abortion rates exceeding 4% [121,122]. Early detection of ectopic pregnancies with this approach is a distinct clinical advantage and contributes to its cost-effectiveness [118,119].

In very early pregnancies, identifying the gestational sac on tissue examination may prove difficult. In one case series of aspiration abortions at less than 6 weeks, gestational tissue was identified in 50% of pregnancies in which the gestational sac was not seen on preprocedure vaginal ultrasound examination [118]. Failure to identify products of conception warrants further workup for possible ectopic pregnancy or continuing pregnancy as described in a later section.

Examining tissue

Examination of the uterine aspirate is an integral aspect of aspiration abortion and has numerous benefits. It allows the provider to ascertain that the major elements of the pregnancy are removed and helps to distinguish intrauterine from ectopic pregnancies. The clinician may also detect abnormalities that warrant microscopic evaluation. For example, while villous edema is quite common with nonviable or genetically abnormal pregnancies, this finding requires evaluation by a pathologist to rule out hydatidiform mole or choriocarcinoma (Chapter 19). Systematic and thorough inspection of the tissue minimizes delayed complications of abortion.

Identifying villi alone in the absence of membranes or a gestational sac is insufficient to confirm an intrauterine gestation or complete abortion. Sometimes the provider can obtain a sampling of villi without removing the gestational sac. Villi may be present in the uterine aspirate in about half of interstitial ectopic pregnancies; this unusual type constitutes about 2% of all ectopic pregnancies. It is not known whether ectopic pregnancies that are located more distally (e.g., ampullary, isthmic) are capable of shedding villi through the uterotubal junction where they can be captured by aspiration. Moreover, identification of products of conception does not rule out the rare case of heterotopic pregnancy.

Typically, the surgeon or appropriately trained clinic staff carries out the tissue examination. Useful items for tissue examination include a standard kitchen strainer, a clear glass dish (e.g., glass baking dish), backlighting, and when necessary, microscopic magnification. Placing the glass dish on an x-ray view box or a photographic slide viewer provides excellent backlighting of the tissue (Fig. 10.4).

Often, the examiner suspends the tissue in water to assist visualization. To accomplish this, transfer the tissue from the vacuum bottle or syringe to the strainer. Rinse the tissue under running water. Float the tissue in a backlit glass dish that is filled with $^{1}/_{4}$ to $^{1}/_{2}$ inch of water. Some practitioners use an isotonic solution (normal saline) or add acetic acid (household vinegar) to enhance identification of the tissue or prevent osmotic damage when pathologic or genetic analysis is planned. Light shining up through the bottom of the container helps distinguish the following elements:

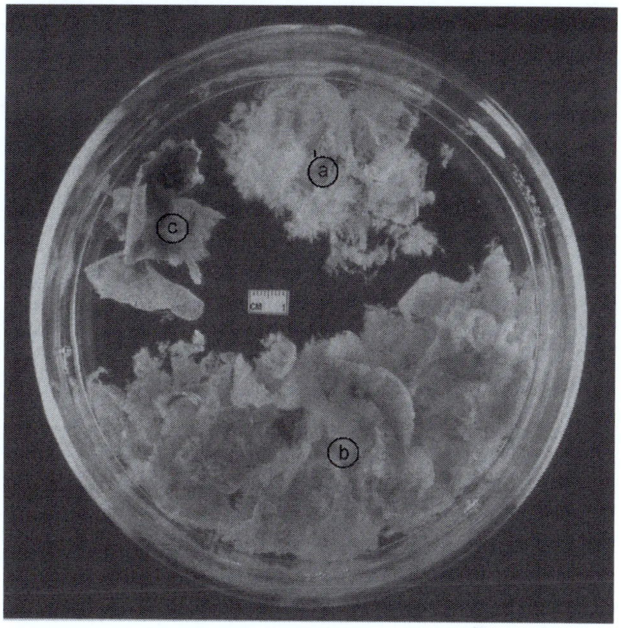

Figure 10.9 Postabortion examination of the uterine aspirate from an 8-week pregnancy. Suspending the tissue in water helps distinguish the various pregnancy elements. Note the thin, transparent gestational sac lined by frond-like villi (a). The decidual tissue is reddish brown or gray and heavier, sinking to the bottom of the dish (b). The decidua capsularis appears as an opaque sheet with hemorrhagic areas (c). See Plate 10.1.

decidual tissue, which is clear, light-colored, or reddish brown; the decidua capsularis, an opaque sheet with hemorrhagic areas; the thin and transparent gestational sac; and chorionic villi, which are transparent with frond-like projections (Fig. 10.9). Very small embryo-fetal parts may be apparent at 9 weeks' gestation and become easier to identify thereafter. Typically, a 6-week intact sac is about the size of a dime (Fig. 10.10); a 7-week sac, a nickel; and an 8-week sac,

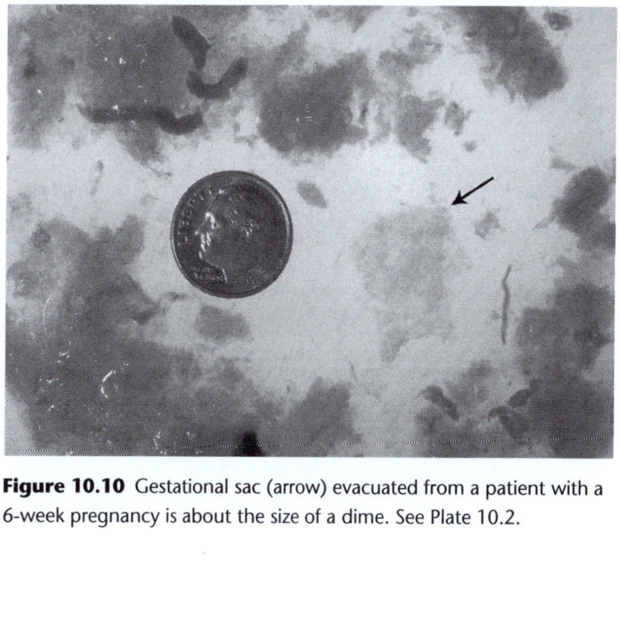

Figure 10.10 Gestational sac (arrow) evacuated from a patient with a 6-week pregnancy is about the size of a dime. See Plate 10.2.

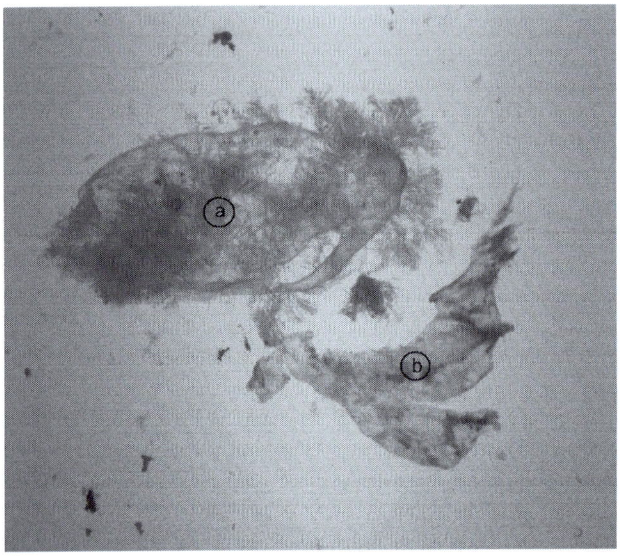

Figure 10.11 Eight-week gestational sac (a) adjacent to a sheet of decidua capsularis (b), floated in water. See Plate 10.3. (Courtesy of Dr. Jerry Edwards.)

a quarter (Fig. 10.11). Often, however, the sac is fragmented, appearing as separate pieces of transparent membranes.

Rather than straining, rinsing, and floating the tissue, some providers find that they can identify the tissue from early pregnancies easily when the aspirate is placed directly into the dish. The small amount of blood outlines the chorionic villi, and even small degrees of hydropic change present with many nonviable or genetically abnormal pregnancies become visible (Fig. 10.12).

Because of individual variation in the amount of decidua, weighing the tissue is not a good predictor of complete removal of the gestation [123]. Photographing or videotaping the gestational tissue offers an inexpensive way to document what is seen in the aspirate, particularly when the tissue is not sent routinely for pathological examination. The additional use of a handheld lens, colposcope, or dissecting microscope may be helpful, especially in very early gestations [118,124]. The provider can suspend tissue in a drop of saline, apply a coverslip, and examine it microscopically under low power (×100). Villi are usually easy to recognize at this magnification (Figs. 10.13, 10.14, 10.15).

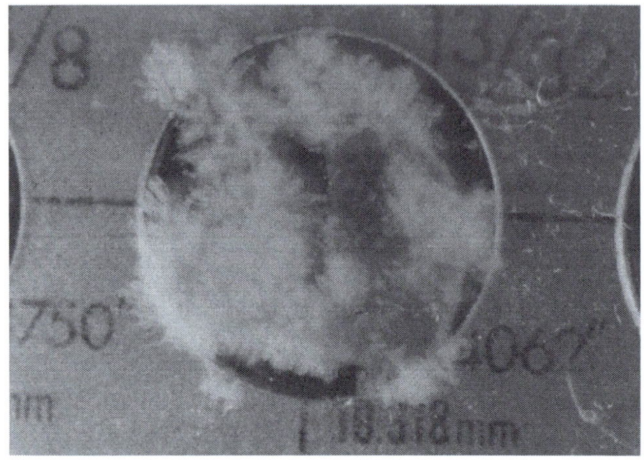

Figure 10.13 Photomicrograph of gestational sac at approximately 4 weeks LMP. Note how delicate and frond-like the villi appear compared to the decidual glands depicted in Plate 10.7. See Plate 10.5. (Courtesy of Dr. Jerry Edwards.)

Unless required by local regulations, many facilities do not routinely send the aspirate for outside pathological examination. With sufficient experience, the expertise of abortion providers in detecting pregnancy elements in fresh aspirates often exceeds that of pathologists who examine the tissue after fixing [125]. However, routine pathological testing provides a permanent record by a dispassionate expert. Pathologic examination is warranted whenever hydropic villi are

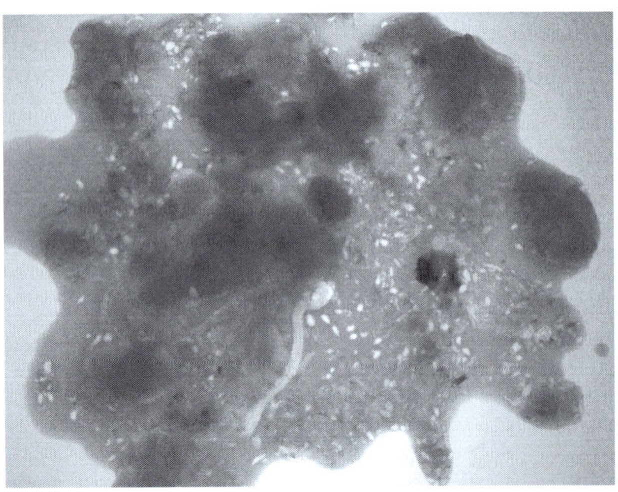

Figure 10.12 Unrinsed hydropic villi from an 11-week pregnancy with trisomy 18. See Plate 10.4.

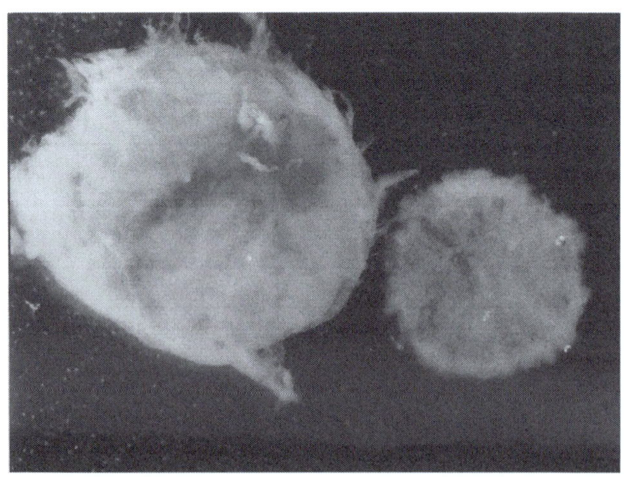

Figure 10.14 Photomicrograph of decidual capsule (left) that has been opened to reveal the early gestational sac (right). See Plate 10.6. (Courtesy of Dr. Jerry Edwards.)

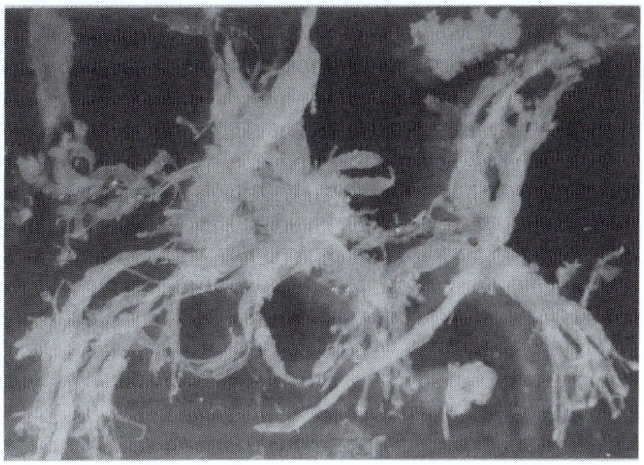

Figure 10.15 Decidual glands as shown in this photomicrograph must not be confused with gestational tissue. See Plate 10.7. (Courtesy of Dr. Jerry Edwards.)

detected and in certain cases of suspected ectopic pregnancy. If necessary, pathologists can use immunochemical stains for human chorionic gonadotropin (hCG), human placental lactogen, and cytokeratin to distinguish trophoblasts from decidua [126] or perform specialized tests to facilitate the diagnosis of early molar pregnancy [127] (Chapter 19).

Procedures for inconclusive tissue examination

Failure to confirm an intrauterine gestation by gross tissue examination warrants evaluation for possible ectopic pregnancy (Chapter 18) or a continuing early pregnancy (Fig. 10.3). If an ultrasound machine is available on-site, perform a sonogram to look for a persistent intrauterine pregnancy, uterine anomalies, or adnexal findings consistent with a tubal pregnancy (Chapters 6 and 18). If a persistent gestation is noted, repeat uterine aspiration.

If intrauterine pregnancy remains unconfirmed, draw an immediate blood sample for determination of hCG level (Fig. 10.3). Patients whose initial serum hCG level exceeds that of the laboratory's discriminatory zone (usually 1500 to 2000 mIU/ml) require prompt evaluation for possible ectopic pregnancy. If the patient has an initial serum hCG below the discriminatory zone and is asymptomatic, she may return for a follow-up hCG measurement 24 to 72 hours later. A decline in hCG levels of 50% or greater during this time period indicates complete abortion, and further testing is unnecessary [118,119]. If the level is increasing, the rate of rise coupled with endovaginal ultrasound helps to distinguish a continuing intrauterine pregnancy from an ectopic gestation. A level that falls by less than 50% warrants evaluation for possible ectopic pregnancy. Most of the ectopic pregnancies detected by this method are early and unruptured, rendering them suitable for treatment with methotrexate rather than surgery (Chapter 18). Some providers send the tissue for a pathological examination in addition to or in lieu of following serum hCG levels [128]. In some settings, this practice may yield results nearly as rapidly as blood draws 2 to 3 days apart. Even detailed pathological examination, however, may not identify an intrauterine pregnancy if a tiny sac adheres to an instrument and is not present in the specimen. In this case, women may be treated unnecessarily for ectopic pregnancy.

Postprocedure care

Patients who have uneventful first-trimester vacuum aspiration abortions with local anesthesia require only short recovery periods; administration of general anesthesia or deep sedation may necessitate longer observation. Key elements of postprocedure care include monitoring of bleeding, pain management, provision of desired contraception, and verbal and written discharge instructions with emergency contact information. Instructions should include when and whom to contact in case of concerning symptoms. Contraception counseling and provision at the time of the abortion help to prevent pregnancies that can occur shortly after abortion and obviates the need for a follow-up visit to obtain contraception (Chapter 14). Although many providers schedule routine follow-up visits 2 to 3 weeks following first-trimester aspiration abortion, the benefits of this practice remain unproven [129]. The NAF *Clinical Policy Guidelines* do not recommend a routine follow-up visit [44]. The Royal College guidelines recommend that providers offer a routine follow-up visit in 2 weeks, although it adds that the visit is optional if complete abortion is confirmed on the day of the procedure [42].

Few data exist to determine the necessity of Rh(D) immunoprophylaxis after early induced abortion [130]. Given its possible advantages and low risks, however, both the ACOG [131] and the RCOG [42] recommend that all unsensitized Rh(D)-negative women receive Rh(D) immune globulin within 72 hours postabortion. Standard practice in the USA includes a 50-μg dose prior to 13 weeks' gestation and a 300-μg dose thereafter.

Periabortal antibiotic prophylaxis reduces the risk of infection after aspiration abortion, regardless of risk factors [132]. Universal prophylaxis costs less and is at least as effective as screen-and-treat strategies [133–135]. Many antibiotic regimens have proven effective for this purpose, and the optimum prophylactic regimen remains unclear [132,136]. The ACOG makes no specific recommendation, although it refers to doxycycline 100 mg orally 1 hour preoperatively followed by 200 mg after the procedure as "one of the most effective and inexpensive regimens reported in a meta-analysis"[136]. The RCOG advises a treatment regimen of metronidazole 1 gm rectally at the time of abortion, followed by a 7-day course of doxycycline or a single 1-gm dose of azithromycin [42]. Doxycycline remains the preferred antibiotic among North American abortion providers with regimens ranging from 1 to 7 days [52].

Conclusion

First-trimester aspiration abortion is one of the safest procedures provided for women of reproductive age. Its use in lieu of dilation and sharp curettage has reduced abortion-related morbidity worldwide. Clinicians employ many variations of technique to accomplish first-trimester aspiration abortion safely in clinics, offices, and hospitals. Manual vacuum aspiration is portable, requires less equipment, and equals electric suction in efficacy and safety. Although most providers use mechanical dilation alone for early first-trimester aspiration, cervical preparation with osmotic dilators or pharmacologic ripening agents may facilitate procedures in the later first-trimester or in adolescents. Tissue examination, appropriate follow-up instructions, and contraception counseling are integral to aspiration abortion practice.

References

1 Sedgh G, Henshaw S, Singh S, Åhman E, Shah IH. Induced abortion: rates and trends worldwide. *Lancet* 2007; **370**: 1145–1338.

2 Jones, RK, Zolna MR, Henshaw SK, Finer LB. Abortion in the United States: incidence and access to services, 2005. *Perspect Sexual Reprod Health* 2008; **40**: 6–16.

3 Gamble SB, Strauss LT, Parker WY, Cook DA, Zane SB, Hamdan S. Abortion Surveillance – United States, 2005. *MMWR Surveill Summ* 2008; **56**: SS-13.

4 Cohen SA. New data on abortion incidence, safety illuminate key aspects of worldwide abortion debate. *Guttmacher Policy Review* 2007; **10**(4).

5 Freedman MA, Jillson DA, Coffin RR, Novick LF. Comparison of complication rates in first trimester abortions performed by physician assistants and physicians. *Am J Public Health* 1986; **76**: 550–554.

6 Henderson JT, Hwang AC, Harper CC, Stewart FH. Safety of mifepristone abortions in clinical use. *Contraception* 2005; **72**: 175–178.

7 Iyengar K, Iyengar SD. Elective abortion as a primary health service in rural India: experience with manual vacuum aspiration. *Reprod Health Matters* 2002; **10**: 54–63.

8 Joffe C, Yanow S. Advanced practice clinicians as abortion providers: current developments in the United States. *Reprod Health Matters* 2004; **12**: 198–206.

9 Warriner IK, Meirik O, Hoffman M et al. Rates of complication in first trimester manual vacuum aspiration abortion done by doctors and mid-level providers in South Africa and Vietnam: a randomised controlled equivalence trial. *Lancet* 2006; **368**: 1965–1972.

10 Dean G, Cardenas L, Darney P, Goldberg A. Acceptability of manual versus electric aspiration for first trimester abortion: a randomized trial. *Contraception* 2003; **67**: 201–206.

11 Chowdhury ME, Botlero R, Koblinsky M, Saha SK, Dieltiens G, Ronsmans C. Determinants of reduction in maternal mortality in Matlab, Bangladesh: a 30-year cohort study. *Lancet* 2007; **370**: 1320–1328.

12 Grimes DA, Benson J, Singh S et al. Unsafe abortion: the preventable pandemic. *Lancet* 2006; **368**: 1908–1919.

13 Weitz TA, Foster A, Ellertson C, Grossman D, Stewart FH. "Medical" and "surgical" abortion: rethinking the modifiers. *Contraception* 2004; **69**: 77–78.

14 Simpson JY. *Clinical Lectures of the Diseases of Women*. R Clark, Edinburgh, 1872, 789.

15 Bykov E. Aspiration of the gravid uterus. *Vrachebnoe Delo* 1927; **9**: 21.

16 Novak E. A suction-curet apparatus for endometrial biopsy. *J Am Med Assoc* 1935; **104**: 1497–1498.

17 T'sai KT. Application of electric vacuum suction in artificial abortion: 30 cases. *Chin J Obstet Gynecol* 1958; **6**: 445.

18 Wu YT, Wu HC. Suction in artificial abortion: 300 cases. *Chin J Obstet Gynecol* 1958; **6**: 447.

19 Vojta M. A critical view of vacuum aspiration: a new method for the termination of pregnancy. *Obstet Gynecol* 1967; **30**: 28–34.

20 Kerslake D, Casey D. Abortion induced by means of the uterine aspirator. *Obstet Gynecol* 1967; **30**: 35–45.

21 Karman H, Potts M. Very early abortion using syringe and vacuum source. *Lancet* 1972; **1**: 1051–1052.

22 Cates W Jr, Schulz KF, Grimes DA, Tyler CW Jr. The effect of delay and choice of method on the risk of abortion morbidity. *Fam Plann Perspect* 1977; **9**: 266–273.

23 Grimes DA, Cates W Jr. Complications from legally induced abortion: a review. *Obstet Gynecol Surv* 1979; **34**: 177–191.

24 Kulier R, Fekih A, Hofmeyr GJ, Campana A. Surgical methods for first trimester termination of pregnancy. *Cochrane Database Syst Rev* 2001; **4**: CD002900.

25 World Health Organization. *Safe Abortion: Technical and Policy Guidance for Health Systems*. World Health Organization, Geneva, 2003.

26 Cates W Jr, Grimes DA, Schulz KF. Abortion surveillance at CDC: creating public health light out of political heat. *Am J Prev Med* 2000; **19**: 12–17.

27 Apter AJ, Kinman JL, Bilker WB et al. Represcription of penicillin after allergic-like events. *J Allergy Clin Immunol* 2004; **113**: 764–770.

28 Bartlett LA, Berg CJ, Shulman HB et al. Risk factors for legal induced abortion-related mortality in the United States. *Obstet Gynecol* 2004; **103**:729–737.

29 Saraiya M, Green CA, Berg CJ, Hopkins FW, Koonin LM, Atrash HK. Spontaneous abortion-related deaths among women in the United States, 1981–1991. *Obstet Gynecol* 1999; **94**: 172–176.

30 Christiansen LR, Collins KA. Pregnancy-associated deaths: a 15-year retrospective study and overall review of maternal pathophysiology. *Am J Forensic Med Pathol* 2006; **27**: 11–19.

31 Grimes DA. Risks of mifepristone abortion in context. *Contraception* 2005; **71**: 161.

32 Tietze C, Henshaw SK. *Induced abortion: A worldwide review, 1986*. Third edition. Guttmacher Institute, New York, 1996.

33 Lefebvre Y, Proulx L, Elie R, Poulin O, Lanza E. The effects of RU-38486 on cervical ripening: Clinical studies. *Am J Obstet Gynecol* 1990; **162**: 61–65.

34 Moreau C, Kaminski M, Ancel PY et al. Previous induced abortions and the risk of very preterm delivery: results of the EPIPAGE study. *BJOG* 2005; **112**: 430–437.

35 Henriet L, Kaminski M. Impact of induced abortions on subsequent pregnancy outcome: the 1995 French national prenatal survey. *BJOG* 2001; **108**: 1036–1042.

36 Martius JA, Steck T, Oehler MK, Wolf KH. Risk factors associated with preterm (<37 + 0 weeks) and early preterm birth (<32 + 0 weeks): univariate and multivariate analysis of 106,345 singleton births from the 1994 statewide perinatal survey of Bavaria. *Eur J Obstet Gynecol Reprod Biol* 1998; **80**: 183–189.

37 Boonstra HD, Gold RB, Richards CL, Finer LB. *Abortion in Women's Lives*. Guttmacher Institute, New York, 2006.

38 Charles VE, Polis CB, Sridhara SK, Blum RW. Abortion and long-term mental health outcomes: a systematic review of the evidence. *Contraception* 2008; **78**: 436–450.

39 Grimes DA, Cates W Jr, Selik RM. Abortion facilities and the risk of death. *Fam Plann Perspect* 1981; **13**: 30–32.

40 Limacher JJ, Daniel I, Isaacksz S et al. Early abortion in Ontario: options and costs. *J Obstet Gynaecol Can* 2006; **28**: 142–148.

41 Harper CC, Henderson JT, Darney PD. Abortion in the United States. *Annu Rev Public Health* 2005; **26**: 501–512.

42 Royal College of Obstetricians and Gynaecologists. *The Care of Women Requesting Induced Abortion: Evidence-Based Clinical Guideline No. 7*. RCOG Press, London, 2004.

43 American Society for Anesthesiologists. Statement on granting privileges for administration of moderate sedation to practitioners who are not anesthesia professionals. American Society of Anesthesiologists – Standards, Guidelines, and Statements. American Society of Anesthesiologists, Chicago, 2006.

44 National Abortion Federation [Online]. Washington (DC): National Abortion Federation; 2008. Clinical policy guidelines; 2008 [cited 2008 Jun 5]. Available from: URL:http://www.prochoice.org/pubs_research/publications/downloads/professional_education/CPG2008.pdf

45 Slade P, Heke S, Fletcher J, Stewart P. A comparison of medical and surgical termination of pregnancy: choice, emotional impact, and satisfaction with care. *Br J Obstet Gynaecol* 1998; **105**: 1288–1295.

46 Henshaw RC, Naji SA, Russell IT, Templeton AA. Comparison of medical abortion with surgical vacuum aspiration: women's preferences and acceptability of treatment. *BMJ* 1993; **307**: 714–717.

47 von Hertzen H, Baird D, Bellagio Study and Conference Center. Frequently asked questions about medical abortion. *Contraception* 2006; **74**: 3–10.

48 Buckshee K, Dhond AJ. A new nonsurgical technique for termination of intrauterine pregnancy associated with large multiple uterine leiomyomas. *Int J Gynaecol Obstet* 1992; **37**: 297–299.

49 Creinin MD. Medical abortion in a woman with a large myomatous uterus. *Am J Obstet Gynecol* 1996; **175**: 1379–1380.

50 Schaff EA, Wortman M, Eisinger SH, Franks P. Methotrexate and misoprostol when surgical abortion fails. *Obstet Gynecol* 1996; **87**: 450–452.

51 Allen RH, Westhoff C, de Nonno L, Fielding S, Schaff EA. Curettage after mifepristone-induced abortion: frequency, timing, and indications. *Obstet Gynecol* 2001; **98**: 101–106.

52 O'Connell K, Jones HE, Simon M, Saporta V, Paul M, Lichtenberg ES. First-trimester surgical abortion practices: A survey of National Abortion Federation members. *Contraception*, in press.

53 Schulz KF, Grimes DA, Cates W Jr. Measures to prevent cervical injury during suction curettage abortion. *Lancet* 1983; **1**: 1182–1185.

54 Grimes DA, Schulz KF, Cates WJ Jr. Prevention of uterine perforation during curettage abortion. *JAMA* 1984; **251**: 2108–2111.

55 Hakim-Elahi E, Tovell HM, Burnhill MS. Complications of first-trimester abortion: a report of 170,000 cases. *Obstet Gynecol* 1990; **76**: 129–135.

56 Allen RH, Goldberg AB, Board of Society of Family Planning. Cervical dilation before first-trimester surgical abortion (<14 weeks' gestation). SFP Guideline 20071. *Contraception* 2007; **76**: 139–156.

57 Ekerhovd E, Radulovic N, Norström A. Gemeprost versus misoprostol for cervical priming before first-trimester abortion: a randomized controlled trial. *Obstet Gynecol* 2003; **101**: 722–725.

58 Platz-Christensen JJ, Nielsen S, Hamberger L. Is misoprostol the drug of choice for induced cervical ripening in early pregnancy termination? *Acta Obstet Gynecol Scand* 1995; **74**: 809–812.

59 Swahn ML, Bygdeman M. The effect of the antiprogestin RU 486 on uterine contractility and sensitivity to prostaglandin and oxytocin. *Br J Obstet Gynaecol* 1988; **95**: 126–134.

60 Ngai SW, Yeung KC, Lao T, Ho PC. Oral misoprostol versus mifepristone for cervical dilatation before vacuum aspiration in first trimester nulliparous pregnancy: a double blind prospective randomised study. *Br J Obstet Gynaecol* 1996; **103**: 1120–1123.

61 Clark K, Ji H, Feltovich H, Janowski J, Carroll C, Chien EK. Mifepristone-induced cervical ripening: structural, biomechanical, and molecular events. *Am J Obstet Gynecol* 2006; **194**: 1391–1398.

62 Ashok PW, Flett GM, Templeton A. Mifepristone versus vaginally administered misoprostol for cervical priming before first-trimester termination of pregnancy: a randomized, controlled study. *Am J Obstet Gynecol* 2000; **183**: 998–1002.

63 MacIsaac L, Grossman D, Balistreri E, Darney P. A randomized controlled trial of laminaria, oral misoprostol, and vaginal misoprostol before abortion. *Obstet Gynecol* 1999; **93**: 766–770.

64 Goldberg AB, Drey EA, Whitaker AK, Kang MS, Meckstroth KR, Darney PD. Misoprostol compared with laminaria before early second-trimester surgical abortion: a randomized trial. *Obstet Gynecol* 2005; **106**: 234–241.

65 Carbonell JL, Velazco A, Rodríguez Y et al. Oral versus vaginal misoprostol for cervical priming in first-trimester abortion: a randomized trial. *Eur J Contracept Reprod Health Care* 2001; **6**: 134–140.

66 Fong YF, Singh K, Prasad RN. A comparative study using two dose regimens (200 microg or 400 microg) of vaginal misoprostol for pre-operative cervical dilatation in first trimester nulliparae. *Br J Obstet Gynaecol* 1998; **105**: 413–417.

67 Singh K, Fong YF, Prasad RN, Dong F. Randomized trial to determine optimal dose of vaginal misoprostol for preabortion cervical priming. *Obstet Gynecol* 1998; **92**: 795–798.

68 Singh K, Fong YF, Prasad RN, Dong F. Evacuation interval after vaginal misoprostol for preabortion cervical priming: a randomized trial. *Obstet Gynecol* 1999; **94**: 431–434.

69 Singh K, Fong YF, Prasad RN, Dong F. Vaginal misoprostol for pre-abortion cervical priming: Is there an optimal evacuation time interval? *Br J Obstet Gynaecol* 1999; **106**: 266–269.

70 Burnett MA, Corbett CA, Gertenstein RJ. A randomized trial of laminaria tents versus vaginal misoprostol for cervical ripening in first trimester surgical abortion. *J Obstet Gynaecol Can* 2005; **27**: 38–42.

71 Carbonell Esteve JL, Marí JM, Valero F et al. Sublingual versus vaginal misoprostol (400 microg) for cervical priming in first-trimester abortion: a randomized trial. *Contraception* 2006; **74**: 328–333.

72 Patel A, Talmont E, Morfeisis J et al. Adequacy and safety of buccal misoprostol for cervical preparation prior to termination of second-trimester pregnancy. *Contraception* 2006; **73**: 420–430.

73 Todd CS, Soler M, Castleman L, Rogers MK, Blumenthal PD. Buccal misoprostol as cervical preparation for second trimester pregnancy termination. *Contraception* 2002; **65**: 415–418.

74 Li CF, Wong CY, Chan CP, Ho PC. A study of co-treatment of nonsteroidal anti-inflammatory drugs (NSAIDs) with misoprostol for cervical priming before suction termination of first trimester pregnancy. *Contraception* 2003; **67**: 101–105.

75 Olund A, Jonasson A, Kindahl H, Fianu S, Larsson B. The effect of cervical dilatation by laminaria on the plasma levels of 15-keto-13,14-dihydro-PGF2 alpha. *Contraception* 1984; **30**: 23–27.

76 Jonasson A, Larsson B. Contractile activity in the human uterine cervix and corpus during cervical dilatation by laminaria tent in first trimester legal abortions. *Acta Obstet Gynecol Scand* 1989; **68**: 401–404.

77 Johnson B, Benson J, Leibson-Hawkins B. Reducing resource use and improving quality of care with MVA. *Adv Abortion Care* 1992; **2**: 1–6.

78 Wen J, Cai QY, Deng F, Li YP. Manual versus electric vacuum aspiration for first-trimester abortion: a systematic review. *BJOG* 2008; **115**: 5–13.

79 Goldberg AB, Dean G, Kang MS, Youssof S, Darney PD. Manual versus electric vacuum aspiration for early first-trimester abortion: a controlled study of complication rates. *Obstet Gynecol* 2004; **103**: 101–107.

80 Bird ST, Harvey SM, Beckman LJ, Nichols MD, Rogers K, Blumenthal PD. Similarities in women's perceptions and acceptability of manual vacuum aspiration and electric vacuum aspiration for first trimester abortion. *Contraception* 2003; **67**: 207–212.

81 Bird ST, Harvey SM, Nichols MD, Edelman A. Comparing the acceptability of manual vacuum aspiration and electric vacuum aspiration as methods of early abortion. *J Am Med Womens Assoc* 2001; **56**: 124–126.

82 Edelman A, Nichols MD, Jensen J. Comparison of pain and time of procedures with two first-trimester abortion techniques performed by residents and faculty. *Am J Obstet Gynecol* 2001; **184**: 1564–1567.

83 EngenderHealth [Online]. New York: EngenderHealth; 2008. Practical Guide for Selection of MVA Instruments; 2004 [cited 2008 Jul 27]. Available from: URL: http://www.engenderhealth.org/files/pubs/pac/mva_instruments_guide.pdf

84 Hulka JF, Lefler HT Jr, Anglone A, Lachenbruch PA. A new electronic force monitor to measure factors influencing cervical dilation for vacuum curettage. *Am J Obstet Gynecol* 1974; **120**: 166–173.

85 Novak F, Andolsek L. (1974) Comparison of the medical effects of induced abortion by two methods, curettage and vacuum aspiration. In: Andolsek L, ed. *The Ljubljana Abortion Study, 1971–1973*. National Institutes of Health, Center for Population Research, Bethesda, MD, 1974: 1–57.

86 Orbach D, Schaff E. Which cannulae fit the Ipas manual vacuum aspiration syringe? *Contraception* 2004; **69**: 171–173.

87 Clark S, Krishna U, Kallenbach L, Mandlekar A, Raote V, Ellertson C. Women's preferences for general or local anesthesia for pain during first trimester surgical abortion in India.*Contraception* 2002; **66**: 275–279.

88 Allen RH, Kumar D, Fitzmaurice G, Lifford KL, Goldberg AB. Pain management of first-trimester surgical abortion: effects of selection of local anesthesia with and without lorazepam or intravenous sedation. *Contraception* 2006; **74**: 407–413.

89 Wiebe ER. Comparison of the efficacy of different local anesthetics and techniques of local anesthesia in therapeutic abortions. *Am J Obstet Gynecol* 1992; **167**: 131–134.

90 Suprapto K, Reed S. Naproxen sodium for pain relief in first-trimester abortion. *Am J Obstet Gynecol* 1984; **150**: 1000–1001.

91 Romero I, Turok D, Gilliam M. A randomized trial of tramadol versus ibuprofen as an adjunct to pain control during vacuum aspiration abortion. *Contraception* 2008; **77**: 56–59.

92 Wiebe E, Podhradsky L, Dijak V. The effect of lorazepam on pain and anxiety in abortion. *Contraception* 2003; **67**: 219–221.

93 Suliman S, Ericksen T, Labuschgne P, de Wit R, Stein DJ, Seedat S. Comparison of pain, cortisol levels, and psychological distress in women undergoing surgical termination of pregnancy under local anaesthesia versus intravenous sedation. *BMC Psychiatry* 2007; **7**: 24.

94 Wong CY, Ng EH, Ngai SW, Ho PC. A randomized, double blind, placebo-controlled study to investigate the use of conscious sedation in conjunction with paracervical block for reducing pain in termination of first trimester pregnancy by suction evacuation. *Hum Reprod* 2002; **17**: 1222–1225.

95 Schulz KF, Grimes DA, Cates W Jr. Measures to prevent cervical injury during suction curettage abortion. *Lancet* 1983; **1**: 1182–1185.

96 Eastwood KL, Kacmar JE, Steinauer J, Weitzen S, Boardman LA. Abortion training in United States obstetrics and gynecology residency programs. *Obstet Gynecol* 2006; **108**: 303–308.

97 Osborne NG, Wright RC. Effect of preoperative scrub on the bacterial flora of the endocervix and vagina. *Obstet Gynecol* 1977; **50**: 148–151.

98 Lundh C, Meirik O, Nygren KG. Vaginal cleansing at vacuum aspiration abortion does not reduce the risk of postoperative infection. *Acta Obstet Gynecol Scand* 1983; **62**: 275–277.

99 Varli IH, Lindelius A, Bergström A. Is preoperative vaginal cleansing necessary for control of infection after first trimester vacuum curettage? *Acta Obstet Gynecol Scand* 2005; **84**: 650–653.

100 Beric BM, Kupresanin M. Vacuum aspiration, using pericervical block, for legal abortion as an outpatient procedure up to the 12th week of pregnancy. *Lancet* 1971; **2**: 619–621.

101 Chen LH, Lai SF, Lee WH, Leong NK. Uterine perforation during elective first trimester abortions: a 13-year review. *Singapore Med J* 1995; **36**: 63–67.

102 Molin A. Risk of damage to the cervix by dilatation for first-trimester-induced abortion by suction aspiration. *Gynecol Obstet Invest* 1993; **35**: 152–154.

103 Forna F, Gülmezoglu AM. Surgical procedures to evacuate incomplete miscarriage. *Cochrane Database Syst Rev* 2001; Record No: CD001993.

104 Acharya G, Morgan H, Paramanantham L, Fernando R. A randomized clinical trial comparing surgical termination of pregnancy with and without ultrasound guidance. *Eur J Obstet Gynecol Reprod Biol* 2004; **114**: 69–74.

105 Hodgson J, Portmann KC. Complications of 10,453 consecutive first-trimester abortions: a prospective study. *Am J Obstet Gynecol* 1974; **120**: 802–807.

106 Debby A, Malinger G, Harow E, Golan A, Glezerman M. Transvaginal ultrasound after first-trimester uterine evacuation reduces the incidence of retained products of conception. *Ultrasound Obstet Gynecol* 2006; **27**: 61–64.

107 Durfee SM, Frates MC, Luong A, Benson CB. The sonographic and color Doppler features of retained products of conception. *J Ultrasound Med* 2005; **24**: 1181–1186.

108 Dillon EH, Case CQ, Ramos IM, Holland CK, Taylor KJ. Endovaginal US and Doppler findings after first-trimester abortion. *Radiology* 1993; **186**: 87–91.

109 Maslovitz S, Almog B, Mimouni GS, Jaffa A, Lessing JB, Many A. Accuracy of diagnosis of retained products of conception after dilation and evacuation. *J Ultrasound Med* 2004; **23**: 749–756.

110 Timor-Tritsch IE, Masch RJ, Goldstein SR, Ng E, Monteagudo A. Transvaginal ultrasound-assisted gynecologic surgery: evaluation of a new device to improve safety of intrauterine surgery. *Am J Obstet Gynecol* 2003; **189**: 1074–1079.

111 Lauersen NH, Conrad P. Effect of oxytocic agents on blood loss during first trimester suction curettage. *Obstet Gynecol* 1974; **44**: 428–433.

112 Ali PB, Smith G. The effect of syntocinon on blood loss during first trimester suction curettage. *Anesthesia* 1996; **51**: 483–485.

113 de Groot AN, van Dongen PW, Vree TB, Hekster YA, van Roosmalen J. Ergot alkaloids. Current status and review of clinical pharmacology and therapeutic use compared with other oxytocics in obstetrics and gynaecology. *Drugs* 1998; **56**: 523–535.

114 Schulz KF, Grimes DA, Christensen DD. Vasopressin reduces blood loss from second-trimester dilatation and evacuation abortion. *Lancet* 1985; **2**: 353–356.

115 Dean CL, Chez RA. Using vasopressin in paracervical block. *Contemporary OB/GYN* 1993; October: 42–44.

116 Phillips DR, Nathanson HG, Milim SJ, Haselkom JS. The effect of dilute vasopressin solution on the force needed for cervical dilatation: a randomized controlled trial. *Obstet Gynecol* 1997; **89**: 507–511.

117 Sands RX, Burnhill MS, Hakim-Elahi E. Postabortal uterine atony. *Obstet Gynecol* 1974; **43**: 595–598.

118 Edwards J, Carson SA. (1997) New technologies permit safe abortion at less than six weeks' gestation and provide timely detection of ectopic gestation. *Am J Obstet Gynecol* 176: 1101–1106.

119 Creinin MD, Edwards J. Early abortion: surgical and medical options. *Curr Prob Obstet Gynecol Fertil* 1997; **20**: 1–32.

120 Paul ME, Mitchell CM, Rogers AJ, Fox MC, Lackie EG. Early surgical abortion: efficacy and safety. *Am J Obstet Gynecol* 2002; **187**: 407–411.

121 Brenner WE, Edelman DA, Kessel E. Menstrual regulation in the United States: a preliminary report. *Fertil Steril* 1975; **26**: 289–295.

122 Kaunitz AM, Rovira EZ, Grimes DA, Schulz KF. Abortions that fail. *Obstet Gynecol* 1985; **66**: 533–537.

123 Felding C, Mikkelsen AL, Villerslev L. First-trimester legally induced abortions. The amount of aspirated tissue in relation to gestational age. *Arch Gynecol Obstet* 1991; **249**: 149–151.

124 Burnhill MS, Armstead JW. Reducing the morbidity of vacuum aspiration abortion. *Int J Gynaecol Obstet* 1978; **16**: 204–209.

125 Paul M, Lackie E, Mitchell C, Rogers A, Fox M. Is pathology examination useful after early surgical abortion? *Obstet Gynecol* 2002; **99**: 567–571.

126 Gruber K, Gelven PL, Austin RM. Chorionic villi or trophoblastic tissue in uterine samples of four women with ectopic pregnancies. *Int J Gynecol Pathol* 1997; **16**: 28–32.

127 Crisp H, Burton JL, Stewart R, Wells M. Refining the diagnosis of hydatidiform mole: image ploidy analysis and p57^{KIP2} immunohistochemistry. *Histopathology* 2003; **43**: 363–373.

128 Benson J, Clark KA, Gerhardt A, Randall L, Dudley S. Early abortion services in the United States: a provider survey. *Contraception* 2003; **67**: 287–294.

129 Grossman D, Ellertson C, Grimes DA, Walker D. Routine follow-visits after first-trimester induced abortion. *Obstet Gynecol* 2004; **103**: 738–745.

130 Jabara S, Barnhart KT. Is Rh immune globulin needed in early first-trimester abortion? A review. *Am J Obstet Gynecol* 2003; **188**: 623–627.

131 American College of Obstetricians and Gynecologists, Committee on Practice Bulletins. Prevention of Rh D alloimmunization. ACOG Practice Bulletin, No. 4, May 1999. American College of Obstetricians and Gynecologists, Washington (DC).

132 Sawaya GF, Grady D, Kerlikowske K, Grimes DA. Antibiotics at the time of induced abortion: the case for universal prophylaxis based on a meta-analysis. *Obstet Gynecol* 1996; **87**: 884–890.

133 Cameron ST, Sutherland S. Universal prophylaxis compared with screen-and-treat for *Chlamydia trachomatis* prior to termination of pregnancy. *BJOG* 2002; **109**: 606–609.

134 Chen S, Li J, van den Hoek A. Universal screening or prophylactic treatment for *Chlamydia trachomatis* infection among women seeking induced abortions: which strategy is more cost effective? *Sex Transm Dis* 2007; **34**: 230–236.

135 Penney GC, Thomson M, Norman J et al. A randomised comparison of strategies for reducing infective complications of induced abortion. *Br J Obstet Gynaecol* 1998; **105**: 599–604.

136 American College of Obstetricians and Gynecologists, Committee on Practice Bulletins. Antibiotic prophylaxis for gynecologic procedures. ACOG Practice Bulletin No. 74, July 2006. American College of Obstetricians and Gynecologists, Washington, (DC).

11

CHAPTER 11 Dilation and evacuation

Cassing Hammond MD, and Stephen Chasen MD

LEARNING POINTS

- Dilation and evacuation (D&E) is a safe and effective method of induced abortion.
- Compared to labor-induction abortion, D&E offers more predictable timing of evacuation, greater cost savings, and safety advantages for patients with certain serious medical conditions. D&E also allows women to avoid the labor-like process of a medical induction.
- Cervical preparation using osmotic dilating devices prior to D&E decreases the risk of complications. Substantial research has documented the safety and efficacy of misoprostol as a cervical ripener in the first trimester; data regarding its use before D&E abortion are limited, but suggest positive outcomes.
- Preoperative injection to cause fetal demise may facilitate completion of D&E abortion, although published data are still limited. It also helps providers in the USA ensure compliance with the Partial-Birth Abortion Ban Act of 2003 and related state laws.
- Surgical skill and experience are paramount in assuring patient safety during D&E.

Introduction

The proportion of US abortions performed in the second trimester has varied little since 1992. According to surveillance data from the Centers for Disease Control and Prevention (CDC), roughly 12% of abortions occur at or after 13 weeks' gestation. Only 3.8% of abortions occur at 16 to 20 weeks and 1.4% at or after 21 weeks [1]. Ninety-six per cent of the more than 140,000 second-trimester abortions performed annually in the USA [1,2] are accomplished by the technique of dilation and evacuation (D&E), primarily in outpatient settings [3,4]. In many other countries, such as Canada, Cuba, the United Kingdom, and most other European nations, medical methods comprise a larger proportion, or the sole option, for second-trimester abortion (Chapter 12).

Where it is available, D&E offers a highly effective method of pregnancy termination. After providing some background information on the safety and benefits of D&E, this chapter focuses on the use of D&E in clinical practice including methods of cervical preparation, variations in surgical techniques, and postoperative care. Because of the plethora of legal requirements governing abortion provision in the USA, including the federal Partial-Birth Abortion Ban Act of 2003 [5] and related state laws, US physicians embarking on second-trimester abortion practice are advised to read Chapter 4 and consult with legal counsel as needed.

Management of Unintended and Abnormal Pregnancy, 1st edition. By M Paul, ES Lichtenberg, L Borgatta, DA Grimes, PG Stubblefield, MD Creinin
 ISBN: 9781405176965.

Historical perspective: Surgical innovation and evolution

In 1973, at the time of nationwide legalization of abortion in the USA, vacuum aspiration was generally available only through 12 weeks' gestation. Women requiring abortion in the second trimester either had hysterotomies or delayed abortion until 16 weeks in order to undergo intra-amniotic instillation [6]. The fundamental challenge to a transvaginal surgical approach was to find an atraumatic means to dilate the uterine cervix that would permit successful extraction of the enlarging second-trimester fetus. During the 1970s, European physician-innovators pioneered methods of dilation and extraction that overcame these barriers and remain cornerstones of today's D&E procedure [7].

Advances in methods of cervical dilation greatly facilitated uterine evacuation. Sir Arthur Finks recognized the advantage of cervical ripening for midtrimester abortion at a time prior to the importation of osmotic dilators to Great Britain. His innovation was to sever the umbilical cord overnight, resulting in fetal demise and cervical ripening, before attempting surgical extraction the following day [8]. Japanese and

European physicians had used hygroscopic, processed seaweed tents (*Laminaria japonica* or *digitata*) for more than a century to deliver compromised pregnancies [9] before their adoption in Eastern and then Western Europe.

Although use of a sizable suction cannula permitted fetal extraction through 14–16 weeks' gestation, it did not suffice for removing the larger fetus of later gestations. European innovators, such as Van Lith [10], fashioned sturdy, slim instruments similar to enlarged and reinforced ovum forceps with elongated jaws. These instruments enabled Dutch and other European surgeons to perform D&E abortion beyond 20 weeks of gestation.

The emergence of gradual overnight cervical dilation encouraged the development of larger instruments for fetal and placenta extraction. Sopher and Bierer [11] fashioned forceps of greater weight and surface area to enable more rapid removal of fetal parts at later gestations. American innovators, such as Hern, developed variants of extraction instruments specifically suited to rotate fetal parts prior to their removal. Variations in instrument length, size of extraction tip, contour, and location of instrument fulcrum permitted increasingly sophisticated extraction maneuvers resulting in safer, more efficient uterine evacuation.

The US adoption of laminaria tents in the 1970s [12] to dilate the cervix before uterine evacuation represented a landmark in abortion care, permitting safe D&E later in pregnancy. The advent of synthetic osmotic dilators, such as Dilapan® and Lamicel® devices, used alone or in combination with laminaria and applied as multiple serial treatments, facilitated even greater atraumatic cervical dilation, virtually eliminating the cervical barrier to second-trimester abortion [13].

Prevalence and safety

The proportion of US abortions performed by D&E at or after 13 weeks' gestation increased from 31% in 1974 to 96% in 2005, while the percentage performed by intrauterine instillation decreased from 57 to 0.4% [1]. This trend reflects D&E's safety and popularity as well as the proliferation of well-trained D&E surgeons and dedicated outpatient facilities offering specialized care in a cost-effective manner. In addition, physicians trained in the D&E procedure routinely employ and adapt the technique to treat women experiencing second-trimester pregnancy loss, such as intrauterine fetal demise, preterm premature rupture of membranes, and preterm labor with irreversible cervical dilation.

Observational data and several retrospective cohort trials in the 1980s consistently confirmed the safety advantages of D&E versus available methods of medical induction throughout much of the second trimester [7,14,15]. These studies included comparison with older induction agents, such as oxytocin, prostaglandin $F_{2\alpha}$, and urea. In a 2002 retrospective observational study by Autry that compared efficacy and side effects of induction using misoprostol with D&E abortion, the reported major disadvantage of induction abortion was a 30% incidence of retained placenta [16]. Subsequent use of higher dosages of misoprostol, or a combination of mifepristone and misoprostol, with prolonged observation until natural expulsion of the placenta lowered the incidence of retained placenta to 3 to 6% [17,18] (Chapter 12). Using modern techniques and drugs, complication rates of both second-trimester medical and surgical abortion are low; major complications occur in less than 1% of D&E cases [7,15,19,20].

Mortality associated with D&E abortion has dropped steadily over time in the USA. Lawson and colleagues at the CDC noted a reduction from 10.4 deaths per 100,000 procedures during 1972 to 1976 to 3.3 deaths per 100,000 cases during 1977 to 1982 [21]. Unfortunately, the CDC could not calculate national abortion case-fatality rates for 1998 to 2002, the most recent study interval, because a substantial number of the abortions occurred in states not reporting data to the CDC. Thus, the total number of abortions (denominator) is unknown.

Because of its impressive safety record as well as patient preference, D&E remains the most prevalent method of second-trimester pregnancy termination in the USA, accounting for 96% of all second-trimester abortions [1]. The British Royal College of Obstetricians and Gynaecologists (RCOG) recognizes D&E as a safe and effective option for abortion beyond 15 weeks' gestation when performed by practitioners with the requisite instruments and skills [22].

Procedure selection

Given the favorable safety profile of both medical induction and surgical abortion, patients would ideally select an abortion procedure based on their personal preference and medical circumstances. When Grimes and colleagues attempted to perform a randomized clinical trial in the USA comparing D&E with medical induction, most women did not consent to randomization because of the many apparent advantages of D&E [3]. Some of the advantages are discussed next.

Timing and predictability

D&E affords both patients and clinicians more predictable timing of the procedure. The patient typically undergoes 1 to 2 days of preoperative cervical preparation with osmotic dilators, chemical ripening agents, or a combination of the two. Experienced clinicians can usually accomplish D&E in less than 30 minutes as an outpatient procedure. Patients commonly return to work the day following the procedure, minimizing disruption at home and at work.

Psychosocial advantages

Many patients find that the predictability of surgical abortion and avoidance of prolonged labor make D&E less emotionally burdensome than medically induced abortion [23–25]. In contrast to D&E, most inductions occur in hospital settings. Women having induction abortions are often confined to a unit where obstetrical patients are also lying-in. Here, they may be exposed to women laboring and delivering highly desired pregnancies and to hospital staff with a strong moral antipathy to pregnancy termination.

Cost

Many patients in the USA incur the immediate cost of abortions themselves. In addition, indirect costs, such as those associated with treatment of complications and utilization of limited health system resources, are of increasing concern to hospital administrators and third-party payers. Cowett used decision tree analysis to compare the cost-effectiveness of hospital-based D&E versus misoprostol induction of labor (assumed induction-abortion interval 20 hours) during the second trimester [26]. No variation in the probabilities of morbidity or the costs made induction of labor a cost-effective alternative to D&E. Medical regimens using mifepristone taken orally at home 24 to 48 hours before induction and then followed by misoprostol result in substantially shorter induction-to-abortion intervals than regimens studied by Cowett. These regimens should reduce the cost of second-trimester induction abortion. Nonetheless, D&E can be performed as an outpatient procedure whereas induction abortion almost always entails either hospitalization or internment at an intermediate facility, thereby increasing costs substantially.

Prenatal diagnosis

Patients undergoing pregnancy termination because of fetal anomalies often prefer D&E to the longer and less predictable methods of labor induction. Shulman demonstrated that abortion by D&E does not necessarily prevent anatomic diagnosis of suspected fetal anomalies [27]. An advantage of the intact variant of D&E (sometimes called *dilation and extraction* or D&X) is to permit more complete morphologic evaluation of an extracted fetus.

Specific medical concerns

Experienced clinicians can safely achieve accelerated cervical preparation before D&E abortion up to 24 weeks' gestation in 12 to 16 hours without subjecting patients in perilous medical or obstetrical condition to appreciable metabolic or physical stress. In addition, D&E is an important option in cases of failed medical induction (Box A).

The availability of trained and experienced providers may affect a woman's choice of second-trimester abortion methods. A 2002 survey of members of the National Abortion Federation (NAF) found that two-thirds of clinician respondents who performed D&E abortions were aged 50 years or older [28]. Whether current levels of training will meet the need for second-trimester service provision in the USA as aging providers retire is unclear. Although abortion training has increased in recent years because of advocacy efforts and more explicit guidelines from the Accreditation Council on Graduate Medical Education, the relative lack of training in second-trimester D&E remains a concern. A survey of US obstetrics and gynecology residency program directors found that 51% of programs offered routine abortion training in 2004 compared to only 12% in 1992. In programs offering routine training, however, most (64%) trained less than half of their residents in D&E techniques, and very few offered the volume of procedures necessary to attain competence [29]. Notwithstanding these limitations, the increase in abortion-training curricula and establishment of fellowships and divisions of family planning at many academic centers of excellence will augment training, research, and availability of the full range of abortion services, including D&E [30].

Preprocedure preparation

Clinical setting and medical screening

Most women seeking abortion are young and healthy. This fact, coupled with the favorable safety profile of D&E, makes the procedure amenable to a variety of clinical settings, including licensed surgical centers, most outpatient clinics, and many physician offices. Pain management options, ranging from cervical anesthesia with or without oral medication to intravenous sedation or general anesthesia, depend on facility resources, patient and provider preferences, gestational age, and other factors (Chapter 8). Although a woman's medical history or physical examination findings can influence choice of procedure and clinical setting, the skill and experience of the D&E provider are paramount in assuring patient safety [14].

Requirements for a safe D&E program include:

- surgeons skilled and experienced in D&E provision;
- adequate pain control options with appropriate monitoring;
- requisite instruments, including aspirating cannulae and extraction forceps;
- staff skilled in patient education and counseling, procedural care, and patient recovery; and
- established procedures at freestanding facilities for transferring patients who require emergency hospital-based care.

Preoperative evaluation of the patient includes a pertinent history, targeted physical examination (including measurement of height and weight as well as pelvic examination), and an ultrasound scan to verify gestational age and to assess placental location as indicated. Pertinent history should include current medications; pertinent allergies; acute and

Box A

The patient is a 32-year-old nulliparous female with a history of chronic hypertension at 22 weeks' gestation who presented to the high-risk obstetric service complaining of increasing upper abdominal pain. Laboratory studies eventually confirmed HELLP syndrome* with liver enzymes three times the normal value and a platelet count of 60,000. Given poor maternal prognosis associated with continuation of the pregnancy, the patient chose to proceed with abortion by induction of labor. The patient's cervix was uneffaced and undilated when maternal fetal medicine consultants began induction using misoprostol 400 μg every 6 hours. Twelve hours after initiation of induction, the patient experienced spontaneous rupture of membranes and became increasingly uncomfortable but her cervix remained only minimally dilated. Her temperature had risen to 39.1°C (102.4°F), prompting initiation of ampicillin and gentamicin for chorioamnionitis. Meanwhile, her platelet count had decreased to 24,000 and her liver function had deteriorated. Obstetricians consulted family planning service staff who placed laminaria ×10 in the patient's cervix. Although the institutional protocol usually called for serial laminaria treatments over 24 hours between 20 and 24 weeks' gestation, the patient's pretreatment with misoprostol had already achieved considerable cervical ripening. Six hours after laminaria insertion, the patient underwent D&E with general anesthesia. The uncomplicated operation required approximately 20 minutes and resulted in estimated blood loss of 200 cc. The patient's medical condition progressively improved following uterine evacuation, and she was discharged home in stable condition a few days later.

* A severe form of pre-eclampsia characterized by hemolysis, elevated liver enzymes, and low platelet count.

chronic medical conditions; and gynecological factors such as uterine scarring, prior pelvic surgery, or uterine fibroids.

Low-risk D&E patients require minimal preoperative laboratory evaluation. Providers can benefit from knowing preoperative hemoglobin or hematocrit, particularly in the relatively uncommon event that a patient's surgical blood loss exceeds 500 cc. Unless their Rh(D) status is documented in writing, all patients should have Rh(D) antigen testing and receive anti-D immune globulin when indicated. Glucometer testing on the day of surgery for patients with labile insulin diabetes is helpful (Chapter 7).

Patient education and counseling

As with any medical procedure, providers must assure that women presenting for abortion after the first trimester have all the information they need to make informed decisions about their care. In addition, some women may desire further counseling to address emotional, logistical, or psychological issues (Chapter 5). Women who terminate wanted pregnancies because of maternal health issues or detection of fetal anomalies may benefit from counseling by staff well versed in perinatal loss.

Second-trimester patients in the USA undergo termination for a variety of reasons, but most often because of delay in recognizing pregnancy or obtaining necessary funds and support [31,32]. This type of delay may reflect inadequate access to health services, ambivalence about the decision to terminate the pregnancy, familial conflict, or peer-group pressure. Teenagers are likelier than older women to delay abortion until the second trimester [1,33,34] (Chapter 3).

Occasionally, women undergoing preparation for second-trimester pregnancy termination reverse their decision to abort and request removal of osmotic dilators. Although data are inadequate to determine risks of infection or preterm delivery in these circumstances, patients need to be informed of possible sequelae. A case series from Israel described 17 women (gestational age range 6–18 weeks) who chose to continue pregnancies after laminaria removal [35]. Fourteen of these patients delivered at term, one delivered prematurely at 36 weeks, one was induced at 35 weeks for severe preeclampsia, and one had a first-trimester spontaneous abortion. Although chlamydia tests were positive in four women, none experienced amnionitis or preterm delivery despite discontinuation of antibiotic prophylaxis after laminaria removal.

Misoprostol, increasingly used to enhance dilation before second-trimester abortion, might also increase the risk of premature fetal expulsion or anomaly should a patient change her decision to undergo uterine evacuation. Although misoprostol exposure in the first trimester has been associated with Möbius syndrome, a constellation of craniofacial and other abnormalities, no current data confirm or refute teratogenicity following second-trimester exposure [36,37].

Several states in the USA require that women receive information related to so-called fetal "pain" before obtaining an abortion. In 1997, an expert panel convened by RCOG concluded that minimal sensory input reaches the fetal brain before 26 weeks' gestation and that fetal reactions to noxious stimuli could not be interpreted as pain perception [38]. Requisite US courses in research-related human subjects' protection cite 28 weeks of gestation as the earliest time in fetal development when cognition may be present. In a recent thorough review of published studies addressing this subject, Lee and colleagues concluded that fetal perception of pain is unlikely before the third trimester [39]. At this time, available evidence demonstrates that the second-trimester fetus lacks the capacity to perceive pain.

Cervical preparation

Adequate cervical preparation decreases the morbidity associated with second-trimester surgical abortion, including the risk of cervical injury, uterine perforation, and incomplete abortion [40,41]. Knowledge of methods to achieve adequate cervical preparation is important to provision of safe D&E abortion.

Osmotic dilators

Types

Three types of osmotic dilators are or have recently been in current use in modern settings: *Laminaria japonica* and *digitata*, Lamicel®, and Dilapan-S™ (Appendix, Fig. A-13).

Laminaria tents (MedGyn: Lombard, IL, USA, and Norscan: Westlake Village, CA, USA), the oldest and most commonly used osmotic dilator, are dried, compressed Japanese seaweed tents derived from *japonica* or *digitata* plants. Laminaria come in at least 11 diameters ranging from 2 to 10 mm, in the standard 60-mm length as well as an extra long 85-mm model. Their dimensions are far more varied than those of synthetic dilators, which can be a distinct advantage. When exposed to fluid, laminaria swell to three to four times their dry weight without changing length. They achieve cervical dilation by exerting direct radial pressure outwardly against surrounding cervical stroma and by causing the release of F-series prostaglandins, fostering a disruption in the collagen matrix of cervical tissue. Laminaria thereby both soften and dilate the cervix, making them an effective primary dilating agent as well as an effective adjunctive agent in combination with other types of osmotic dilators or prostaglandins. They achieve most of their clinical effect in 3 hours but reach maximal diameter in 24 hours [42,43].

Lamicel® are dry polyvinyl alchohol sponges impregnated with 450 mg of magnesium sulfate. They measure 67 mm in length and come in two diameters, 3 mm and 5 mm. Lamicel® work by absorbing fluid from the surrounding cervix, reversibly decoupling collagen cross-linkages and increasing sensitivity to E-series prostaglandins within the cervical stroma. They begin working within 2 hours and achieve maximal clinical effect by 4 to 6 hours [44]. Lamicel® devices dilate to 8 mm when placed 6 hours before D&E, and they provide adequate dilation for most D&Es at 17 weeks' gestation or less [45]. Although Lamicel® exert little radial force, they have great utility in early second-trimester procedures, particularly by ripening the cervix before using rigid osmotic dilators. Unfortunately, in 2008 Lamicel® were no longer commercially available in the USA.

Dilapan™ devices (J.C.E.C. Co., Inc., Kendall Park, NJ) are synthetic, hygroscopic polyacrylonitrile rod-shaped dilators. The original model, Dilapan®, was retooled in 1998, underwent several years of clinical testing outside the USA, and is now available as Dilapan-S™. Each Dilapan-S™ rod comes in two lengths, 55 mm or 65 mm, and two diameters, 3 mm or 4 mm. Whereas Lamicel® work primarily chemically and laminaria® work both chemically and mechanically, Dilapan-S™ devices cause cervical dilation predominantly by exerting radial pressure. A 4-mm Dilapan-S™ tent swells to nearly 15 mm, shortening its length by about one-fifth in the process (Appendix, Fig. A-13). Although the device continues to expand up to 24 hours following placement, significant effect is noted in 2 hours and most dilation is achieved within 4 to 6 hours. Many providers use Dilapan-S™ following an initial treatment with laminaria or in combination with Lamicel® or laminaria to soften or predilate the cervix.

In the past, Dilapan™ devices occasionally fractured, leaving plastic debris in the endometrial cavity; these bits could be confoundingly difficult to remove and reconstitute [46]. The retooled Dilapan-S™ model became commercially available in 2002, but its distribution is limited to a few countries. The retooled version is cast longitudinally, conferring increased tensile strength when stretched during a difficult removal and resulting in far fewer instances of fragmentation.

Insertion techniques

Most clinicians can easily learn how to insert osmotic dilators, and techniques and protocols for use are quite varied. Experienced providers gradually acquire dexterity and acumen in tailoring the use of osmotic dilating devices to the great variety of cervical responses they encounter. A general technique of insertion is described here:

- After inserting a speculum into the vagina and optionally cleansing the cervix, grasp the cervix with a single-tooth or vulsellum tenaculum, long Allis clamp, or similar device. This maneuver permits stabilization of the cervix during insertion. Some providers prefer to inject local anesthetic into the cervical lip before grasping it; others prefer to administer full cervical anesthesia prior to osmotic dilator placement. Patient anxiety and sensitivity to pain may govern these choices;
- Before placing the first set of osmotic devices, many providers like to "test" the cervix by passing one or a series of small-caliber rigid plastic or metal dilators past the internal os. This maneuver defines the angle and length of the cervical canal while permitting initial assessment of tissue resistance at the internal os. Modest dilation with rigid mechanical dilators prior to insertion of osmotic devices also permits placement of more osmotic dilators, thereby increasing the width of dilation eventually achieved;
- Grasp the end of the osmotic device with a ring or packing-style forceps and insert it into the endocervical canal such that the tip extends just beyond the internal os (Fig. 11.1). Coating the osmotic dilator with lubricant jelly often eases insertion. Some providers also bathe the devices in a disinfectant such as iodine-povidone solution, although this step is of unproven value as a safety or performance-enhancing technique;
- Osmotic dilators are usually placed in "sets" by sequentially inserting one device after the other until several

devices fit snuggly, but not tightly, within the cervix. Ideally, the distal end of laminaria should extend a few millimeters beyond the external os in order to facilitate removal (Fig. 11.1). Lamicel® are inserted full length up to the flared knob. Similarly, the provider should see the end or knob of the Dilapan-S™ device protruding from the external os;

- Digital examination after insertion of osmotic dilators confirms that the devices have not slipped out of the cervix and are not packed too tightly;
- Most providers place one or more gauze sponges in the vagina following osmotic device insertion to absorb blood and vaginal fluid. The sponges also may help prevent dilators from sliding out prior to swelling. The clinician can hold the sponge(s) in place with packing forceps while removing the vaginal speculum;
- Document in the patient's record the number, size, and type of osmotic dilators placed. These devices are packaged as single units, so counting the wrappers before discarding them or attaching the wrappers to the chart helps assure an accurate account of placed devices.

Women whose osmotic dilators will remain in place overnight can be discharged after receiving appropriate instructions. Patients can resume normal activity following placement. Many will experience mild to moderate cramping, especially in the first few hours postinsertion, but the pain usually responds to low dose nonsteroidal analgesics. Many providers begin antibiotic prophylaxis at the time of osmotic dilator placement. Forewarn patients about the rare possibility that the gauze sponge(s), as well as some of the dilators, might dislodge prior to surgery. Asking patients to track the number of devices expelled or to bring them to the facility helps to account for all devices. Occasionally, patients will experience spontaneous rupture of membranes during or after osmotic dilator insertion. This event is not an emergency and rarely requires additional therapy prior to surgical evacuation of the uterus. However, these patients should be monitored closely for fever, especially if multiple-day cervical preparation is planned. If fever should ensue, some clinicians add parenteral antibiotics or a second antibiotic orally. Finally, clinicians should stress the importance of returning as scheduled for the D&E procedure

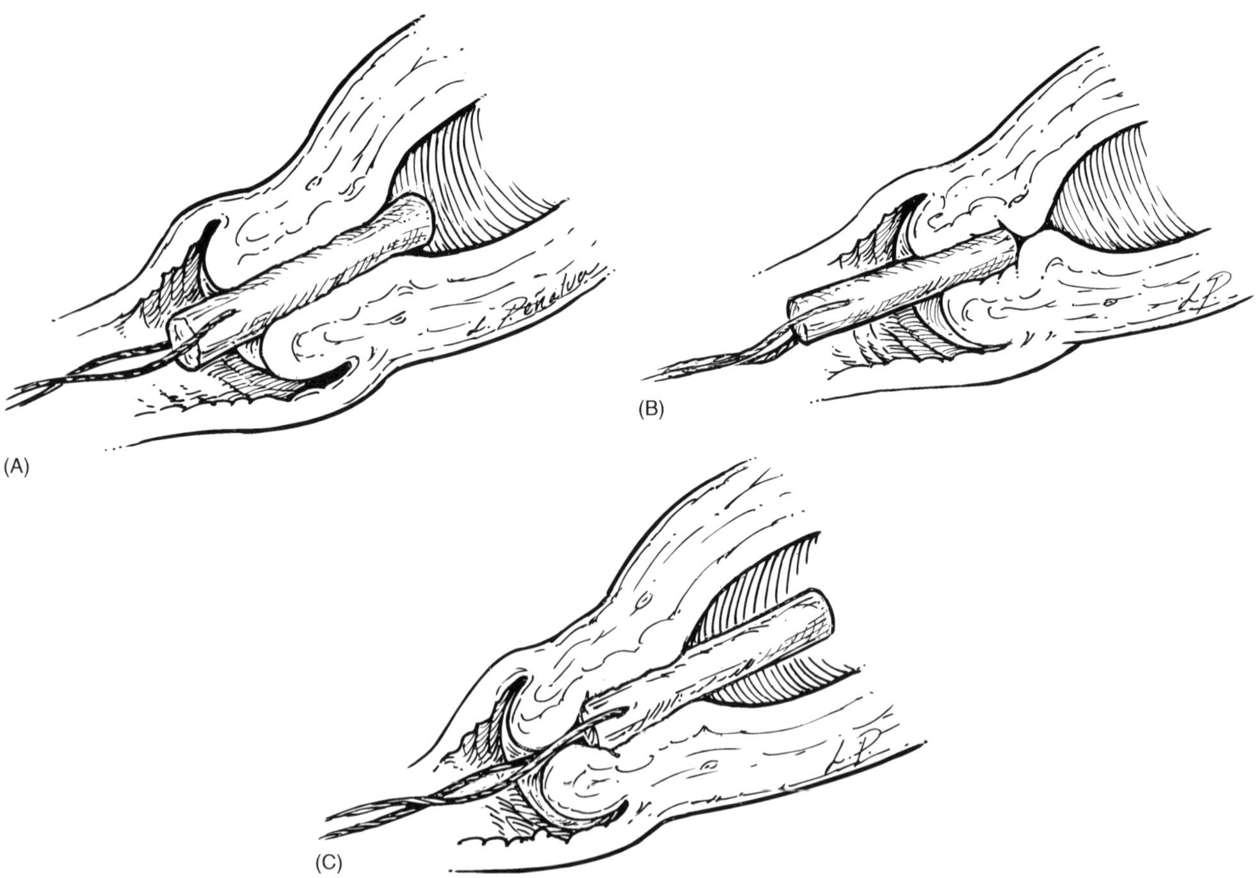

Figure 11.1 Osmotic dilator insertion. (A) Laminaria placed appropriately through the internal os. (B) Laminaria does not pass through the internal os. Swelling results in funneling of the endocervical canal and inadequate dilation of the internal os. (C) Laminaria inserted too far into the endocervical canal. This placement may result in rupture of the membranes and difficult removal.

to avoid the risk of infection from prolonged retention of the dilators.

Addressing challenges

Many special issues and problems can complicate osmotic dilator insertion, particularly for less experienced clinicians. Helpful strategies are addressed next as well as in Chapter 13.

Placing an adequate number of dilators

Obtaining sufficient dilation for an effective "first set" of osmotic dilating devices frequently requires predilation with rigid mechanical dilators, particularly at later gestational ages. Although predilation protocols vary, many clinicians dilate sequentially to 10 to 12 mm when feasible before inserting osmotic devices. To minimize the risk of traumatizing the cervix or creating a false channel, experienced clinicians avoid dilating the cervix too aggressively or packing it too tightly. Performing a digital examination of the endocervical canal before placing the first tent helps to assess its angle, path, and integrity. When placing multiple dilators, consider using devices without plastic stops or remove the stops prior to insertion.

Devices "falling out" of a partially dilated cervix

When the cervix is widely dilated, especially if placental membranes have entered the endocervical canal, the dilators may persistently extrude from the cervix. The problem is exacerbated if the patient bears down, changes position, or is experiencing uterine contractions. In such circumstances, clinicians often digitally insert osmotic devices in a cluster. Using gauze pads to build a "dam" against the cervix helps to prevent extrusion of already placed devices. Exceptionally uncomfortable or anxious patients may benefit from parenteral analgesics or anxiolytics; in rare instances (e.g., some cases of sexual assault), women may require deeper levels of anesthesia in order to tolerate an osmotic dilator treatment.

Strategies for difficult removal

The assumption that more is better can backfire when inserting osmotic dilators. Osmotic dilating devices frequently "hourglass," particularly in resistant or stenotic cervices, and multiple laminaria wedged together have a tendency to meld into a uniform, intractable mass. Because laminaria are neither pliable nor easily transected, they can be difficult to remove after swelling ensues (Fig. 13.5). Dilapan-S™ devices can stretch to remarkable lengths before fragmenting, but on occasion they too can become incarcerated. All types of osmotic dilators can migrate into the uterine cavity resulting in ongoing pain, bleeding, or infection before removal [47].

Several strategies can aid removal of incarcerated devices (Chapter 13). The most effective approach is to exercise caution when choosing how many devices to place, although hourglassing can still occur if the cervix is noncompliant. Slow extraction of device(s) from the middle of the set often aids removal of the entire pack. Many clinicians place one osmotic dilating device near the center of the set, leaving it slightly more extended from the external os than the others. Should difficulties arise when removing the devices, extracting this "key" device first facilitates removal of the remainder.

Because even the reformulated Dilapan-S™ devices can occasionally fragment during removal, many providers use them in combination with laminaria. Laminaria achieve their ripening effect partly through direct contact with the cervix, so they should be placed at the periphery of the bundle.

Protocols for insertion

The amount of dilation required before D&E varies based on gestational age and fetal size, the latter sometimes magnified as a result of certain fetal anomalies such as hydrocephaly. In order to obtain adequate dilation, clinicians usually place sets of osmotic dilating devices over 1 to 2 days preceding uterine evacuation. Cervical response to osmotic dilation can vary considerably, however. Some patients have stenotic cervices that barely admit a first "set" of two or three laminaria but then soften and dilate easily thereafter. Alternatively, a clinician may encounter a multiparous patient whose cervix appears pliable with the first set but then fails to ripen as anticipated with several sets of assorted osmotic dilators.

Providers use a variety of osmotic dilation protocols that dictate the number of devices, number of sets, and the timing of reinsertions (Table 11.1). Protocols may entail laminaria alone, in combination with other osmotic dilators, or in combination with pharmacologic agents such as misoprostol. Package labeling for Lamicel® and laminaria references use of a single device only, although it does not countermand multiple device placement. Package labeling for Dilapan-S™ recommends two tents between 13 and 15 weeks' gestation, three between 16 and 18 weeks, and four at 18 weeks or more [37]. Notwithstanding various recommendations, providers must constantly adapt to individual variations in anatomy in order to optimize patient safety.

The number of devices included in a "set" varies but usually entails the maximum number of devices the clinician can place without undue force. A first "set" in a typical patient after 14 weeks' gestation might consist of three to seven laminaria (Table 11.1). After placing the initial set of devices, the patient returns for insertion of more devices either by the withdrawal of all the previous devices (the "replacement method") or the addition of new devices alongside the previously placed set (the "addition method"). Placing all new osmotic devices enhances dilation but incurs higher cost. No studies address whether the addition method poses greater risk of infection; however, consistent evidence

Table 11.1 Sample osmotic dilator protocols.

Gestational Age in Weeks	Family Planning Associates Medical Group, Ltd. (Chicago, IL)	Northwestern University Section of Family Planning
12.0–13.5		3–5 laminaria
>13.5–14.0	1–2 laminaria[a]	
>14.0–15.5	2–3 laminaria	
>15.5–17.0	4–5 laminaria	
>17.0–19.5	5–8 laminaria	Two sets of 3–5 laminaria. Second set placed 6–8 hours following first set. *[Minimum number of laminaria = Gestational age minus 10]*
>19.5–20.5	6–9 laminaria or 4 Dilapan-S™	Day 1: • First set: 3–5 laminaria • Second set: 7–20 laminaria Day 2: • 20 laminaria *[Minimum number of laminaria = Gestational age minus 10]*
>20.5–22.0	7–10 laminaria or 5–6 Dilapan-S™	
>22.0–23.5	Day 1: 5 laminaria Day 2: 20 laminaria	

[a] The standard size laminaria used by Family Planning Associates Medical Group, Ltd. is a 5-mm tent, with exceptions as clinically indicated for extremes of cervical noncompliance or cervical laxity.

indicates that, overall, osmotic dilating device treatments do not increase infection risk in patients having second-trimester abortions [37].

In most circumstances, all three types of hygroscopic dilators achieve considerable, although not maximum, dilation by about 8 hours. Thus, most devices can be added or replaced in 4 to 8 hours. When the cervix is exceedingly stiff, a second dilator treatment in a single day is a prudent and often effective strategy. This approach can also reduce by 1 day the duration needed to achieve cervical ripening in late D&E abortion (20 weeks' gestation or greater). These protocols often use Dilapan-S™ to take advantage of its greater radial force for cervical dilation compared to laminaria and Lamicel® models.

A single set of osmotic devices placed for several hours or overnight usually suffices for gestations in the early second trimester, but clinicians often insert serial sets of laminaria over 1 to 2 days for later gestational ages. Stubblefield performed a randomized trial of 60 patients comparing a 1-day and 2-day laminaria protocol preceding D&E at 17 to 19 weeks' gestation. Although the 2-day protocol resulted in greater dilation (22.4 mm vs. 18.2 mm diameter; $p < 0.001$), the authors questioned whether the additional dilation justified the patient inconvenience and discomfort associated with an additional day of preparation [48].

The minimal cervical dilation required to complete a given D&E varies somewhat based on gestational age, parity, the patient's cooperation, and the provider's skill and equipment. Digital examination of the cervix, similar to that performed among laboring patients, may mislead a less experienced examiner, because the second-trimester cervix can feel underdilated while having become pliable enough to admit required instruments easily. Therefore, part of the digital examination should involve testing the pliability of the cervix when subject to gentle stretch (Box B).

General safety of osmotic dilators

Osmotic dilators decrease the risk of cervical trauma [37,41] and increase the safety of second-trimester D&E abortion [37,49]. Like all medical devices, however, they may carry some risk.

Several minor, short-term risks are associated with insertion of any osmotic dilator. Five to 20% of women may develop vasovagal symptoms during insertion [37]. Dilators may create a false passage in the cervix or, when placed forcefully, result in cervical fracture, a stretch-induced injury of the internal os (Chapter 15). On some occasions, placement of osmotic dilators results in spontaneous rupture of membranes or otherwise facilitates the onset of labor and fetal expulsion before scheduled surgery.

Laminaria, the most frequently used osmotic dilator, are a natural product and can theoretically harbor potential genital pathogens, even after gas sterilization [50]. Fortunately, infection attributable solely to osmotic devices occurs infrequently. Reported rates of infection following abortion with laminaria use are comparable or lower than those associated with abortion without osmotic dilation [46,51]. No studies document whether the initiation of antibiotics concurrent

Box B

The cervix's ability to permit the entry, expansion, and free mobility of extraction forceps offers the most practical gauge of cervical adequacy.

with insertion of osmotic dilators changes rates of infection [37]. Serious infections have occurred in association with retained devices, making it essential that providers document successful removal of all devices at the time of surgical evacuation [52]. Localizing a retained osmotic dilator using conventional radiography is difficult, because osmotic dilators are not radiopaque. Ultrasound often assists in localization, although dilated laminaria can still resemble blood clots even on endovaginal scan [53]. Sonohysterography remains unstudied for this purpose but theoretically is a promising modality.

Anaphylaxis has been reported in response to laminaria placement [54,55]. Lichtenberg has described effective substitution of Lamicel® in this situation [46], but Dilapan-S™ are an alternative if the cervical stroma is minimally pliable.

Most recent studies suggest that use of osmotic dilators followed by D&E exerts no deleterious effect on cervical integrity or subsequent rates of spontaneous abortion or preterm birth. Postoperative studies examining laxity of the internal cervical os following second-trimester D&E suggest no persistent laxity when pretreatment occurs with osmotic dilators. In a small study involving women at 17 to 19 weeks' gestation who were treated with single or multiple insertions of laminaria before D&E, the mean diameter of the internal cervical os 2 weeks postoperatively was less than that before initial treatment [48]. In Kalish's retrospective review of 600 patients who had undergone D&E between 14 and 24 weeks' gestation, the overall rate of preterm birth in subsequent pregnancies was lower than that for the general US population (6.5% vs. 12.5%)[56]. Similarly, Jackson et al compared subsequent pregnancy outcomes among 317 women undergoing second-trimester D&E with 170 matched controls who had no history of midtrimester D&E. Although patients with a history of prior D&E delivered slightly earlier in gestation than controls (38.9 weeks vs. 39.5 weeks, $p = 0.001$), the researchers found no statistically significant difference in birth weight, spontaneous preterm delivery, abnormal placentation, or the frequency of overall perinatal complications [57].

Misoprostol for cervical ripening

Although many studies document the safety and efficacy of misoprostol for cervical ripening before first-trimester aspiration abortion (Chapter 10), Goldberg et al have performed the only randomized, double-blinded, controlled trial to date comparing misoprostol with the traditional practice of overnight laminaria before second-trimester surgical abortion [58]. Subjects at 13 to 16 weeks' gestation ($n = 84$) received either 400 μg of vaginal misoprostol 3 to 4 hours preoperatively or overnight laminaria. The primary outcome was procedure time; secondary outcomes included completion of the procedure on the first attempt, procedural difficulty, and patients' pain scores and preferences. Second-trimester abortions following same-day misoprostol took approximately 4 minutes longer and were technically more challenging (particularly in nulliparas) than those following overnight laminaria. Dilation effect was greater with laminaria (43F vs. 33F, $p < 0.001$). Patients, however, preferred a same-day procedure to overnight treatment. The vast majority of procedures in both groups were accomplished safely and with adequate dilation. No D&E trial has yet compared same-day presurgical use of osmotic dilators versus misoprostol.

Patel and colleagues analyzed data from 2,218 D&E procedures between 12 and 23 completed weeks of gestation in which providers at multiple clinic sites applied cervical preparation consisting of various regimens of buccal misoprostol with or without osmotic dilators [59]. The dose of misoprostol ranged from 400 to 800 μg, but most patients received 400 μg buccally at least 90 minutes preoperatively. Cervical preparation was considered adequate if the cervix did not require additional dilation before D&E or the physicians rated additional dilation as "not difficult." Adequacy was generally greater for laminaria versus no laminaria regardless of misoprostol use. For instance, patients receiving buccal misoprostol but no laminaria had *inadequate* cervical preparation 18% of the time, whereas those receiving both buccal misoprostol and laminaria failed to achieve adequate cervical preparation only 2% of the time. When misoprostol was used alone, the 800-μg dose achieved adequacy significantly more often than lower doses but at a cost of more frequent side effects. In the misoprostol-only group, a strong association emerged between need for additional dilation and lower gestational age. Providers completed the D&E procedures as scheduled in all but five patients, and complication rates were low. Patel and coworkers concluded that buccal misoprostol is safe and holds promise as a primary cervical ripening agent in the second trimester. Given the study's limitations, further research is needed to define the optimal role of misoprostol in second-trimester cervical preparation protocols.

To determine whether adjuvant buccal misoprostol improves cervical preparation with laminaria, Edelman et al performed a randomized double-blinded, placebo-controlled trial comparing overnight laminaria and either placebo or misoprostol 400 μg administered buccally 90 minutes before D&E at 16 to 21 weeks' gestation [60]. Although some surgeons subjectively reported easier dilation following misoprostol priming, this study recorded no objective differences in cervical dilation measured by passage of rigid dilators, need for additional dilation, or duration of procedures at less than 19 weeks' gestation. However, for procedures at 19 to 21 weeks, preoperative use of misoprostol had a positive effect on dilation (54F vs. 49F, $p = 0.01$). As in the study by Goldberg [58], patients receiving misoprostol experienced more discomfort than those in the nonmisoprostol arm.

Where cost and availability permit its use for cervical ripening, mifepristone has clinical value either alone or in combination with misoprostol or laminaria. Carbonell and colleagues [61] evaluated the efficacy of mifepristone among 900 women undergoing D&E at 12 to 20 weeks' gestation. They randomized patients to one of four groups: 200-mg mifepristone plus 600-μg sublingual misoprostol; 200-mg mifepristone plus 600-μg vaginal misoprostol; 600-μg sublingual misoprostol alone; or 600-μg vaginal misoprostol alone. Mifepristone was administered 48 hours before D&E, and misoprostol was given 1.5 to 2.5 hours preoperatively. The combination of mifepristone and misoprostol before D&E decreased operating time and the risk of cervical injury. However, mifepristone increased cost by approximately 25 euros per procedure, the total number of patient visits, and the number of pre-D&E fetal expulsions. Noted advantages of adjuvant mifepristone included decreased waiting time after administering misoprostol (1.7 ± 0.6 hours vs. 2.1 ± 0.7 hours, $p < 0.001$), a significant reduction in the number of osmotic dilators used, and greater preoperative cervical dilation. The difference in degree of mean cervical dilation obtained following mifepristone was noted in both the sublingual misoprostol groups (12.6 ± 2.1 mm vs. 8.9 ± 3.0 mm) and the vaginal groups (12.4 ± 3.3 mm vs. 8.1 ± 3.3 mm).

Injections to cause fetal demise

Indications

Injections to cause fetal demise prior to operative evacuation may have certain benefits. At gestational ages when a live birth is possible, these injections avoid that possibility, including in patients who experience labor following cervical preparation [62]. Some clinicians believe that the process of cortical bone softening, which begins within 24 hours of fetal death and makes fetal tissue more pliable, may facilitate evacuation and avoid lacerations caused by sharp fragments of fetal bone. Some patients may find solace in knowing that fetal death occurred prior to operative evacuation.

US abortion providers may prefer using these injections to ensure compliance with the federal Partial-Birth Abortion Ban Act of 2003 [5] and related state laws. The act is an intentionally imprecisely worded statute prescribing criminal sanctions against offending physicians but applicable only when a "living fetus" is present at the outset of evacuation [5] (Chapter 4). The federal law bans abortions in which the physician first intentionally removes a "living fetus" to the point at which either its entire head or any part of its trunk above the navel is outside the woman's body, and then performs an overt act, separate from delivery, that kills the fetus. According to the US Supreme Court, it does not apply to "most" nonintact D&Es [63]. Injection to cause fetal demise is one of many ways to assure compliance with this law. Whatever method is chosen, providers who intend to remove (or who know there is a strong possibility of removing) the fetus in a way that would violate the ban if the fetus were still living must ensure fetal demise before the fetal head or any part of the trunk above the navel is outside the woman's body.

Precautions

The two agents used to cause fetal demise are digoxin and potassium chloride (KCl). The only known contraindications to digoxin are Wolff-Parkinson-White syndrome and allergy to the medication. Cardiac auscultation should be performed prior to administration of digoxin, followed by electrocardiogram (EKG) if the clinician detects evidence of arrhythmia. Potassium chloride has no known contraindications.

The safety of administration of digoxin or KCl for this purpose depends on injection of the agent in the desired location and avoiding maternal intravascular injection. Factors such as morbid obesity or oligohydramnios can limit sonographic visualization of the needle, thereby increasing the risk of maternal complications. The practitioner should consider foregoing the injection if technical limitations prevent safe administration of digoxin or KCl.

Agents

Digoxin, which decreases conduction of electric impulses through the atrioventricular node, is administered via intra-amniotic or intrafetal injection. KCl requires direct fetal intracardiac or intraumbilical (funic) injection. In toxic doses, KCl results in depolarization of the membrane potential of cells and impairment of impulses in the cardiac conduction system, ventricular tachycardia, and asystole.

Techniques

Overview

To minimize the risk of chorioamnionitis, use of sterile technique is standard practice. The abdomen is cleansed with an antiseptic solution, and a sterile cover (e.g., a sterile glove) is placed over the ultrasound probe. Arranging sterile supplies (a prefilled syringe containing the digoxin or KCl, spinal needle[s], and gauze sponges) on a nearby tray facilitates access. Most providers use a 20-gauge or a 22-gauge spinal needle, but having available needles of different lengths will accommodate women with varying abdominal wall thickness.

Whichever technique is used, ultrasound evaluation prior to needle insertion permits the clinician to confirm gestational age, evaluate amniotic fluid volume and placental location, and identify uterine abnormalities that can complicate the procedure, such as large leiomyomata. Although amniocentesis can be accomplished without it, real-time ultrasound guidance helps to confirm proper needle placement and direct the injection of digoxin or KCl to a precise location. The injection of the solution causes a turbulent stream that may be visible sonographically, aiding confirmation of proper placement.

Physicians experienced at ultrasound-guided obstetric procedures, including genetic amniocentesis, chorionic villus sampling, and injections to cause fetal demise, use a variety of techniques of needle insertion based on training and experience. Differences include ultrasound imaging techniques (longitudinal vs. transverse placement of the ultrasound probe), needle placement (at the end of the probe vs. in the middle of the probe), and needle angle (straight and close to the probe vs. angled and farther from the probe). Inserting the needle while holding the ultrasound transducer allows the clinician to estimate the required angle and depth of insertion, although some clinicians prefer to have an assistant hold the probe. No evidence suggests that any single technique is safer than others, and individual practitioners should adopt methods based on ease, experience, and personal outcomes.

Some ultrasound machines contain a probe and attachments for a needle guide. This method involves placing the needle through a slot attached to the probe. Prior to needle placement, the probe is angled so that the needle pathway appearing on the screen will intersect the desired target. Needle guidance may be helpful for funic or intracardiac placement. It is not required for intra-amniotic needle placement but may be useful in the presence of morbid obesity or oligohydramnios.

Injection sites

Intra-amniotic digoxin

For intra-amniotic digoxin injection, a dose of 1.0 mg undiluted or in 3 to 5 ml of saline [64] is a common regimen, but doses in the 1.0- to 2.0-mg range are acceptable. Aspiration of amniotic fluid confirms appropriate placement of the needle. Fetal death does not occur immediately after intra-amniotic injection.

Intrafetal digoxin

Based on large published series of outpatient abortion procedures after the first trimester, intrafetal injection of digoxin in doses of 1.0 to 1.5 mg appears to effect fetal demise [65,66]. Providers may feel a change in resistance at the needle tip as it enters the fetus. Unless the needle is in the fetal cardiac chambers, aspiration will not usually yield fetal blood. Haskell, in a personal case series of 67 consecutive patients receiving 2.0 mg of intrafetal digoxin, reported that sonographically confirmed fetal demise occurred in 43% at 2 hours; 75% at 3 hours, and 98% in 5 hours (Haskell M, 2008, personal communication). Fetal cardiac asystole may be visible on ultrasound within 1 to 2 minutes of intracardiac injection.

Intracardiac or funic potassium chloride

Potassium chloride will not achieve fetal demise when injected into the amniotic fluid; injection into the fetal heart or umbilical cord is required. To achieve fetal death, 5 to 10cc of KCl at a concentration of 2 mEq/ml (10–20 mEq total) suffice. Injection of KCl into the fetal heart or umbilical cord typically causes cardiac asystole within 1 minute. Needle placement should be maintained until fetal death is confirmed sonographically.

These technically challenging procedures are performed most commonly for multifetal pregnancy reduction or selective termination of an abnormal fetus (Chapter 21), and a relatively small number of physicians possess the requisite skill and experience. Expertise in performing intracardiac or funic injections may not be available in many outpatient settings that offer midtrimester abortion services.

Confirmation of fetal demise

Clinicians typically administer agents to cause fetal demise 1 to 2 days before D&E, often in conjunction with cervical preparation. Because intra-amniotic or intrafetal digoxin does not result in immediate fetal death, ultrasound can be used prior to uterine evacuation to confirm absence of fetal cardiac motion. If demise has not occurred, the advisability of a repeat injection will require weighing the putative benefits of fetal death prior to evacuation with the risks of another injection, possible maternal anxiety and discomfiture, and the possible need to delay uterine evacuation. Intracardiac or intrafunic injection, if feasible, will accomplish immediately verifiable fetal death and avoid surgical delay. If US providers decide to proceed with D&E after an injection fails to cause fetal demise, they will have to consider alternative means of complying with the Partial-Birth Abortion Ban Act of 2003 [5] and related state laws.

Monitoring

Based on available data, routine monitoring of the patient's vital signs or EKG is not necessary during or after digoxin or KCl injections. Specific patient complaints should be investigated as clinically indicated.

Safety and efficacy

Published data on the use of injections to cause preoperative fetal demise are limited primarily to retrospective case series. Although most of these studies report no maternal complications, their small size does not permit evaluation of uncommon complications or side effects attributable to these injections. Moreover, most studies are uninformative about the putative surgical benefits of preoperative fetal demise, because they did not include a control group for comparison.

One small observational study assessed maternal side effects of intra-amniotic digoxin. Drey and colleagues examined maternal serum digoxin levels and EKG changes following intra-amniotic injection of 1 mg of digoxin in eight patients at 19 to 23 weeks' gestation [67]. Peak serum digoxin levels occurred approximately 11 hours after administration. The peak concentrations were in the low therapeutic range, and no level approached the potentially toxic concentration of 2 ng/ml. EKG monitoring did not identify any patterns indicative of digoxin toxicity. Reported side effects associated with digoxin toxicity (e.g., nausea, blurred vision, and light-headedness) were uncommon, and they did not correlate with peak digoxin levels in the affected patients. No laboratory evidence of coagulopathy was observed.

Research suggests that maternal serum digoxin levels are far higher than maternal tissue levels after injections to cause fetal demise, conferring an extra measure of safety. Haskell and Kade recorded serial maternal serum digoxin levels in 60 consecutive women undergoing intrafetal injection with 2.0 mg of digoxin (Haskell M, 2008, personal communication). Single values in two women substantially exceeded the reference range of 0.8 to 2.0 ng/ml (6 ng/ml and 7 ng/ml, respectively) within 1 hour of injection, but neither patient exhibited clinical signs of cardiac toxicity. The investigators attributed this lack of serum and clinical correlation to the fact that digoxin takes at least 8 hours to redistribute from serum to tissues. Because of digoxin's long half-life of 30 hours, a steady state concentration is not achieved for 5 days or more. Published reference ranges for digoxin apply to serum levels observed after redistribution, and samples taken within 8 hours of digoxin administration will falsely imply elevated tissue levels [68].

Spontaneous abortion prior to operative evacuation has been reported in women who received intra-amniotic or intrafetal digoxin. Jackson and colleagues, in a pilot study preceding a subsequent randomized controlled trial, described an "unacceptably high rate of spontaneous abortion" with digoxin injected 48 hours prior to evacuation. However in their randomized study, in which the injection was performed 24 hours prior to abortion, they reported no cases of spontaneous abortion [64]. In Molaei's series of 1,795 women receiving intra-amniotic or intrafetal digoxin the day before D&E, nine patients (0.5%) were sent to the hospital for "spontaneous contractions" prior to their scheduled return visit [66]. It is not clear whether spontaneous abortion is related to fetal death or possibly to the presence of digoxin in the amniotic fluid, which is known to increase muscular contractility. If spontaneous abortion is due to fetal death, similar risks would be expected with the use of intracardiac or funic KCl. Although this occurrence has not been reported, preinduction fetal intra-cardiac KCl did result in more rapid delivery in patients undergoing second-trimester medical abortion using prostaglandin agents [69].

One case report described maternal cardiac arrest within 1 minute of attempted fetal intracardiac injection with 5 mEq of KCl. The case involved a patient with advanced cervical dilation at 23 weeks' gestation who declined further tocolysis. The administration of KCl occurred on a labor and delivery suite using a bedside ultrasound machine that lacked magnification. According to the authors of the case report, this arrangement deviated from their normal protocol for effecting fetal demise. Cardiac arrest was attributed to direct rapid injection of KCl into the maternal circulation [70].

Any procedure associated with transabdominal needle placement into the uterine cavity can result in maternal infection. Although this complication is extremely uncommon given the large number of amniocenteses performed in obstetric practice, a few case reports describe maternal sepsis following genetic amniocentesis [71,72]. A single case of maternal sepsis following funic KCl administration has been reported [73]. Although no report has described sepsis following intracardiac KCl or intra-amniotic digoxin, the similarities between these procedures and amniocentesis suggest that they may carry a small risk.

Although many providers believe that fetal bone and joint softening induced by fetal demise facilitates uterine evacuation, only one published study has evaluated the medical benefit of these injections. Jackson et al randomized 126 women at a mean gestational age of 22.5 weeks to receive 1 mg of intra-amniotic digoxin or placebo. The study found no differences in procedure duration, estimated blood loss, operator-perceived procedure difficulty, or frequency of complications. Intra-amniotic digoxin induced fetal death in 57 (92%) of the 62 patients in the study group. Women who received digoxin reported vomiting significantly more often than those who did not (16% vs. 3%) [64].

Molaei and coworkers examined the efficacy of digoxin to cause fetal demise in a retrospective cohort analysis of 1,795 women at 17 to 24 weeks' gestation who received the drug before laminaria placement on the day prior to D&E [66]. Most patients (n = 1,665; 93%) in this study had intrafetal (described as "in the fetal heart region") digoxin injections with doses ranging from 0.125 to 1.0 mg; the remaining patients received intra-amniotic digoxin in doses ranging from 0.125 to 0.50 mg. In the intrafetal digoxin group, the overall rate of failure to achieve fetal demise was 4.7% (95% CI 3.7, 5.8%); the failure rate decreased from 14.3% (95% CI 8.0, 22.8%) in patients who received the lowest dose of digoxin (0.125 mg, $n = 98$) to 0 (95% CI 0.0, 3.4%) in those who received a 1-mg dose (n = 107). Failure occurred in nearly one-third of the 131 women who had intra-amniotic injections, most likely because of the low doses of digoxin used. No patients experienced palpitations or visual changes suggestive of digoxin toxicity; rates of nausea and vomiting were not reported. To date, no study has examined efficacy by site of injection in the fetus.

Data on the efficacy of KCl to cause fetal demise are limited. In the largest study of 239 patients at a median gestational age of 22 weeks, no failures or complications occurred using an average fetal intracardiac dose of 4.7 ml (15% KCl; 20 mM/10 ml) [74]. In a smaller series of 106 patients,

Bhide et al found that funic injection required lower doses of KCl compared to intracardiac injection, although the average doses used exceeded those reported in more recent studies. However, the failure rate was higher with funic injection [75]. Gill and colleagues attempted funic KCl injection in 60 patients. In eight cases (13%), funipuncture either could not be achieved or did not result in fetal cardiac asystole, mirroring the higher rate of failure reported by Bhide. These cases required intracardiac administration to accomplish fetal demise [76].

In conclusion, injection to cause fetal demise appears to be a safe procedure with low complication rates based on the limited data available. Intra-amniotic or intrafetal digoxin is likely to be the procedure of choice in most settings, as funic or intracardiac KCl administration is technically much more difficult. Fetal death is not inevitable with intra-amniotic or intrafetal digoxin, however. Published data confer no clear medical benefit of causing fetal demise, although individual practitioners may want to consider it if: (1) in their experience fetal cortical bone softening makes the procedure easier; (2) a patient expresses a preference for fetal death prior to operative evacuation; (3) they desire to avoid the possibility of unscheduled delivery of a live fetus; or (4) they are concerned about compliance with the Partial-Birth Abortion Ban Act of 2003 [5]. To minimize the risk of spontaneous abortion prior to surgical evacuation, providers should avoid performing the injection longer than 24 hours prior to planned evacuation if possible. Clinicians who use these injections should consider monitoring outcomes, including rates of success and complications such as chorioamnionitis or spontaneous abortion prior to operative evacuation.

D&E procedures

Instruments

A variety of specula, tenacula, and extracting forceps are available for surgical abortion after the first trimester. Although many surgeons base these choices on their exposure during training and their practical experience, certain instruments may be useful in particular circumstances.

Specula

A speculum allows the surgeon to have access to the cervix. Its length should not impede the clinician's effort to draw the cervix toward the vaginal introitus. The speculum should provide sufficient room to manipulate extracting forceps during fetal removal. The blades of the speculum can also be used as a fulcrum, to change the angle of the endocervical canal and ease entry into the endometrial cavity.

The two basic types of specula are the Graves and weighted versions. Several modifications of the Graves speculum have foreshortened blades of varying width, number, and design (e.g., the Klopfer model) (Appendix, Figs. A-2 and A-3). A juvenile or pediatric speculum may prove useful in patients with a narrow introitus. In patients with converging vaginal walls, a tri-blade design (e.g., the Guttmann vaginal retractor) can allow for appropriate visualization of the cervix.

Despite their apparent size and forbidding appearance, patients generally tolerate weighted specula well, particularly if they receive intravenous sedation along with cervical anesthesia. Late in the second trimester, when forceps extraction is likely to be necessary, a weighted speculum accommodates larger fetal parts and allows more angulation of the forceps, particularly in patients with considerable vaginal depth. Weighted specula can be modified by beveling any sharp edges of the blade and by increasing the angle between blade and stem to reduce the chance of their spontaneous release from the vagina, especially when awake or semiconscious patients exhibit guarding or uncontrolled movements.

Tenacula

Traction on the lip of the cervix brings the cervix closer to the vaginal introitus and straightens the endocervical canal. The tenaculum chosen must maintain its attachment through strong and steady traction. A long instrument facilitates access to the cervix, and many surgeons prefer models with a pelvic curve (vulsellum design). If the cervix is firm and not very dilated, a tenaculum with teeth can be especially useful. With a soft dilated cervix, instruments with an Allis tip or ring-forceps design can maintain traction while minimizing the risk of cervical mucosal laceration (Appendix, Fig. A-6). These superficial lacerations or bleeding puncture sites are treated easily with tamponade, cauterizing agents (e.g., silver nitrate or ferric subsulfate [Monsel's] solution) or, in the last resort, one or two absorbable sutures.

Forceps

The choice of forceps depends on cervical dilation and gestational age, as well as provider preference. Available models vary in length, size of the jaws, and grasping surfaces (Appendix, Fig. A-11). Experienced surgeons may use a combination of forceps in individual cases to accommodate changes in uterine size as the emptying cavity contracts or to remove retained portions of fetal anatomy when other forceps do not suffice.

Ring forceps require minimal cervical dilation (10–12 mm), and they can be used early in the second trimester to extract fetal parts that are not easily removed with large-bore suction. Because of their relatively short length, small grasping area, and minimal serrations, they do not suffice for most gestations beyond 17 to 18 weeks. After this gestational age, longer and weightier forceps are essential. Sopher forceps have weightier, longer shafts with bulkier grasping surfaces. About 13 and 15 mm of cervical dilation are required to open widely the jaws of the small and large Sopher forceps, respectively. Sopher forceps lack a pelvic curve, limiting their ability to explore the uterine cornua.

Of the commonly used types of forceps, Bierer forceps are the weightiest and largest-jawed. The fenestrated and sharply serrated jaws provide the most traction, and the pelvic curve and long length maximize access to all aspects of most uterine cavities in the later second trimester. Bierer forceps require more than 15 mm of cervical dilation to permit maximal expansion of the jaws. Hern forceps are longer than either Sopher or Bierer forceps and, like Blumenthal forceps, they are useful in cases of extreme uterine depth. The jaws of Hern forceps have fewer and smaller teeth, making them especially useful when traction or rotation of an intact fetus, is desired (e.g., when attempting intrauterine version of the fetus to a more favorable lie).

Uterotonic agents

As the fetus and placenta are removed during surgical abortion, contraction of the uterine cavity is necessary to prevent hemorrhage. The most important step in minimizing the risk of uterine atony, which is more common with advancing gestational age, is to ensure complete removal of fetal and placental tissue. Limited data suggest that prophylactic use of uterotonics for surgical abortion beyond the first trimester also helps to lessen blood loss [77]. Oxytocin can be given in concentrated form intramuscularly, intracervically, or intravenously (10–20 units) or in diluted form as an intravenous infusion (20–80 units/500–1000 cc). Some surgeons administer oxytocin at the beginning of the procedure, whereas others prefer to wait until complete removal of the fetus because of a concern about entrapment of fetal parts. No data or clinical consensus address this issue of timing. Giving dilute oxytocin as an intravenous drip allows clinicians to discontinue the infusion during surgery if increased myometrial tone is preventing safe completion of the procedure. Continuing oxytocin infusion for 30 to 60 minutes after the abortion procedure may help to maintain uterine tone and prevent postoperative uterine atony.

When cervical anesthesia is used, dilute vasopressin (1–6 units/20 ml) can be added to the anesthetic solution (Chapter 8). In one randomized controlled trial, paracervical injection of vasopressin lessened blood loss compared to placebo, particularly after 15 weeks of gestation [77]. A recent study randomized 36 women at a mean gestational age of 16 weeks to paracervical injection of saline with or without 4 units of vasopressin, with the primary objective of evaluating hemodynamic changes in blood flow through the uterine artery. In these early second-trimester patients, vasopressin was not associated with changes in uterine blood flow or in estimated blood loss [78]. Vasopressin also can be administered as a dilute intravenous infusion, similar to the use of oxytocin. One protocol uses 4–8 units per 500 ml of crystalloid prior to 20 weeks' gestation, and 8–16 units per liter of crystalloid at or beyond 20 weeks' gestation.

Other agents used to improve uterine tone after vaginal or cesarean birth, such as methylergonovine, misoprostol, or tromethamine carboprost (Hemabate®) may be used during D&E as well [79]. No controlled studies have evaluated their efficacy in women undergoing surgical abortion after the first trimester. Ergot derivatives (e.g., methylergonovine) should be avoided in women with poorly controlled hypertension and used cautiously, perhaps primarily intramuscularly, in women with well-controlled hypertension. Carboprost tromethamine, an F-series prostaglandin, is contraindicated in asthmatics.

Risk factors for uterine atony include advancing gestational age, chorioamnionitis, grand multiparity, multiple pregnancy, prior uterine scarring, and general anesthesia using halogenated gases [79]. In the presence of any of these risk factors, clinicians should strongly consider the use of uterotonic agents. If uterotonic agents are not used routinely, they must be readily available in the event of hemorrhage resulting from uterine atony or other causes.

Most physicians employ a stepwise approach to uterotonic medications. Dilute infusions of oxytocin or vasopressin or direct injection of methylergonovine (0.2 mg intramuscularly or intracervically) are commonly administered routinely or as an initial step in managing uterine atony. Refractory cases of uterine atony may respond to treatment with misoprostol (400–1,000 μg per rectum), or direct injection of carboprost (250 μg) or vasopressin (10–20 units/20ml) into the cervix or endomyometrium. The different classes of uterotonic medications (oxytocin, vasopressin, ergot alkaloids, and prostaglandin derivatives) are complementary in their action (different gene sites) and can thus be used concurrently or sequentially.

Patient positioning

Some D&E procedures are technically challenging even under optimum circumstances. If the patient is not positioned properly, the speculum may not permit adequate visualization and mobilization of the cervix. Optimum patient positioning enhances the surgeon's ability to straighten and negotiate the cervical canal and maneuver the forceps into all areas of the endometrial cavity. When difficulty is encountered in a procedure, particularly in the presence of obesity or a narrow pelvis, the surgeon's success may depend on having achieved proper positioning at the outset of the case.

Standard examination tables are suitable for performing D&E. Hydraulic operating tables, if available, allow greater control and variety in customizing the height and angle of the table. The patient's hips should extend slightly beyond the table's edge, tilting the vagina posteriorly and providing room for angling the forceps acutely in all directions.

Removing osmotic dilators

Remove osmotic dilators by inserting two fingers into the vagina, grasping the gauze and strings, and pulling gently. If a "keyhole" dilator has been placed, taking out this device first usually facilitates removal of the remaining dilators. If gentle traction on the strings does not extract the dilators easily, then exposing the cervix with a speculum and grasping the end of one dilator at a time with a ring forceps usually works. Some patients require cervical anesthesia or intravenous sedation to accomplish this step.

The number of dilators removed should equal the number inserted. If a discrepancy exists, one or more of the first devices placed may be intrauterine, having been pushed beyond the internal os by subsequent dilators. In this case, the surgeon must inspect closely all material removed from the uterine cavity to identify missing dilators. To avoid searching for devices that the patient may have passed spontaneously, the clinician should ask the patient if any dilators fell out beforehand. Numerous approaches are available for addressing the problem of retained osmotic dilator fragments (Chapter 13).

Once the osmotic dilators are removed, a digital examination is often highly instructive. With this maneuver the surgeon can assess the degree of cervical dilation and pliability; the presence in the endocervical canal of any niches, fossae, or lacerations created by improper insertion of osmotic dilating devices; and often, fetal presentation.

Ultrasound guidance

For decades, experienced providers have been performing surgical abortion after the first trimester without routine ultrasound guidance and with very low complication rates. Regardless of the surgeon's skills and experience, however, ultrasonic monitoring can help in performing D&E abortions in certain circumstances.

One study in a residency training program assessed the frequency of uterine perforation during D&E performed at 16 to 24 weeks' gestation before and after adopting routine use of intraoperative ultrasound. In 353 cases performed without routine ultrasound, five perforations (1.4%) occurred. In the subsequent 457 procedures accomplished with routine intraoperative ultrasound, only one uterine perforation (0.2%) occurred [80]. Although these data have been used to support a policy of routine intraoperative ultrasound, the use of a historical cohort as a control is not ideal and a teaching setting is not necessarily representative of community practice at dedicated facilities staffed with highly experienced D&E surgeons.

Imaging in a sagittal plane enables the surgeon to visualize the entire depth of the uterus, from cervix to fundus. Imaging in a transverse plane provides circumferential visualization at a specific depth and can help the provider guide the jaws of the forceps around a fetal part. In cases that require a considerable degree of force to remove fetal parts, visualizing movement of fetal tissue caused by traction without concomitant movement of the uterine wall can reassure the surgeon that myometrium has not been grasped. Intraoperative sonographic views are not three-dimensional; thus, sagittal and transverse planes cannot be seen at the same time. Additionally, extracting forceps shift constantly during uterine evacuation. These movements cause moment-by-moment repositioning of visual landmarks, making continuous monitoring a moving target and explaining in part why intraoperative ultrasound cannot prevent all occurrences of iatrogenic injury.

When not employed routinely, ultrasound imaging should be readily available in facilities offering D&E, and the surgeon should have a low threshold for using it. A 2002 NAF-member survey found that approximately half of respondents routinely use intraoperative ultrasound during D&E, and most of the remaining respondents use it selectively. Younger physicians were more likely to use ultrasound routinely [28]. Clinicians should strongly consider ultrasound guidance in patients with uterine abnormalities, such as large leiomyomata; in morbidly obese patients, in whom the uterine fundus is not palpable; and when repeated insertion of forceps fails to grasp or remove fetal parts. If the surgeon has difficulty identifying some fetal parts following evacuation, ultrasound may help to rule out retention of large fragments containing fetal bone.

Although ultrasound is extremely useful in some cases, it is not a substitute for good judgment. Ultrasound does not provide continuous visualization of the entire uterus or of all fetal or placental tissue. The surgeon must not ignore other important crucial information, such as the sensation of tissue contacting the forceps blades, the degree of resistance encountered in removing fetal tissue, the patient's pain response, an inventory of pregnancy elements already removed, and direct visualization of tissue emerging from the cervix.

Operative technique: Standard D&E[1]

Early in the second trimester, suction may suffice to remove the fetus and placenta without the use of forceps (suction D&E). This technique is similar to vacuum aspiration for first-trimester abortion. A 12- or 13-mm cannula is often adequate to evacuate a gestation of approximately 14 weeks, and a 14- or 15-mm cannula is typically used at 15 weeks. A 16-mm suction cannula usually removes a fetus of 16 weeks' size, although forceps may be needed to extract some fetal parts such as the calvarium or spine. The suction-only approach poses problems when a stiff cervix limits dilation or when the intact calvarium becomes incarcerated in the cornua or lower uterine segment. In most of these cases, some form of forceps extraction becomes necessary. After about 16 weeks' gestation, the 16-mm suction cannula alone is not sufficient, and forceps extraction is necessary [81].

---

[1]While the authors here adopt the term "standard D&E" as the US Supreme Court used it in *Gonzales v. Carhart*, 127 S. Ct. 1610 (2007), to refer to non-intact D&Es, the term is not medical, and the authors in no way suggest that any one variation of D&E is more or less standard than another.

Skill in utilizing forceps to remove fetal tissue requires special apprenticeship training and ongoing operative experience. Before performing procedures late in the second trimester, the surgeon should be comfortable performing surgical abortion at earlier gestational ages. Providers vary in their approaches to fetal extraction, as with any common surgical procedure. Nonetheless, the following suggestions may facilitate evacuation and minimize the risk of complications:

- Prior to inserting the forceps, determine the location of fetal tissue by ultrasound or digital examination. The digital examination involves placing one or two fingers through the cervical canal while applying gentle pressure on the uterine fundus in an attempt to palpate fetal parts. This maneuver usually does not require removing the speculum (especially a weighted speculum) or the tenaculum.
- When inserting forceps, stabilize and straighten the endocervical canal by applying firm, steady traction with the tenaculum. Once the forceps has passed through the internal os, open the jaws as widely as possible to encircle the fetal tissue and avoid pushing fetal parts deeper into the fundus (Fig. 11.2).
- The uterine cavity can be explored with forceps by rotating the jaws to explore the anterior and posterior walls. After 16 weeks' gestation, fetal skeletal development is such that the surgeon can manually sense the presence of fetal parts within the closed jaws. If fetal parts are not present, open the jaws once again and rotate them to explore other areas of the uterine cavity.
- Removing the fetus from the lower uterine segment, rather than the fundus, lessens the risk of uterine perforation (Fig. 11.2). After grasping a fetal part, withdraw the forceps while gently rotating it. This maneuver brings the fetus into the lower uterine segment before the grasped fetal part is separated (if necessary) and removed from the cervix.
- Minimizing the number of forceps passes into the uterus may lessen the risk of surgical trauma. Ample cervical dilation helps to achieve this objective. If a fetal extremity is brought through the cervix without separation, advance the forceps beyond the extremity to grasp part of the fetal trunk. Bringing the fetal trunk into the lower segment markedly reduces the number of instrument passes into the fundus.

When fetal tissue must be removed from the uterine fundus, take care to avoid perforation. If ultrasound guidance is not used to visualize the relationship of the forceps to fetal tissue, placing an abdominal hand on the fundus, as described by Hanson, may be of value [82] (Fig. 11.3). The abdominal hand accomplishes two goals. It allows the clinician to palpate the movements of the forceps against the uterine wall, providing reassurance that perforation has not occurred (or immediate evidence that it has). By manipulating the uterine fundus, the abdominal hand also helps to bring fetal tissue into contact with the forceps.

During the procedure, try to identify and keep track of fetal parts as they are removed. A "pouch" or surgical pan at the edge of the table to catch fetal parts can assist this process. Knowledge of what fetal parts remain in utero may affect decisions regarding selection of forceps and administration of uterotonic and anesthetic medications.

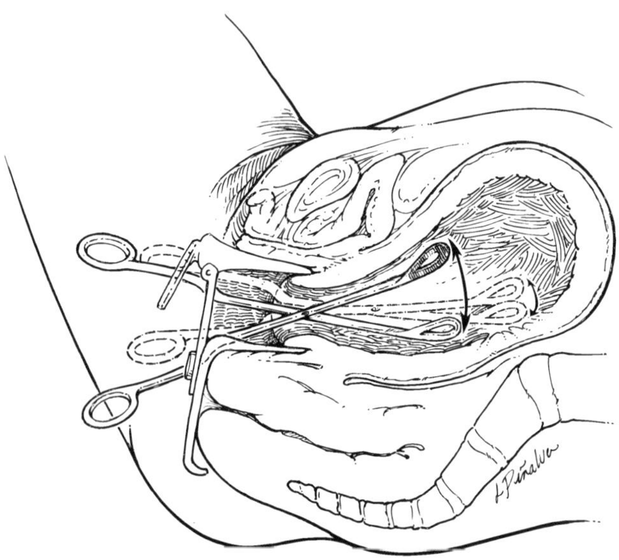

Figure 11.2 Placement of forceps in the lower uterine segment. Hinge remains at the level of the cervix, allowing maximum range of motion of the jaws to extract pregnancy elements from the lower uterine segment. When deeper insertion of the forceps is necessary to explore the fundus and cornua, care must be taken to apply cervical traction and follow the axis of the uterus to minimize the risk of trauma to the uterine wall.

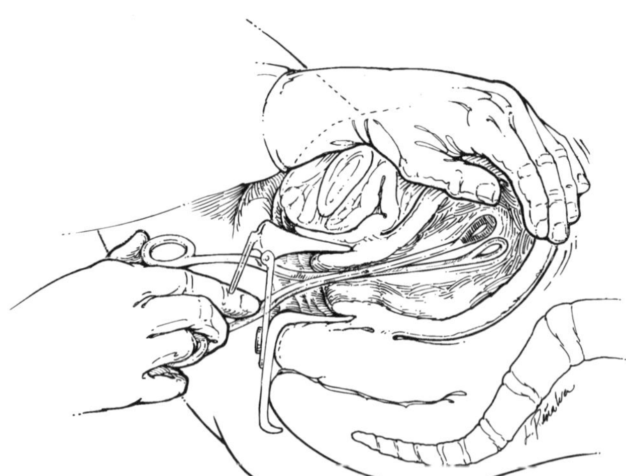

Figure 11.3 Hanson maneuver. By palpating the uterus with the nonoperating hand, the provider may be able to decipher the location of fetal parts relative to the jaws of the forceps. Also shown is a proper method for holding the extraction forceps. Placing the thumb outside the ring on the handle allows the jaws to open wider.

This inventory also will prevent patient injury resulting from fruitless attempts to remove fetal parts that have already been evacuated.

The timing of placental delivery depends on placental position and ease of fetal extraction. The placenta typically feels softer and bulkier than fetal tissue when grasped with forceps. After the placenta is grasped, light traction with the forceps accompanied by vigorous fundal massage will help the placenta detach from the myometrium. Once placental tissue is brought through the cervix, the surgeon can regrasp it until it delivers completely. Intact delivery of the placenta is preferable, as it obviates the need for repeated instrument passes and vigorous curettage. No evidence supports the contention that selective removal of the placenta at the outset of a D&E prevents amniotic fluid embolism or disseminated intravascular coagulopathy, and this strategy is often impossible to execute.

After extracting the fetus and placenta, some surgeons routinely explore the uterine cavity with a blunt-edged rake or large curette to remove any residual placental tissue and confirm complete evacuation. This gentle exploration ("check" curettage) also can confirm the integrity of the myometrium and help rule out an unrecognized perforation. Most providers perform suction curettage as a last evacuating step to remove blood clots and any residual tissue. Although the endocervical canal may accommodate a cannula greater than 12 mm in diameter, a smaller device (8–12 mm) may improve the surgeon's ability to explore the entire uterine cavity, particularly when the uterus is well contracted. After removal of the tenaculum and speculum, digital examination of the uterine cavity, with particular attention to the integrity of the entire length of the endocervical canal just beyond the internal cervical os, can confirm absence of injury.

Tissue examination

Even when the surgeon inventories fetal parts during their removal, tissue examination at the end of the procedure helps to verify complete evacuation. Identify major fetal parts, including the calvarium, pelvis, spine, and extremities, and confirm that the volume of placental tissue is adequate for gestational age. If not all major fetal parts are present, examine surgical drapes and sponges thoroughly before considering reexploration of the uterine cavity. Ultrasound examination of the uterine cavity can identify fetal tissue, although blood clots may on occasion obscure nonbony fetal tissue or decidua.

Measurement of fetal foot length has been used to estimate gestational age after abortion, and refined formulae provide greater accuracy [83,84]. Routine postoperative measurement of foot length is not necessary in most settings, but it may be useful when the surgeon perceives a size-dates discrepancy or elects documentation for medicolegal purposes.

Operative technique: Intact D&E

The challenge of removing a large volume of tissue through a small opening is not unique to abortion after the first trimester. Obstetrician-gynecologists, for example, may encounter similar challenges during vaginal birth and vaginal hysterectomy. In both instances, the risk of injury increases with the extensive use of instruments. In obstetrics, use of operative forceps is associated with higher rates of vaginal and perineal injury, making unassisted or manual delivery preferable. Similarly in vaginal hysterectomy, morcellation of tissue can cause bladder, bowel, or vascular injury, and intact removal of the uterus is preferred.

Similar principles apply to D&E. As a general rule, when cervical dilation is sufficient, fewer instrument passes are needed to remove the fetus. In some cases, intact delivery is feasible. Because the cranium represents the largest and least compressible structure, it often requires decompression. This situation has precedent in obstetrics, as cranial decompression has long been used to facilitate delivery in the presence of obstructed labor with fetal death or severe fetal brain anomalies associated with hydrocephalus and hydranencephaly [85].

In addition to a potentially safer fetal extraction, intact extraction may have other advantages. Removal of an intact or near-intact fetus minimizes the risk of retained tissue. When abortion is performed for fetal anomalies, an intact fetal specimen can improve the quality of autopsy. The opportunity to view or hold an intact fetus may facilitate the grieving process for some patients and their partners.

Intact D&E is generally accomplished with serial laminaria insertion over 2 or more days, with the goal of achieving adequate cervical dilation. Although some clinicians use this variant only when the fetus presents as a breech, others perform manual or instrumental conversion of the fetus to a breech presentation if necessary, followed by breech extraction. Decompression of the calvarium is necessary if it becomes lodged in the cervix. Decompression can be accomplished with forceps or by making an incision at the base of the skull through which the intracranial contents are suctioned. If the fetus is in cephalic presentation with the calvarium well-applied to the cervix, the surgeon can pierce the calvarium with a sharp instrument and collapse it externally with forceps or internally with suction. Provided cervical dilation is sufficient, the physician can then extract the fetus otherwise intact.

In 1995, McMahon presented a personal series of 1,362 intact D&E procedures, with only four major complications (McMahon J, 1995, personal communication). This low rate (2.94 per 1,000 cases) of complications was comparable to that reported in a large series of D&Es performed at earlier gestational ages [14]. In addition, Haskell described his experience of more than 1,500 consecutive intact D&E procedures at 20 to 26 weeks' gestation without any serious complications (Haskell M, 1992, personal communication).

One study retrospectively compared outcomes in 383 women undergoing surgical abortion at or after 20 weeks' gestation; in this study, the surgeon intended to perform intact D&E when technically feasible. A total of 263 women underwent standard D&E[1] and 120 women had intact D&E procedures. Compared to standard D&E[1] intact D&E was associated with higher parity, later gestational age (median 23 weeks vs. 21 weeks), and more preoperative cervical dilation (median 5 cm vs. 3 cm). No differences were found in estimated blood loss or operative time between the two groups. The overall rate of minor and major complications was 5% in both groups. Four major complications (i.e., complications requiring blood transfusion, laparotomy, or hospitalization) occurred in the patients who had standard D&E[1] versus none in those who underwent intact D&E [86].

Based on available data, intact D&E is a safe procedure associated with a low rate of complications. In the second trimester, intact extraction minimizes or eliminates the need for forceps and is a reasonable consideration when sufficient cervical dilation can be achieved.

Postoperative care

In women undergoing surgical abortion after the first trimester, not all complications occur or are apparent during the procedure. In the immediate postoperative period, staff must observe patients for bleeding or pain that may signal uterine atony, retained tissue, disseminated intravascular coagulopathy, or uterine perforation. For patients who have abortions early in the second trimester using cervical anesthesia, an observation period of 45 minutes to 1 hour usually suffices. Women having abortions at later gestational ages or those requiring sedation during the procedure may need a longer period of observation. Patients often require analgesia for cramps, and they generally respond well to low doses of narcotics or nonsteroidal antiinflammatory agents. Serial temperature and red cell determinations, abdominal palpation to elicit rebound tenderness, orthostatic vital signs, and crude bleeding times are useful adjuncts to clinical diagnosis of potential complications in patients whose full recovery is prolonged. They can be performed swiftly and accurately within the recovery area of facilities with a minimally equipped laboratory.

Conclusion

D&E is a safe and effective method of second-trimester abortion, and it may be preferable to labor induction for some patients. Adequate cervical dilation achieved with osmotic dilators clearly decreases the risks of complications. Although the efficacy of misoprostol for first-trimester cervical preparation is well documented, further study is necessary to evaluate its role in cervical ripening before second-trimester D&E abortion. Data regarding the benefits and risks of injection to cause preoperative fetal demise are limited. Some surgeons feel that fetal demise facilitates operative evacuation by softening fetal cortical bone, and providers in the USA may use these injections to ensure compliance with various laws. Although variations in operator techniques are numerous, these aspects are less important than intraoperative judgment and operator experience in assuring the safety of D&E abortion.

References

1 Gamble S, Strauss L, Parker W, Cook D, Zane SB, Hamdan S; Centers for Disease Control and Prevention (CDC). Abortion Surveillance-United States, 2005. *MMWR Surveill Summ* 2008; **57**: SS–13.

2 Jones RK, Zolna MRS, Henshaw SK, Finer LB. Abortion in the United States: Incidence and access to services, 2005. *Perspect Sex Reprod Health* 2008; **40**: 6–16.

3 Grimes DA, Smith MS, Witham AD. Mifepristone and misoprostol versus dilation and evacuation for midtrimester abortion: a pilot randomized controlled trial. *BJOG* 2004; **111**: 148–153.

4 Stubblefield PG, Carr-Ellis S, Borgatta L. Methods for induced abortion. *Obstet Gynecol* 2004; **104**: 174–185.

5 Partial-Birth Abortion Ban Act of 2003. 18 U.S.C. §1531. (2003).

6 Stubblefield PG. Surgical techniques of uterine evacuation in first- and second-trimester abortion. *Clin Obstet Gynaecol* 1986; **13**: 53–70.

7 Grimes DA, Schulz KF, Cates W Jr, Tyler CW Jr. Mid-trimester abortion by dilatation and evacuation: a safe and practical alternative. *N Engl J Med* 1977; **296**: 1141–1145.

8 Finks AA. Mid-trimester abortion. *Lancet* 1973; **1**: 263–264.

9 Manabe Y. Laminaria tent for gradual and safe cervical dilatation. *Am J Obstet Gynecol* 1971; **110**: 743–745.

10 Van Lith DAF, Beekhuizen W, van Schie KJ. Complications of aspirotomy (AT): a modified dilatation and curettage procedure for termination of early second-trimester pregnancies. In: Zatuchni GI, Sciarra JJ, Speidel JJ, eds. *Pregnancy Termination: Procedures, Safety, and New Developments*. Harper and Row, Hagerstown, 1979.

11 Bierer I, Steiner V. Termination of pregnancy in the second trimester with the aid of laminaria tents. *Med Gynaecol Sociol* 1972; **6**: 9–10.

12 Hale RW, Pion RJ. Laminaria: an underutilized clinical adjunct. *Clin Obstet Gynecol* 1972; **15**: 829–850.

13 Hern WM, Oakes A. Multiple laminaria treatment in early midtrimester outpatient suction abortion. *Adv Plann Parent* 1977; **12**: 93–97.

14 Hern WM Serial multiple laminaria and adjunctive urea in late outpatient dilatation and evacuation abortion. *Obstet Gynecol* 1984; **63**: 543–549.

15 Peterson WF, Berry N, Grace MR, Gulbranson CL. Second-trimester abortion by dilatation and evacuation: an analysis of 11,747 cases. *Obstet Gynecol* 1983; **62**: 185–190.

16 Autry AM, Hayes EC, Jacobson GF, Kirby RS. A comparison of medical induction and dilation and evacuation for second-trimester abortion. *Am J Obstet Gynecol* 2002; **187**: 393–397.

17 Kapp N, Borgatta L, Stubblefield P, Vragovic O, Moreno N. Mifepristone in second trimester medical abortion: a randomized controlled trial. *Obstet Gynecol* 2007; **110**: 1304–1310.

18 Green J, Borgatta L, Sia M et al. Intervention rates for placental removal following induction abortion with misoprostol. *Contraception* 2007; **76**: 310–313.

19 Jacot FR, Poulin C, Bilodeau AP et al. A five-year experience with second-trimester induced pregnancy terminations: no increase in complication rate as compared to the first trimester. *Am J Obstet Gynecol* 1993; **168**: 633–637.

20 Goldberg AB, Greenberg MB, Darney PD. Misoprostol and pregnancy. *N Engl J Med* 2001; **344**: 38–47.

21 Lawson HW, Frye A, Atrash HK, Smith JC, Shulman HB, Ramick M. Abortion mortality, United States, 1972–1987. *Am J Obstet Gynecol* 1994; **171**: 1365–1372.

22 Royal College of Obstetricians and Gynaecologists. The care of women requesting abortion. *National Evidence-based Clinical Guideline No. 7* [Online]. London: Royal College of Obstetricians and Gynaecologists Press; 2004 [cited 2008 Aug 11]. Available from: URL:http://www.rcog.org.uk/resources/Public/pdf/abortion_summary.pdf

23 Freeman EW. Abortion: subjective attitudes and feelings. *Fam Plann Perspect* 1978; **10**: 150–155.

24 Rooks JB, Cates W Jr. Abortion methods: morbidity, costs, and emotional impact. 3. Emotional impact of D&E vs. instillation. *Fam Plann Perspect* 1977; **9**: 276–277.

25 Kaltreider NB, Goldsmith S, Margolis AJ. The impact of midtrimester abortion techniques on patients and staff. *Am J Obstet Gynecol* 1979; **135**: 235–238.

26 Cowett AA, Golub RM, Grobman WA. Cost-effectiveness of dilation and evacuation versus the induction of labor for second-trimester pregnancy termination. *Am J Obstet Gynecol* 2006; **194**: 768–773.

27 Shulman LP, Ling FW, Meyers CM, Shanklin DR, Simpson JL, Elias S. Dilation and evacuation for second-trimester genetic pregnancy termination. *Obstet Gynecol* 1990; **75**: 1037–1040.

28 O'Connell K, Jones HE, Lichtenberg ES, Paul M. Second-trimester surgical abortion practices: a survey of National Abortion Federation Members. *Contraception* 2008; **78**: 492–499.

29 Eastwood KL, Kacmar JE, Steinauer J, Weitzen S, Boardman LA. Abortion training in United States obstetrics and gynecology residency programs. *Obstet Gynecol* 2006; :**108**: 303–308.

30 Landy U. Is family planning a subspecialty of obstetrics and gynecology? *Contraception* 2005; **72**: 399–401.

31 Drey EA, Foster DG, Jackson RA, Lee SJ, Cardenas LH, Darney PD. Risk factors associated with presenting for abortion in the second trimester. *Obstet Gynecol* 2006; **107**: 128–135.

32 Finer LB, Frohwirth LF, Dauphinee LA, Singh S, Moore AM. Timing of steps and reasons for delay in obtaining abortions in the United States. *Contraception* 2006; **74**: 334–344.

33 Bracken MB, Swigar ME. Factors associated with delay in seeking induced abortions. *Am J Obstet Gynecol* 1972; **113**: 301–309.

34 Fielding WL, Sachtleben MR, Friedman LM, Friedman EA. Comparison of women seeking early and late abortion. *Am J Obstet Gynecol* 1978; **131**: 304–310.

35 Schneider D, Golan A, Langer R, Caspi E, Bukovsky I. Outcome of continued pregnancy after first- and second-trimester cervical dilatation by laminaria tents. *Obstet Gynecol* 1991; **78**: 1121–1123.

36 Pastuszak AL, Schuler L, Speck-Martins CE et al. Use of misoprostol during pregnancy and Möbius syndrome in infants. *N Engl J Med* 1998; **338**: 1881–1885.

37 Fox MC, Hayes JL; Society of Family Planning. Cervical preparation for second-trimester surgical abortion prior to 20 weeks of gestation. *Contraception* 2007; **76**: 486–495.

38 Royal College of Obstetricians and Gynaecologists. *Fetal Awareness. Report of a Working Party.* Royal College of Obstetricians and Gynaecologists Press, London, 1997.

39 Lee SJ, Ralston HJ, Drey EA, Partridge JC, Rosen MA. Fetal pain: a systematic multidisciplinary review of the evidence. *JAMA* 2005; **294**: 947–954.

40 Grimes DA, Schulz KF, Cates WJ Jr. Prevention of uterine perforation during curettage abortion. *JAMA* 1984; **251**: 2108–2111.

41 Schultz KF, Grimes DA, Cates WJ Jr. Measures to prevent cervical injury during suction curettage abortion. *Lancet* 1983; **1**: 1182–1185.

42 Eaton CJ, Cohn F, Bollinger CC. Laminaria tent as a cervical dilator prior to aspiration-type therapeutic abortion. *Obstet Gynecol* 1972; **39**: 535–537.

43 Krammer J, O'Brien WF. Mechanical methods of cervical ripening. *Clin Obstet Gynecol* 1995; **38**: 280–286.

44 Norstrom A, Bryman I, Hansson HA. Cervical dilatation by Lamicel before first trimester abortion: a clinical experimental study. *Br J Obstet Gynaecol* 1988; **95**: 372–376.

45 Tan SL, Cheng H, Ho KK, Mitra R, Hii J, Yeo KC. Lamicel is more effective in preparing the cervix for midtrimester termination of pregnancy than *Laminaria japonicum*. *Aust N Z J Obstet Gynaecol* 1988; **28**: 49–52.

46 Lichtenberg ES. Complications of osmotic dilators. *Obstet Gynecol Surv* 2004; **59**: 528–536.

47 Borgatta L, Barad D. Prolonged retention of laminaria fragments: an unusual complication of laminaria usage. *Obstet Gynecol* 1991; **78**: 988–990.

48 Stubblefield PG, Altman AM, Goldstein SP. Randomized trial of one versus two days of laminaria treatment prior to late midtrimester abortion by uterine evacuation: a pilot study. *Am J Obstet Gynecol* 1982; **143**: 481–482.

49 Newmann S, Dalve-Endres A, Drey EA; Society of Family Planning. Clinical Guidelines. Cervical preparation for surgical abortion from 20 to 24 weeks' gestation. *Contraception* 2008; **77**: 308–314.

50 Evaldson GR, Fianu S, Jonasson A, Larsson B, Nord CE, Olund AR. Does the hydroscopic property of the laminaria tent imply a risk for ascending infection in legal abortion? A microbiological study. *Acta Obstet Gynecol Scand* 1986; **65**: 257–261.

51 Jonasson A. Contractile activity in the human uterine cervix and corpus during cervical dilatation by laminaria tent in first trimester legal abortions. *Acta Obstet Gynecol Scand* 1989; **68**: 401–404.

52 Gusdon JP Jr, May WJ. Complications caused by difficult removal of laminaria tents. *Am J Obstet Gynecol* 1975; **121**: 286–287.

53 Hirsh MP, Levy HM. The varied ultrasonographic appearance of laminaria. *J Ultrasound Med* 1988; **7**: 45–47.

54 Nguyen MT, Hoffman DR. Anaphylaxis to Laminaria. *J Allergy Clin Immunol* 1995; **95**: 138–139.

55 Cole DS, Bruck LR. Anaphylaxis after laminaria insertion. *Obstet Gynecol* 2000; **95**: 1025.

56 Kalish RB, Chasen ST, Rosenzweig LB, Rashbaum WK, Chervenak FA. Impact of midtrimester dilation and evacuation on subsequent pregnancy outcome. *Am J Obstet Gynecol* 2002; **187**: 882–885.

57 Jackson JE, Grobman WA, Haney E, Casele H. Mid-trimester dilation and evacuation with laminaria does not increase the risk for severe subsequent pregnancy complications. *Int J Gynaecol Obstet* 2007; **96**: 12–15.

58 Goldberg AB, Drey EA, Whitaker AK, Kang MS, Meckstroth KR, Darney PD. Misoprostol compared with laminaria before early second-trimester surgical abortion: a randomized trial. *Obstet Gynecol* 2005; **106**: 234–241.

59 Patel A, Talmont E, Morfesis J et al. Planned Parenthood Federation of America Buccal Misoprostol Waiver Group. Adequacy and safety of buccal misoprostol for cervical preparation prior to termination of second-trimester pregnancy. *Contraception* 2006; **73**: 420–430.

60 Edelman AB, Buckmaster J, Goetsch MF, Nichols MD, Jensen JT. Cervical preparation using laminaria with adjunctive buccal misoprostol before second-trimester dilation and evacuation procedures: a randomized clinical trial. *Am J Obstet Gynecol* 2006; **194**: 425–430.

61 Carbonell JL, Gallego FG, Llorente MP et al. Vaginal vs. sublingual misoprostol with mifepristone for cervical priming in second-trimester abortion by dilation and evacuation: a randomized clinical trial. *Contraception* 2007; **75**: 230–237.

62 Fletcher JC, Isada NB, Pryde PG, Johnson MP, Evans MI. Fetal intracardiac potassium chloride injection to avoid the hopeless resuscitation of an abnormal abortus: II. Ethical issues. *Obstet Gynecol* 1992; **80**: 310–313.

63 *Gonzales v. Carhart*, 127 S. Ct. 1610, 1629 (2007).

64 Jackson RA, Teplin VL, Drey EA, Thomas LJ, Darney PD. Digoxin to facilitate late second-trimester abortion: a randomized, masked, placebo-controlled trial. *Obstet Gynecol* 2001; **97**: 471–476.

65 Hern WM, Zen C, Ferguson KA, Hart V, Haseman MV. Outpatient abortion for fetal anomaly and fetal death from 15–34 menstrual weeks' gestation: techniques and clinical management. *Obstet Gynecol* 1993; **81**: 301–306.

66 Molaei M, Jones HE, Weiselberg T, McManama M, Bassell J, Westhoff CL. Effectiveness and safety of digoxin to induce fetal demise prior to second-trimester abortion. *Contraception* 2008; **77**: 223–225.

67 Drey EA, Thomas LJ, Benowitz NL, Goldschlager N, Darney PD. Safety of intra-amniotic digoxin administration before late second-trimester abortion by dilation and evacuation. *Am J Obstet Gynecol* 2000; **182**: 1063–1066.

68 Barclay M, Begg E. The practice of digoxin therapeutic drug monitoring. *N Z Med J* 2003; **116**: U704.

69 Elimian A, Verma U, Tejani N. Effect of causing fetal cardiac asystole on second-trimester abortion. *Obstet Gynecol* 1999; **94**: 139–141.

70 Coke GA, Baschat AA, Mighty HE, Malinow AM. Maternal cardiac arrest associated with attempted fetal injection of potassium chloride. *Int J Obstet Anesth* 2004; **13**: 287–290.

71 Erez Y, Ben-Shushan A, Elchalal U, Ben-Meir A, Rojansky N. Maternal morbidity following routine second trimester genetic amniocentesis. *Fetal Diagn Ther* 2007; **22**: 226–228.

72 Elchalal U, Shachar IB, Peleg D, Schenker JG. Maternal mortality following diagnostic 2nd-trimester amniocentesis. *Fetal Diagn Ther* 2004; **19**: 195–198.

73 Li Kim Mui SV, Chitrit Y, Boulanger MC, Maisonneuve L, Choudat L, de Bièvre P. Sepsis due to *Clostridium perfringens* after pregnancy termination with feticide by cordocentesis: a case report. *Fetal Diagn Ther* 2002; **17**: 124–126.

74 Pasquini L, Pontello V, Kumar S. Intracardiac injection of potassium chloride as method for feticide: experience from a single UK tertiary centre. *BJOG* 2008; **115**: 528–531.

75 Bhide A, Sairam S, Hollis B, Thilaganathan B. Comparison of feticide carried out by cordocentesis versus cardiac puncture. *Ultrasound Obstet Gynecol* 2002; **20**: 230–232.

76 Gill P, Cyr D, Afrakhtah M, Mack L, Easterling T. Induction of fetal demise in advanced pregnancy terminations: report on a funic potassium chloride protocol. *Fetal Diagn Ther* 1994; **9**: 278–282.

77 Schulz KF, Grimes DA, Christensen DD. Vasopressin reduces blood loss from second-trimester dilatation and evacuation abortion. *Lancet* 1985; **2**: 353–356.

78 Crawford JT, Edelman AB, Pereira L, Bednarek P, Buckmaster J. The effects of vasopressin injection on uterine artery blood flow during dilation and evacuation. *Am J Obstet Gynecol* 2007; **196**: e38–e39.

79 American College of Obstetricians and Gynecologists, Committee on Practice Bulletins – Obstetrics. *ACOG Practice Bulletin 76: Postpartum Hemorrhage*. The American College of Obstetricians and Gynecologists, Washington (DC), 2006.

80 Darney PD, Sweet RL. Routine intraoperative ultrasonography for second trimester abortion reduces incidence of uterine perforation. *J Ultrasound Med* 1989; **8**: 71–75.

81 Stubblefield PG, Albrecht BH, Koos B, Frederiksen MC, Williford JF, Kayman DJ. A randomized study of 12-mm and 15.9 mm cannulas in midtrimester abortion by laminaria and vacuum curettage. *Fertil Steril* 1978; **29**: 512–517.

82 Hanson MS. Discussion: medical aspects of abortion. In: Hern WM, Andrikopoulos B, eds. *Abortion in the Seventies*. National Abortion Federation, New York, 1977, p.52.

83 Mercer BM, Sklar S, Shariatmadar A, Gillieson MS, D'Alton ME. Fetal foot length as a predictor of gestational age. *Am J Obstet Gynecol* 1987; **156**: 350–355.

84 Drey EA, Kang MS, McFarland W, Darney PD. Improving the accuracy of fetal foot length to confirm gestational duration. *Obstet Gynecol* 2005; **105**: 773–778.

85 World Health Organization. (2008) Craniotomy and craniocentesis. In: *Managing Complications in Pregnancy and Childbirth: A Guide for Midwives and Doctors* [Online]. Geneva: World Health Organization; 2003 [cited 2008 12 Aug]. Available from: URL: http://www.who.int/reproductive-health/impac/index.html

86 Chasen ST, Kalish RB, Gupta M, Kaufman JE, Rashbaum WK, Chervenak FA. Dilation and evacuation at > or = 20 weeks: comparison of operative techniques. *Am J Obstet Gynecol* 2004; **190**: 1180–1183.

12

CHAPTER 12

Medical methods to induce abortion in the second trimester

Nathalie Kapp MD, MPH, and Helena von Hertzen MD, DDS

LEARNING POINTS

- Regimens of inducing abortion in the midtrimester that are most efficient, efficacious, and safe use mifepristone in combination with misoprostol or gemeprost.
- Where mifepristone is less available, induction using a prostaglandin E_1 analog alone is the preferable alternative.
- Cervical preparation with osmotic dilators placed simultaneously with initiation of the inductive agent does not decrease the induction time interval or complication rates in protocols using prostaglandin E_1 analogs.
- Complications such as retained placenta occur infrequently with the combination regimen of mifepristone and gemeprost or misoprostol; hence, routine uterine curettage is unwarranted.

Introduction

Second-trimester pregnancies can be terminated surgically by dilation and evacuation (D&E) (Chapter 11) or medically by use of various agents. Induction abortion is the termination of pregnancy by stimulation of labor-like contractions that cause eventual expulsion of the fetus and placenta from the uterine cavity [1]. Ideally, women should be given the choice between a surgical and medical procedure in the second trimester; however, this is possible only where clinicians are trained to provide both methods.

In the hands of an experienced provider, a D&E is likely to have few complications; it is a relatively short procedure, close to 100% effective in ending a pregnancy, and does not generally require inpatient bed space. The procedure may be easier for the woman when compared to medical methods, but it may be more difficult technically or emotionally for some clinicians [2]. Provision of D&E requires a number of resources not available in all settings, including specialized training and the maintenance of an adequate caseload to maintain surgical skills, specialized forceps, and the ability to adequately dilate the cervix by mechanical or pharmacologic means. Although comparative studies are lacking between surgical and currently used medical techniques because of the practical difficulties of conducting such a study [3], the published safety data of both methods are excellent. Because D&E is safe only in the hands of well-trained experienced providers, however, many institutions offering second-trimester abortion services use medical protocols for pregnancy termination.

Medical methods can be safely offered with less provider training than surgical procedures. They are the standard method of effecting second-trimester abortion in most European and in many developing countries, such as India and China. However, medical abortion in the second trimester takes more time for completion than surgical procedures and requires available hospital beds and supportive staff. Medical methods of pregnancy termination are preferable to surgical methods for women who are poor surgical candidates. They also permit more comprehensive fetal autopsy, although D&E (particularly the intact variant [Chapter 11]) may suffice for this purpose [4]. In some cases, providers or women themselves prefer the induction process over a surgical procedure.

This chapter describes the efficacy, safety, and clinical use of various agents to induce abortion in the second trimester. In addition to reviewing some historical or rarely used methods, this chapter focuses on contemporary regimens using the prostaglandin E_1 analogs, misoprostol and gemeprost, alone or in combination with mifepristone. Special considerations include counseling for women undergoing second-trimester medical abortion, management of specific complications, and postprocedure care, including contraceptive initiation. Physicians in the USA providing

Management of Unintended and Abnormal Pregnancy, 1st edition. By M Paul, ES Lichtenberg, L Borgatta, DA Grimes, PG Stubblefield, MD Creinin
 ISBN: 9781405176965.

second-trimester abortion care must comply with the federal Partial-Birth Abortion Ban Act of 2003, [5] which is addressed in Chapter 4.

History

Abortion by induction has been practiced since the earliest recorded times; it is discussed in the writings of Plato and Aristotle, in medical prescriptions by Hippocrates, and referenced in religious texts such as the Bible and the Talmud. Agents utilized in modern times in various parts of the world include those injected into the amniotic cavity (hypertonic saline, urea, ethacridine lactate, or prostaglandins); instilled into the extra-amniotic space using a catheter (ethacridine lactate, prostaglandins, or inflation of a Foley balloon); or administered intramuscularly (prostaglandins) or intravenously (prostaglandins or oxytocin). Additional administration routes for prostaglandin analogs may include vaginal, sublingual, and oral routes, depending on the analog.

The naturally occurring prostaglandins used for pregnancy termination included the prostaglandins E_1, E_2, and $F_{2\alpha}$. Their use in second-trimester abortion was limited by their side effects, particularly on the gastrointestinal system (diarrhea and vomiting) and respiratory system (bronchoconstriction with prostaglandin $F_{2\alpha}$) and serious, although rare, effects on the cardiovascular system. Therefore, these prostaglandins were rapidly replaced by their analogs, which are more slowly metabolized, offer noninvasive administration, and have a lower rate of side effects.

The advent of the prostaglandin analogs and the synthesis of mifepristone significantly improved induction abortion techniques. The current regimen recommended by the World Health Organization [6] and the Royal College of Obstetricians and Gynaecologists (RCOG) [7] consists of mifepristone followed by either misoprostol or gemeprost. When this combination is used, the induction-to-abortion interval is significantly shorter than with any other medical method to induce abortion. A number of published large series of second-trimester medical termination using mifepristone and misoprostol regimens demonstrate that it is safe: no maternal deaths and only rare complications were reported in these series [8,9].

Epidemiology

Of the 42 million abortions that occur yearly worldwide [10], approximately 10 to 15% take place in the second trimester. In 2005 induction techniques for termination comprised approximately 10% of the total number of abortions in the USA [11], and about 18% of the total in European countries such as Sweden, where surgical abortion is not provided in the second trimester [12]. Global rates are difficult to estimate, given the manner in which the data on abortion procedures are collected. Doing so accurately in the USA is also challenging, as data collected by the two agencies that report abortion statistics, the Centers for Disease Control and Prevention (CDC) and the Guttmacher Institute, are incomplete [13]. Notwithstanding these limitations, the CDC reports a relatively stable proportion of second-trimester abortions from 1980 to 2005 (the last report available): 3.8% of abortions took place between 16 and 20 weeks in 2005, while 1.4% occurred after 20 weeks. From 35 reporting areas that submitted data on medical procedures, approximately 2% of all reported second-trimester abortions in the year 2005 were medical procedures [11].

Although second-trimester abortion accounts for a small percentage of all induced abortions, it is associated with a disproportionate occurrence of morbidity. Two-thirds of major abortion-related complications and half of abortion-related mortality occur in pregnancies terminated after 13 weeks of gestation [14]. In addition to increasing gestational age, the risk of complications is influenced by the method of the termination procedure, the skill and experience of the abortion practitioner, the age and general health of the woman, and the availability and quality of the backup facilities should complications occur.

Preprocedure issues

Counseling and information provision

Counseling needs may be greater for women in the second trimester because of psychosocial issues, limited access to care, and/or a higher degree of internal conflict resulting in a later presentation for abortion. The reasons for seeking abortion in the second trimester seem to be similar globally, across health care systems and social constructs [15–17]:

- Women may fail to recognize their pregnancy during the first trimester or admit to themselves that they are pregnant;
- Women may struggle with confronting the reality of an unwanted pregnancy and the decision to terminate it;
- Some women need time to sort through social pressures, religious attitudes, and their relationship status to decide to seek abortion;
- Changed circumstances (e.g., abandonment by partner) cause many women to seek an abortion after initially planning to carry to term;
- Second-trimester abortions are more costly, and finding the resources may be difficult and time-consuming;
- Barriers to accessing health care services may cause delays; difficulty locating an abortion provider may cause the pregnancy to advance to an even later gestational age;
- Because of legal restrictions, many women are forced to travel, including to other states or countries, and these arrangements and financial considerations take time to arrange; and

- More women terminate wanted pregnancies for maternal conditions or fetal indications (after detection of anomalies by ultrasound or prenatal screening) during the second trimester (Chapter 20).

Addressing the varying circumstances in which women present for second-trimester abortion may require a range of staff, from doctors and nurses to genetic counselors and social workers.

Information provision prior to midtrimester abortion includes a review of the benefits and risks of available procedures. For women having medical abortions, the discussion should include the components of the procedure (amniotic injection, if applicable; administration and the route of the inductive agent), average length of the procedure, the labor-like course of the induction, options for pain control, and whether the woman wishes to view or not view the fetus (particularly after termination of a wanted pregnancy for fetal indications). Risks of the procedure include the possible need for postdelivery curettage, prolonged induction time, failed abortion requiring surgical completion, and hemorrhage with possible need for transfusion. Reviewing follow-up care, return to normal activities (including sexual intercourse), and contraceptive options is also important (Chapter 14).

Providers should consider the possibility of a live-born fetus, particularly if fetal death is not induced prior to the procedure and the gestational age is 18 to 20 weeks or more. Before this gestational age, uterine contractions reliably initiate fetal death. Besides the emotional and ethical difficulties for patients, their partners, and staff, a delivery with signs of life may have legal implications. This situation necessitates a clearly defined protocol for resuscitation that involves neonatal intensive care staff, abortion providers, ancillary staff, and legal consultation.

Eligibility

Worldwide, a range of second-trimester induction methods is currently used. In general, the medical eligibility criteria for a woman to undergo either a first- or second-trimester medical abortion are similar and include [18]:

- intrauterine pregnancy;
- confirmed gestational age no greater than the highest gestational age lawfully and institutionally permitted;
- no allergies to the inductive agents;
- hemodynamic stability;
- absence of severe coagulopathies; and
- no history of chronic adrenal failure or inherited porphyria (in regimens using mifepristone).

The current WHO guidance advises caution in women considering medical abortion who have a history of long-term systemic corticosteroid use, renal failure, or liver failure. Whether mifepristone may be used in women with these medical problems is not established. Women with a retained intrauterine device (IUD) warrant close observation for signs of infection throughout the procedure. Additionally, the medical conditions listed in the next section require consideration but are not necessarily contraindications to medical abortion.

Current breastfeeding

Small amounts of misoprostol are present in breast milk and mifepristone most likely passes through breast milk as well; however, no adverse clinical effects on infants have been recorded [19]. As a precaution, women may be advised to pump and discard their milk when undergoing a medical termination [20].

Multifetal pregnancy

No evidence suggests that failure rates are higher or that a dose-adjustment of the inductive agent is required in the case of multifetal pregnancies.

Human immunodeficiency virus (HIV)

Theoretically, women with HIV might experience more complications when compared to women who are HIV-negative, given a possible higher susceptibility to infection and anemia [21]. In the obstetrics literature, postpartum morbidity after vaginal and cesarean delivery for women with HIV occurs more frequently with more advanced disease [22,23]. Complications as a result of medical abortion have not been studied in this population.

Uterine scar

Women with prior hysterotomies deserve special consideration when presenting for midtrimester termination. Use of misoprostol for third-trimester labor induction warrants caution because of its association with uterine rupture in women with prior cesarean deliveries [24]. Uterine response to oxytocin is diminished in the early midtrimester, however, and the rarity of uterine rupture may be an acceptable risk for women with a uterine scar.

Both retrospective and prospective studies of women with a scarred uterus undergoing midtrimester induction abortion have been conducted [25–30]. These studies report outcomes of protocols using gemeprost or misoprostol, either alone or with mifepristone. Misoprostol regimens used 200 to 400 μg every 3 to 6 hours, depending on the study. A total of 554 women with at least one prior hysterotomy were included; sample sizes ranged from 50 to 108 per study. One uterine rupture was reported at 16 weeks' gestation in a woman with a scarred uterus [29], and one rupture occurred in a woman with an unscarred uterus [27]. Other case reports of rupture in an unscarred uterus have been documented in women undergoing prostaglandin analog or ethacridine lactate induction terminations [31,32].

The absolute risk of uterine rupture with or without a uterine scar during induction abortion is not known, as the data are derived from case reports. However, the available information suggesting a rate of occurrence that is less than 0.5% is reassuring for the use of prostaglandin analogs in the midtrimester. Included in these studies were women with average gestational ages from 16 to 21 weeks; more advanced gestational ages may result in different rates of adverse events. Whether the total prostaglandin analog dose or dosing frequency should be decreased to reduce the risk of uterine rupture in women with a uterine scar is not established.

Techniques for induction abortion

Successful medical abortion depends upon adequate uterine contractions and cervical dilation to expel both the fetus and placenta in a timely manner. Contractions that are too vigorous can cause uterine or cervical damage, whereas those that are inadequate can lead to excessive bleeding, prolonged induction time, and uterine infection. Additionally, the side effect profiles and routes of administration of all of the agents used must be acceptable to women and providers. Induction times, side effects, and complications of various induction methods are listed in Table 12.1.

In general, the existing efficacy and safety data on medical methods apply to healthy women undergoing elective terminations. In the case of septic abortions, uterine receptors are less reliable in their response to stimulation, so surgical removal of the pregnancy is the preferred method of treatment provided a trained surgeon is available.

Table 12.1 Compounds to induce second-trimester abortion.

Agents	Induction-Abortion Interval (hours)	Reported Adverse Effects (% occurrence)	Comments
Mifepristone and PGE_1	6–11	Vomiting and diarrhea rates related to PGE product and dose	Combination allows lower total dose of PGE_1 Low rate of retained placenta (<10%)
Misoprostol (PGE_1)	9–20	Vomiting (4–10%) Diarrhea (4–15%)	Oral, sublingual, or vaginal routes Inexpensive
Gemeprost (PGE_1)	15	Vomiting (1–14%) Diarrhea (2–20%)	Vaginal pessary Not available in the USA
Dinoprostone (PGE_2)	11–13 (6–7 hours with cervical ripening)	Fever, nausea, vomiting, diarrhea (majority of patients experience at least one side effect)	Vaginal suppositories Must be refrigerated
Ethacridine lactate (Rivanol)	20–40	Headache, vomiting (more than with saline)	Requires extraovular placement Shorter induction intervals with oxytocin augmentation
Historical methods			
Sulprostone (PGE_2)	11	Vomiting (12–46%) Diarrhea (6–17%)	Given intramuscularly or intravenously Not available in USA
15 methyl $PGF_{2\alpha}$ (carboprost)	8–16	Vomiting, diarrhea, and fever (2–3 episodes per patient)	Intramuscular (has also been used via intra-amniotic, extra-amniotic, and vaginal routes)
$PGF_{2\alpha}$	14–37 (dose dependent)	Incomplete abortion Hemorrhage Live-born fetus Nausea, vomiting, and diarrhea (30%)	Intra-amniotic instillation; majority of patients require oxytocin augmentation No longer available in the USA in form used for induction Potent bronchoconstrictor
Oxytocin	8–18	Water intoxication (rare) Nausea and vomiting	Significantly fewer gastrointestinal side effects than with prostaglandins Requires IV infusion
Saline	20–46	Fever/vomiting (5–12%) Hemorrhage (6% transfusion rate) Disseminated intravascular coagulopathy (DIC) (0.8%) Rare seizures and intramuscular injection causing myometrial necrosis	Intra-amniotic injection following amniotic fluid aspiration; frequently used with oxytocin augmentation Inexpensive

Box A Commonly Used Mifepristone Plus Prostaglandin Analog Regimens After 12 Weeks' Gestation (WHO 2003 [6])

200 mg mifepristone followed after 36 to 48 hours by:
800 μg vaginal misoprostol followed by 400 μg oral misoprostol every 3 hours up to a maximum of four doses, ***OR***
1 mg vaginal gemeprost, repeated every 6 hours up to maximum of four doses, and if necessary every 3 hours up to four additional doses.

Mifepristone

Mifepristone is a 19-norsteroid that specifically blocks the receptors for progesterone and glucocorticosteroids. It is active when given by mouth and peak plasma levels are reached within 2 hours. Its half-life in plasma is 24 to 48 hours but nanomolar concentrations persist for several days [33]. Progesterone is necessary for the maintenance of a pregnancy, and its presence increases uterine relaxation; therefore, antagonizing this effect leads to uterine contractions and pregnancy disruption as well as dilating and softening of the uterine cervix [34].

The blockage of progesterone receptors results in the breakdown of maternal capillaries in the decidua [35], the synthesis of prostaglandins by the epithelium of the decidual glands [36], and inhibition of prostaglandin dehydrogenase [37]. Mifepristone increases the sensitivity of the uterus to prostaglandin analogs by an approximate factor of five [38]. This effect develops over 24 to 48 hours and is the basis of the regimen for medical abortion in which mifepristone is followed 36 to 48 hours later by a prostaglandin analog.

The addition of mifepristone to a prostaglandin analog regimen shortens the abortion time interval and reduces the number of doses of misoprostol or gemeprost required for successful induction, without increasing side effects of the procedure. In combination with either misoprostol or gemeprost, mifepristone's effect is dramatic: the abortion interval is shortened by up to 50% [39] and the rate of successful abortion in 24 hours is increased up to 95% [40]. Therefore, the total dose needed of the prostaglandin analog and the subsequent occurrence of side effects are decreased.

Based on available evidence and expert opinion, the following regimen is recommended by RCOG for midtrimester medical abortion [7]: mifepristone 200 mg orally, followed 36 to 48 hours later by misoprostol, 800 μg vaginally, then misoprostol 400 μg orally every 3 hours to a maximum of four oral doses (Box A). Because 200 mg of mifepristone has demonstrated equal effectiveness to 600 mg [41], the recommended regimen differs from the licensed regimen in the UK of 600 mg of mifepristone followed 36 to 48 hours later by gemeprost, 1 mg vaginally every 3 hours to a maximum of five vaginal pessaries. If the woman has not aborted within 3 hours of the last dose, the mifepristone dose is repeated and the misoprostol regimen is restarted the following day. In the case of failure of the primary method of termination, further treatment depends on the clinician's preference. A randomized trial confirmed that when the first dose of misoprostol after mifepristone pretreatment was given vaginally, the efficacy was not affected if the subsequent doses were administered orally [42].

The combination of mifepristone and gemeprost is also effective for second-trimester medical abortion. The regimen of 200 mg mifepristone followed by misoprostol administration, as described in the RCOG guidelines [7], was compared to 200 mg mifepristone followed by gemeprost, administered every 6 hours, in a randomized study including 100 women [43]. Complete abortion rates, induction-to-abortion intervals, surgical evacuation rates, and side effects were similar in the two groups.

When the interval between mifepristone and misoprostol administration was reduced to 24 hours, the induction-to-abortion interval was somewhat longer than after a 48-hour interval. In a retrospective study, the time to fetal expulsion was 9.8 hours in the 24-hour interval group compared to 7.5 hours when the interval was 48 hours ($p < 0.01$), and in a randomized study it was 7.3 hours versus 6.2 hours ($p < 0.05$), respectively [44,45]. This latter study also reported a higher rate of uterine curettage with the 24-hour interval ($p < 0.001$).

Today, mifepristone is registered in over 35 countries, primarily for the termination of pregnancy early in the first trimester [46]. Although availability of mifepristone is increasing globally, expense still prohibits its use in many settings. Moreover, consideration must be given to the need to administer mifepristone 1 to 2 days prior to induction when introducing its use to existing protocols.

The short induction times seen with mifepristone and prostaglandin E_1 analog combinations accentuate biologic differences among women undergoing termination procedures. Studies using this combination have demonstrated statistically shorter induction-to-abortion intervals among parous when compared to nulliparous women (Fig. 12.1) [8,9,47], whereas this finding is not typical with singular prostaglandin E_1 analog or ethacridine lactate induction abortions.

Misoprostol

Misoprostol is a synthetic prostaglandin E_1 analog that differs from other analogs in the following qualities: it is inexpensive, orally active with multiple effective routes of administration, and it can be stored at room temperatures without losing effectiveness [48]. Additionally, misoprostol is equally or more effective as other prostaglandin analogs, with a low rate of dose-dependent side effects. Misoprostol is effective at initiating uterine contractions and cervical ripening at any gestational age (unlike agents such as oxytocin), and it is used in decreasing doses as the pregnancy advances [24]. Its pharmacokinetics and uterine effects are discussed in detail in Chapter 9.

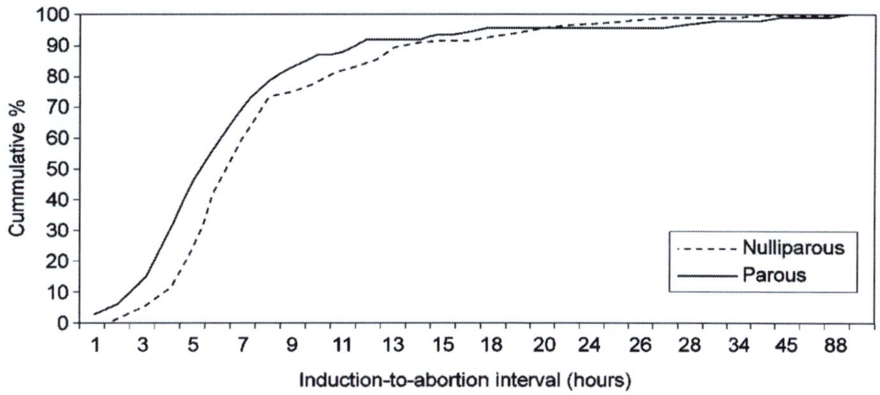

Figure 12.1 Combination mifepristone and misoprostol induction-to-abortion interval in parous versus nulliparous women. The 1-hour difference between the groups is statistically significant ($p < 0.001$). (Reprinted with permission from Rose et al [9].)

Misoprostol may be administered by different routes; vaginal administration appears to be the most effective, followed by sublingual administration. Oral administration is associated with higher rates of diarrhea and longer induction times when compared to vaginal administration [49]. However, some women prefer nonvaginal dosing, and sublingual administration may be preferable in women with vaginal bleeding [49–51]. For regimens using mifepristone followed by vaginal misoprostol initially, with repeat dosing by oral administration, efficacy and the abortion time interval are similar to regimens using all vaginal dosing [8,42,52]. Several randomized trials using misoprostol alone for second-trimester medical abortion demonstrate that the vaginal route of administration is more effective with a lower incidence of side effects than oral administration [51,53] or sublingual administration [54].

Although the combination of mifepristone and misoprostol is the regimen of choice for midtrimester pregnancy terminations, misoprostol may be used alone when mifepristone is less available. The recommended evidence-based regimen is 400 μg of vaginal misoprostol every 3 hours, up to five doses, in pregnancies between 13 and 22 weeks [55]. After 22 weeks' gestation, the misoprostol dose and frequency of administration should be reduced.

In regimens using misoprostol alone, the median induction to abortion interval is 10 to 15 hours, with an 80 to 90% rate of successful abortion within 24 hours [56–59]. The abortion time interval is decreased with more frequent dosing: two randomized clinical trials demonstrate a significantly shorter induction time with vaginal administration of 400 μg misoprostol every 3 hours than with administration every 6 hours, without a significant increase in side effects [57,59].

Finally, misoprostol regimens are easy to provide and teach, as is evident by its widespread global use. In a recent study, use of misoprostol also demonstrates high acceptability and uptake among providers of midtrimester termination in settings unfamiliar with evidence-based medicine [60].

Other prostaglandin analogs

Prostaglandins have been used to induce abortion since the mid-1970s [61,62]. The most commonly used of the prostaglandin analogs have been carboprost, sulprostone, gemeprost, and misoprostol. Carboprost, an $F_{2\alpha}$ prostaglandin analog, is infrequently used because of its relatively high side-effect profile when compared to the E analogs [63]. Sulprostone, an E_2 analog, was uniquely associated with coronary spasm. Myocardial infarctions occurred in 3 out of 60,000 women who received the drug; one woman, a heavy smoker over age 30, died as a result. Sulprostone is no longer used [64,65].

Gemeprost and misoprostol, both E_1 analogs, are by far the most common of the prostaglandin analogs currently utilized for induction abortion. Both have demonstrated higher efficacy and shorter induction intervals when compared to intra-amniotic $PGF_{2\alpha}$ and extra-amniotic PGE_2 [66–69].

When the prostaglandin E_1 analogs are directly compared, misoprostol is equivalent to or more efficacious than gemeprost [58,70,71]. A meta-analysis of randomized trials compared misoprostol to gemeprost in midtrimester abortion, using various regimens of each. Compared to gemeprost vaginal suppositories, vaginal misoprostol was associated with reduced need for narcotic analgesia and surgical evacuation of the uterus [72]. No other statistically significant differences were observed.

Gemeprost is still used in some settings for cervical preparation prior to surgical uterine evacuation, midtrimester medical abortion, and treatment after intrauterine fetal death [28,73]. Widespread use of gemeprost is limited by its expense, instability at room temperatures, and singular route of administration (vaginal pessary) when compared to misoprostol [63].

Ethacridine lactate (Rivanol)

Before prostaglandin analogs became available, ethacridine lactate was the agent most frequently used for second-trimester abortion globally. This method is currently used in

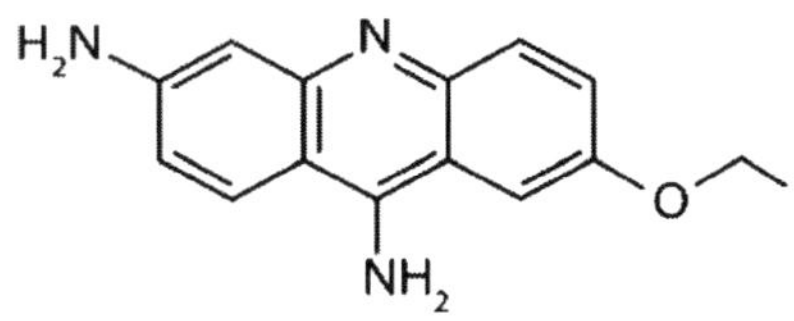

Figure 12.2 Chemical structure of ethacridine lactate.

such settings as China, India, and Mongolia, as it is inexpensive, efficacious, and relatively safe (Fig. 12.2).

Ethacridine lactate is commonly used as a 0.1% solution (1 mg/ml) that is instilled transcervically into the extra-amniotic space in a volume corresponding to 10 ml per gestational week up to a maximum of 150 ml. A number 16 rubber Foley catheter (filled with the solution) is placed transcervically, taking care that the tip is placed only minutely beyond the internal os. This technique avoids accidental intravascular injection of the solution [74]. The instillation is carried out by gravity without forceful injection. The catheter is usually removed after 4 to 24 hours. The abortion process may be slow, and augmentation with an intravenous oxytocin infusion (50 mU/min) is common [75]. Ethacridine lactate, when used alone, offers a success rate of about 90% in 72 hours with a mean induction time of less than 24 hours [76]. Intra-amniotic injection of the drug has been reported in some settings, with a mean abortion interval of 37 to 41 hours [77–79].

Ethacridine lactate has weak antiseptic properties, resulting in low rates of infection. Data collected from eight gynecological departments in Sweden of 2,058 consecutive women undergoing ethacridine lactate midtrimester abortions demonstrated no fatal or life-threatening complications [76].

Historical techniques

Hypertonic saline was first used for induction termination in the 1940s. A typical regimen involved aspiration of up to 200 ml of amniotic fluid followed by instillation of a similar volume of 20% saline [80]. Although efficacious, safety concerns (primarily the risk of hypernatremia, coagulopathy, and consequent massive hemorrhage) have rendered this method obsolete. When compared directly to misoprostol in a randomized trial, hypertonic saline had longer induction times and higher rates of required blood transfusion and retained placenta [60]. When compared to PGE_2 gel, hypertonic saline had higher rates of retained placenta (63% vs. 25%), fever, and coagulopathy leading to disseminated intravascular coagulation (DIC) (0.8% vs. 0%) [81].

Similar to saline procedures, instillation of hyperosmolar urea required aspiration of amniotic fluid followed by instillation of the agent (59.7% urea). Augmentation of uterine contractions with oxytocin or prostaglandins was common. Procedures using urea were less likely to be associated with the serious complications of hypernatremia or coagulopathy when compared to the use of hypertonic saline, and they were better tolerated than $PGF_{2\alpha}$ regimens [82]. The use of hyperosmolar urea has not been directly compared to prostaglandin analogs.

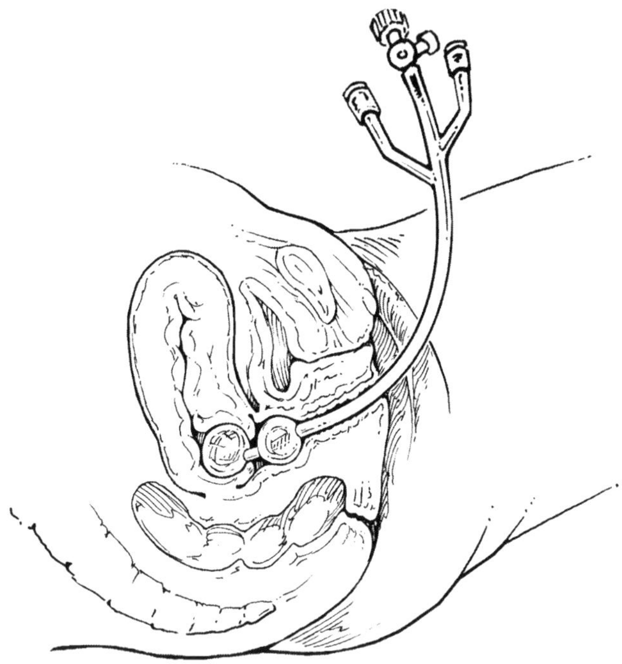

Figure 12.3 Extraovular placement of Foley catheter.

Oxytocin is less effective at initiating uterine contractions in the midtrimester than in the third trimester, as the number of oxytocin receptors in the myometrium increases over the length of the gestation. When compared to misoprostol, use of oxytocin is associated with longer induction times [83] and higher rates of serious side effects such as water intoxication. To avoid water intoxication, high-dose protocols have incorporated regular interruptions of oxytocin administration (1 hour for every 4 hours of treatment) [84]. Oxytocin still plays a role in induction abortion, as it is frequently used after fetal expulsion to augment uterine contractility and facilitate placental delivery [56].

Mechanical methods of inducing abortion also have been utilized. Devices such as a Foley balloon or double-balloon catheter placed transcervically to separate the amniotic sac from the uterine wall while placing pressure on the internal os (when the catheter is weighted) result in contractions, cervical change, and eventual fetal expulsion (Fig. 12.3). The mechanism of action is created by the myometrial cells themselves, which release prostaglandins in response to manipulation. Mean induction intervals using the balloon alone, or in combination with extra-amniotic infusion of prostaglandin E_2, range from 13 to 18 hours [85,86]. In one series, use of the double-balloon device to instill prostaglandin E_2 resulted in successful abortion in 91% of subjects after 24 hours with very few side effects [85].

Direct comparisons to pharmacologic agents for induction abortion have not been reported. Given that catheters may be reused after sterilization, mechanical devices to induce abortion have played an important role in resource-poor areas of developing countries.

When compared to regimens using prostaglandin analogs, these historical methods result in longer induction times and higher rates of retained placenta requiring postdelivery curettage. The historical methods also have associated serious morbidities such as coagulopathy and DIC, water intoxication, hypernatremia, uterine myonecrosis, and amniotic fluid embolism (with techniques requiring amniotic instillation). Given the advances in pharmacologic agents for medical abortion, these methods need no longer be used.

Adjunctive procedures

Inducing preprocedure fetal demise

Clinicians have used various agents to cause fetal death before midtrimester abortion for many reasons, including the belief that softened fetal tissue may facilitate the D&E procedure [87]. More commonly, some patients or clinicians prefer initiating the abortion procedure with a nonliving fetus for emotional reasons or to avoid the problem of a transiently living neonate at the time of fetal expulsion [88].

Historical inductive agents such as hyperosmolar urea, hypertonic saline, or $PGF_{2\alpha}$ to induce abortion had the secondary effect of initiating fetal death. Prostaglandin analogs alone, or in combination with mifepristone, do not have this effect. With sufficiently short induction intervals, transient fetal survival may occur, particularly in pregnancies with gestational ages greater than 18 to 20 weeks [63]. Agents that may be administered to cause fetal death prior to second-trimester surgical or medical abortion include digoxin administered into the amniotic fluid or fetus or 20% potassium chloride injected through the umbilical cord or into the fetal cardiac chambers (Chapter 11).

Digoxin prior to induction abortion has been reported, but its use in this setting has not been the subject of randomized trials. Hern et al reported its use in a paper demonstrating the safety of late abortion, as a 1.5- to 2.0-mg intrafetal dose injected 1 to 2 days prior to induction [89]. The overall rate of complications of the termination procedure was low; however, side effects attributable to the digoxin (between the time of the injection and initiation of the induction) were not reported. Other studies include the use of 1.5 mg of digoxin intra-amniotically at the time of mifepristone (or placebo) administration, 1 day prior to induction with misoprostol [47]. Women in these studies reported low rates of nausea during the 24 hours before the first misoprostol dose, and no other side effects were noted. No fetuses were delivered with signs of life.

A few reports have included intracardiac injection of potassium chloride to effect fetal death before induction. In a retrospective study of the effect of day-prior feticide with potassium chloride on induction abortion using vaginal prostaglandin E_2, successful abortion required less prostaglandin and time for the 17 of 68 women who received intracardiac potassium chloride [90]. The two groups had similar rates of side effects, both gastrointestinal and febrile, throughout the procedure. In a separate report, 21 women underwent fetal cardiac injection of potassium chloride the day prior to induction with prostaglandin $F_{2\alpha}$. No maternal complications were noted; immediate cardiac asystole occurred in 20 of 21 cases, and no fetuses were live-born [88].

Cervical preparation

Cervical preparation is an integral part of safe provision of second-trimester surgical abortion (Chapter 11). Early reports of the use of osmotic dilators prior to induction abortion using prostaglandin E_2 or $F_{2\alpha}$ demonstrated decreased induction-to-abortion intervals [91–93]. In induction protocols using prostaglandin $F_{2\alpha}$, placement of Dilapan™ approximately 12 hours prior to induction significantly reduced the time-to-abortion interval when compared to laminaria [92]; laminaria inserted 4 hours prior was similarly superior to placement at the time of injection and to no laminaria [93]. A greater reduction in induction time was found when laminaria placement occurred 14 to 24 hours prior to induction [94–96]. Similarly, laminaria placement 24 hours prior to prostaglandin E_2 induction decreased induction times [91], although placement 3 to 6 hours prior was not found to be beneficial [97].

For the current prostaglandin analogs or ethacridine lactate induction abortions, placement of osmotic dilators at the time of the inductive agent's initiation does not shorten the induction-to-abortion interval or decrease complication rates of the procedure. Two randomized trials examined the use of cervical preparation with laminaria at the time of misoprostol induction [56,98]; in addition, one study included day-prior administration of hypertonic saline to effect fetal death. The results were concordant: for induction regimens using misoprostol alone, placement of laminaria did not decrease the abortion interval. In fact, both trials demonstrated longer median abortion intervals, although in only one trial was this difference significant [56]. A secondary outcome reported was that women who received laminaria had increased analgesic needs during the induction procedure [56]. Although simultaneous placement of laminaria with initiation of misoprostol administration does not decrease the abortion interval, the effect of pretreatment with laminaria on the induction-to-abortion interval has not been studied.

Laminaria use also has been compared to mifepristone, which has cervical ripening properties, in randomized trials. Ho et al first compared mifepristone given 36 hours prior to induction to laminaria placement 12 hours prior to induction with gemeprost. Mifepristone was more effective than laminaria at shortening the induction interval [99]. In a second trial, Prairie et al found that administration of mifepristone, when compared to laminaria, 24 hours prior to misoprostol induction resulted in a significantly shorter induction interval. However, cervical dilation, as measured by palpation by the clinician, was greater in those who received laminaria [100].

Pretreatment with Dilapan™ for 6 hours prior to an induction regimen using gemeprost demonstrated no benefit when compared to gemeprost alone, while mifepristone significantly shortened the induction interval when compared with Dilapan™ [101]. In the setting of ethacridine lactate-induced abortion, use of Lamicel® at the time of ethacridine lactate initiation demonstrated no beneficial effect of cervical preparation on the induction time interval when compared to no cervical preparation [102].

Management of problems and complications

Retained placenta

Early reports of retained placenta after saline and PGE_2-induced abortion demonstrated that complication rates increased with passing time after fetal expulsion; therefore, routine curettage between 30 minutes and 2 hours after fetal expulsion was recommended [103,104]. In contrast, outcomes after misoprostol inductions reveal that expectant management of the placenta, as opposed to routine intervention, does not increase complications such as transfusion rates [50].

In a large, retrospective study of misoprostol second-trimester inductions, 59% of women experienced spontaneous placental expulsion within 1 hour, and the overall rate of surgical intervention for retained placenta was 6% [50]. Similar rates are found in studies that use the combination mifepristone with misoprostol, demonstrating rates of needed surgical intervention between 2.5 and 10% [43,52,105]. Therefore, routine surgical intervention for removal of the placenta is not required following midtrimester induction termination using misoprostol or gemeprost alone or in combination with mifepristone. Interventions to remove the placenta need only be performed for excessive bleeding or fever [63].

Pain management

Abdominal pain and cramping are the most common side effects of induced medical abortion [106, 107]; however, pain is highly subjective, difficult to quantify, and therefore difficult to study. Effective treatment for abortion-related pain is not well-established, and analgesic regimens vary widely. Regimens usually include combinations of paracetamol or acetaminophen, nonsteroidal antiinflammatory agents (NSAIDs), and narcotics (often by intravenous administration). RCOG recommends that a wide range of oral and parenteral analgesics be available to women undergoing a midtrimester medical abortion [7]. In one small randomized trail, prophylactic use of NSAIDs reduced opiate requirements among women undergoing midtrimester medical abortions [108]. Despite the fact that NSAIDs inhibit the production of endogenous prostaglandins, they do not attenuate the effect of the exogenous prostaglandins [108–110].

No studies have directly compared different analgesic regimens for the relief of medical abortion pain in the midtrimester, and analgesic use typically varies widely by treatment center [111]. However, predictors of severe pain are well-established and fairly consistent across studies of medical abortion. In women undergoing midtrimester medical abortion, higher analgesic needs are reported by younger women, those with longer induction intervals and higher cumulative doses of misoprostol, and those at more advanced gestational ages [112]. Similarly, in women undergoing first-trimester medical abortion, severe pain is more likely to be reported by younger women, women of lower parity, and by those with higher levels of anxiety or a history of dysmenorrhea [113].

Postprocedure care

Complications

After induction abortion, women should be monitored for the most common complications: hemorrhage and infection. The risk of hemorrhage increases with gestational age (0.88 in 1,000 at less than 13 weeks; 4.0 in 1,000 at more than 20 weeks) [7]. Heavy bleeding requiring a transfusion is reported to occur in less than 1% of midtrimester medical abortions [8]. Heavy vaginal bleeding warrants investigation into the following etiologies: lower genital tract lacerations, uterine atony, and retained placenta. Their respective treatments include laceration repair, administration of uterotonic agents, and uterine curettage (Chapter 15). In the rare case of hemorrhage prior to fetal expulsion, surgical evacuation of the uterus and assessment for uterine rupture are indicated.

Infection in the setting of midtrimester medical termination occurs rarely. A large series of more than 1,000 women reported a 2.6% rate of infections requiring antibiotic administration [8]. Signs and symptoms of infection may include lower quadrant abdominal pain, bleeding, foul-smelling discharge, fever, and chills. In addition to antibiotic treatment, surgical evacuation of the uterus is warranted in the case of incomplete abortion.

Although few studies report subsequent medical regimens for women who fail to abort within the first 24 hours of induction, many practitioners repeat the initial regimen or switch to another prostaglandin analog [8]. Failure to abort by the second or third day of a medical induction may be an appropriate indication for surgical completion with a D&E

[63]. The D&E procedure is facilitated by the effects of the failed medical induction: fetal maceration and cervical shortening and dilation [114].

Delayed postprocedure care for women is similar to recommended care for women after first-trimester abortion, with a few particular considerations for contraception, lactation, and postprocedure counseling.

Contraception

Contraceptive counseling for women having midtrimester abortions is similar to counseling for women having first-trimester abortions (Chapter 14), with some exceptions. The WHO recommends that women delay the next pregnancy after an induced abortion for 6 months to improve maternal and fetal health outcomes [115].

A woman may begin ovulating as soon as 2 weeks following an abortion, thus conception can occur as early as 10 to 14 days postabortion [116]. Therefore, a contraceptive plan is important for a woman's postabortion care. With the exception of cervical barriers, all contraceptive methods may be safely initiated immediately following an uncomplicated second-trimester abortion, including hormonal contraception and insertion of the IUD [117]. The hypercoagulability associated with third-trimester pregnancy is not a factor after second-trimester pregnancy; therefore, hormonal contraception may be initiated immediately. The fitting of a cervical diaphragm or cap should be delayed until uterine involution occurs. Special considerations when initiating contraception after a second-trimester abortion are as follows [117]:

IUD

An IUD may be safely inserted immediately following a second-trimester abortion. However, expulsion rates are higher than after a first-trimester abortion or in the nonpregnant state [118]. IUDs should not be placed immediately following a septic abortion.

Surgical sterilization

Following an uncomplicated second-trimester abortion, a woman may safely undergo sterilization. The surgical procedure immediately following the abortion may be completed by mini-laparotomy. For a laparoscopic procedure, women usually wait for complete uterine involution, around 4 to 6 weeks postabortion, although open laparoscopic techniques may allow for earlier procedures. No data are available to guide recommendations for hysteroscopic sterilizations, but a similar 6-week interval between the termination and sterilization procedure is a reasonable time frame.

Cervical cap or diaphragm

Although the Lea's Shield® is a one-size-fits-all device, the FemCap and diaphragm must be sized to fit a woman's cervix. After a second-trimester pregnancy, a fitting will not be reliable until uterine involution is complete.

Fertility awareness-based methods

Use of fertility awareness-based methods relies on either symptoms of ovulation or regular menstrual cycles. Generally, women may start using these methods immediately following the first postabortion menses. Patients who wish to use fertility awareness-based methods may be advised to abstain from intercourse or to use a method such as condoms until regular menses are established [117].

Lactation

Following second-trimester abortion, particularly at more advanced gestational ages, a small percentage of women may experience milk secretion, primarily between 3 to 7 days postabortion [119]. Management of these symptoms includes the routine methods to suppress lactation: breast compression, ice packs, avoidance of breast stimulation, or medical therapy with a prolactin-suppressing drug such as bromocriptine [119].

Follow-up counseling

For most women, the induction abortion procedure is stressful. After completion of the abortion, women generally report a great sense of relief [120]. Postprocedure counseling differs from woman to woman; those who have terminated wanted pregnancies for maternal or fetal indications may have a greater need for counseling. The decision to terminate a pregnancy, particularly for an anomaly that is not lethal, may be an overwhelming emotional experience for some women and couples. Consideration of an individual woman's needs and situation should guide clinical care, including possible counseling referrals.

Conclusion

Over the last decade, midtrimester medical abortion protocols have adapted to accommodate the emerging information on the effective and safe use of prostaglandin analogs and the antiprogestin mifepristone. Currently, recommended protocols using the combination mifepristone with either gemeprost or misoprostol result in the safest and most efficient termination procedures; they offer an approximate 50% reduction in the induction-to-abortion time interval when compared to singular agent induction regimens. Where mifepristone is less available, gemeprost or misoprostol may be used alone, although the total prostaglandin analog dose, the induction-to-abortion time interval, and subsequent occurrence of side effects are greater than when the regimen is combined with mifepristone. With these regimens, additional cervical preparation with osmotic dilators, placed at the time of the inductive agent, does not decrease complication rates or the induction time interval.

Additionally, as retained placenta occurs infrequently with recommended regimens, routine curettage is unwarranted in the absence of evidence of incomplete abortion.

Ongoing and future research in midtrimester medical abortion is likely to include assessing the induction procedure in women with medical problems, such as HIV; exploring ways to further minimize side effects, such as pain during the procedure; and examining the feasibility of expanding levels of providers and services, such as in outpatient clinics for 1-day procedures. Unquestionably, provision of medical methods of pregnancy termination is an important component of comprehensive abortion care, and it may play an increasingly important role as prenatal screening for fetal anomalies continues to advance.

Acknowledgment

The views expressed are those of the authors and may not necessarily reflect those of Special Programme of Research, Development, and Research Training in Human Reproduction (HRP), World Health Organization, or of its cosponsors.

References

1 Blumenthal PD, Castleman LD, Jain JK. (1999) Abortion by labor induction. In: Paul M, Lichtenberg ES, Borgotta L, Grimes DA, Stubblefield PG, eds. *A Clinician's Guide to Medical and Surgical Abortion*. Churchill Livingstone, New York, 1999.

2 Kaltreider NB, Goldsmith S, Margolis AJ. The impact of midtrimester abortion techniques on patients and staff. *Am J Obstet Gynecol* 1979; **135**: 235–238.

3 Grimes DA, Smith MS, Witham AD. Mifepristone and misoprostol versus dilation and evacuation for midtrimester abortion: a pilot randomised controlled trial. *BJOG* 2004; **111**: 148–153.

4 Shulman LP, Ling FW, Meyers CM, Shanklin DR, Simpson JL, Elias S. Dilation and evacuation for second-trimester genetic pregnancy termination. *Obstet Gynecol* 1990; **75**: 1037–1040.

5 Partial-Birth Abortion Ban Act of 2003. 18 U.S.C. §1531 (2003).

6 World Health Organization. *Safe Abortion: Technical and Policy Guidance for Health Systems*. World Health Organization, Geneva, 2003.

7 Royal College of Obstetricians and Gynaecologists. *The Care of Women Requesting Induced Abortion*. Royal College of Obstetricians and Gynaecology Press, London, 2004.

8 Ashok PW, Templeton A, Wagaarachchi PT, Flett GM. Midtrimester medical termination of pregnancy: a review of 1002 consecutive cases. *Contraception* 2004; **69**: 51–58.

9 Rose SB, Shand C, Simmons A. Mifepristone- and misoprostol-induced mid-trimester termination of pregnancy: a review of 272 cases. *Aust N Z J Obstet Gynaecol* 2006; **46**: 479–485.

10 Sedgh G, Henshaw S, Singh S, Ahman E, Shah IH. Induced abortion: estimated rates and trends worldwide. *Lancet* 2007; **370**: 1338–1345.

11 Gamble SB, Strauss LT, Parker WY et al. Abortion surveillance – United States, 2005. *MMWR Surveill Summ* 2008; **56**: SS–13.

12 Socialstyrelsen [Online]. Stockholm: 2005. Aborter 2005 [cited 2009 Jan 2]. Available from: URL: http://www.socialstyrelsen.se/NR/rdonlyres/A15D144C-EE18-4CA0-B141-48EED8D6F7B6/5496/Publ200506422.pdf

13 Guttmacher Institute [online]. Issues in Brief: The Limitations of U.S. Statistics on Abortion; 1997 [cited 2009 Jan 2]. Available from: URL: http://www.guttmacher.org/pubs/ib14.html

14 World Health Organization. *Medical Methods for Termination of Pregnancy*. World Health Organization, Geneva, 1997: 871.

15 Finer LB, Frohwirth LF, Dauphinee LA, Singh S, Moore AM. Timing of steps and reasons for delays in obtaining abortions in the United States. *Contraception* 2006; **74**: 334–344.

16 Guilbert E, Marcoux S, Rioux JE. Factors associated with the obtaining of a second-trimester induced abortion. *Can J Public Health* 1994; **85**: 402–406.

17 Jones RK, Darroch JE, Henshaw SK. Patterns in the socioeconomic characteristics of women obtaining abortions in 2000–2001. *Perspect Sex Reprod Health* 2002; **34**: 226–235.

18 World Health Organization. *Frequently Asked Questions about Medical Abortion*. World Health Organization, Geneva, 2006.

19 Vogel D, Burkhardt T, Rentsch K et al. Misoprostol versus methylergometrine: pharmacokinetics in human milk. *Am J Obstet Gynecol* 2004; **191**: 2168–2173.

20 Fiala C, Gemzell-Danielsson K. Review of medical abortion using mifepristone in combination with a prostaglandin analog. *Contraception* 2006; **74**: 66–86.

21 Delvaux T, Nöstlinger C. Reproductive choice for women and men living with HIV: contraception, abortion, and fertility. *Reprod Health Matters* 2007; **15**: 46–66.

22 Marcollet A, Goffinet F, Firtion G et al. Differences in postpartum morbidity in women who are infected with the human immunodeficiency virus after elective cesarean delivery, emergency cesarean delivery, or vaginal delivery. *Am J Obstet Gynecol* 2002; **186**: 784–789.

23 Duarte G, Read JS, Gonin R et al. Mode of delivery and postpartum morbidity in Latin American and Caribbean countries among women who are infected with human immunodeficiency virus-1: the NICHD International Site Development Initiative (NISDI) Perinatal Study. *Am J Obstet Gynecol* 2006; **195**: 215–229.

24 Blanchard K, Clark S, Winikoff B, Gaines G, Kabani G, Shannon C. Misoprostol for women's health: a review. *Obstet Gynecol* 2002; **99**: 316–332.

25 Bhattacharjee N, Ganguly RP, Saha SP. Misoprostol for termination of mid-trimester post-Caesarean pregnancy. *Aust N Z J Obstet Gynaecol* 2007; **47**: 23–25.

26 Daponte A, Nzewenga G, Dimopoulos KD, Guidozzi F. The use of vaginal misoprostol for second-trimester pregnancy

termination in women with previous single cesarean section. *Contraception* 2006; **74**: 324–327.

27 Daskalakis GJ, Mesogitis SA, Papantoniou NE, Moulopoulos GG, Papapanagiotou AA, Antsaklis AJ. Misoprostol for second trimester pregnancy termination in women with prior caesarean section. *BJOG* 2005; **112**: 97–99.

28 Marinoni E, Santoro M, Vitagliano MP, Patella A, Cosmi EV, Di Iorio R. Intravaginal gemeprost and second-trimester pregnancy termination in the scarred uterus. *Int J Gynaecol Obstet* 2007; **97**: 35–39.

29 Mazouni C, Provensal M, Porcu G et al. Termination of pregnancy in patients with previous cesarean section. *Contraception* 2006; **73**: 244–248.

30 Shammas AG, Momani MD. Misoprostol for termination of second trimester pregnancy in a scarred uterus. *Saudi Med J* 2006; **27**: 1173–1176.

31 Bagga R, Chaudhary N, Kalra J. Rupture in an unscarred uterus during second trimester pregnancy termination with mifepristone and misoprostol. *Int J Gynaecol Obstet* 2004; **87**: 42–43.

32 Malhotra N, Chanana C. Silent rupture of unscarred uterus: an unusual presentation at second trimester abortion. *Arch Gynecol Obstet* 2007; **275**: 283–284.

33 Lähteenmäki P, Heikinheimo O, Croxatto H et al. Pharmacokinetics and metabolism of RU486. *J Steroid Biochem* 1987; **27**: 859–863.

34 Swahn ML, Bygdeman M. The effect of the antiprogestin RU 486 on uterine contractility and sensitivity to prostaglandin and oxytocin. *Br J Obstet Gynaecol* 1988; **95**: 126–134.

35 Johannisson E, Oberholzer M, Swahn ML, Bygdeman M. Vascular changes in the human endometrium following the administration of the progesterone antagonist RU 486. *Contraception* 1989; **39**: 103–117.

36 Smith SK, Kelly RW. The effect of the antiprogestins RU 486 and ZK 98734 on the synthesis and metabolism of prostaglandins F2 alpha and E2 in separated cells from early human decidua. *J Clin Endocrinol Metab* 1987; **65**: 527–534.

37 Cheng L, Kelly RW, Thong KJ, Hume R, Baird DT. The effects of mifepristone (RU486) on prostaglandin dehydrogenase in decidual and chorionic tissue in early pregnancy. *Hum Reprod* 1993; **8**: 705–709.

38 Bygdeman M, Swahn ML. Progesterone receptor blockage: effect on uterine contractility and early pregnancy. *Contraception* 1985; **32**: 45–51.

39 Tang OS, Chan CC, Kan AS, Ho PC. A prospective randomized comparison of sublingual and oral misoprostol when combined with mifepristone for medical abortion at 12–20 weeks' gestation. *Hum Reprod* 2005; **20**: 3062–3066.

40 Thong KJ, Baird DT. Induction of second trimester abortion with mifepristone and gemeprost. *Br J Obstet Gynaecol* 1993; **100**: 758–761.

41 Webster D, Penney GC, Templeton A. A comparison of 600 and 200 mg mifepristone prior to second trimester abortion with the prostaglandin misoprostol. *Br J Obstet Gynaecol* 1996; **103**: 706–709.

42 el-Refaey H, Templeton A. Induction of abortion in the second trimester by a combination of misoprostol and mifepristone: a randomized comparison between two misoprostol regimens. *Hum Reprod* 1995; **10**: 475–478.

43 Bartley J, Baird DT. A randomised study of misoprostol and gemeprost in combination with mifepristone for induction of abortion in the second trimester of pregnancy. *BJOG* 2002; **109**: 1290–1294.

44 Heikinheimo O, Suhonen S, Haukkamaa M. One- and two-day mifepristone-misoprostol intervals are both effective in medical termination of second-trimester pregnancy. *Reprod Biomed Online* 2004; **8**: 236–239.

45 Nilas L, Glavind-Kristensen M, Vejborg T, Knudsen UB. One- or two-day mifepristone-misoprostol interval for second trimester abortion. *Acta Obstet Gynecol Scand* 2007; **86**: 1117–1121.

46 Gynuity Health Projects [Online]. New York: Gynuity Health Projects; 2007. Resources: medical abortion; 2007 [cited 2008 Aug 7]. Available from: URL:http://www.gynuity.org/pub_b.html

47 Kapp N, Borgatta L, Stubblefield PG, Vragovic O, Moreno N. Mifepristone in midtrimester medical abortion: a randomized controlled trial. *Obstet Gynecol* 2007; **110**: 1304–1310.

48 Goldberg AB, Greenberg MB, Darney PD. Misoprostol and pregnancy. *N Engl J Med* 2001; **344**: 38–47.

49 Ngai SW, Tang OS, Ho PC. Randomized comparison of vaginal (200 microg every 3 h) and oral (400 microg every 3 h) misoprostol when combined with mifepristone in termination of second trimester pregnancy. *Hum Reprod* 2000; **15**: 2205–2208.

50 Green J, Borgatta L, Sia M et al. Intervention rates for placental removal following induction abortion with misoprostol. *Contraception* 2007; **76**: 310–313.

51 Ho PC, Ngai SW, Liu KL, Wong GC, Lee SW. Vaginal misoprostol compared with oral misoprostol in termination of second-trimester pregnancy. *Obstet Gynecol* 1997; **90**: 735–738.

52 Ashok PW, Templeton A. Nonsurgical mid-trimester termination of pregnancy: a review of 500 consecutive cases. *Br J Obstet Gynaecol* 1999; **106**: 706–710.

53 Nigam A, Singh VK, Prakash A. Vaginal vs. oral misoprostol for mid-trimester abortion. *Int J Gynaecol Obstet* 2006; **92**: 270–271.

54 Tang OS, Lau WN, Chan CC, Ho PC. A prospective randomised comparison of sublingual and vaginal misoprostol in second trimester termination of pregnancy. *BJOG* 2004; **111**: 1001–1005.

55 Ho PC, Blumenthal PD, Gemzell-Danielsson K, Gómez Ponce de León R, Mittal S, Tang OS. Misoprostol for the termination of pregnancy with a live fetus at 13 to 26 weeks. *Int J Gynaecol Obstet* 2007; **99**: S178–S181.

56 Borgatta L, Chen AY, Vragovic O, Stubblefield PG, Magloire CA. A randomized clinical trial of the addition of laminaria to misoprostol and hypertonic saline for second-trimester induction abortion. *Contraception* 2005; **72**: 358–361.

57 Pongsatha S, Tongsong T. Intravaginal misoprostol for pregnancy termination. *Int J Gynaecol Obstet* 2004; **87**: 176–177.

58 Wong KS, Ngai CS, Wong AY, Tang LC, Ho PC. Vaginal misoprostol compared with vaginal gemeprost in termination of second trimester pregnancy. A randomized trial. *Contraception* 1998; **58**: 207–210.

59 Wong KS, Ngai CS, Yeo EL, Tang LC, Ho PC. A comparison of two regimens of intravaginal misoprostol for termination of second trimester pregnancy: a randomized comparative trial. *Hum Reprod* 2000; **15**: 709–712.

60 Kapp N, Todd CS, Yadgarova KT et al. A randomized comparison of misoprostol to intrauterine instillation of hypertonic saline plus a prostaglandin F2alpha analogue for second-trimester induction termination in Uzbekistan. *Contraception* 2007; **76**: 461–466.

61 Bygdeman M. Comparison of prostaglandin and hypertonic saline for termination of pregnancy. *Obstet Gynecol* 1978; **52**: 424–429.

62 Karim SM, Ratnam SS. Termination of abnormal intrauterine pregnancies with intramuscular administration of dihomo 15 methyl prostaglandin F2 alpha. *Br J Obstet Gynaecol* 1976; **83**: 885–889.

63 Lalitkumar S, Bygdeman M, Gemzell-Danielsson K. Mid-trimester induced abortion: a review. *Human Reprod Update* 2007; **13**: 37–52.

64 Peyron R, Aubény E, Targosz V et al. Early termination of pregnancy with mifepristone (RU 486) and the orally active prostaglandin misoprostol. *N Engl J Med* 1993; **328**: 1509–1513.

65 Ulmann A, Silvestre L, Chemama L et al. Medical termination of early pregnancy with mifepristone (RU 486) followed by a prostaglandin analogue. Study in 16,369 women. *Acta Obstet Gynecol Scand* 1992; **71**: 278–283.

66 Andersen LF, Poulsen HK, Sørensen SS, Christensen BM, Sponland G, Skjeldestad FE. Termination of second trimester pregnancy with gemeprost vaginal pessaries and intra-amniotic PGF2 alpha. A comparative study. *Eur J Obstet Gynecol Reprod Biol* 1989; **31**: 1–7.

67 Cameron IT, Baird DT. The use of 16,16-dimethyl-trans delta 2 prostaglandin E_1 methyl ester (gemeprost) vaginal pessaries for the termination of pregnancy in the early second trimester. A comparison with extra-amniotic prostaglandin E_2. *Br J Obstet Gynaecol* 1984; **91**: 1136–1140.

68 Makhlouf AM, Al-Hussaini TK, Habib DM, Makarem MH. Second-trimester pregnancy termination: comparison of three different methods. *J Obstet Gynaecol* 2003; **23**: 407–411.

69 Su LL, Biswas A, Choolani M, Kalaichelvan V, Singh K. A prospective, randomized comparison of vaginal misoprostol versus intra-amniotic prostaglandins for midtrimester termination of pregnancy. *Am J Obstet Gynecol* 2005; **193**: 1410–1414.

70 Nor Azlin MI, Abdullah HS, Zainul Rashid MR, Jamil MA. Misoprostol (alone) in second trimester terminations of pregnancy: as effective as Gemeprost? *J Obstet Gynaecol* 2006; **26**: 546–549.

71 Nuutila M, Toivonen J, Ylikorkala O, Halmesmäki E. A comparison between two doses of intravaginal misoprostol and gemeprost for induction of second-trimester abortion. *Obstet Gynecol* 1997; **90**: 896–900.

72 Dodd JM, Crowther CA. Misoprostol versus cervagem for the induction of labour to terminate pregnancy in the second and third trimester: a systematic review. *Eur J Obstet Gynecol Reprod Biol* 2006; **125**: 3–8.

73 Neilson JP, Hickey M, Vasquez J. Medical treatment for early fetal death (less than 24 weeks). *Cochrane Database Syst Rev* 2006; **3**: CD002253.

74 Gustavii B. Studies on accidental intravascular injection in extra-amniotic saline induced abortion and a method for reducing this risk. *J Reprod Med* 1972; **8**: 70–74.

75 Toppozada M, Ismail AA. Intrauterine administration of drugs for termination of pregnancy in the second trimester. *Baillieres Clin Obstet Gynaecol* 1990; **4**: 327–349.

76 Ingemanson CA. Legal abortion by extra-amniotic instillation of Rivanol in combination with rubber catheter insertion into the uterus after the twelfth week of pregnancy. *Am J Obstet Gynecol* 1973; **115**: 211–215.

77 Berg C, Ludwig M, Sturm N, Diedrich K, Gembruch U, Geipel A. Intra-amniotic ethacridine lactate instillation versus vaginal PGE1 in second trimester termination of pregnancy. *Eur J Obstet Gynecol Reprod Biol* 2006; **126**: 193–196.

78 Gardó S, Nagy M. Induction of second trimester abortion by intra-amniotic instillation of Rivanol (ethacridine) combined with oxytocin infusion. *Arch Gynecol Obstet* 1990; **247**: 39–41.

79 Tien KH. Intra-amniotic injection of ethacridine for second-trimester induction of labor. *Obstet Gynecol* 1983; **61**: 733–736.

80 Allahbadia G. Comparative study of midtrimester termination of pregnancy using hypertonic saline, ethacridine lactate, prostaglandin analogue, and iodine-saline. *J Indian Med Assoc* 1992; **90**: 237–239.

81 Herabutya Y, O-Prasertsawat P. Mid-trimester abortion using hypertonic saline or prostaglandin E2 gel: an analysis of efficacy and complications. *J Med Assoc Thai* 1994; **77**: 148–152.

82 Binkin NJ, Schulz KF, Grimes DA, Cates W Jr. Urea-prostaglandin versus hypertonic saline for instillation abortion. *Am J Obstet Gynecol* 1983; **146**: 947–952.

83 Nuthalapaty FS, Ramsey PS, Biggio JR, Owen J. High-dose vaginal misoprostol versus concentrated oxytocin plus low-dose vaginal misoprostol for midtrimester labor induction: a randomized trial. *Am J Obstet Gynecol* 2005; **193**: 1065–1070.

84 Winkler CL, Gray SE, Hauth JC, Owen J, Tucker JM. Mid-second-trimester labor induction: concentrated oxytocin compared with prostaglandin E2 vaginal suppositories. *Obstet Gynecol* 1991; **77**: 297–300.

85 Abramovici H, Bornstein J, Ben-David Y, Yishai D, Rofe A, Atad J. Double-balloon instillation device for second-trimester abortion. Outcome in 340 consecutive cases. *J Reprod Med* 1995; **40**: 56–62.

86 Toppozada MK, Shaala SA, Anwar MY, Haiba NA, Abdrabbo S, el-Absy HM. Termination of pregnancy with fetal death in

the second and third trimesters—the double balloon versus extra-amniotic prostaglandin. *Int J Gynaecol Obstet* 1994; **45**: 269–273.

87 Drey EA, Thomas LJ, Benowitz NL, Goldschlager N, Darney PD. Safety of intra-amniotic digoxin administration before late second-trimester abortion by dilation and evacuation. *Am J Obstet Gynecol* 2000; **182**: 1063–1066.

88 Isada NB, Pryde PG, Johnson MP, Hallak M, Blessed WB, Evans MI. Fetal intracardiac potassium chloride injection to avoid the hopeless resuscitation of an abnormal abortus: 1. Clinical issues. *Obstet Gynecol* 1992; **80**: 296–299.

89 Hern WM, Zen C, Ferguson KA, Hart FV, Haseman MV. Outpatient abortion for fetal anomaly and fetal death from 15–34 menstrual weeks' gestation: techniques and clinical management. *Obstet Gynecol* 1993; **81**: 301–306.

90 Elimian A, Verma U, Tejani N. Effect of causing fetal cardiac asystole on second-trimester abortion. *Obstet Gynecol* 1999; **94**: 139–141.

91 Atlas RO, Lemus J, Reed J III, Atkins D, Alger LS. Second trimester abortion using prostaglandin E2 suppositories with or without intracervical Laminaria japonica: a randomized study. *Obstet Gynecol* 1998; **92**: 398–402.

92 Blumenthal PD. Prospective comparison of Dilapan and laminaria for pretreatment of the cervix in second-trimester induction abortion. *Obstet Gynecol* 1988; **72**: 243–246.

93 Strauss JH, Wilson M, Caldwell D, Otterson W, Martin AO. Laminaria use in midtrimester abortions induced by intra-amniotic prostaglandin F2alpha with urea and intravenous oxytocin. *Am J Obstet Gynecol* 1979; **134**: 260–264.

94 Karim SM, Ratnam SS, Lim AL, Yeo KC, Choo HT. Termination of second trimester pregnancy with laminaria and intramuscular 16 phenoxy-omega-17, 18, 19, 20 tetranor PGE2 methylsulfonylamide (sulprostone)–A randomized study. *Prostaglandins* 1982; **23**: 257–263.

95 Papageorgiou I, Minaretzis D, Tsionou C, Michalas S. Late midtrimester medical pregnancy terminations: three different procedures with prostaglandin F2 alpha and laminaria tents. *Prostaglandins* 1991; **41**: 487–493.

96 Stubblefield PG, Naftolin F, Frigoletto F, Ryan KJ. Laminaria augmentation of intra-amniotic PGF2 for midtrimester pregnancy termination. *Prostaglandins* 1975; **10**: 413–422.

97 Surrago EJ, Robins J. Mid-trimester pregnancy termination by intravaginal administration of prostaglandin E2. *Contraception* 1982; **26**: 285–294.

98 Jain JK, Mishell DR Jr. A comparison of misoprostol with and without laminaria tents for induction of second-trimester abortion. *Am J Obstet Gynecol* 1996; **175**: 173–177.

99 Ho PC, Tsang SS, Ma HK. Reducing the induction to abortion interval in termination of second trimester pregnancies: a comparison of mifepristone with laminaria tent. *Br J Obstet Gynaecol* 1995; **102**: 648–651.

100 Prairie BA, Lauria MR, Kapp N, MacKenzie T, Baker ER, George KE. Mifepristone versus laminaria: a randomized controlled trial of cervical ripening in midtrimester termination. *Contraception* 2007; **76**: 383–388.

101 Thong KJ, Baird DT. A study of gemeprost alone, dilapan or mifepristone in combination with gemeprost for the termination of second trimester pregnancy. *Contraception* 1992; **46**: 11–17.

102 Schubert W, Cullberg G. Second trimester abortion by Rivanol with or without cervical dilatators. A randomized comparison. *Acta Obstet Gynecol Scand* 1987; **66**: 549–550.

103 Berger GS, Kerenyi TD. Analysis of retained placenta associated with saline abortion: clinical considerations. *Am J Obstet Gynecol* 1974; **120**: 484–488.

104 Kirz DS, Haag MK. Management of the third stage of labor in pregnancies terminated by prostaglandin E2. *Am J Obstet Gynecol* 1989; **160**: 412–414.

105 Hamoda H, Ashok PW, Flett GM, Templeton A. A randomized trial of mifepristone in combination with misoprostol administered sublingually or vaginally for medical abortion at 13–20 weeks' gestation. *Hum Reprod* 2005; **20**: 2348–2354.

106 Honkanen H, Piaggio G, Hertzen H et al. WHO multinational study of three misoprostol regimens after mifepristone for early medical abortion. II: Side effects and women's perceptions. *BJOG* 2004; **111**: 715–725.

107 Spitz IM, Bardin CW, Benton L, Robbins A. Early pregnancy termination with mifepristone and misoprostol in the United States. *N Engl J Med* 1998; **338**: 1241–1247.

108 Fiala C, Swahn ML, Stephansson O, Gemzell-Danielsson K. The effect of nonsteroidal antiinflammatory drugs on medical abortion with mifepristone and misoprostol at 13–22 weeks' gestation. *Hum Reprod* 2005; **20**: 3072–3077.

109 Creinin MD, Shulman T. Effect of nonsteroidal antiinflammatory drugs on the action of misoprostol in a regimen for early abortion. *Contraception* 1997; **56**: 165–168.

110 Li CF, Wong CY, Chan CP, Ho PC. A study of co-treatment of nonsteroidal antiinflammatory drugs (NSAIDs) with misoprostol for cervical priming before suction termination of first trimester pregnancy. *Contraception* 2003; **67**: 101–105.

111 Westhoff C, Dasmahapatra R, Winikoff B, Clarke S. Predictors of analgesia use during supervised medical abortion. *Contraception* 2000; **61**: 225–229.

112 Hamoda H, Ashok PW, Flett GM, Templeton A. Analgesia requirements and predictors of analgesia use for women undergoing medical abortion up to 22 weeks of gestation. *BJOG* 2004; **111**: 996–1000.

113 Wiebe E. Pain control in medical abortion. *Int J Gynaecol Obstet* 2001; **74**: 275–280.

114 Burkman RT, Atienza MF, King TM, Burnett LS. The management of midtrimester abortion failures by vaginal evacuation. *Obstet Gynecol* 1977; **49**: 233–236.

115 World Health Organization. *Report of a Technical Consultation on Birth Spacing*. World Health Organization, Geneva, 2005.

116 Boyd EF Jr, Halmstrom EG. Ovulation following therapeutic abortion. *Am J Obstet Gynecol* 1972; **113**: 469–473.

117 World Health Organization Department of Reproductive Health and Research & Johns Hopkins Bloomberg School of

Public Health Center for Communication Programs, INFO Project. *Family Planning: A Global Handbook for Providers*. CCP and WHO, Baltimore and Geneva, 2007.

118 Grimes D, Schulz K, Stanwood N. Immediate postabortal insertion of intrauterine devices. *Cochrane Database Syst Rev* 2004; **4**: CD001777.

119 Nyboe Andersen A, Damm P, Tabor A, Pedersen IM, Harring M. Prevention of breast pain and milk secretion with bromocriptine after second-trimester abortion. *Acta Obstet Gynecol Scand* 1990; **69**: 238.

120 Talluri-Rao S, Baird TL. *Information and Training Guide for Medical Abortion Counseling*. Ipas, Chapel Hill, 2003.

13

CHAPTER 13
The challenging abortion

Lynn Borgatta MD, MPH, and Phillip G. Stubblefield, MD

LEARNING POINTS

- Vaginal anomalies and scarring may require additional procedures prior to successful uterine aspiration.
- In many instances, cervical stenosis can be overcome by surgical or pharmacological approaches.
- Key complications associated with extreme uterine flexion or uterine anomalies include perforation and failed attempted abortion.
- Uterine leiomyomas may be managed by a number of individualized approaches.
- Identifying risk factors for a more difficult abortion procedure allows the provider to customize care and minimize complications.

Introduction

Although most abortion procedures are uncomplicated, some abortions present technical and management challenges. These challenges may result from the physical characteristics of the woman or the pregnancy or social or emotional circumstances. By identifying potentially difficult situations, providers can adapt the abortion procedure to minimize the risks of clinical complications, invasive or extirpative procedures, and/or medical or emotional sequelae.

Like other technical skills, clinicians learn abortion techniques by didactic teaching, observation, apprenticeship, study, and experience. Because most abortions are straightforward, novice providers typically perform numerous procedures before encountering a challenging situation. Knowing one's limits and when to seek advice are fundamental tenets of safe abortion care.

Sometimes the challenge is appreciated ahead of time (e.g., a woman with a known uterine duplication); more commonly, an unanticipated problem arises during a procedure. In general, these situations involve the inability to visualize or dilate the cervix, access the pregnancy, evacuate the uterus, or identify products of conception.

Experienced practitioners can handle most of these challenging situations with adequate planning, forethought, and improvisation. However, consultation or referral is occasionally necessary for optimal care of the woman. In this circumstance, the guiding principle should be to *refer, rather than refuse, care*. Simply informing a woman that she cannot obtain service at one location does not help her to select a more suitable site. Major delay increases the risks of the abortion procedure, because abortion-related morbidity rises with gestational age (Chapter 15).

This chapter describes infrequent but important challenges that abortion providers may encounter. We focus on surgical procedures in part because the complications of medical abortion, such as failed or incomplete abortion, are often treated surgically (Chapter 8). Some management approaches are not addressed in the scientific literature and derive from the personal experience of the authors or other expert providers.

Anatomically challenging abortions

Abnormalities of the vagina

Vaginal septae

Vaginal septae are either transverse or longitudinal. Transverse septae are rare, with a reported incidence of 1 in 30,000 to 1 in 84,000 women [1]. Nearly half are located in the upper third of the vagina where the constituent embryologic precursors of the upper and lower vagina meet [2], and they may be thin and elastic or thick and vascular. Pregnancy is only possible if the transverse septum is perforate or incomplete; however, the opening may be microscopic. Low, thin transverse septae can be incised transvaginally. Resection of thick transverse septae or those located high in the vagina requires special expertise, and in rare

Management of Unintended and Abnormal Pregnancy, 1st edition. By M Paul, ES Lichtenberg, L Borgatta, DA Grimes, PG Stubblefield, MD Creinin
 ISBN: 9781405176965.

instances necessitates an abdominoperineal approach and split-thickness skin grafts [3]. Longitudinal septae are vestiges of incomplete midline fusion of embryological uterine precursors and usually coexist with uterine anomalies, most commonly uterus didelphys (complete uterine duplication) [4]. The septum may extend a short distance from the cervix or run the length of the vagina to the introitus [3]. A longitudinal septum may remain undetected until examination. Because of the association with uterine duplication anomalies, ascertaining the anatomy of the cervix and uterus before beginning a surgical procedure is advisable. If a bimanual examination and gentle probing of the uterine cavity are not conclusive, conventional sonography usually suffices to identify major anomalies. Magnetic resonance imaging (MRI) is required in some cases [4,5].

If the septum allows introduction of a speculum and visualization of the cervix, the provider can usually perform a surgical abortion without modification in technique. If the cervix cannot be visualized, however, dilation or resection of the septum is necessary [2]. Medical abortion is an alternative in early pregnancy without division of the septum, but a small number of these women (typically $\leq 5\%$) will still require a surgical procedure for failed or incomplete abortion.

Longitudinal septae are divided vaginally using simple incision with suture ligation or electrocautery. If the longitudinal septum is in the lower vagina, local anesthesia should suffice, but intravenous sedation or general anesthesia may be indicated for septae that require manipulation high in the vagina. The provider should complete the surgical abortion at the same time, if possible.

Intact hymeneal orifice

Rarely, a woman requesting abortion may have an intact hymen with only a small fenestration. In this case, pregnancy presumably resulted from ejaculation at the introitus without vaginal penetration.

If the hymeneal orifice does not admit even the smallest (pediatric) speculum, dilation or incision of the hymen is necessary. A motivated woman, given instruction and encouragement, may accomplish sufficient manual or instrumental dilation (graduated mechanical dilators) in a week or two to allow speculum insertion. Sometimes, adequate anesthesia permits the provider to stretch the hymen without incision. Otherwise, hymenotomy will be necessary, a procedure that may require general anesthesia. In this case, the abortion should be performed at the same time, if possible.

Vaginal scarring

Vaginal and introital scarring may follow trauma, radiation, surgery, female genital cutting, skin disease, or other conditions. The scar tissue may be unresponsive to estrogen and less distensible than normal tissue. When the scarring is severe, medical abortion may be preferable to surgical abortion.

Patients who experience intolerable discomfort with speculum insertion will require sedation or general anesthesia for surgical abortion. Sometimes, a releasing incision of the introitus is necessary to complete the abortion. In contrast to normal labial and perineal skin, which generally heals very well despite constant exposure to vaginal and anal bacteria, the scarred skin may be far more calloused and avascular.

Female genital cutting/mutilation

Physicians working in certain countries or those caring for immigrant women may encounter patients who have undergone forms of female genital mutilation resulting in a tightly constricted vaginal opening [6]. It may be possible to insert a long narrow speculum (e.g., a Smith-Pedersen) to visualize the cervix and perform the abortion. In the most extreme form of female genital mutilation, infibulation, the labia have been sewn together in the midline, leaving only a small opening [7]. Clinicians can perform limited deinfibulation sufficient to allow for surgical abortion by separating the fused labia anterior to this small opening. Care must be taken to incise only the midline labial tissue to avoid injury to the urethral meatus and clitoris.

Abnormalities of the cervix

Cervical anomalies

Congenital anomalies of the cervix often accompany vaginal or uterine malformations but may exist in isolation. They range from complete atresia of the cervix (extremely rare) to complete duplication, as well as anatomic changes caused by intrauterine exposure to diethylstilbestrol (DES). Because use of DES began in the 1950s and was discontinued by 1970 in developed countries, many women who were exposed in utero are beyond their reproductive years. Women may still inadvertently be exposed to exogenous estrogen from either medications or diet, but DES-type severe anatomic distortion of the uterus from these exposures has not been reported.

The provider needs to evaluate medical and surgical abortion options in light of the particular anomaly. For instance, a hypoplastic cervix typical of DES exposure may be difficult to grasp with a tenaculum; in addition, the columnar epithelium is more vascular and may be friable. These factors might shift the optimum method toward a medical abortion. For surgical abortion, using an atraumatic tenaculum (e.g., a Bierer tenaculum) or placing one or two tenacula on the lateral cervix rather than on the cervical hood may help. These measures also apply to cases of iatrogenic cervical hypoplasia such as that resulting from extensive cold-knife conization, loop electrosurgical excision procedures (LEEP), or inadequately repaired cervical injury accompanying childbirth.

Cervical duplication can result in a double external os but a single canal, two separate canals within the matrix of one cervix, or two completely separate cervices. Having a single cervix and two functionally separate uterine cavities is possible. In such cases, the uterine anomaly may remain undetected until the provider fails to enter the uterine cavity containing the pregnancy, resulting in failed attempted abortion. Intraoperative ultrasound guidance can aid in completing the procedure in these circumstances [8].

Duplicate cervices are usually not symmetric. Typically, one cervix is larger than the other; and rather than being side by side, one can lie posterior to the other (Box A). The posterior cervical os is easy to miss, as it is usually smaller and often distorted.

Box A

A 21-year-old nulliparous woman at 7 weeks' gestation was referred to a family planning specialty clinic after her primary care physician (PCP) could not complete an aspiration abortion. The PCP performed dilation and aspiration but noted no products of conception on tissue examination. A persistent gestational sac was evident on postprocedure ultrasound. The patient refused the option of medical abortion. The specialist noted a normal-appearing cervix on speculum examination. She was able to pass the dilator through the external os easily, but met resistance at the internal os. Gentle probing with a small dilator, and then an os finder, was unsuccessful. Although ultrasound guidance was used during these maneuvers, the ultrasound technician had persistent problems visualizing the cervix. Just as the provider was about to abandon her attempts, she noted a dimple in the vaginal vault posterior to the cervix. She was able to pass a small dilator easily through the dimple and into the uterine cavity. Under continued ultrasound guidance, she enlarged the opening and evacuated the uterus expeditiously using a 7-mm cannula and manual vacuum aspiration. Unlike most duplication anomalies, the atretic cervical opening was the true passage into the uterus.

Contributed by Maureen Paul MD, MPH

When the cervix is small and misshapen, digital palpation may be the most efficient way to locate it initially. Techniques that create more exposure may help the provider visualize the os. Examples include using a sponge-stick, abdominal pressure on the fundus, and "walking" a tenaculum consecutively along the cervix until the os comes into view. If cervical distortion makes the os hard to see, gentle probing with a blunt dilator or cotton swab may locate it.

Despite the appearance of a tiny os, the cervical canal may be soft and patulous, easily admitting a small dilator such as a 15-mm Pratt. If not, the clinician can use a smaller dilator or probe to establish the direction and course of the cervical canal, followed by progressive mechanical dilation. Commercially available "os finders" of flexible plastic may be safer than metal dilators or lacrimal probes for this purpose (Appendix, Fig. A-7). If the direction of the canal is not obvious, abdominal ultrasound guidance may allow the provider to target the internal os visually and direct the dilator toward it. As always in such cases, gentle but firm traction on the cervix, with adequate pain control, is invaluable.

Several approaches are available if mechanical dilation is unusually difficult. Delaying the procedure by a week allows for more softening of the cervix. A more immediate option involves cervical preparation with osmotic dilators or misoprostol. A small laminaria tent can be placed and left overnight as long as minimal dilation is possible. Alternatively, cervical priming with 400 μg of misoprostol for 3 to 4 hours may suffice (Chapter 10). The same dose of misoprostol can be used overnight, allowing more time for effect, as long as the patient accepts the small possibility of an unscheduled expulsion of the pregnancy during the night. Mifepristone 200 mg orally given 24 to 48 hours before surgical abortion also results in cervical softening (Chapter 10). Finally, medical abortion is a consideration.

Cervical scarring and stenosis

Cervical scars may result from obstetrical trauma; cryotherapy; cautery; cervical biopsy, including cold-knife cone biopsy and electrosurgical excision; vaginal reconstructive surgery; radiation; or traumatic gynecological injuries. Reported rates of stenosis range from 2 to 15% after laser or electrosurgical excisions [9]. The scarring may be visible grossly or may not be evident until the clinician attempts dilation. The cervix can appear normal or be virtually absent (Box B).

Box B

A 35-year-old G_2P_0 woman with a history of a cervical LEEP procedure requested an abortion at 18 weeks' gestation. Following the LEEP, she had an early spontaneous abortion. Although the provider could palpate some cervical tissue on bimanual examination, no cervix was visible on speculum examination. A pinpoint dimple did not allow even a tiny dilator to pass. The patient consented to induction or hysterotomy (as a last resort) if D&E was infeasible. After intra-amniotic injection of digoxin 1.5 mg to induce fetal demise, the patient received a single dose of buccal misoprostol 400 μg. She had moderate cramping and a small amount of bleeding overnight. On pelvic examination the upper vagina was slightly ballooned, and blood was coming from the dimple seen the day before. A small clamp passed through the dimple into the cervical canal, which then dilated easily. The pregnancy was evacuated without difficulty using a 14-mm cannula and forceps.

Contributed by Lynn Borgatta, MD, MPH

The management of prior cervical injury is similar to the management of an anomalous cervix and includes assessment of the location and degree of the injury, ease of visualization, and the risks and benefits of each method of abortion. When the cervix is clearly identified but no dimple is apparent to pinpoint the external os, the problem may be stenosis or agglutination of the external cervical os. Often the rest of the canal is patent; if so, the clinician can attempt to open the stenotic external os mechanically using the following technique: Place two single-tooth tenacula, one on the anterior lip and one on the posterior lip of the cervix. Some providers prefer to use Allis or Bierer clamps

Box C Technical Note: Early Demised Pregnancies May Disappear

Once pregnancy growth has either stopped spontaneously or by means of pharmacologic agents, early pregnancies may wither. This process is similar to the spontaneous resorption occasionally seen with ectopic and 'vanishing' twin pregnancies.

with the choice suggested by the size and shape of the cervix (Appendix, Fig. A-6). With the cervix on traction, place the point of a closed hemostat against the central area of the cervix and spread laterally. Pretreating with misoprostol for 3 to 4 hours as described earlier may help. If the pregnancy is early, medical abortion can be offered as an alternative [10] (Box C).

Cervical lesions

The pelvic examination prior to abortion may reveal a cervical lesion such as a neoplasm of the cervix, inflammation, or recent trauma. Cervical intraepithelial lesions, including carcinoma *in situ*, do not interfere with the performance of abortion. A vascular friable lesion may be a carcinoma, and tenaculum placement or dilation can result in hemorrhage that is difficult to control. A suspicious cervical lesion warrants biopsy, and if feasible, delaying the procedure until the diagnosis is established. Treatment of the cancer by radical hysterectomy or radiation will end the pregnancy. Misoprostol has been used successfully to expel a dead fetus after radiation therapy for advanced cervical cancer [11].

Condyloma acuminata can involve the vulva extensively, but they do not usually prevent exposure of the cervical os. Occasionally a large vaginal or cervical condyloma requires excision to allow access to the cervix.

Acute herpes simplex vulvitis is severely painful, and women with acute outbreaks involving the perineum usually cannot tolerate speculum placement. They can be treated with an antiviral agent (acyclovir, valacyclovir) and rescheduled for the abortion in a week or so, after the lesions have resolved. Alternatively, the abortion can proceed using deep sedation or general anesthesia.

Cervical chlamydia or gonococcal infections [12–14] increase the risk of postabortal endometritis. Antibiotic treatment of the patient and her partner(s) is warranted. No randomized trials have compared outcomes in women treated concurrent with the abortion versus those who complete treatment before the procedure (Chapter 7). The role of bacterial vaginosis as a risk factor for postabortal infection is unclear.

Abnormalities of the uterus

Positional abnormalities: extreme flexion

Extreme degrees of flexion can make a surgical abortion difficult. The cervical canal may lie at a right angle to the uterine cavity when the uterus is very anteflexed or very retroflexed (Fig. 13.1). Bimanual pelvic examination is frequently superior to ultrasound in detecting this condition. With acute retroflexion, the cervix is often markedly anterior and recessed beneath the pubic symphysis. Rarely, a severely retroflexed uterus becomes incarcerated as the pregnancy enlarges, causing the vagina to elongate and resulting in a cervix that is almost cephalad to the uterus, seated high in the anterior fornix behind the pubic symphysis. Ultrasound may be necessary to locate the cervix [15]. Immobility of the uterine corpus or fundus because of surgical scarring, as sometimes occurs after cesarean sections, can cause or exacerbate extreme flexion.

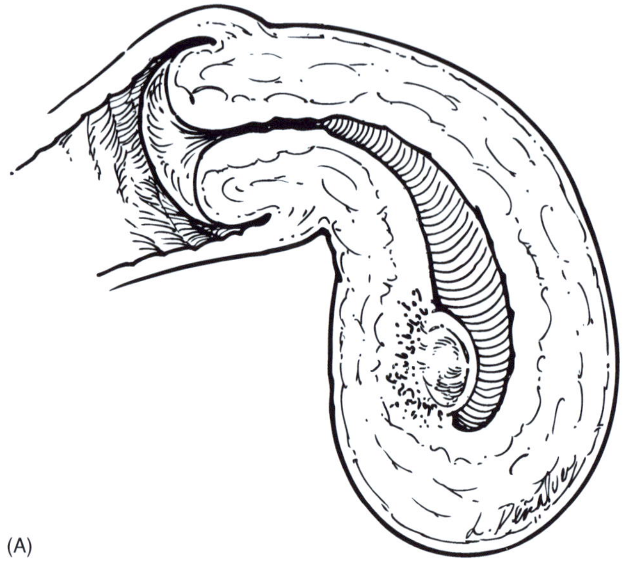

(A)

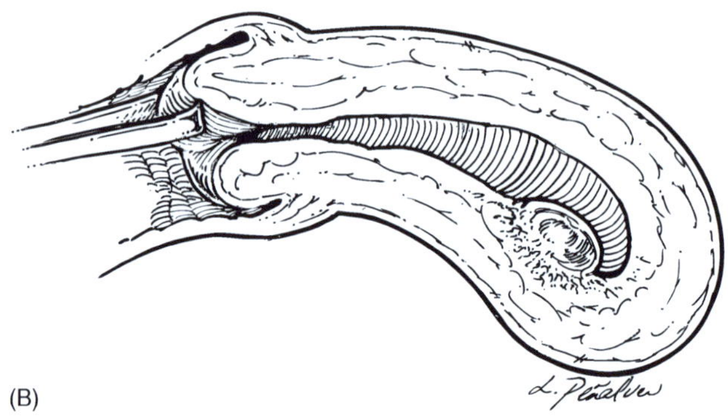

(B)

Figure 13.1 A retroflexed uterus is shown, but the comments also apply to a very anteflexed uterus. (A) The uterus is retroflexed, and the endometrial cavity forms a right angle with the cervical canal. The pregnancy is on the posterior wall and is impossible to reach in this position. (B) Traction on one (or both) cervical lips results in straightening of the angle between the cervix and the endometrial cavity, facilitating access to the pregnancy.

Key complications with extreme flexion include failed attempted abortion and perforation. In two case series of failed first-trimester surgical abortion reported by Fielding [16] and Gürkan Zorlu [17], marked anteversion or retroversion was present in 20 and 17% of patients, respectively. The risk of perforation increases when the degree of flexion is not recognized preoperatively. A likely site of perforation is

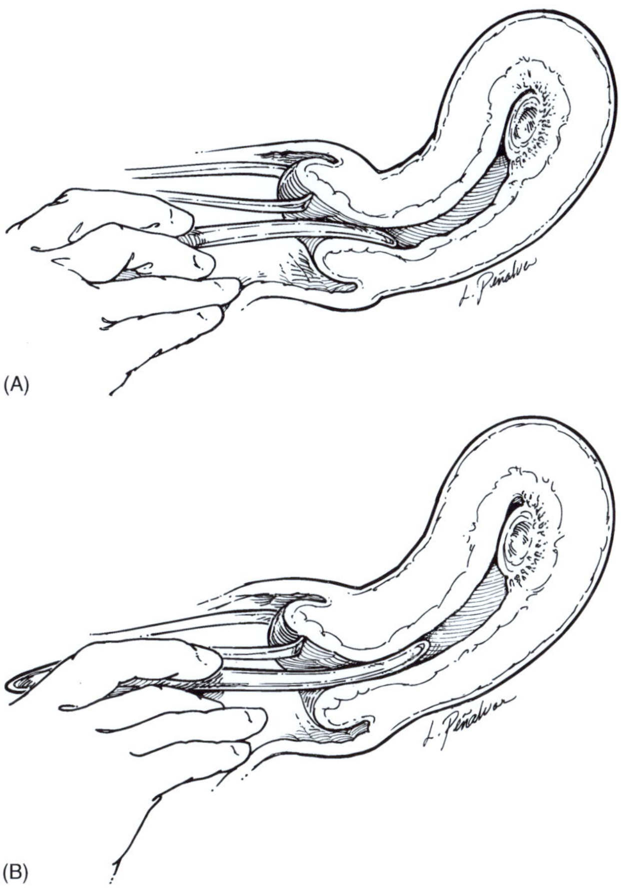

(A)

(B)

Figure 13.2 Rotating the dilator to negotiate the cervix. (A) An anteflexed uterus is shown. The dilator slips into the cervical canal, which is oriented posteriorly. (B) Once inside the cervical canal, the dilator is rotated gently to find the path of least resistance. Gentle but firm traction on the cervix is continued.

at the junction of the cervix and lower uterine segment or corpus. Because a perforation can be asymptomatic even in awake patients, the first sign of this complication may be lack of products of conception on postprocedure tissue examination.

Identifying the degree of flexion beforehand and straightening the cervico-uterine angle to the extent possible by gentle and continuous traction help to minimize complications. The provider may need to rotate and conjure the dilator in the canal in order to negotiate the cervix (Fig. 13.2). When difficulty is encountered in dilating or passing instruments through the canal, the following approaches may help:

- Use a type of speculum that permits more surgical exposure, such as a side-opening or weighted speculum. Paradoxically, a short speculum, such as a Moore-Graves model, may be useful because it does not push the cervix higher into the pelvis (Appendix, Fig. A-2);
- Alter patient positioning (e.g., Trendelenburg or reverse Trendelenburg and/or forward flexion of the trunk);
- Use ultrasound guidance; and/or
- Reshape a flexible cannula by inserting a metal uterine sound through the cannula and bending it to conform to the extreme angularity of the cervical canal and lower segment.

If in doubt about the location of the cannula, do not initiate suction until confirming correct placement by ultrasound.

If repeated attempts fail, the provider should stop the procedure and plan another course of action rather than risk perforation. Regardless of the direction of extreme flexion, treating the patient with misoprostol 400 μg for 3 to 4 hours may soften the cervix and produce uterine contractions that help to straighten the cervico-uterine angle. Other alternatives include using misoprostol with or without mifepristone overnight; referral; or waiting a week or two, because flexion usually decreases as the uterus enlarges.

Uterine anomalies

Congenital uterine malformations encompass a spectrum that ranges from partial or total agenesis to complete duplication (Fig. 13.3). Complex anomalies involving combinations of duplication and atresia are rare. Renal or ureteral anomalies frequently accompany abnormal uterine development, especially when the anomaly results in an asymmetrical configuration. A study by Jurkovic et al [5] of 1,046 women undergoing three-dimensional ultrasonography for a variety of gynecologic conditions revealed an overall rate of uterine malformations of 5%, including a 2% frequency of major anomalies. In addition, women with a history of in utero DES exposure may have a characteristic T-shaped uterus or irregular constrictions of the uterine cavity [18].

Transvaginal ultrasound is superior to transabdominal scanning in delineating uterine malformations, and its accuracy exceeds that of hysterosalpingogram for some anomalies [19]. Although advanced radiographic modalities are seldom needed for purposes of surgical abortion, MRI or three-dimensional sonography enables noninvasive and accurate diagnosis in complex cases [4,5].

A completely duplicated uterus (uterine didelphys) is usually evident on examination, as two cervices are present (Fig. 13.3). This symmetrical anomaly is unlikely to be associated with genitourinary anomalies. Ultrasound typically reveals an intrauterine pregnancy in one horn and decidual reaction in the other. A single pregnancy in one uterine horn does not usually require any change in abortion technique. Some providers aspirate the contralateral horn to avoid heavy bleeding when the decidualized endometrium sheds, but no data support this practice.

Some uterine anomalies increase the risk for failed surgical abortion [8,17,20,21] (Chapter 16). A failed abortion may, in fact, trigger the first suspicion of an anatomic abnormality. A septate uterus (Fig. 13.3), for example, may not be suspected until suction curettage is unsuccessful, because the uterus usually feels normal during bimanual palpation. Although transvaginal ultrasound may reveal the pregnancy and a separate endometrial stripe, the septum

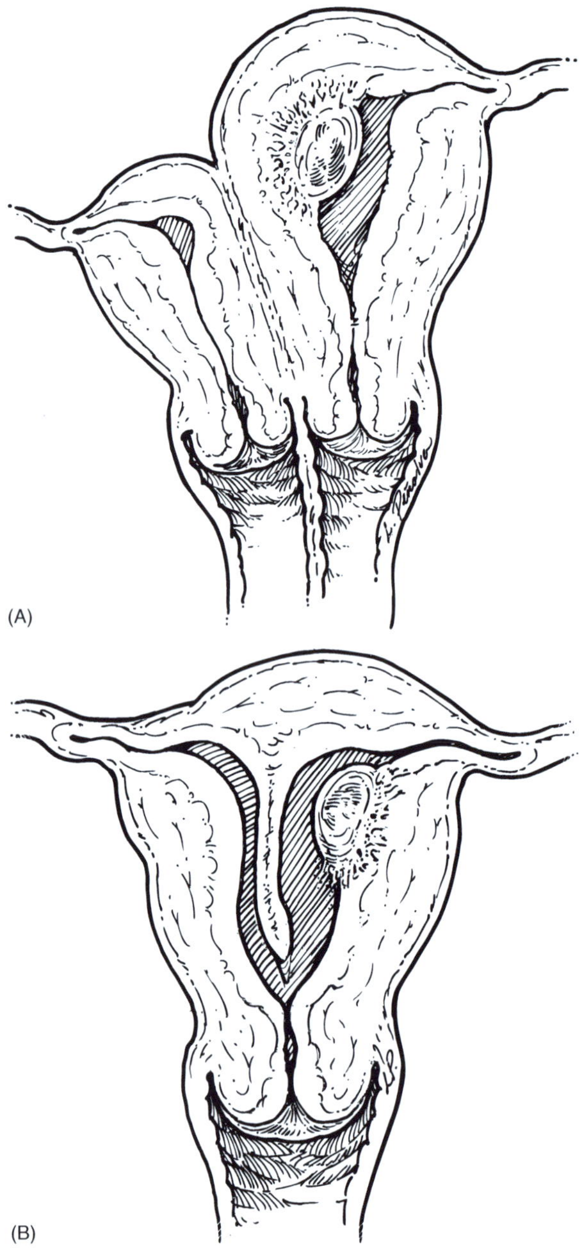

(A)

(B)

Figure 13.3 Uterine duplications: frontal view. There are many types of uterine duplication; some are associated with vaginal and urinary tract anomalies. Two examples are shown. (A) A completely duplicated uterus and cervix (uterus didelphys). Both uterine cavities are unicornuate. A longitudinal vaginal septum is also present. (B) A septate uterus with a single cervix. If a suction cannula is introduced into the left cavity only, the pregnancy will not be evacuated.

may be compressed by the gestational sac and easily missed. Intraoperatively, the provider sometimes senses the septum with a suction cannula or other instrument. Cervical dilation and evacuation of the pregnancy present challenges, as the fundus bearing the pregnancy is often located at an extremely lateralized angle. Ultrasound may help to guide the suction cannula into the gestational sac. Some cases require hysteroscopy to diagnose the condition and evacuate the pregnancy [20]. As with a double uterus, once the pregnancy is evacuated, aspirating the other side of the septum is unnecessary. Similar modifications of technique often apply to a bicornuate uterus; the gravid horn is also frequently extremely lateralized.

Anomalies that are known ahead of time may warrant modifications of technique. For instance, occurrence of pregnancy in a noncommunicating rudimentary uterine horn mandates laparotomy with excision of the horn if the patient is beyond the gestational age limit for medical abortion. Early pregnancies in a blind horn have been successfully aborted with methotrexate [10], but medical treatment failed in another case that subsequently required laparotomy [22]. Samuels [23] reported a case of rupture of an 18-week pregnancy in an unsuspected rudimentary horn during induction with misoprostol.

Uterine scarring

Sometimes after one or more cesarean sections, the uterus adheres to the anterior abdominal wall and the cervix becomes elongated and sequestered behind the pubic symphysis. Placing the patient in steep Trendelenburg position may facilitate visualization of the cervix. If the cervix can be palpated, an atraumatic tenaculum (Bierer or similar model) can be blindly advanced along the examiner's fingers to grasp the cervix and pull it into view after placement of a side-opening speculum. The extreme anterior position of the uterus may render evacuation difficult (Box D).

Box D

A 34-year-old primiparous woman requested abortion at 14 weeks. She had a history of one cesarean section. The day before the procedure, three laminaria were inserted. After removing the laminaria the next day, the provider had trouble grasping the cervix securely. It was small, high in the vault, and very anterior. Using a combination of Trendelenburg position and a long speculum, the clinician was able to grasp the cervix with a tenaculum. However, the cervix did not move at all when traction was applied. The cervix was well-dilated, allowing the provider to insert a #13 curved cannula. The fetus was removed, but the cannula could not reach the placenta. On ultrasound the placenta was high on the anterior wall out of reach of the cannula, curette, or forceps. The patient received misoprostol overnight, but she did not expel the placenta. In the operating room the following day, the provider still could not reach the placenta through the cervix. Laparotomy was performed. Dense adhesions from the uterus to the abdominal wall required extensive dissection. Once the uterus was freed up, a "mini-hysterotomy" was performed. After placing two stay sutures in the uterine fundus, the provider made a small puncture site to accommodate a 12-mm suction cannula and removed the placenta. The puncture site was closed with two sutures.

Contributed by Phillip Stubblefield, MD

Intracervical or intrauterine scarring (both of which are variations of Asherman syndrome) may also obscure access to the pregnancy (Box E). Most cases are mild in severity and respond well to mechanical dilation of affected areas. One report described termination of an intrauterine pregnancy only after hysteroscopic excision of scarring under laparoscopic guidance made uterine entry possible [24].

Box E

A 36-year-old G_2P_1 woman with a history of endometrial ablation for menorrhagia was referred for termination of pregnancy at 8 weeks' gestation after two failed attempted abortions. The initial attempt at an outpatient surgical clinic was abandoned when the provider had difficulty dilating the cervix. A subsequent medical abortion using mifepristone and misoprostol also failed, and the pregnancy remained viable. At the hospital, the patient received multidose methotrexate, which rendered the pregnancy nonviable, but the products did not expel even after two doses of misoprostol. She was brought to the operating room where she received general anesthesia. A band of scar tissue had to be "punctured" in order to gain access to the pregnancy. After this maneuver, the pregnancy was evacuated successfully with suction.

Contributed by Paula Bednarek, MD, MPH

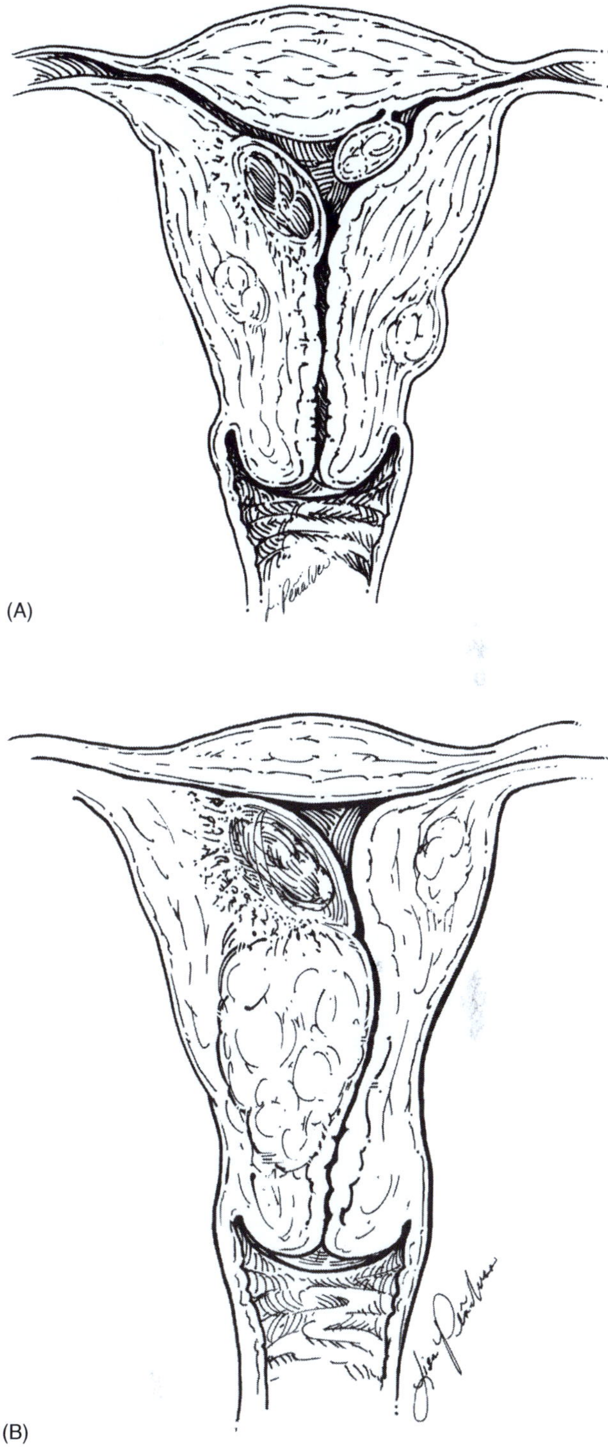

(A)

(B)

Figure 13.4 Leiomyomas can enlarge and distort the uterine cavity and obstruct the lower uterine segment or cervix. (A) Small intramural fibroids are usually not problematic. (B) A submucous fibroid may result in increased bleeding. (C) A large fundal fibroid does not distort the uterine cavity, and despite its size, may not change the procedure at all. (D) Lower segment intramural or submucous fibroids may obstruct or distort the uterine cavity. It may not be possible for instruments to negotiate the uterine cavity to reach the pregnancy.

Fibroids (Leiomyomas)

Uterine leiomyomas are the most common pelvic tumors in women. Uterine or cervical fibroids may enlarge and deform the uterine cavity and obstruct the lower uterine segment or cervix (Fig. 13.4). During physical examination, the enlarged fibroid uterus can be mistaken for a more advanced pregnancy. Ultrasound identifies the gestational age as well as the location, size, and number of leiomyoma and their relationship to the gestational sac. Isolated fundal fibroids usually do not impede the abortion procedure, although they can increase the amount of cramping and bleeding. Infrequently, large fibroids undergo sudden degeneration or infarction after evacuation, producing severe pain and symptoms indistinguishable from endometritis or colitis.

Obstruction or distortion of the cervix or uterine cavity by fibroids presents a technical challenge (Box F). If the cervix is noncompliant, the provider can use osmotic dilators instead of, or before, mechanical dilation or administer pharmacologic agents to soften the cervix. Relative "overdilation" of the cervix for the gestational age may facilitate manipulation of the cannula around individual fibroids, using ultrasound guidance if necessary. Some models of flexible cannulae are longer than rigid cannulae and may reach a gestational sac that sits high in a distorted fundus [25]. Providers have also improvised devices using other tubes, such as a large-bore nasogastric tube (for additional length) or an endotracheal tube with or without a stylet (for additional stiffness and maneuverability). Telescoping a flexible cannula inside the barrel of a rigid cannula creates a makeshift instrument of considerable length and efficiency. When a large submucous fibroid prevents the cannula from reaching the pregnancy, a curved polyp or extracting (e.g.,

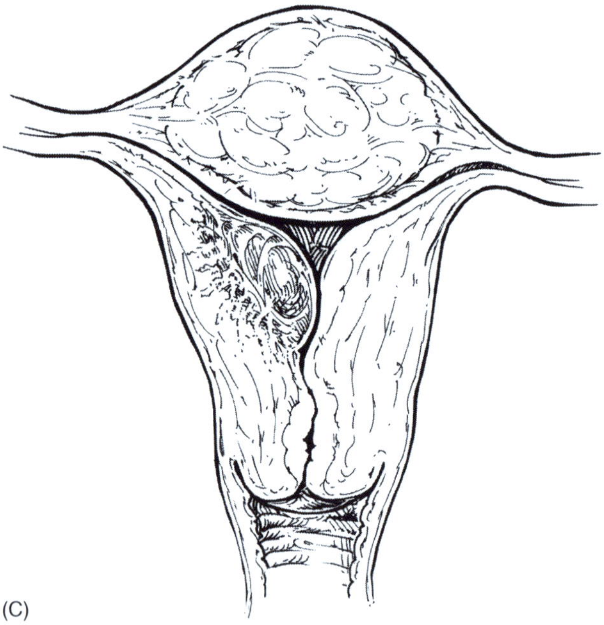

(C)

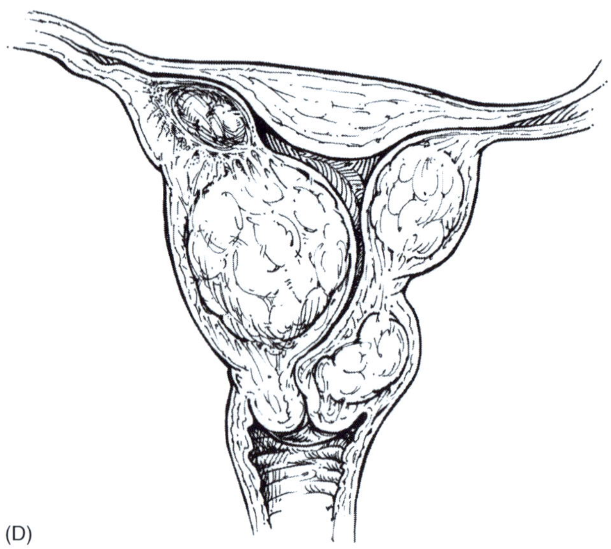

(D)

Figure 13.4 *(Continued)*

Van Lith) forceps may work. Successful medical abortions using methotrexate or mifepristone regimens have also been reported when massive leiomyomas render small gestational sacs inaccessible to surgical evacuation [10,26–28]. Uncommonly, the provider may accidentally extract a submucous fibroid during aspiration or instrumental tissue extraction. Although disconcerting and momentarily puzzling, this event rarely results in heavy or uncontrollable bleeding.

Fetal abnormalities

Therapeutic abortion for fetal abnormalities seldom necessitates a change in abortion technique. Multiple gestation itself, by increasing the size of the uterus and the placental mass relative to a singleton pregnancy, may result in more atony and bleeding. Because evacuation may require more time and manipulation, adequate pain control is important.

Conjoined twins in the second trimester can be difficult to remove by dilation and evacuation (D&E). Measures to facilitate evacuation include serial laminaria treatments over 2 or more days and induction of fetal demise over 12 to 24 hours to soften fetal cortical bone and joints. Because of the increase in tissue mass, conjoined twins may not be easy to abort by labor induction methods either.

Pronounced hydrocephaly (including hydranencephaly) may complicate induction or surgical abortion because of the need for greater dilation. If fetal death occurs before abortion, the fetal cranium begins to soften within 12 to 24 hours and may pass more easily. Alternatively, the provider can aspirate the central nervous system fluid by ultrasound-guided transabdominal or transvaginal needle puncture. During surgical abortion, the provider can collapse the cranium bluntly or by puncture with a needle, trocar, or scissors if necessary (Chapters 11 and 20).

Polyhydramnios sometimes accompanies fetal anomalies and is a concern in the second trimester. Sudden decompression of a very large uterus increases the risk of uterine atony. In cases of severe polyhydramnios, transabdominal or transvaginal amniocentesis allows for controlled removal of the fluid prior to abortion.

Box F

A 38-year-old multiparous woman requested abortion. She had a fibroid uterus enlarged to 28 weeks' size with a 12-week pregnancy at the fundus, which was palpable well above the umbilicus. We discussed medical treatment, hysterotomy, and hysterectomy. The patient wanted to try to expel the pregnancy, if possible. She did not intend to have any more children. Under ultrasound guidance, the fetal thorax was injected with potassium chloride, which caused cessation of fetal cardiac activity. Demise was confirmed by ultrasound the following day. The patient was given a single dose of vaginal misoprostol. She had some light bleeding over the next few days but did not pass the pregnancy. Five days later, she started to bleed heavily and decided to proceed with hysterectomy rather than hysterotomy. At hysterectomy, multiple large leiomyomas were noted. The pregnancy was in the fundus about 2 cm from the serosal surface, surrounded by fibroids, and completely detached (abrupted) from the uterine wall. Although a channel from the pregnancy to the cervical os was apparent, the pregnancy was still 15 to 20 cm from the cervix. The patient's surgery was uncomplicated, and she did well postoperatively. Given the location of the pregnancy in a uterus distorted by large fibroids, it is unclear whether she would have expelled the pregnancy given more time. Heavy bleeding from the abruption warranted prompt intervention. The patient was well prepared for a hysterectomy and was satisfied with her care.

Contributed by Sacheen Carr-Ellis, MD, MPH

The obese woman

Currently, almost 40% of women in the USA are overweight and 33% are obese (body mass index ≥ 30) [29]. Obesity increases the risks of pregnancy, surgery, and anesthesia. Following ultrasound examination and prior to any cervical ripening, an experienced provider and airway manager should assess the feasibility of performing the procedure in the proposed facility (Chapter 8). Some considerations include surgical and airway management experience, the availability of specialized surgical instruments and equipment, and proximity to the nearest tertiary hospital. In contrast, medical abortion has not been shown to carry additional risks for obese women when compared to women of normal weight [30]. Even so, providers must consider the small possibility of the need for vacuum aspiration in the event of heavy bleeding or failed abortion.

Exposure to the cervix can represent a key challenge in obese women. In some obese women the cervix is close to the introitus, but others (particularly those with prior uterine incisions) have a very recessed cervix than can be identified only by palpation. Moreover, protruding lateral vaginal walls sometimes obscure visualization of the cervix.

Numerous approaches are available in these circumstances, including use of specialized instruments. An elongated bivalve speculum facilitates access to the cervix, but it also decreases the mobility of the uterus during the procedure. Alternatives include using a specially designed, foreshortened Klopfer speculum (Appendix, Fig. A-3) or having assistants hold two Sims specula. One or two assistants can hold the thighs and/or labia apart to facilitate speculum placement. Because increased intra-abdominal pressure can push out the speculum, an assistant may need to hold the speculum in place, making adequate pain control essential. If protruding vaginal walls compromise visualization, the clinician can place a condom or finger cut from an examining glove over the speculum to create a tube or use a retracting vaginal speculum or a self-retaining vaginal wall retractor (Appendix, Fig. A-5). Other maneuvers include facilitating descent of the cervix by asking the patient to cough or having an assistant apply fundal pressure. If all else fails, identifying the cervix on bimanual exam and guiding an atraumatic tenaculum to grasp the cervix may work.

Even with the cervix visualized and placed on tension with a tenaculum, standard instruments may not be long enough to reach the uterine fundus during evacuation. Flexible vacuum cannulae are longer than standard rigid cannulae. Extension tubes also can be purchased. In the midtrimester, longer extracting forceps are available, including a 15-inch version of the Sopher forceps specifically designed with the obese patient in mind (Appendix, Fig. A-11).

Trendelenburg positioning, as steep as the patient can tolerate without respiratory discomfort, is helpful. A patient may tolerate Trendelenburg position better by allowing some forward flexion of her trunk. In some difficult cases, the provider can consider asking the patient to remove her legs from the stirrups, flex her widely-separated thighs onto her abdomen and bear down, much as the McRoberts maneuver is used for difficult obstetric deliveries. Vaginal ultrasound usually is both feasible and helpful for obese women, as virtually no fat tissue is deposited in the vaginal walls and vault. Abdominal ultrasound, if needed for intraoperative guidance, may provide adequate albeit suboptimal imaging. An assistant may need to elevate the patient's panniculus so that the sonographer can place the ultrasound transducer just above the pubic symphysis where the abdominal wall is thinnest.

The woman with physical handicaps

Some physical handicaps require modification of surgical abortion technique. Women with neuromuscular disease or paraparesis (e.g., muscular dystrophy) may find the lithotomy position difficult to maintain. Limited mobility of the hips or knees may preclude the lithotomy position as well. This problem can occur in women with congenital skeletal anomalies (e.g., dwarfism), contractures, traumatic injuries, and conditions such as rheumatoid arthritis or sickle cell disease. Having assistants hold the patient's legs may be more comfortable than usual knee or foot stirrups. Elevation of the legs may permit access to the cervix with only minimal abduction of the thighs. If spasm or discomfort occurs, the assistant can move the leg without necessarily disrupting the procedure. A side-lying (Sims) position is another alternative.

General anesthesia may be advantageous for some women with neuromuscular disease; however, it may be less safe if the woman has limited neck mobility, greater risk of aspiration, or other anesthesia risk factors. Because sleep anesthesia does not allow the woman to express discomfort if a stressful or potentially injurious position occurs, placing the patient in a comfortable position prior to induction of deep sedation or general anesthesia is important.

Technical problems

Difficult removal of osmotic dilating devices

Laminaria and Dilapan™ soften as they swell and are usually constricted by the internal os. They may resist removal if the innermost portion of the dilator swells above the internal cervical os ("dumbbelling," Fig. 13.5). This problem is less likely to occur if the clinician inserts multiple smaller dilating devices rather than a single tent. Removing the smallest device first usually makes room for the others (Chapter 11).

At times the cervix is so resistant that none of the dilators can be removed. This problem can occur with or without dumbbelling. Several options for management exist:

- Treat the patient with one or more doses of misoprostol (e.g., 400 μg vaginally or buccally every 4 hours) until the cervix begins to soften and expand.

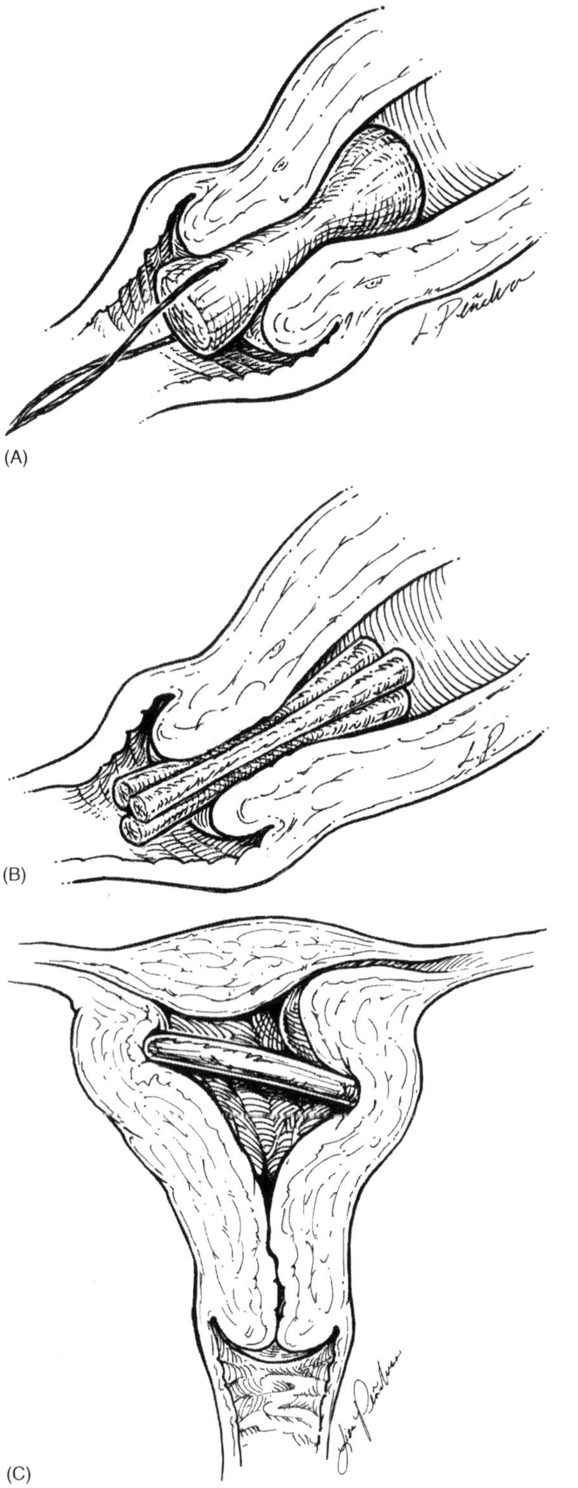

Figure 13.5 Osmotic dilator problems. (A) A single large osmotic dilator is "dumbbelled" by the stiff internal os. Removal of this dilator may be difficult. (B) Several small dilators achieve the same diameter as one large dilator. Each is dumbbelled; but because they are smaller, removing one may be possible, thereby freeing the others. (C) A dilator that has been pushed in the uterine cavity may lodge transversely, making removal difficult.

- Place paracervical anesthesia for patient comfort, apply a tenaculum to the cervix with one blade as far up the cervical canal as possible, and attempt to pass a small Pratt dilator alongside the osmotic dilators. Exercise great caution to avoid perforation.
- If the osmotic dilators have been in place for only a few hours, postpone the procedure until the next day to allow for more softening and dilation of the cervix, when misoprostol may also be given.

Sometimes one or several dilating devices are not visible at the external os at the time of removal because of displacement into the cervical canal or uterine cavity (Fig. 13.5). Migration or incorrect placement of a dilator may result in inadequate cervical dilation. The clinician can attempt to remove a displaced dilator by grasping the string, but the string may break if the dilator is tightly wedged in the internal os. Cervical ripening with misoprostol may help in this circumstance. A dilator that has migrated into the uterine cavity may come out during suctioning; a 13-mm suction cannula usually suffices to remove an entire device, but the requisite degree of mechanical dilation can be difficult to achieve if the cervix is stiff. The provider also can try using forceps to retrieve the device under ultrasound guidance; a large dilator may need to be crushed with a strong extracting clamp (e.g., a Sopher forceps) prior to removal. Use of the smallest grasping forceps usually requires a minimum of 12 mm of cervical dilation. Immediate removal of the device is not paramount and may be delayed for 24 to 48 hours rather than risk uterine injury.

Sometimes laminaria or Dilapan™ devices fracture after persistent efforts at removal with forceps, with the fragments coming to lie in the uterine cavity. Fracture is less likely with the retooled Dilapan-S™ device because the polymer is oriented longitudinally (Chapter 11). If the cervix is adequately dilated, the provider can complete the abortion as usual and remove the fragments through the vacuum cannula or with a thin retrieval clamp. Even with the use of ultrasound, however, certifying that all fragments have been removed may prove difficult. Large fragments of retained osmotic dilators are usually visible under ultrasound as homogeneous, geometric masses of medium echogenicity, but smaller fragments may not be apparent. Occasionally, fragments of laminaria remain in the uterine cavity long after the abortion and require removal via hysteroscopy [31]. Hysterography or sonohysterography can be helpful in locating small fragments [32].

Fracture of equipment, such as plastic suction cannulae, is extremely rare [33]. Extraction of such pieces should follow the same principles as extraction of osmotic dilators.

Completion of a procedure with known or suspected uterine injury

When an injury to the uterus or cervix is suspected, the provider must consider whether to proceed with the abortion. This decision depends on many factors such as the nature of the injury, the skill of the clinician, the available equipment, and the patient's wishes and concerns. Less experienced operators may need to obtain assistance or refer the woman to a provider with more expertise. In most cases, the remaining pregnancy tissue does not cause acute vaginal bleeding, allowing transport to another site for completion if necessary. Completion in a timely manner is beneficial if perforation is known or highly suspect, because the retained products can become a nidus of infection that has a portal (via the perforation) into the abdominal cavity, raising the prospect of peritonitis.

False passage

The provider may create a false passage with instruments or devices that burrow into the matrix of the cervix instead of following the true cervical canal (Fig. 13.6). One way to recognize this condition is by a change in consistency of the cervix: it may feel tough and dry rather than the smooth,

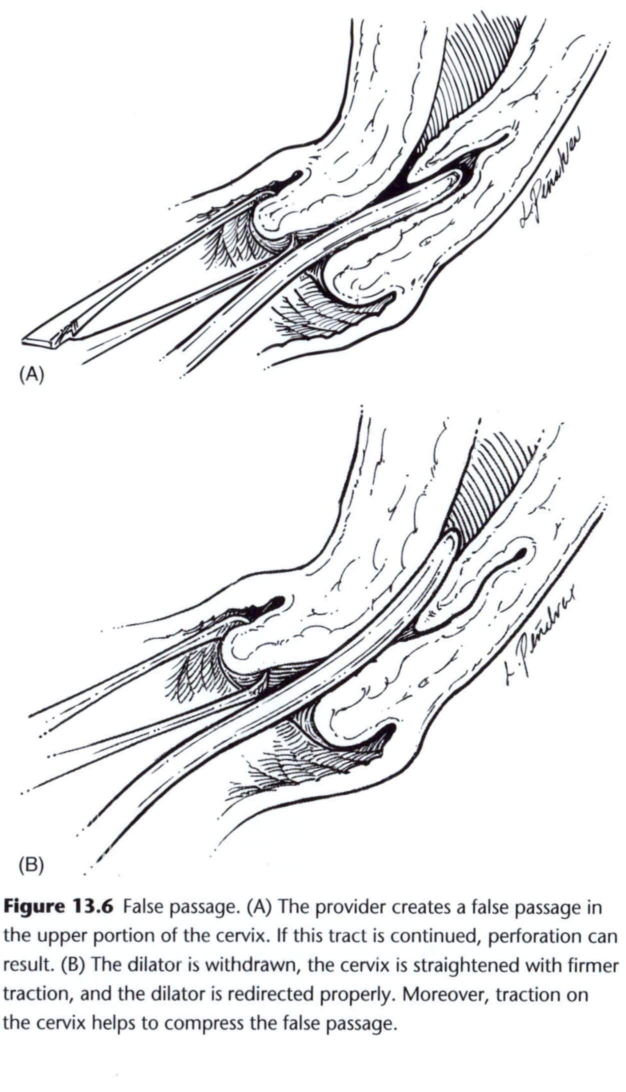

Figure 13.6 False passage. (A) The provider creates a false passage in the upper portion of the cervix. If this tract is continued, perforation can result. (B) The dilator is withdrawn, the cervix is straightened with firmer traction, and the dilator is redirected properly. Moreover, traction on the cervix helps to compress the false passage.

moist texture typical of the mucus-laden endocervical canal. Also common is the sensation of a dead-end after the dilator advances only 2 to 3 centimeters. At times, the surgeon may feel a shearing or shredding sensation as instruments pass through cervical stroma or myometrium. A tract into the cervix that does not perforate into other organs or structures will most likely heal without incident and often does not interfere with completion of the abortion.

If the provider suspects a false passage, repeating the pelvic examination and performing ultrasound help to reassess the relationship of the cervix to the uterine corpus before proceeding. When completing the procedure, make sure that the tenaculum is well applied and that analgesia is adequate. Try to assess where the tract deviated from the cervical canal. A frequent location is anterior, in the upper half of the cervix. Straighten the cervix as much as possible using slow, firm but gentle traction. This maneuver tends to compress a false channel in the cervical tissue (Fig. 13.6). Paradoxically, a slightly larger dilator or an instrument with a blunter tip (e.g., a uterine sound or small Hegar dilator) may slip through the canal more easily. A small, flexible, lubricated suction cannula may also pass. The cervical canal may have a corkscrew or tortuous route that requires a soft touch with the mechanical dilator or aspiration device to allow it to wind through the natural course of the canal. Ultrasound guidance may help. Once the direction and shape of the canal are clear, expanding the canal with larger dilators as indicated is usually feasible. Occasionally the clinician will be forced to evacuate the cavity with a narrower-than-customary cannula.

In managing a false passage, the following points are important:

- Do not assume that an osmotic dilating device will necessarily solve the problem. The device, being firm and rigid, can perforate the cervix as can a mechanical dilator or sound.
- Do not assume that a small dilator is the safest. The smallest dilator is also the sharpest, and sometimes a larger diameter device makes it easier to sense the correct direction of the canal.
- Do not assume that the ability to pass larger dilators assures the correct position. Dilating a false passage is possible. Ultrasound monitoring can help in this context.

Another option is to delay the procedure for a week with close observation and follow-up. The tract will probably close and the cervix may soften further, facilitating identification of the canal. Together with the patient, the provider must assess the advantages of proceeding versus the harm of delay, including any social, personal, and financial risks to the woman.

Uterine perforation

Uterine perforations that involve injury to major blood vessels or organs adjacent to the uterus, such as bowel or omentum, require in-hospital surgical management. Lateral perforations are of special concern, as they may injure branches of the uterine artery [34] (Chapter 15, Fig. 15.4).

Some low-risk perforations can be managed in the office or clinic setting. A small midline perforation in the first trimester, without suspicion of other injury, may be handled conservatively [35,36]. These perforations typically occur at either the lower uterine segment or the fundus, and extensive bleeding is unusual [37]. If the perforation occurred with a dilator or a cannula without suction, injury of other organs is unlikely. Completion of the abortion allows the uterus to contract and may seal off a small perforation. The decision to use intraoperative ultrasound or laparoscopy to complete the abortion depends on the comfort and skill of the operator [38]. If the provider has emptied the uterus and the patient has no excessive bleeding or sign of other injury, hospitalization is not necessary. Most of these perforations heal without incident [39]. However, close observation in the immediate postoperative period is essential along with close outpatient follow-up.

Situational challenges

Performing abortion in other than the usual environment

On occasion, a provider is asked to perform an abortion in an unusual setting. For instance, a woman with severe skeletal trauma, acute organ failure, multisystem illness, or terminal illness may be confined to an intensive care setting.

For the woman whose health is severely compromised, consent may need to be obtained from family members. Various local and state laws may govern the counseling and consent process for the emergent care of the incapacitated patient. Education and support for the assisting medical staff also may be crucial. Many medical staff members are unfamiliar with abortion procedures, and they may have received information (or misinformation) about abortion from lay or religious sources.

Facilities that do not customarily perform abortions are not likely to have optimum equipment. An equipment deficiency or failure can endanger the patient and raise the anxiety level of the provider, assistants, and ancillary staff. Therefore, the provider may need to bring appropriate equipment and supplies to the treatment site including suitable sizes of cannulae, mechanical dilators, specialty specula, and medications such as uterotonic agents. Manual vacuum aspirators, which are portable, less bulky, and quieter than electric suction, may be more convenient and less disturbing to staff. A gynecologic operating table is the least necessary piece of equipment. Abortions can be performed at the end or side of a bed, using assistants to position and support the patient.

Addressing common fears of the pelvic examination or abortion procedure

Many women dislike pelvic examinations and vaginal procedures under any circumstance, and induced abortion may involve additional fears and tensions. Some women perceive pelvic examinations and procedures as embarrassing or sexually threatening [40]. If a woman has avoided routine pelvic examinations because of fear, embarrassment, or modesty, she may have her first adult contact with obstetrical or gynecological care because of pregnancy. Likewise, in many countries, gynecologic care is seldom sought until pregnancy occurs.

Some medical schools teach pelvic examination with attention to the patient's experience; others do not. In one study, medical students trained by a laywoman had better communication skills and equal technical skills compared to those trained by an attending physician [41]. Even after years of experience, pelvic examination technique can always be improved. Research suggests that stress during a pelvic examination is decreased by the following factors [42]:

- informed communication;
- sensitive positioning during the examination;
- integrity during nakedness;
- trust in the clinician; and/or
- female gender of clinician.

The management of women having their first examination does not differ substantially from that of other women of similar age and social circumstances, except for the benefit of a more detailed explanation of the examination itself. In one study, the circumstance of a first examination was not associated with increased discomfort during abortion [43]. No evidence indicates that these women require additional sedation or anesthesia.

One aversive response to pelvic examination is vaginismus, also called penetration phobia, an involuntary spasm of the perineal musculature. Some women will report a history of abuse (often with the comment that no one has ever asked them before). Severe vaginismus can prevent vaginal intercourse, even after term vaginal delivery [44]. It may occur only in certain situations; for example, the woman may be able to tolerate a pelvic examination but not be able to have vaginal intercourse, or the reverse. Some women are unable to tolerate any vaginal manipulation. Treatment of vaginismus includes psychotherapy, desensitization, and relaxation techniques. Desensitization with vaginal mold insertion can achieve pelvic relaxation in 2 to 6 weeks [45], but this therapy delays the abortion. Women with severe vaginismus may require deep sedation or general anesthesia for abortion.

We suggest the following examination and procedural techniques to improve the patient's experience:

- Meet the patient while she is dressed and upright. Introduce yourself in a professional manner with your medical title. Use language and movements that cannot be construed as sexual in content.

- Wear clean clothes; patients may mistake iodine splashes for blood.
- Take your time, no matter how busy your schedule.
- Address any questions or concerns that the woman may have.
- Make sure that the patient's body is adequately covered during the examination and abortion procedure.
- Explain the position for the examination using nonsexual language. For example, "Please move your knees to the side" is preferable to "Please spread your legs."
- Describe what you are going to do before each step of the examination and abortion procedure, as well as the sensations that the patient might feel. Use neutral words such as pressure instead of those that suggest an unpleasant experience, such as pain.
- Use warm jelly and instruments.
- Announce when you will first touch the patient. Avoid immediately inserting the speculum if the patient has tensed her introital muscles. Try touching a less threatening area first, such as the medial aspect of the patient's knee or lower thigh, with your hand and then the speculum. Sometimes, brief muscle-awareness exercises can help. Gently place one finger inside the vaginal introitus and ask the patient to contract her muscles as if stopping the flow of urine. After a few cycles of contracting and then loosening these muscles, insertion of the speculum is often successful.
- Give positive suggestions to anxious patients, such as to breathe slowly and concentrate on the breathing. Using "if... then" statements encourages the patient to participate in a successful examination and enhances her sense of control (Chapter 5). For example, "If you breathe deeply and keep your abdomen loose, then the examination will be over much more quickly."
- If obtaining a Pap test for a woman having her first pelvic examination, let her know precisely when you are taking the test and when it is over. Realizing that it is a brief and painless procedure may decrease her anxiety about the abortion and about future well-woman examinations.
- Ask the patient if she wants the assistant to hold her hand. Most patients do better when the assistant maintains eye contact, tells them what they might feel, guides their breathing, and converses during the procedure.
- Congratulate the patient on her cooperation in completing the procedure.

Emotionally challenging patients

Women who have been abused and who have dread of vaginal penetration may perceive vaginal procedures as invasive. The defenses women have established to protect themselves, whether anger, fear of doctors and needles, alcoholism, or dissociation, need special attention. Women who responded to childhood sexual trauma by dissociation may abstract themselves from their current surroundings when they feel threatened [46]. Some may experience pelvic examinations, abortion, or childbirth as a replay of their original trauma. At the conclusion of the abortion, anxiety and other manifestations of unease often markedly diminish [47].

Some psychiatric illnesses are especially difficult for physicians and staff, as when a delusional patient perceives the physician or staff to be a perpetrator. These conditions may include co-morbidities such as posttraumatic stress disorder, substance abuse, homelessness, and personality disorders. The patients may identify themselves in the waiting room: they may abuse the medical staff verbally, fight loudly with their partners, challenge office routines, or threaten lawsuits. Others sit quietly crying in a corner, act withdrawn, or have extreme difficulty making decisions.

Some problems do not become apparent until the patient is in the procedure room. For example, if a woman holds her knees tightly together in the stirrups or tries valiantly to cover herself with the drape, these signs may reflect overwhelming shame and/or previous abuse or a desire, conscious or otherwise, to defer the procedure. Other signs of emotional distress may include crying, screaming, rocking from side to side, or calling for people who are not there. In these situations, the provider should stop the procedure, invite the patient to sit up, assist her, and cover her fully. Simply telling the patient to relax is ineffective ("relax" is also a word used frequently by perpetrators of childhood sexual abuse and may provoke terror) [48]. If the clinician or the patient needs a few minutes to regain composure, the provider can leave the room temporarily. If the patient has an understanding chaperone, reuniting them for a brief time may be consoling. Further counseling may be necessary to explore the woman's feelings and concerns and to provide appropriate support. Do not restart the procedure until the patient indicates that she is willing to do so, both explicitly and through her body language.

Like all women seeking abortion, women with emotional issues or psychiatric illness benefit from care that is compassionate, professional, and tailored to meet their needs. Identifying potential risk factors or behaviors (Table 13.1) before the abortion increases the opportunity to customize care (Chapter 5). Many facilities have trained counseling staff to assist in this process; occasionally, consultation or referral is indicated. All staff can participate in providing optimum care by treating the patient with respect and offering support throughout the visit. Providing an opportunity for the patient to make even seemingly inconsequential choices, such as which arm she prefers for an injection, enhances her sense of control. Clinicians can also use breathing exercises, visualization (Chapter 8), ongoing conversation, and expectation of successful outcome. Many women are surprised,

Table 13.1 Factors and behaviors that may indicate a more difficult abortion procedure.

HISTORICAL RISK FACTORS
Previous difficulty with pelvic examination
Victim of incest or sexual abuse
Victim of physical or verbal assault
Posttraumatic stress disorder
Substance abuse
Religious conflict
Antiabortion stance
Shame-based family
Mood, affective, or personality disorder
Psychosis
Secret sexual relationship
BEHAVIORAL RISK FACTORS
Uncommunicative affect
Extreme ambivalence
Difficulty in trusting decisions
Agitation
Anger
Crying without resolution during the intake interview
Argumentative with a chaperone or staff member
Extreme fear or phobia, specifically of pain, needles, or consciousness-altering anesthesia
Resistance to use of contraception

gratified, and strengthened by their ability to negotiate their decision to abort and maintain their composure and dignity during the procedure.

Conclusion

Although most surgical abortions are uncomplicated, providers must remain vigilant of conditions that can increase the technical complexity of the procedure. When a clinician is uncomfortable proceeding with the abortion, obtaining the assistance of a more experienced colleague or referring the patient is the best course. Some of these conditions are evident on preabortion evaluation of the patient, whereas others arise during the abortion procedure itself. Clinicians with the requisite skills and experience can manage most challenging situations safely, compassionately, and expeditiously.

References

1 Wenof M, Reyniak JV, Novendstern J, Castadot MJ. Transverse vaginal septum. *Obstet Gynecol* 1979; **54**: 60–64.

2 Polasek PM, Erickson LD, Stanhope CR. Transverse vaginal septum associated with tubal atresia. *Mayo Clin Proc* 1995; **70**: 965–968.

3 Meyers RL. Congenital anomalies of the vagina and their reconstruction. *Clin Obstet Gynecol* 1997; **40**: 168–180.

4 Wagner BJ, Woodward PJ. Magnetic resonance evaluation of congenital uterine anomalies. *Semin Ultrasound CT MR* 1994; **15**: 4–17.

5 Jurkovic D, Gruboeck K, Tailor A, Nicolaides KH. Ultrasound screening for congenital uterine anomalies. *Br J Obstet Gynaecol* 1997; **104**: 1320–1321.

6 Kelly E, Hillard PJ. Female genital mutilation. *Curr Opin Obstet Gynecol* 2005; **17**: 490–494.

7 World Health Organization. *A systematic review of the health complications of female genital mutilation including sequelae in childbirth*. World Health Organization, Geneva, 2000.

8 Pennes DR, Bowerman RA, Silver TM, Smith SJ. Failed first trimester pregnancy termination: uterine anomaly as etiologic factor. *J Clin Ultrasound* 1987; **15**: 165–170.

9 Baldauf JJ, Dreyfus M, Ritter J, Meyer P, Philippe E. Risk of cervical stenosis after large loop excision or laser conization. *Obstet Gynecol* 1996; **88**: 933–938.

10 Schaff EA, Wortman M, Eisinger SH, Franks P. Methotrexate and misoprostol when surgical abortion fails. *Obstet Gynecol* 1996; **87**: 450–452.

11 Ostrom K, Ben-Arie A, Edwards C, Gregg A, Chiu JK, Kaplan AL. Uterine evacuation with misoprostol during radiotherapy for cervical cancer in pregnancy. *Int J Gynecol Cancer* 2003; **13**: 340–343.

12 Westergaard L, Philipsen T, Scheibel J. Significance of cervical *Chlamydia trachomatis* infection in postabortal pelvic inflammatory disease. *Obstet Gynecol* 1982; **60**: 322–325.

13 Barbacci MB, Spence MR, Kappas EW, Burkman RC, Rao T, Quinn TC. Postabortal endometritis and isolation of *Chlamydia trachomatis*. *Obstet Gynecol* 1986; **68**: 686–690.

14 Sorensen JL, Thranov I, Hoff G, Dirach J. Early- and late-onset pelvic inflammatory disease among women with cervical *Chlamydia trachomatis* infection at the time of induced abortion: a follow-up study. *Infection* 1994; **22**: 242–246.

15 Lettieri L, Rodis JF, McLean DA, Campbell WA, Vintzileos AM. Incarceration of the gravid uterus. *Obstet Gynecol Surv* 1994; **49**: 642–646.

16 Fielding WL, Lee SY, Friedman EA. Continued pregnancy after failed first trimester abortion. *Obstet Gynecol* 1978; **52**: 56–58.

17 Gürkan Zorlu CG, Aral K, Ekici E, Yalçin H, Turan C, Gökmen O. Causative factors in first trimester abortion failure. *Adv Contracept* 1996; **12**: 63–67.

18 Kaufman RH, Noller K, Adam E et al. Upper genital tract abnormalities and pregnancy outcomes in diethylstilbestrol-exposed progeny. *Am J Obstet Gynecol* 1984; **148**: 973–984.

19 Pellerito JS, McCarthy SM, Doyle MB, Glickman MG, DeCherney AH. Diagnosis of uterine anomalies: relative accuracy of MR imaging, endovaginal sonography, and hysterosalpingography. *Radiology* 1992; **183**: 795–800.

20 Valle RF, Sabbagha RE. Management of first trimester pregnancy termination failures. *Obstet Gynecol* 1980; **55**: 625–629.

21 Kaunitz AM, Rovira EZ, Grimes DA, Schulz KF. Abortions that fail. *Obstet Gynecol* 1985; **66**: 533–537.

22 Lazenby GB, Huang C, Rahall AM, Fogelson NS. Pregnancy termination via laparotomy in a woman with bicornuate uterus. *Contraception* 2007; **75**: 241–243.

23 Samuels TA, Awonuga A. Second-trimester rudimentary uterine horn pregnancy: rupture after labor induction with misoprostol. *Obstet Gynecol* 2005; **106**: 1160–1162.

24 Luk J, Allen RH, Schantz-Dunn J, Goldberg AB. Intrauterine adhesions as a risk factor for failed first-trimester pregnancy termination. *Contraception* 2007; **76**: 331–333.

25 Dalton VK, Lebovic DI. Use of a flexible cannula to bypass an obstructing fibroid during a first-trimester surgical abortion: a case report. *J Reprod Med* 2003; **48**: 551–552.

26 Buckshee K, Dhond AJ. A new nonsurgical technique for termination of intrauterine pregnancy associated with large multiple uterine leiomyomas. *Int J Gynaecol Obstet* 1992; **37**: 297–299.

27 Fenwick DK, Divers MJ. Medical pregnancy termination in the presence of a massive uterine fibroid. *Br J Clin Pract* 1995; **49**: 332–333.

28 Creinin MD. Medically induced abortion in a woman with a large myomatous uterus. *Am J Obstet Gynecol* 1996; **175**: 1379–1380.

29 Reece EA. Perspectives on obesity, pregnancy, and birth outcomes in the United States: the scope of the problem. *Am J Obstet Gynecol* 2008; **198**: 23–27.

30 Strafford M, Mottl-Santiago J, Savla A, Soodoo N, Borgatta L. Relationship of obesity to outcome of medical abortion. *Am J Obstet Gynecol* 2008; Dec 23 [Epub ahead of print]

31 Borgatta L, Barad D. Prolonged retention of laminaria fragments: an unusual complication of laminaria usage. *Obstet Gynecol* 1991; **78**: 988–990.

32 Bussey LA, Laing FC. Sonohysterography for detection of a retained laminaria fragment. *J Ultrasound Med* 1996; **15**: 249–251.

33 Edelman A, Jensen J, Nelson E, Nichols M. Cannula fracture in first trimester abortion: a case report and survey of NAF providers. *Contraception* 2003; **67**: 49–51.

34 Berek JS, Stubblefield PG. Anatomic and clinical correlates of uterine perforation. *Am J Obstet Gynecol* 1979; **135**: 181–184.

35 Goldchmit R, Zalel Y, Elchalal U, Matzkel A, Dgani R. Management of uterine perforation complicating first-trimester termination of pregnancy. *Isr J Med Sci* 1995; **31**: 232–234.

36 Lindell G, Flam F. Management of uterine perforations in connection with legal abortions. *Acta Obstet Gynecol Scand* 1995; **74**: 373–375.

37 Mittal S, Misra SL. Uterine perforation following medical termination of pregnancy by vacuum aspiration. *Int J Gynaecol Obstet* 1985; **23**: 45–50.

38 Kohlenberg CF, Casper GR. The use of intraoperative ultrasound in the management of a perforated uterus with retained products of conception. *Aust N Z J Obstet Gynecol* 1996; **36**: 482–484.

39 Kaali SG, Szigetvari IA, Bartfai GS. The frequency and management of uterine perforations during first-trimester abortions. *Am J Obstet Gynecol* 1989; **161**: 406–408.

40 Kaplan HS, Fyer AJ, Novick A. The treatment of sexual phobias: the combined use of antipanic medication and sex therapy. *J Sex Marital Ther* 1982; **8**: 3–28.

41 Kleinman DE, Hage ML, Hoole AJ, Kowlowitz V. Pelvic examination instruction and experience: a comparison of laywoman-trained and physician-trained students. *Acad Med* 1996; **71**: 1239–1243.

42 Larsen M, Oldeide CC, Malterud K. "Not so bad after all": women's experiences of pelvic examinations. *Fam Pract* 1997; **14**: 148–152.

43 Borgatta L, Nickinovich D. Pain during early abortion. *J Reprod Med* 1997; **42**: 287–293.

44 Drenth JJ, Andriessen S, Heringa MP, Mourits MJ, van de Wiel HB, Weijmar Schultz WC. Connections between primary vaginismus and procreation: some observations from clinical practice. *J Psychosom Obstet Gynecol* 1996; **17**: 195–201.

45 Biswas A, Ratnam SS. Vaginismus and outcome of treatment. *Ann Acad Med Singapore* 1995; **24**: 755–758.

46 Spiegel D. (1996) Dissociative disorders. In: Hales RE, Yudofsky SC, eds. *Synopsis of Psychiatry*. American Psychiatric Press, Washington (DC), 1996: 583–604.

47 Lowenstein L, Deutsch M, Gruberg R et al. Psychological distress symptoms in women undergoing medical vs. surgical termination of pregnancy. *Gen Hosp Psychiatry* 2006; **28**: 43–47.

48 Holz K. A practical approach to clients who are survivors of childhood sexual abuse. *J Nurse Midwifery* 1994; **39**: 13–18.

14

CHAPTER 14

Contraception and surgical abortion aftercare

Eve Espey MD, MPH, and Laura MacIsaac MD, MPH

LEARNING POINTS

- All unsensitized Rh(D) negative women undergoing abortion should receive anti-D immune globulin, and all women should receive perioperative antibiotics.
- Providing women with instructions about home care, medications, contraceptive initiation, warning signs for complications, and emergency contact information may obviate the need for a routine follow-up visit after surgical abortion.
- Although many women are motivated to initiate effective contraception after an abortion, women with a history of abortion remain at high risk of another unintended pregnancy; 47% of abortions are repeat procedures.
- Long-acting reversible contraceptive methods, including intrauterine devices (IUDs) and implants, are highly effective and can be initiated immediately after an abortion in nulliparous women and teenagers as well as in older parous women.
- IUDs and implants are good contraceptive choices for most women with concurrent medical problems.

Introduction

Care of women after surgical abortion varies depending on the type of procedure, gestational age, type of anesthesia or analgesia, and the presence of complicating medical or psychosocial variables. A critical component of abortion aftercare is contraceptive initiation. Incorporating evidence-based contraceptive care into abortion practice offers the opportunity to reduce future unplanned pregnancy and improve long-term family planning, an essential component of preventive care for women and families.

Contraceptive education, initiation, and continuation strategies should be emphasized at the first and subsequent clinical encounters for several reasons:

- Previous abortion is consistently observed as a risk for recurrent unintended pregnancy [1,2];
- Women who seek abortion because of unintended pregnancy may be particularly motivated to initiate an effective contraceptive [3–5];
- If not addressed at the abortion visit, loss of continuity of care may compromise implementation and maintenance of long-term contraception; and
- Follow-up care after abortion varies by country; in the USA at least 35% of women do not attend a follow-up visit [6].

Regardless of procedure type, clinical setting, or gestational age at the time of abortion, an emphasis on immediate initiation of long-acting reversible contraceptives (LARCs), specifically intrauterine devices (IUDs) and implants, has the potential to increase contraceptive uptake [7,8], improve method continuation [7,9,10], reduce repeat adolescent pregnancy [11,12], and reduce repeat abortion [8].

Postprocedure care

The elements of recovery from an abortion procedure include surveillance for short- and long-term complications (Chapters 15 and 16) as well as observation and support related to analgesia and anesthesia (Chapter 8). Research to develop practice guidelines for postabortion care is scant, likely because of the wide range of settings, anesthesia, and procedure types. Women undergoing early aspiration procedures in the office with local cervical anesthesia and oral nonsteroidal antiinflammatory agents may require only 15 to 20 minutes of recovery. Women undergoing moderate to deep sedation or general anesthesia for first- or second-trimester surgical abortion warrant more prolonged and skilled postprocedure surveillance that usually occurs in

Management of Unintended and Abnormal Pregnancy, 1st edition. By M Paul, ES Lichtenberg, L Borgatta, DA Grimes, PG Stubblefield, MD Creinin

a specified recovery area. Postprocedure policies related to sedation are frequently determined by anesthesia or nursing protocols. For safe postprocedure monitoring in the office setting, emergency equipment and supplies for intravenous access and emergency medications are recommended [13]. The addition of uterotonic medications to the standard emergency cart is important for quickly treating uterine atony [14].

Immediate complications

Although serious complications are unusual in the immediate recovery period, facilities and personnel must be prepared for the range of problems. Complications include uterine atony, retained products of conception (POCs), hematometra, low and high cervical tears, uterine perforation, syncope, and cardiovascular and respiratory disorders (Chapter 15). These adverse events most often arise during the procedure or in the recovery area. Providers should be knowledgeable about approaches to diagnosis and rapid treatment. The facility and staff should maintain a well-rehearsed plan for urgent transfer of a patient to a more intensive level of care if needed.

Delayed complications

Delayed complications occur within a few hours to 2 weeks after the procedure and usually present with symptoms similar to those of immediate complications: abnormal bleeding, fever, and/or pain [13,15]. The same differential diagnosis for immediate pain and bleeding applies to these delayed problems. Excessive or prolonged bleeding may result from retained POCs, hematometra, infection, injury, or incomplete abortion. Pain and uterine tenderness, with or without fever or abnormal bleeding, are prominent features of postabortal pelvic infection. When a woman has the delayed complication of pain and persistent symptoms of pregnancy, she may have an ongoing intrauterine pregnancy or ectopic pregnancy. Careful inspection of the products of conception at the time of uterine evacuation helps to minimize this rare event (Chapter 10).

Discharge from the facility and home care

To confirm absence of immediate complications, recovery staff should assess and document the following at least once prior to discharge [14,15]:

- normal mental status;
- ability to ambulate independently;
- adequate pain control;
- normal, stable vital signs; and
- absence of excessive vaginal bleeding.

Additional assessments for women who received sedation include:

- ability to void and to take oral liquids;
- absence of severe or persistent nausea and vomiting; and
- escort available to accompany the woman home.

In addition, nonsensitized Rh(D) negative women should receive anti-D immune globulin.

All women require discharge instructions about antibiotics and other medications, contraceptives, warning signs for complications, and emergency contact information for the provider or the clinic. In women who receive sedation, counseling about home care and contraception may be more appropriately accomplished prior to the abortion procedure.

Anti-D immune globulin

Rh(D) sensitization may occur when D-positive fetal red blood cells enter the circulation of an Rh(D)-negative woman. Although sensitization most commonly occurs in the third trimester of pregnancy, induced and spontaneous abortions confer a risk of up to 5% in susceptible women [16]. Debate continues about the need to use prophylaxis in all Rh(D)-negative women undergoing early induced abortion [17]. A transfusion of 0.25 cc is considered the lower estimate of blood volume required to cause isoimmunization. Studies examining this association are plagued by methodological flaws such as small sample sizes or use of the Kleihauer-Betke test as a surrogate for isoimmunization. At 8 weeks' gestation, approximately 0.33 cc of fetal red blood cells may be transfused [17]. Whether this small amount of fetal-maternal transfusion actually increases the risk of isoimmunization is unclear.

In the USA, practice guidelines recommend that all women undergoing abortion have Rh status documented and that all Rh(D)-negative women receive anti-D immune globulin or sign an informed waiver [14,18]. The American College of Obstetricians and Gynecologists (ACOG) recommends anti-D immune globulin prophylaxis within 72 hours of an abortion, either medical or surgical, with no lower gestational age limit. Standard dosages in the USA include 50 micrograms of anti-D immune globulin through 12 weeks' gestation (covers up to 2.5 cc of fetal-maternal transfusion), and 300 micrograms for abortions after 12 weeks [18]. In the UK, Rh isoimmunization prophylaxis is also standard for all women undergoing abortion, but recommended dosages differ [13]. Patients undergoing medical abortion may receive anti-D immune globulin on the day medications are initiated. When using a regimen with mifepristone or methotrexate combined with misoprostol, anti-D immune globulin may be given instead on the day of misoprostol administration. Although anti-D immune globulin is ideally administered within 72 hours of the abortion, evidence suggests that it remains at least partially effective as long as 13 days after exposure to D-positive red cells. Therefore, administering prophylaxis beyond 72 hours may afford some protection with minimal risk.

Antibiotics

Postabortion infection is uncommon and depends on a variety of factors including prevalence of sexually transmitted infections (STIs) in the population, protocols for testing and treating women with positive results prior to procedures, and consistency of diagnostic criteria for pelvic infection. Despite the variability of these factors, most studies demonstrate a protective effect of perioperative antibiotics, regardless of regimen. A meta-analysis of 12 randomized controlled trials using a variety of antibiotics suggests a substantial reduction in postabortion infection [19]. The mostly European studies in the meta-analysis demonstrated wide variation in the background rate of postabortal infection, ranging from 5 to 20%. The background rate of postabortal infection in the USA is less than 1% [20] (Chapter 15). In a randomized study comparing outcomes of medical abortion and surgical aspiration in Scotland, the infection rate was similar in both groups at 0.9% [21]. Efficacy of routine preventative antibiotics may be overstated for populations with a low background prevalence of postabortal infection; however, the authors demonstrate cost-effectiveness and prevention of numerous infections even given the assumption of a low (1%) incidence of postabortal infection.

Most studies in the meta-analysis included tetracyclines or nitroimidazoles, such as metronidazole, both of which were effective. Four placebo-controlled trials using oral doxycycline, a well-tolerated and inexpensive drug, showed similar reductions in infection [22–25]. Both ACOG and the National Abortion Federation (NAF) guidelines recommend the use of perioperative antibiotics for all women undergoing surgical abortion, but do not endorse a specific regimen [14,26]. The two prophylactic regimens described in the ACOG bulletin include: 1) doxycycline 100 mg orally 1 hour before the procedure and 200 mg orally after the procedure; and 2) metronidazole 500 mg orally twice daily for 5 days. In high-risk women, NAF recommends treatment with therapeutic doses of antibiotics consistent with Centers for Disease Control and Prevention (CDC) guidelines [14].

Consistent with surgical principles of perioperative infection prophylaxis, antibiotics may be initiated before the abortion or immediately after first-trimester procedures that occur in a single visit. For second-trimester procedures that include a day of cervical preparation with osmotic dilators, antibiotics are often initiated at the time of dilator insertion. Optimal antibiotic choices and dosing regimens remain open fields for further investigation.

Postprocedure uterotonic medications

Few studies have examined ideal ways of reducing blood loss during abortion procedures or preventing it afterwards. Knowledge of uterotonic medications, including dosages, routes, and intervals of administration, is crucial to successful management of problem bleeding during or after surgical abortion (Chapter 15). Uterotonic medications are primarily used to treat atony, and they may assist in resolving or temporarily modulating excessive bleeding from other sources, such as injury or abnormal placentation.

Methylergonovine

Methylergonovine is an ergot derivative that causes uterine contractions. It may be given orally or, for more rapid onset, as an intramuscular or intracervical injection. Doses may be repeated at intervals when serious bleeding occurs. An observational study found a reduced risk of hematometra when intramuscular ergonovine was administered after first-trimester abortion [27]. A common oral regimen is 0.2 mg every 4 to 6 hours for six doses, but little evidence supports the routine use of this medication after abortion.

Prostaglandin analogs

Many prostaglandins have a contractile effect on uterine smooth muscle. Carboprost tromethamine (Hemabate® in the USA), a prostaglandin $F_{2\alpha}$ derivative, is a potent uterotonic available for intramuscular administration. It is used frequently for postpartum hemorrhage in a dose of 0.25 mg every 15 to 90 minutes, with a maximum dose of 2 g (Hemabate® package insert). Carboprost can also cause contractile effects on bronchial smooth muscle and is therefore contraindicated in women with reactive airway disease. Misoprostol, a synthetic prostaglandin E_1 analog, has several uses in medical and surgical abortion. No studies have examined its use to treat bleeding at the time of abortion. However, favorable pharmacokinetic data [28] and its successful application in postpartum hemorrhage [29,30] make the use of misoprostol a consideration for postabortal bleeding resulting from atony, particularly in the setting of a large uterus. Misoprostol is often administered rectally in a dose of 800 to 1,000 μg for postabortal bleeding [14].

Oxytocin

Oxytocin is a drug administered parenterally. It has a short half-life and can be used intravenously or intramuscularly. Oxytocin also can be added to the cervical anesthetic [14]. The number of oxytocin receptors in the uterus rises as gestational age advances. Because the uterus is not very sensitive to oxytocin during the first trimester [31], routine use of this uterotonic medication in early abortion is unlikely to be effective. Oxytocin is used more commonly during and immediately after second-trimester procedures, based on experience with postpartum hemorrhage.

Instructions for home care

Patients typically recover quickly after abortion and usually resume normal daily activities immediately or shortly after the procedure. If a woman received sedation or general anesthesia, she should be warned of transient mental impairment [14]; advising her to refrain from driving or operating heavy machinery until the following day is prudent. Although no evidence is available to guide recommendations, most clinicians advise at least a few days to a week of pelvic rest. Discharge instructions are most important in advising women about return to fertility, initiation and maintenance of contraception, managing postprocedure discomfort, recognizing warning signs of common complications, and accessing emergency treatment if needed.

Cramping

Cramping is common and expected following an abortion procedure. Bothersome cramping generally lasts for a day or less and usually responds to over-the-counter analgesics or local measures, such as heat or back/uterine massage. Nonsteroidal antiinflammatory agents (NSAIDs), such as ibuprofen 400 to 800 mg every 4 to 8 hours, may help reduce cramping. Acetaminophen can be given in oral doses up to 1,000 mg every 4 hours, with the total dose not to exceed 4 g in 24 hours. Some patients require oral narcotic agents for pain relief. Commonly used agents include codeine or its derivative, oxycodone (with or without acetaminophen) in a dose of one or two tablets every 3 to 4 hours. Patients may take narcotics along with NSAIDs, as they have different mechanisms of action.

Nausea and vomiting

Occasionally, nausea and vomiting from analgesia associated with the procedure persist and require treatment. Several medications are available for this purpose including droperidol (Inapsine®) 1.25 mg given intravenously or intramuscularly, promethazine (Phenergan®) 25 mg administered parenterally or via rectal suppository, and prochlorperazine (Compazine®) 10 mg given parenterally or via rectal suppository. Women who have received misoprostol for cervical priming may experience gastrointestinal side effects; the symptoms are usually self-limiting and seldom require treatment.

Psychosocial problems

In the month following abortion, quality of life measures and mood improve in women who undergo abortion [32,33]. Depression is no more likely to occur in women after an abortion than in women of reproductive age in the general population [34]. Some women experience persistent or worsening depression or other mental health disorders after a pregnancy event, regardless of outcome of pregnancy, including abortion [35]. Clinicians should be trained to identify women in need of further counseling or referral (Chapter 5).

Complications

Written postoperative instructions should provide directions for telephone contact with specific phone numbers and instructions about when to call. Careful attention to the general literacy and health literacy of patients will ensure that women understand the print materials given to them. A clinician must be available to provide the patient with information, triage, and when possible, any necessary treatment [14]. Documentation of phone calls is important for follow-up, continuity of care, and for medical-legal purposes (Chapter 23).

Bleeding

Women should receive both oral and written instructions that include parameters for when to call in the case of excess bleeding. These instructions should include contact information for the provider or the clinic [14]. A commonly used guideline for medical abortion is to call the provider or clinic after fully saturating two sanitary pads per hour for 2 hours in a row; some providers also use this recommendation following surgical abortion. Prompt phone contact and communication may forestall unnecessary visits to the office or an emergency department. Clinicians use many factors to judge when an office or emergency room visit is necessary including the reported amount of bleeding, time until next available visit, the patient's medical co-morbidities, and available assistance in the home.

Fever

Women who experience fever (temperature >38 °C on two separate occasions), severe or persistent pelvic pain, chills, whole body aches, or general malaise require prompt evaluation for possible postabortal complications, especially infection (Chapter 15).

Pain

Severe persistent pain warrants evaluation. Possible diagnoses include infection, ectopic pregnancy, incomplete abortion, hematometra, ruptured ovarian cyst, or uterine injury (Chapter 15).

Abortion follow-up

Minimal evidence is available to guide best practices for follow-up after abortion. Clinicians traditionally have recommended a routine follow-up appointment 2 to 4 weeks after surgical abortion [36–38], although evidence supporting the utility of a follow-up examination is lacking [6]. The RCOG guidelines consider a 2-week follow-up visit optional if complete abortion is confirmed on the day of the procedure [13]. The traditional follow-up visit was recommended to accomplish several objectives including:

- detection of complications;
- detection of ongoing intrauterine or ectopic pregnancy;
- provision of contraception;
- provision of psychosocial counseling, if indicated; and
- performance of health maintenance services, such as STI and Pap testing.

In the USA, however, between 35 and 60% of women do not attend the follow-up appointment [39–41]. Given the safety and efficacy of both surgical and medical abortion, women who do not return for follow-up are unlikely to have complications. Additionally, the timing of the visit at 2 to 4

Table 14.1 Contraceptive efficacy. Percentage of women experiencing an unintended pregnancy during the first year of typical use of contraception and the percentage continuing use at the end of the first year, USA. (Adapted with permission from Trussel J [49].)

Method	% of Women Experiencing an Unintended Pregnancy within the First Year of Use: Typical Use[a]	% of Women Continuing Use at 1 Year[b]
No method[c]	85	
IUD		
ParaGard® (copper T)	0.8	78
Mirena® (LNG-IUS)	0.2	80
Implanon™	0.05	84
Female sterilization	0.5	100
Male sterilization	0.15	100
Combined pill and progestin-only pill	8	68
Evra® patch	8	68
NuvaRing®	8	68
Depo-Provera	3	56
Diaphragm[d]	16	57
Condom[e]		
Female (Reality®)	21	49
Male	15	53
Spermicides[f]	29	42
Withdrawal	27	43
Sponge		
Parous women	32	46
Nulliparous women	16	57

Emergency Contraceptive Pills: Treatment initiated within 72 hours after unprotected intercourse reduces the risk of pregnancy by at least 75%.[g]
Lactational Amenorrhea Method: LAM is a highly effective, *temporary* method of contraception.[h]

Notes:

[a] Among *typical* couples who initiate use of a method (not necessarily for the first time), the percentage that experience an accidental pregnancy during the first year if they do not stop use for any other reason.

[b] Among couples attempting to avoid pregnancy, the percentage that continues to use a method for 1 year.

[c] The percentages becoming pregnant in column 2 are based on data from populations where contraception is not used and from women who cease using contraception in order to become pregnant. Among such populations, about 89% become pregnant within 1 year. This estimate was lowered slightly (to 85%) to represent the percentage who would become pregnant within 1 year among women now relying on reversible methods of contraception if they abandoned contraception altogether.

[d] With spermicidal cream or jelly.

[e] Without spermicides.

[f] Foams, creams, gels, vaginal suppositories, and vaginal film.

[g] The treatment schedule is one dose within 120 hours after unprotected intercourse and a second dose 12 hours after the first dose. Both doses of Plan B can be taken at the same time. Plan B (1 dose is 1 white pill) is the only dedicated product specifically marketed for emergency contraception. The US Food and Drug Administration has declared 22 brands of combined oral contraceptives to be safe and effective for emergency contraception, in addition to Plan B.

[h] However, to maintain effective protection against pregnancy, another method of contraception must be used as soon as menstruation resumes, the frequency or duration of breastfeeds is reduced (such as infant sleeping through the night), bottle feeds are introduced, or the baby reaches 6 months of age.

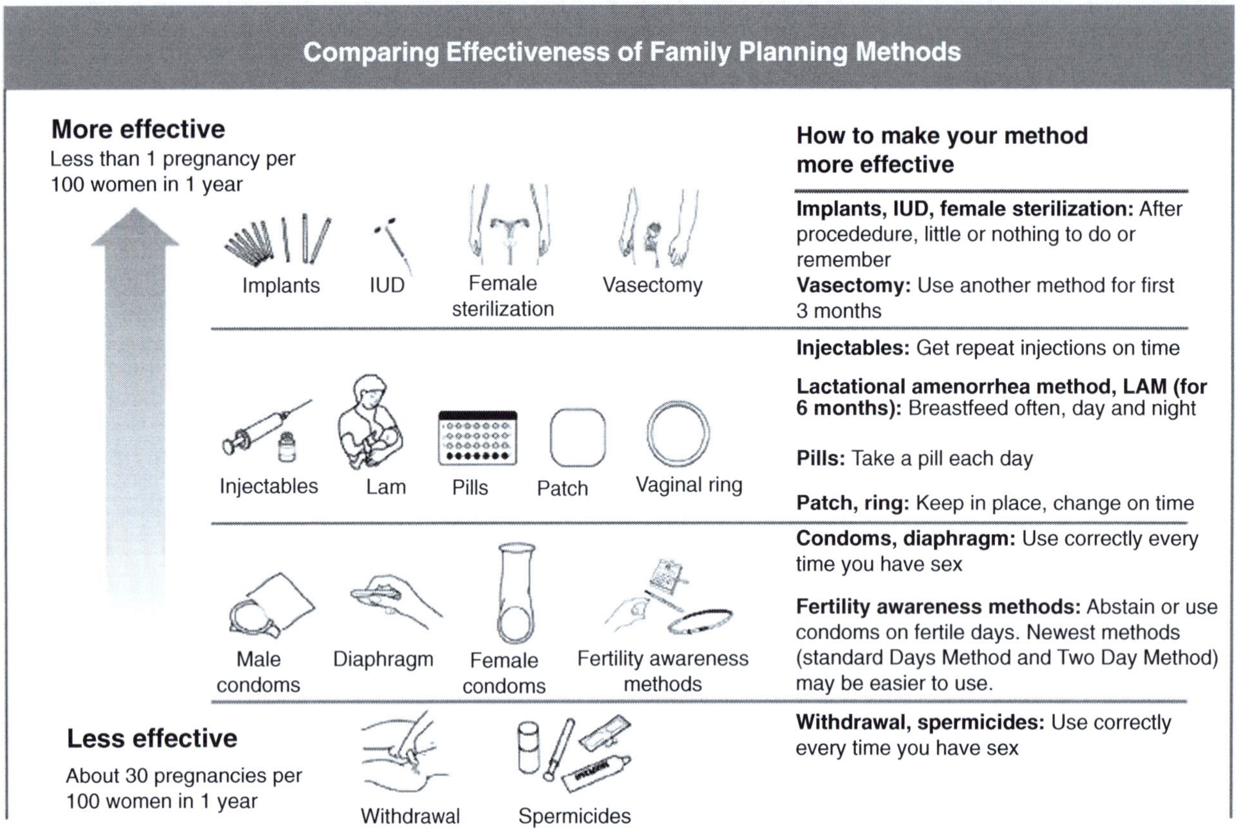

USAID World Health Organization

Sources:
Steiner MJ, Trussell J, Mehta N, Condon S, Subramaniam S, Bourne D. Communicating contraceptive effectiveness: a randomized controlled trial to inform a World Health Organization family planning handbook. *Am J Obstert Gynecol* 2006,195(1):85–91.
World Health Organization/Department of Reproductive Health and Research (WHO/RHR), Johns Hopkins Bloomberg School of Public Health (JHSPH)/Center for Communication Programs (CCP). *Family Planning: A Global Handbook for Providers.* Baltimore, MD and Geneva: CCP and WHO, 2007.
Trussell J. Choosing a contraceptive: efficacy, safety, and personal considerations. In: Hatcher RA, Trussell J, Nelson A, Cates W Jr, Stewart FH, Kowal D, eds. Contraceptive Technology, 19th edn. Ardent Media, New York, 2007 [49].

Figure 14.1 World Health Organization chart comparing the effectiveness of family planning methods (From USAID, WHO [50].).

years was initiation of the contraceptive implant [11]. Currently, only a small percentage of female contraceptors in the USA use implants and IUDs. The high rate of unintended pregnancy in the USA as compared to other developed countries suggests that more extensive use of top-tier methods might lower this rate [8,10].

Women are commonly sexually active within days to weeks after an abortion [9]. Because ovulation resumes quickly (as early as 10 days) following abortion [50], initiating a method at the time of abortion or very shortly thereafter is critical in preventing repeat unplanned pregnancy. Most contraceptive methods can be safely initiated at the time of the abortion [6,52].

Intrauterine contraception methods

Intrauterine contraception is the most widely used method of reversible contraception in the world, but it is underutilized in the USA where only 2% of women contraceptors currently use IUDs [53]. Globally, a large array of copper and hormonal devices is available, and more are in development. The copper IUD (ParaGard®, Duramed, Pomona NY) and the levonorgestrel-releasing intrauterine system (LNG-IUS, Mirena®, Bayer, Montville, NJ) are the two devices approved in the USA. Other copper IUDs are also available in other countries. IUDs provide top-tier contraception (Table 14.1), have excellent safety profiles [52,54,55] and offer protection against endometrial cancer [56]. IUDs have the

Box A Determinants of Real Life Contraceptive Effectiveness [59]

$$\text{Contraceptive Effectiveness} = \frac{\text{Efficacy} \times \text{Compliance} \times \text{Continuation}}{\text{Fecundability} \times \text{Coital Frequency}}$$

(Adapted from Grimes 2007) [59]

highest continuation rate of all reversible methods (Table 14.1). The LNG-IUS has noncontraceptive benefits to prevent and treat many common gynecologic conditions [57]; in several countries, the system is approved for treatment of menorrhagia and protection of the uterus against development of endometrial hyperplasia in women taking exogenous estrogen.

The *real-life contraceptive effectiveness equation* puts the effectiveness of contraceptive methods in perspective, factoring in not only efficacy, but also compliance and continuation (Box A) [58]. All three of these factors are maximized with the IUD.

Placing an IUD immediately after abortion is both safe and practical [59]. An evidence-based decision analysis of immediate versus delayed insertion of IUDs after abortion estimated that 20% of women would choose an IUD at the time of abortion [60]. With this assumption, the model estimated a reduction of 20,000 repeat abortions in the first year for the immediate insertion group. Several studies [9,61,62] demonstrate the safety and effectiveness of immediate insertion of a copper IUD or LNG-IUS. Risks for serious complications such as perforation and infection are small and similar to those reported for interval insertion. The risk of IUD expulsion has been compared in women who obtained the IUD immediately after first-trimester abortion versus those who obtained the IUD 2 or more weeks later. The results of these studies, conducted outside the USA, were reassuring [61,62]. For medication abortion and surgical abortion at more advanced gestational ages, more data are needed. Several randomized studies are ongoing in the USA to determine optimal timing of IUD insertion.

Although an increased expulsion risk would be a disadvantage of immediate insertion, many women may decide that the benefit of timely placement outweighs this risk. The WHO Medical Eligibility Criteria and the copper IUD package insert support immediate IUD insertion at the time of first-trimester surgical abortion (ParaGard® package insert)[52,59]. Unfortunately, nonclinical issues sometimes dictate immediate versus delayed insertion. These obstacles include reimbursement problems and logistics (e.g., when contraceptive supplies are not stored in close proximity to the abortion procedure room)[60,63].

Technique of immediate insertion after abortion is similar to that of interval insertion. After confirming that the abortion is complete (by inspection of the products of conception, ultrasound, or both), the clinician inserts the IUD with the applicator just as in interval insertion. After second-trimester abortion, ultrasound guidance is employed to assure fundal placement. Second-trimester insertion techniques include placement with the inserter, manual insertion with a sterile gloved hand, or placement with a ring forceps; the optimal method is unclear.

As one of the top-tier contraceptive methods, IUDs represent an excellent option for women seeking highly effective and reliable contraception after abortion. Facilitating the placement of a postabortion IUD through accommodating protocols, adequate access for all women, timely reimbursement, and ready availability of devices in all clinical settings could have a major impact on reducing unintended pregnancy [64].

Implants

Hormonal implants are highly effective, long-acting, reversible contraceptives that are considered top-tier methods because they do not require user adherence. They also offer an excellent safety record and rapid return to fertility. Implants currently available globally include the six-rod Norplant® system, the two-rod Jadelle® system, both with levonorgestrel, and the single-rod Implanon™, with etonogestrel. Implanon®, the only FDA-approved implant in the USA, is highly effective for 3 years. Implanon™ may be inserted within 5 days of abortion, as noted on the package insert.

A recent cohort study followed women who had an implant contraceptive placed within 15 minutes of an aspiration abortion procedure [9]. Ninety-eight of 100 women continued the method at 6 months. The main reason for early discontinuation of implants is menstrual irregularity, a characteristic common to all progestin-only methods (Implanon™ package insert)[65–67]. Other reported but infrequent side effects include weight gain, acne, breast pain, mood changes, and headache [68]. Still, continuation rates are high (Table 14.1). Anticipatory guidance and counseling prior to implant insertion may be the most important factor in reducing discontinuation because of side effects [69].

Sterilization

Female sterilization is the most common contraceptive method worldwide and in the USA for women over age 35 years. Permanent contraception with sterilization is an excellent choice for women who have completed childbearing. The two main sterilization procedures after abortion include laparoscopic tubal ligation (which may also be performed concurrently with early abortion) and hysteroscopic tubal occlusion.

Laparoscopic tubal ligation, most often performed under general anesthesia, includes a variety of techniques including bands, clips, and cautery. Overall, the failure rate of laparoscopic tubal ligation is 1 to 2% over 10 years [70]. Failure rates are lower in older women and those who have unipolar cautery. Hysteroscopic tubal occlusion may be performed in the office or operating room using local anesthesia. No studies have examined an appropriate time interval between abortion and subsequent hysteroscopic sterilization.

A serious disadvantage of all sterilization procedures, male and female, is the potential for regret. The overall likelihood of regret is relatively high, between 12 and 14%[71]. Risk factors for regret include age under 30 at the time of sterilization as well as divorce and remarriage [71]. Given the similar failure rates, IUDs and implants can be considered reversible sterilization [72]. The association between timing of postabortal tubal ligation and risk of regret has not been studied.

Although small cohort studies have not identified differences in medical outcomes [73,74], concurrent sterilization and abortion is not routinely performed in the USA. The RCOG cites a concern with higher sterilization failure rates when the procedures are performed concurrently [75]. A 1979 international trial [76] randomized 406 women to aspiration abortion and mini-laparotomy tubal ligation under epidural anesthesia versus aspiration abortion with paracervical anesthesia and mini-laparotomy tubal ligation under epidural anesthesia 6 weeks later. Complications were similar in both groups. All women in the concurrent group underwent sterilization. Thirty-three per cent of women ($n = 64$) in the delayed group changed their minds and did not undergo interval sterilization. Investigators were later able to contact 51 of the 64 women. Of these 51 women, seven became pregnant again: six terminated the pregnancy and underwent concurrent sterilization, and one carried the pregnancy and had a postpartum sterilization. Overall, 22% of the 51 women eventually underwent sterilization and 78% remained unsterilized. Whether women who did not undergo sterilization would have regretted it if they had been sterilized is unclear. Certainly, the permanence of sterilization must be emphasized and a reversible method encouraged when a woman shows any possible desire for future childbearing.

Injectable Contraception

Depo-medroxyprogesterone acetate (DMPA), given as an intramuscular injection of 150 mg every 3 months or as a subcutaneous dose of 104 mg every 3 months, can be administered the day of the abortion visit. Advantages of DMPA include its high effectiveness; relatively convenient dosing schedule; and, for women who wish to keep their method confidential, the lack of "evidence" such as pills or patches. Use of DMPA has been increasing in the USA since its FDA approval as a contraceptive in 1993, contributing in part to the reduction in teen pregnancies over the last decade [77].

Despite a very low failure rate, DMPA is plagued by poor continuation rates, mainly because of side effects. Irregular bleeding is the reason most often cited for discontinuation. In an attempt to decrease irregular bleeding and improve continuation, a study of women receiving DMPA immediately after abortion randomized users to a low cyclic dose of transdermal estrogen versus placebo [78]. Cyclic estrogen did not improve bleeding patterns during the initial 3 months or have an impact on continuation through 1 year, which was 19.4% in the study group and 23.9% in the placebo group. Overall, 21.9% of women had a repeat unintended pregnancy within a year of the abortion. The low continuation rates with DMPA and the high rate of repeat unintended pregnancy are perhaps the most important findings of the study, suggesting that alternative contraceptive methods may be more compatible with long-term use in some populations of women seeking abortion.

Combination hormonal contraceptives (pills, patch, and ring)

Combination hormonal methods are popular and prevalent. The combined oral contraceptive pill, the contraceptive patch, and the contraceptive ring all contain both estrogen and progestin and work primarily by preventing ovulation. Combination hormonal methods have numerous advantages including effectiveness (Table 14.1), independence of coital activity, as well as the noncontraceptive benefits of cycle control, improvement in acne, and a major reduction in uterine and ovarian cancer. The biggest disadvantage of these methods is the need for continued adherence. Because of the need for daily, weekly, or monthly acts of motivation, the real-life effectiveness and continuation rates vary widely depending on the population, and gaps in contraceptive protection are frequent.

Women having surgical or medical abortion procedures can initiate oral contraceptive pills, the ring, or the patch on the day of the abortion. Bednarek et al [79] evaluated method continuation in women who started their hormonal method on the day of medical abortion follow-up versus those who started their method the following Sunday. Continuation rates were exceptionally high (>90%) and equal at 6 weeks in both groups. Fine et al [80] have shown that women who begin using the contraceptive ring within a week of surgical or medical abortion do not have increased signs of infection or serious adverse events; moreover, women report a high level of satisfaction and intention to continue the method.

Progestin-only pills

Progestin-only pills (POPs) are appropriate for women who desire an oral contraceptive but have contraindications to the estrogen component in combination methods. Whereas the estrogen component is prothrombotic, progestin-only methods have no effect on the clotting system and may attenuate estrogen effects. Unfortunately, the package labels of certain POPs include the same contraindications as those on combination hormonal contraceptives. No clinical evidence supports such restrictive labeling. POPs can be a good option for women with contraindications to estrogen, particularly as a bridge method to a more effective choice.

Depending on the type and dose of progestin, POPs do not consistently inhibit ovulation [81]. Although POPs have several independent mechanisms of action, the primary mechanism is thickening of cervical mucus [82].

Progestin-only pills may be initiated on the day of surgical abortion. POPs in typical use are assumed to have real-life effectiveness similar to that of combined hormonal methods. The primary side effect is spotting between periods or irregular bleeding. Because the progestin content in POPs is lower than that in combined methods, the pills must be taken no more than 27 hours apart before efficacy wanes. Women using progestin-only pills may benefit from anticipatory guidance emphasizing the importance of strict adherence to their pill-taking schedule.

Barrier methods

Barrier methods have relatively low efficacy with routine use. A major disadvantage is the requirement for placement of barriers with each act of intercourse. Condom use confers protection against STIs, but it does not provide top-tier protection from pregnancy because of breakage, slippage, inconsistent use, and low continuation rates (Table 14.1). Although the probability of pregnancy should theoretically be lower with the simultaneous use of a male condom and female vaginal spermicide, clinical trial data demonstrating improved effectiveness are lacking [83].

The diaphragm and cervical cap (FemCap or Lea's Shield®) may be used after abortion. Although Lea's Shield® comes in a single size, current female diaphragms require fitting that can be carried out at a postabortion follow-up visit. New one-size-fits-all, over-the-counter diaphragms are in development.

The easy access and affordability of barrier methods make them a popular choice in many populations; male condom use is the second most common choice of reversible contraception among US women. Women who choose barrier methods require instruction on proper use and encouragement to use them consistently. Given the high prevalence of STIs in many women [84,85], condom use should be encouraged where feasible. Actual distribution of condoms may promote usage.

An important strategy to address the impact of unplanned pregnancy and STIs, both internationally and in the USA, is dual-method use. Dual protection, an intervention for pregnancy prevention and a second one for STI protection [86–88], is particularly applicable to young women, among whom STIs are on the rise, serious sequelae are most frequent, and repeat pregnancy and abortion are commonplace [1,2].

The frequency of dual use varies among populations. In a survey of 15-year-old females in 24 countries, dual use of condoms and combined oral contraceptive pills ranged from 2.5% in Croatia to 28.8% in Canada [89]. In Australia, 28% of pill users in a large survey reported using dual protection with condoms [90]. Dual protection in the USA remains low but is increasing. Dual use of a hormonal method and condoms increased in women aged 15 to 19 years from 7.5% in 1995 to 17.9% in 2002 [77].

A recent large randomized intervention to increase dual protection in the USA [2] demonstrated increases in self-reported dual use, but no change in the frequency of new STIs or unintended pregnancy. Women who used condoms consistently and continuously (those who reported dual use at more than one follow-up visit) had reduced pregnancy and STI rates. A US prospective study of 1,073 first-time users of either the contraceptive implant or injectable examined the use of dual protection. Condom use declined markedly among women who initiated a long-term hormonal method [91]. However, condom use increased from 25 to 31% in the subgroup of women with more than one sexual partner and those who received a counseling message to continue condom use. A survey of condom use among teenagers [92] found a low prevalence of dual protection. Young people view condoms primarily as a means of pregnancy prevention, identifying prevention of STIs and human immunodeficiency virus (HIV) as unassociated goals.

Emergency contraception

An abortion visit presents an optimal opportunity to educate women about the benefits of emergency contraception as a backup for user-dependent birth control methods, such as barriers, pills, the patch, the ring, and the contraceptive injectable. Education and instruction, prescription, or supplies should be provided as backup contraception to all barrier or hormonal contraception users at the time of abortion. Additionally, some women choose abstinence or do not choose a contraceptive method after abortion. A discussion of emergency contraception, as well as advance provision, for such women increases utilization of emergency contraception without decreasing regular contraceptive use or increasing sexual risk taking behavior [93]. However, research has not yet demonstrated an impact of these interventions on abortion rates [94].

Emergency contraception may be given as a 1.5 mg total dose of levonorgestrel, marketed by various names throughout the world. Alternatively, two doses of a combined estrogen-progestin regimen may be formulated from standard birth-control pills. The levonorgestrel regimen is more effective, taken either in two doses 12 hours apart or as a single dose within 5 days of unprotected intercourse [95]. A large randomized controlled trial found that use of the levonorgestrel regimen reduced expected pregnancies by 85%[96].

Table 14.2 Contraceptives to avoid in women with select medical problems.

Medical problem	Contraceptives to avoid	Comments
Migraine headaches with aura	Combination hormonal contraceptives	Although myocardial infarction (MI) and stroke risk may be increased in women with migraines even without aura, the magnitude of that risk is quite low. Women with migraine without aura who do not have other cardiovascular risk factors may be reasonable candidates for combined hormonal contraceptives.
History of thromboembolism and/or hypercoagulability	Combination hormonal contraceptives	Women with history of unexplained deep venous thrombosis (DVT) or with a known hypercoagulable syndrome should not use combination hormonal contraceptives. Women with a remote history of a single DVT associated with a known risk factor (e.g., lengthy immobilization) may be reasonable candidates for combined hormonal contraceptives.
Systemic lupus erythematosis (SLE)	Combination hormonal contraceptives in SLE complicated by nephritis, vascular disease, or antiphospholipid antibodies	Although data suggest that combination hormonal contraceptives do not increase the number of flares in women with mild SLE, those women with antiphospholipid antibodies still may have significant risk for venous thromboembolic disease. Those with advanced disease should avoid combined hormonal contraceptives.
Depression	None	Limited data show no significant association between hormonal contraceptives and depression, including progestin-only methods.
Risk for STIs	None, but dual protection (condoms + effective contraceptive) favored	Insufficient evidence exists to determine an effect of hormonal contraceptives on HIV transmission.
Smoking	Combination hormonal contraceptives in women over age 35	Younger women using combined hormonal contraceptives have a very low risk of MI and stroke, but this risk may be significantly increased in women aged 35 years and older who smoke at least 10 cigarettes daily.
Concomitant use of antibiotics	Combination and progestin-only hormonal contraceptives only in women taking rifampin	A common misperception is that hormonal contraceptives are less effective when women are also taking antibiotics. Pharmacokinetic evidence of reduced serum levels of steroids in women taking pills occurs only in those taking rifampin. No effects on serum steroid levels occur with the use of most common antibiotics.
Obesity	Combination hormonal contraceptives in obese women with other cardiovascular risk factors	Transdermal hormonal contraceptives are not as highly effective (but are still effective) in obese women, an increasingly common proportion of American women. Cardiovascular health risks with combination hormonal contraceptives in obese women are increased with other risk factors such as smoking, age $\geq$35, and hypertension.

The public remains largely unaware of emergency contraception. Even those who have heard of emergency contraception often confuse it with the abortifacient mifepristone [97–99]. Verbal counseling and fact sheets about emergency contraception help to educate women, but advance provision of emergency contraceptive pills may be most effective in motivating women to actually use the medication after unprotected sex [100]. Removing cost as an obstacle may further increase emergency contraceptive use [101].

Strategies for successful use of contraceptive methods

Contraceptive care is an integral part of abortion services and should be a major focus of the abortion visit. Helping women choose methods from the highest tier of the WHO contraceptive counseling diagram may be particularly helpful in reducing future unintended pregnancies. In low-risk women, immediate initiation of most methods is an important strategy [52]. Additional strategies include the following:

Strategies for clinicians:

- Encourage LARCs (National Institute Health and Clinical Excellence guideline #30, 2005), including use in nulliparous women [8,102,103] and teenagers [11,12];
- Counsel women thoroughly on all contraceptive options, particularly LARCs, even if a preference for a particular contraceptive is given [104];
- Avoid "bundling" of preventive measures, that is, requiring cervical cytology screening or a medical visit in order to prescribe contraception [105];
- Avoid unnecessary delays, such as waiting to initiate a method until a follow-up examination after abortion or miscarriage, or until menses resume [8,60,106];
- Increase the number of units of contraceptives prescribed or dispensed. More supplies may predict better continuation [107];
- Include the male partner in counseling when possible [108,109];
- Encourage dual protection in appropriate women [77,87,110]; and
- Educate about and encourage use of emergency contraception for all women using methods other than the IUD, the implant, or sterilization. Dispense a product if possible; give advance emergency contraception prescriptions to women under age 18 when necessary [100,111].

Strategies for reducing obstacles in private health systems:

- Identify and prescribe the least expensive pills in area pharmacies. Inform women of lower cost pharmacies;
- Examine the woman's insurance and initiate methods before insurance expires. Assess if coverage for supplies will continue;
- Become familiar with local and state programs (including Medicaid) for assisting women with family planning, and develop a process for women to access these programs; and
- Develop strategies to provide "high-cost" LARCs to unfunded or underfunded women. Where possible, avoid advocating alternatives (e.g., oral contraceptives)[101] simply based on cost.

Contraceptive management in women with medical problems

Determining appropriate contraceptive choices is particularly challenging in women with medical problems. Although serious medical problems are unusual in women seeking abortion, clinicians may encounter certain problems frequently. Examples include migraine headaches, history of thromboembolism, hypercoagulability, systemic lupus erythematosis, depression, risk for STIs, smoking, and obesity.

Although identifying a risk-free contraceptive for women with medical problems presents challenges, pregnancy in such women is often the riskier alternative. Initiating almost any contraceptive method in a woman seeking abortion is usually less risky than using no method.

Fortunately, the best performing long-acting reversible contraceptives, IUDs and implants, are rarely contraindicated in women with medical problems. Similarly, sterilization is often an excellent choice in women with medical problems who desire a permanent, nonreversible method.

Optimizing contraceptive choices involves individualizing counseling based on the woman's specific medical condition and needs. Several excellent sources exist to help practitioners identify appropriate contraceptives for women in special categories [52,112,113]. Table 14.2 lists contraceptives to avoid for women in several common risk categories.

Conclusion

Care of women after abortion should emphasize prevention and treatment of albeit uncommon immediate and long-term complications. The cornerstone of postabortion care is counseling and provision of effective contraceptives. Emphasis and resources focused on initiation and continuation of contraceptives, particularly LARCs, provide our best opportunity to reduce recurrent unintended pregnancy.

References

1 Kuroki LM, Allsworth JE, Redding CA, Blume JD, Peipert JF. Is previous unplanned pregnancy a risk factor for a subsequent unplanned pregnancy? *Am J Obstet Gynecol* 2008; **199**: 517. e1–7.

2 Peipert JF, Redding CA, Blume JD et al. Tailored intervention to increase dual-contraceptive method use: a randomized trial to reduce unintended pregnancies and sexually transmitted infections. *Am J Obstet Gynecol* 2008; **198**: 630 e1–8.

3 Garg M, Singh M, Mansour D. Peri-abortion contraceptive care: can we reduce the incidence of repeat abortions? *J Fam Plann Reprod Health Care* 2001; **27**: 77–80.

4 Truong HM, Kellogg T, McFarland W, Kang MS, Darney P, Drey EA. Contraceptive intentions among adolescents after abortion. *J Adolesc Health* 2006; **39**: 283–286.

5 Stanwood NL, Bradley KA. Young pregnant women's knowledge of modern intrauterine devices. *Obstet Gynecol* 2006; **108**: 1417–1422.

6 Grossman D, Ellertson C, Grimes DA, Walker D. Routine follow-up visits after first-trimester induced abortion. *Obstet Gynecol* 2004; **103**: 738–745.

7 Shunmann C, Glasier A. Specialist contraceptive counseling and provision after termination of pregnancy improves uptake of long-acting methods but does not prevent repeat abortion: a randomized trial. *Hum Reprod* 2006; **21**: 2296–2303.

8 Heikinheimo O, Gissler M, Suhonen S. Age, parity, history of abortion, and contraceptive choice affect the risk of repeated abortion. *Contraception* 2008; **78**: 149–154.

9 Ortayli N, Bulut A, Sahin T, Sivin I. Immediate postabortal contraception with the levonorgestrel intrauterine device, Norplant, and traditional methods. *Contraception* 2001; **63**: 309–314.

10 Trussell J, Wynn LL. Reducing unintended pregnancy in the United States. *Contraception* 2008; **77**: 1–5.

11 Stevens-Simon C, Kelly L, Kulick R. A village would be nice but… it takes a long-acting contraceptive to prevent repeat adolescent pregnancies. *Am J Prev Med* 2001; **21**: 60–65.

12 Atkin LC. Pregnant again? Psychosocial predictors of short interval repeat pregnancy among adolescent mothers in Mexico City. *J Adolesc Health* 1992; **13**: 700–706.

13 Royal College of Obstetricians and Gynaecologists. The care of women requesting induced abortion. *Evidence-based Clinical Guideline No 7*. RCOG Press, London, 2004.

14 National Abortion Federation [Online]. Washington (DC): National Abortion Federation; c2008. Clinical policy guidelines; 2008 [cited 2008 Jun 5]. Available from: URL:http://www.prochoice.org/pubs_research/publications/downloads/professional_education/CPG2008.pdf

15 Speroff L, Darney PD. *A Clinical Guide for Contraception*, 4th edn. Williams & Wilkins, Baltimore, MD 2005: 387–416.

16 Howard HL, Martlew VJ, McFadyen IR, Clarke CA. Preventing Rhesus D haemolytic disease of the newborn by giving anti-D immunoglobulin: are the guidelines being adequately followed? *Br J Obstet Gynaecol* 1997; **104**: 37–41.

17 Jabara S, Barnhart KT. Is Rh immune globulin needed in early first-trimester abortion? A review. *Am J Obstet Gynecol* 2003; **188**: 623–627.

18 American College of Obstetricians and Gynecologists. Prevention of Rh D alloimmunization. *ACOG Practice Bulletin No. 4*. American College of Obstetricians and Gynecologists, Washington (DC), 1999.

19 Sawaya GF, Grady D, Kerlikowske K, Grimes DA. Antibiotics at the time of induced abortion: the case for universal prophylaxis based on a meta-analysis. *Obstet Gynecol* 1996; **87**: 884–890.

20 Hakim-Elahi E, Tovell HM, Burnhill MS. Complications of first-trimester abortion: a report of 170,000 cases. *Obstet Gynecol* 1990; **76**: 129–135.

21 Henshaw R, Naji S, Russell I, Templeton A. A comparison of medical abortion (using mifepristone and gemeprost) with surgical vacuum aspiration: efficacy and early medical sequelae. *Hum Reprod* 1994; **9**: 2167–2172.

22 Brewer C. Prevention of infection after abortion with a supervised single dose of oral doxycycline. *Br Med J* 1980; **281**: 780–781.

23 Darj E, Stralin E, Nilsson S. The prophylactic effect of doxycycline on postoperative infection rate after first-trimester abortion. *Obstet Gynecol* 1987; **70**: 755–758.

24 Levallois P, Rioux JE. Prophylactic antibiotics for suction curettage abortion: results of a clinical controlled trial. *Am J Obstet Gynecol* 1988; **158**: 100–105.

25 London RS, London ED, Siegelbaum M, Goldstein P. Use of doxycycline in elective first trimester abortion. *South Med J* 1978; **71**: 672–673.

26 American College of Obstetricians and Gynecologists. Antibiotic prophylaxis for gynecologic procedures. *ACOG Practice Bulletin No. 74*. American College of Obstetricians and Gynecologists, Washington (DC), 2006.

27 Sands RX, Burnhill MS, Hakim-Elahi E. Postabortal uterine atony. *Obstet Gynecol* 1974; **43**: 595–598.

28 Meckstroth KR, Whitaker AK, Bertisch S, Goldberg AB, Darney PD. Misoprostol administered by epithelial routes: drug absorption and uterine response. *Obstet Gynecol* 2006; **108**: 582–590.

29 Villar J, Gülmezoglu AM, Hofmeyr GJ, Forna F. Systematic review of randomized controlled trials of misoprostol to prevent postpartum hemorrhage. *Obstet Gynecol* 2002; **100**: 1301–1312.

30 Goldberg AB, Greenberg MB, Darney PD. Misoprostol and pregnancy. *N Engl J Med* 2001; **344**: 38–47.

31 Ali PB, Smith G. The effect of syntocinon on blood loss during first trimester suction curettage. *Anaesthesia* 1996; **51**: 483–485.

32 Westhoff C, Picardo L, Morrow E. Quality of life following early medical or surgical abortion. *Contraception* 2003; **67**: 41–47.

33 Sit D, Rothschild AJ, Creinin MD, Hanusa BH, Wisner KL. Psychiatric outcomes following medical and surgical abortion. *Hum Reprod* 2007;**22**: 878–884.

34 American Psychological Association, Task Force on Mental Health and Abortion. Report of the Task Force on Mental Health and Abortion [online]. Washington (DC): American Psychological Association; 2008 [cited 2009 Jan 3]. Available from URL: http://www.apa.org/pi/wpo/mental-health-abortion-report.pdf

35 Rees D, Sabia JJ. The relationship between abortion and depression: new evidence from the fragile families and child wellbeing study. *Med Sci Monit* 2007; **13**: CR430–CR436.

36 Darney P, Horbach N, Korn A. First-trimester elective abortion. In: *Protocols for Office Gynecologic Surgery*. Blackwell Science, Cambridge (MA), 1996: 158–193.

37 Keder LM. Best practices in surgical abortion. *Am J Obstet Gynecol* 2003; **189**: 418–422.

38 Paul M. Office management of early induced abortion. *Clin Obstet Gynecol* 1999; **42**: 290–305.

39 Cameron ST, Glasier AF, Logan J, Benton L, Baird DT. Impact of the introduction of new medical methods on therapeutic abortions at the Royal Infirmary of Edinburgh. *Br J Obstet Gynaecol* 1996; **103**: 1222–1229.

40 Paul M, Lackie E, Mitchell C, Rogers A, Fox M. Is pathology examination useful after early surgical abortion? *Obstet Gynecol* 2002; **99**: 567–571.

41 Westfall JM, Sophocles A, Burggraf H, Ellis S. Manual vacuum aspiration for first-trimester abortion. *Arch Fam Med* 1998; **7**: 559–562.

42 Seckl MJ, Gillmore R, Foskett M, Sebire NJ, Rees H, Newlands ES. Routine terminations of pregnancy: should we screen for gestational trophoblastic neoplasia? *Lancet* 2004; **364**: 705–707.

43 Saeed GA, Fakhar S, Rahim F, Tabassum S. Change in trend of contraceptive uptake: effect of educational leaflets and counseling. *Contraception* 2008; **77**: 377–381.

44 Canto De Cetina TE, Canto P, Ordoñez Luna M. Effect of counseling to improve compliance in Mexican women receiving depot-medroxyprogesterone acetate. *Contraception* 2001; **63**: 143–146.

45 Kero A, Lalos A. Increased contraceptive use one year post-abortion. *Hum Reprod* 2005; **20**: 3085–3090.

46 Nobili MP, Piergrossi S, Brusati V, Moja EA. The effect of patient-centered contraceptive counseling in women who undergo a voluntary termination of pregnancy. *Patient Educ Couns* 2007; **65**: 361–368.

47 Moos MK, Bartholomew NE, Lohr KN. Counseling in the clinical setting to prevent unintended pregnancy: an evidence-based research agenda. *Contraception* 2003; **67**: 115–132.

48 Trussell J. Contraceptive failure in the United States. *Contraception* 2004; **70**: 89–96.

49 Trussell J. (2007) Choosing a contraceptive: efficacy, safety, and personal considerations. In: Hatcher RA, Trussell J, Nelson AL, Cates W Jr, Stewart FH, Kowal D, eds. *Contraceptive Technology*, 19th edn. Ardent Media, New York, 2007.

50 United States Agency for International Development, World Health Organization. Comparing effectiveness of family planning methods [chart]. Washington (DC): USAID; 2007.

51 Cameron IT, Baird DT. The return to ovulation following early abortion: a comparison between vacuum aspiration and prostaglandin. *Acta Endocrinol (Copenh)* 1988; **118**: 161–167.

52 World Health Organization. *Medical Eligibility Criteria for Contraceptive Use* [Online]. Geneva: World Health Organization, Reproductive Health and Research; 2004 [cited 2008 Jul 14]. Available from: URL:http://www.who.int/reproductive-health/publications/mec/mec.pdf

53 Turok D. The quest for better contraception: future methods. *Obstet Gynecol Clin North Am* 2007; **34**: 137–166.

54 MacIsaac L, Espey E. Intrauterine contraception: the pendulum swings back. *Obstet Gynecol Clin North Am* 2007; **34**: 91–111.

55 American College of Obstetricians and Gynecologists. (2005) Intrauterine device. *ACOG Practice Bulletin No. 59.* American College of Obstetricians and Gynecologists, Washington (DC), 2005.

56 Beining RM, Dennis LK, Smith EM, Dokras A. Meta-analysis of intrauterine device use and risk of endometrial cancer. *Ann Epidemiol* 2008; **18**: 492–499.

57 Fraser IS. The promise and reality of the intrauterine route for hormone delivery for prevention and therapy of gynecological disease. *Contraception* 2007; **75**(6 Suppl): S112–S117.

58 Grimes D. Intrauterine devices (IUDs). In: Hatcher RA, Trussell J, Nelson AL, Cates W Jr, Stewart FH, Kowal D, eds. *Contraceptive Technology*, 19th edn. Ardent Media, New York, 2007.

59 Grimes DA, Lopez LM, Schulz KF, Stanwood NL. Immediate postabortal insertion of intrauterine devices. *Cochrane Database Syst Rev* 2004; **4**: CD001777.

60 Reeves MF, Smith KJ, Creinin MD. Contraceptive effectiveness of immediate compared with delayed insertion of intrauterine devices after abortion: a decision analysis. *Obstet Gynecol* 2007; **109**: 1286–1294.

61 El-Tagy A, Sakr E, Sokal DC, Issa AH. Safety and acceptability of post-abortal IUD insertion and the importance of counseling. *Contraception* 2003; **67**: 229–234.

62 Göçmen A, Demirpolat N, Aysin H. The efficacy of immediate post-abortion intrauterine device insertion. *Clin Exp Obstet Gynecol* 2002; **29**: 274–276.

63 Goodman S, Hendlish SK, Benedict C, Reeves MF, Pera-Floyd M, Foster-Rosales A. Increasing intrauterine contraception use by reducing barriers to post-abortal and interval insertion. *Contraception* 2008; **78**: 136–142.

64 Goodman S, Hendlish SK, Reeves MF, Foster-Rosales A. Impact of immediate postabortal insertion of intrauterine contraception on repeat abortion. *Contraception* 2008; **78**: 143–148.

65 Affandi B. An integrated analysis of vaginal bleeding patterns in clinical trials of Implanon. *Contraception* 1998; **58**(Suppl.): 99S–107S.

66 Bitzer J, Tschudin S, Alder J. Acceptability and side-effects of Implanon in Switzerland: a retrospective study by the Implanon Swiss Study Group. *Eur J Contracept Reprod Health Care* 2004; **9**: 278–284.

67 Funk S, Miller MM, Mishell DR Jr et al. Safety and efficacy of Implanon, a single-rod implantable contraceptive containing etonogestrel. *Contraception* 2005; **71**: 319–326.

68 Urbancsek J. An integrated analysis of nonmenstrual adverse events with Implanon. *Contraception* 1998; **58**(Suppl.): 109S–115S.

69 Meckstroth KR, Darney PD. Implant contraception. *Semin Reprod Med* 2001; **19**: 339–354.

70 Peterson HB, Xia Z, Hughes JM, Wilcox LS, Tylor LR, Trussell J. The risk of pregnancy after tubal sterilization: findings from the U.S. Collaborative Review of Sterilization. *Am J Obstet Gynecol* 1996; **174**: 1161–1168.

71 Hillis SD, Marchbanks PA, Tylor LR, Peterson HB. Poststerilization regret: findings from the United States Collaborative Review of Sterilization. *Obstet Gynecol* 1999; **93**: 889–895.

72 Grimes DA, Mishell DR Jr. Intrauterine contraception as an alternative to interval tubal sterilization. *Contraception* 2008; **77**: 6–9.

73 Kaali S, Szigetvari I, Bartfai F. The frequency and management of uterine perforations during first-trimester abortions. *Am J Obstet Gynecol* 1989; **161**: 406–408.

74 Chamberlain G. Safety of post-abortion sterilisation. *Lancet* 1979; **2**: 1020.

75 Royal College of Obstetricians and Gynaecologists. Male and female sterilisation. *Evidence-based Clinical Guideline No. 4*. RCOG Press, London, 2004.

76 Cheng MC, Chew SC, Cheong J. Safety of postabortion sterilisation compared with interval sterilisation. A controlled study. *Lancet* 1979; **2**: 682–685.

77 Santelli JS, Lindberg LD, Finer LB, Singh S. Explaining recent declines in adolescent pregnancy in the United States: the contribution of abstinence and improved contraceptive use. *Am J Public Health* 2007; **97**: 150–156.

78 Goldberg AB, Cardenas LH, Hubbard AE, Darney PD. Post-abortion depot medroxyprogesterone acetate continuation rates: a randomized trial of cyclic estradiol. *Contraception* 2002; **66**: 215–220.

79 Bednarek PH, Nichols MD, Carlson N et al. Effect of "observed start" vs. traditional "Sunday start" on hormonal contraceptive continuation rates after medical abortion. *Contraception* 2008; **78**: 26–30.

80 Fine PM, Tryggestad J, Meyers NJ, Sangi-Haghpeykar H. Safety and acceptability with the use of a contraceptive vaginal ring after surgical or medical abortion. *Contraception* 2007; **75**: 367–371.

81 Rice CF, Killick SR, Dieben T, Coelingh Bennink H. A comparison of the inhibition of ovulation inhibition with the desogestrel 75 micrograms and the levonorgestrel 30 micrograms daily. *Hum Reprod* 1999; **14**: 982–985.

82 McCann MF, Potter LS. Progestin-only oral contraception: a comprehensive review. *Contraception* 1994; **50**(Suppl.): S1–S195.

83 Craig S, Hepburn S. The effectiveness of barrier methods of contraception with and without spermicide. *Contraception* 1982; **26**: 347–359.

84 Centers for Disease Control and Prevention. *Sexually Transmitted Disease Surveillance*. US Department of Health and Human Services, Atlanta (GA), 2006.

85 Sangani P, Rutherford G, Wilkinson D. Population-based interventions for reducing sexually transmitted infections, including HIV. *Cochrane Database Syst Rev* 2004; **2**: CD001220.

86 World Health Organization, Joint United Nations Programme on HIV/AIDS, United Nations Population Fund. Joint WHO/UNAIDS/UNFPA Policy Statement: dual protection against unwanted pregnancy and sexually transmitted infections, including HIV [Online]. Geneva: World Health Organization; 2000 [cited 2008 Aug 12]. Available from: URL:http://www.popline.org/docs/164540

87 Cates W Jr, Steiner MJ. Dual protection against unintended pregnancy and sexually transmitted infections: what is the best contraceptive approach? *Sex Transm Dis* 2002; **29**: 168–174.

88 Delvaux T, Nostlinger C. Reproductive choice for women and men living with HIV: contraception, abortion, and fertility. *Reprod Health Matters* 2007; **15**(Suppl.): 46–66.

89 Godeau E, Nic Gabhainn S, Vignes C, Ross J, Boyce W, Todd J. Contraceptive use by 15-year-old students at their last sexual intercourse: results from 24 countries. *Arch Pediatr Adolesc Med* 2008; **162**: 66–73.

90 Parr N, Siedlecky S. Use of 'dual protection' and other combinations of contraceptive methods in Australia. *Aust N Z J Public Health* 2007; **31**: 567–570.

91 Cushman LF, Romero D, Kalmuss D, Davidson AR, Heartwell S, Rulin M. Condom use among women choosing long-term hormonal contraception. *Fam Plann Perspect* 1998; **30**: 240–243.

92 Santelli JS, Warren CW, Lowry R et al. The use of condoms with other contraceptive methods among young men and women. *Fam Plann Perspect* 1997; **29**: 261–267.

93 Harper CC, Cheong M, Rocca CH, Darney PD, Raine TR. The effect of increased access to emergency contraception among young adolescents. *Obstet Gynecol* 2005; **106**: 483–491.

94 Raymond EG, Trussell J, Polis CB. Population effect of increased access to emergency contraceptive pills: a systematic review. *Obstet Gynecol* 2007; **109**: 181–188.

95 von Hertzen H, Piaggio G, Ding J et al. Low-dose mifepristone and two regimens of levonorgestrel for emergency contraception: a WHO multicentre randomised trial. *Lancet* 2002; **360**: 1803–1810.

96 Anonymous. Randomised controlled trial of levonorgestrel versus the Yuzpe regimen of combined oral contraceptives for emergency contraception. Task Force on Postovulatory Methods of Fertility Regulation. *Lancet* 1998; **352**: 428–433.

97 Kaiser Family Foundation. *Women and Health Care: A National Profile* [Online]. Menlo Park (CA): Kaiser Family Foundation; 2005 [cited 2008 Jul 14]. Available from: URL: http://www.kff.org/womenshealth/7336.cfm

98 Kaiser Family Foundation. *Emergency Contraception in California* [Online]. Menlo Park (CA): Kaiser Family Foundation; 2004 [cited 2008 Jul 14]. Available from: URL:http://www.kff.org/womenshealth/7036.cfm

99 Moodley J, Morroni C. Emergency contraception: lack of awareness among women presenting for termination of pregnancy. *S Afr Med J* 2007; **97**: 584–585.

100 Raine TR, Harper CC, Rocca CH et al. Direct access to emergency contraception through pharmacies and effect on unintended pregnancy and STIs: a randomized controlled trial. *JAMA* 2005; **293**: 54–62.

101 Postlethwaite D, Trussell J, Zoolakis A, Shabear R, Petitti D. A comparison of contraceptive procurement pre- and post-benefit change. *Contraception* 2007; **76**: 360–365.

102 Prager S, Darney PD. The levonorgestrel intrauterine system in nulliparous women. *Contraception* 2007; **75**(Suppl.): S12–S15.

103 Hubacher D. Copper intrauterine device use by nulliparous women: review of side effects. *Contraception* 2007; **75**(Suppl.): S8–S11.

104 Lamvu G, Steiner MJ, Condon S, Hartmann K. Consistency between most important reasons for using contraception and current method used: the influence of health care providers. *Contraception* 2006; **73**: 399–403.

105 Schwarz EB, Saint M, Gildengorin G, Weitz TA, Stewart FH, Sawaya GF. Cervical cancer screening continues to limit provision of contraception. *Contraception* 2005; **72**: 179–181.

106 Stanback J, Thompson A, Hardee K, Janowitz B. Menstruation requirements: a significant barrier to contraceptive access in developing countries. *Stud Fam Plann* 1997; **28**: 245–250.

107 Westhoff C, Heartwell S, Edwards S et al. Initiation of oral contraceptives using a quick start compared with a conventional start: a randomized controlled trial. *Obstet Gynecol* 2007; **109**: 1270–1276.

108 Beenhakker B, Becker S, Hires S, Molano Di Targiana N, Blumenthal P, Huggins G. Are partners available for post-abortion contraceptive counseling? A pilot study in a Baltimore City clinic. *Contraception* 2004; **69**: 419–423.

109 Harvey SM, Henderson JT, Casillas A. Factors associated with effective contraceptive use among a sample of Latina women. *Women Health* 2006; **43**: 1–16.

110 Berer M. Dual protection: more needed than practised or understood. *Reprod Health Matters* 2006; **14**: 162–170.

111 Lo SS, Fan SY, Ho PC, Glasier AF. Effect of advanced provision of emergency contraception on women's contraceptive behaviour: a randomized controlled trial. *Hum Reprod* 2004; **19**: 2404–2410.

112 American College of Obstetricians and Gynecologists. Use of hormonal contraception in women with coexisting medical conditions. *ACOG Practice Bulletin No. 73*. American College of Obstetricians and Gynecologists, Washington (DC), 2006, reaffirmed 2008.

113 Teal, SB, Ginosar DM. Contraception for women with chronic medical conditions. *Obstet Gynecol Clin North Am* 2007; **34**: 113–126.

15

CHAPTER 15

Surgical complications: Prevention and management

E. Steve Lichtenberg MD, MPH, and David A. Grimes MD

LEARNING POINTS

- Surgical abortion is one of the safest procedures in contemporary medical practice.
- Prophylactic antibiotics reduce the risk of postabortal infection, although the optimum regimen remains unclear.
- Failed attempted abortion occurs more commonly in women with uterine anomalies, such as a bicornuate uterus.
- Immediate postoperative tissue inspection confirms successful abortion and excludes the remote possibility of an unsuspected ectopic pregnancy in most cases.
- Postoperative hemorrhage, like obstetrical hemorrhage, usually results from atony, retained tissue, uterine trauma, or coagulopathy.

Introduction

Induced abortion is an impressively safe procedure, particularly but not exclusively where it is legal, accessible, and performed under modern medical conditions [1]. The near elimination of abortion-related mortality in most industrialized nations stands in stark contrast to conditions in many developing countries where tens of thousands of women die annually from preventable complications [2] (Chapter 2).

Many of the difficulties encountered during modern induced abortion are not foreseeable or avoidable. The self-limiting nature of most adverse events underscores how remarkably resilient the uterus and other pelvic organs are in circumscribing damage and acute loss of blood. These protective mechanisms, coupled with the astute diagnosis and management of complications that do occur, make serious sequelae of induced abortion rare.

This chapter focuses on surgical abortion complications, addressing the conditions and practices that influence the risk of complications and acceptable approaches to their clinical diagnosis and management. Complications associated with early medical abortion and labor induction abortion are described in Chapters 9 and 12, respectively.

Management of Unintended and Abnormal Pregnancy, 1st edition. By M Paul, ES Lichtenberg, L Borgatta, DA Grimes, PG Stubblefield, MD Creinin

Mortality and morbidity

The risk of death from modern induced abortion is negligible. The US abortion-related mortality rate for 1988 to 1997 (the most recent period for which data are available) was 0.7 per 100,000 legal induced abortions [3]. The nationwide legalization of abortion in 1973 had a dramatic impact on abortion-related deaths; case-fatality rates subsequently declined by 85%, with most of the decrease occurring from 1973 to 1976 [3]. From 1991 to 1999, the risk of dying from live birth was about 12 times higher than that from induced abortion [2]. During that time period, induced or spontaneous abortion accounted for 4% of US maternal mortality whereas pregnancies resulting in live births accounted for 60%[4].

Gestational age is the most important risk factor for abortion-related mortality. Compared to the case-fatality rate for induced abortion at 8 weeks' gestation or less (0.1 per 100,000 procedures or 1 in a million), the risk of death increases by 38% for each successive gestational week [3] (Table 15.1). Race is another risk factor for abortion-related mortality in the USA. Women of races other than White are more than twice as likely to die from induced abortion. About one-fifth of the excess mortality risk among minority-race women is because of their later gestational age at the time of abortion.

The causes of abortion-related mortality have changed over time, and they differ by type of procedure [3]. Compared to the preceding decade, in 1988 to 1997 the

Table 15.1 Legal induced abortion-related deaths, mortality rates, and relative risks, by selected characteristics, USA, 1988–1997 (Reprinted with permission from Bartlett et al [3].)

Characteristic	Legal induced abortion-related deaths	Mortality rate[a]	Relative risk (95% confidence interval)
Gestational age (wk)			
First Trimester			
≤8	8	0.1	Referent
9–10	5	0.2	1.4 (0.5, 4.2)
11–12	6	0.4	3.4 (1.2, 9.7)
Second Trimester			
13–15	15	1.7	14.7 (6.2, 34.7)
16–20	19	3.4	29.5 (12.9, 67.4)
≥21	15	8.9	76.6 (32.5, 180.8)
Unknown	26	Not applicable	Not applicable
Race			
White	38	0.5	Referent
Black or other	56	1.1	2.4 (1.6, 3.6)
Time Period			
1972–1979	163	2.2	3.1 (2.4, 4.0)
1980–1987	80	0.8	1.1 (0.8, 1.4)
1988–1997	94	0.7	Referent
Age (y)			
≤19	20	0.7	1.2 (0.6, 2.2)
20–24	29	0.7	1.1 (0.6, 2.0)
25–29	18	0.6	Referent
30–34	16	0.9	1.5 (0.7, 2.9)
≥35	10	0.8	1.3 (0.6, 2.9)
Parity			
0	16	0.3	Referent
1–2	27	0.5	1.9 (1.0, 3.5)
≥3	7	0.5	2.1 (0.9, 5.2)
Unknown[b]	42	Not applicable	Not applicable

[a] Legal-induced abortion mortality rate is the number of abortion-related deaths per 100,000 legal-induced abortions.

[b] Denominators for calculating rates by parity use previous live births from abortion surveillance data; deaths with unknown parity are excluded.

proportion of abortion-related deaths attributable to anesthesia decreased substantially, as general anesthesia became both safer and less widely used for abortion. This decrease resulted in a proportionate rise in deaths because of hemorrhage and infection. Infection accounted for approximately one-third of deaths among women who had first-trimester vacuum aspiration abortions, whereas hemorrhage and embolism each accounted for 14%. In contrast, hemorrhage was the most common cause of mortality in the second trimester, accounting for about one-third of deaths attributable to labor-induction abortion and nearly 40% of deaths associated with dilation and evacuation (D&E) [3].

Morbidity with surgical abortion is also uncommon. For example, among 170,000 first-trimester surgical abortions performed in low-risk women by experienced providers, minor complications occurred in 8.46 per 1,000 cases and complications requiring hospitalization in 0.71 per 1,000 [5]. More recent reports confirm that fewer than 1 in 1,000 US women are hospitalized for abortion complications annually [6]. As with mortality, the risk of major complications is related to gestational age; it increases from about 2 per 1,000 procedures for abortions performed at 7 to 8 weeks' gestation, to 6 per 1,000 at 13 to 14 weeks, and 15 per 1,000 after 20 weeks [7].

Performing vaginal operations on obese women can be difficult or impossible, and almost half of US women of childbearing age are overweight or obese [8]. In a prospective study of 163 consecutive women having D&E abortion with preoperative laminaria, providers found that the procedures of obese women (body mass index ≥30) were significantly more difficult, took longer, and incurred greater loss of blood than those of women with normal body mass. However, the obese women were also older and had more prior pregnancies [9]. Others have confirmed a significant association between increased blood loss and obesity among D&E patients [10]. Obesity may also present challenges for perioperative pain management (Chapter 8).

In a 2002 survey of members of the National Abortion Federation (NAF), the professional association of abortion providers in the USA and Canada, most respondents imposed no weight or body mass index restrictions on patient eligibility for abortion. Among those with a weight limit, the most common upper boundary (56%) was 300 pounds [11]. Hydraulic operating tables with lateral extensions, surgical assistants to help with retraction and visualization, large-sized surgical instruments, and adequate pain control are helpful in providing surgical abortions for obese women.

Comparison of labor induction versus D&E abortion

Historically in the USA, the method of abortion also has been an important risk factor. In a large prospective study of second-trimester abortion complications published in 1985, D&E was safer than instillation procedures using urea-prostaglandin or hypertonic saline [12]. According to legal abortion mortality data collected by the US Centers for Disease Control and Prevention (CDC) from 1972 to 1987, the number of deaths per 100,000 abortions was 0.5 for first-trimester vacuum curettage procedures, 3.7 for D&E, 7.1 for instillation abortions, and 51.6 for hysterotomy/hysterectomy [13]. At gestational ages of more than 20 weeks the difference in mortality rates for D&E and instillation procedures narrowed and was statistically nonsignificant for the period 1983 to 1987, presaging a trend that has continued in ensuing years.

More recent clinical reports suggest that if the higher rate of retained placenta associated with induction abortion can be overcome, medical procedures and D&E may have similar overall complication rates. Autry et al [14] retrospectively compared 297 pregnant women from 14 to 24 weeks' gestation undergoing either D&E or medical induction by a variety of methods. Apart from failed inductions, the only statistically significant difference was the high incidence of retained placenta (21%) in patients who had medical abortions. Those women who received misoprostol for induction rather than prostaglandin E_2 analogs had markedly fewer complications (OR 0.2, 95% CI 0.1–0.4). In another retrospective analysis of 425 women during the period 1996 to 2001 [15], induction patients experienced more complications than D&E patients in the same institution, but most of these events were associated with prolonged membrane rupture (four of nine cases), retained placenta or hemorrhage associated with prostaglandin E_2 analogs (two of nine cases), or complications unrelated to procedure method (abruption, deep vein thrombosis, one case each). This breakdown suggests that the inherent risk profile of the induction patients was greater than for D&E patients because of underlying obstetrical or maternal conditions, as is often the case in communities where both procedures are readily available.

Three recent induction abortion studies provide encouragement that aggressive regimens of misoprostol can achieve low rates of retained placenta and low overall complication rates, with high procedure success. In a multicenter study in Uzbekistan using vaginal misoprostol 400 μg every 3 hours, the incidence of retained placenta was less than 2% (two of 120 women) [16]. A study from Edinburgh, Scotland, reported curettage in 5% of 386 women using vaginal misoprostol 400 μg every 3 hours following a loading dose of 800 μg vaginally. These women had been primed with 200 mg of mifepristone 36 to 48 hours prior. The mean induction-to-abortion interval was 6.7 hours [17]. Finally, in a retrospective analysis, Green et al [18] reported a frequency of retained placenta of 6% in 233 women who received a loading dose of 400 μg of vaginal or buccal misoprostol plus 200 μg every 6 hours. The authors used a lower dose of misoprostol because they had induced fetal demise with intra-amniotic injection of digoxin 1 day prior to induction. Clinically stable patients were allowed 4 hours for spontaneous placental expulsion before intervening surgically. Patience in permitting natural placental expulsion is an important feature of induction protocols that achieve low rates of retained placenta.

In terms of the emotional burden of undergoing labor induction compared with D&E abortion, a recent prospective study of grief response showed no significant differences in depression and grief scores among 49 women with desired but severely compromised pregnancies who self-selected their method of pregnancy termination. This unique study had low power and a high dropout rate of approximately 40% at 4- and 12-month follow-up intervals [19].

Finally, data regarding risk of future adverse obstetrical outcomes subsequent to abortion are reassuring (Chapter 16). A Danish study found no differences in women who had had a previous first-trimester medical versus surgical abortion [20]. Three US studies [21–23] have described the subsequent obstetrical outcomes of women who underwent D&E abortion with preoperative cervical preparation. Among the collective total of more than 200 subsequent pregnancies, the only adverse outcome that occurred at higher frequency than that in historical or matched controls was preterm delivery in women with prior obstetrical histories of cervical incompetence or premature membrane rupture [22]. Case-control studies of obstetrical outcomes following first-trimester vacuum abortion have been plagued with recall bias. Women with adverse health outcomes are more likely to recall and acknowledge previous induced and spontaneous abortion. Risk of nondisclosure is higher in women subjected to domestic violence and those who regard their intimate relationships as weak [24]. Scandinavian studies largely overcome these methodological limitations by identifying subjects through cross-linked birth and abortion registries. In one such study the authors

[25] matched 670 primiparas with a prior vacuum abortion to 622 primiparas and 626 secundiparas who had had no abortions; they found no significant difference in obstetrical outcomes. In a more recent registry-linked study [26], the frequency of preterm delivery was significantly higher in women with histories of induced or spontaneous abortion only when the interpregnancy interval exceeded 12 months; this study did not control for socioeconomic status or smoking during pregnancy.

Hysterotomy as a means of pregnancy termination is generally regarded as an outmoded operation and has been associated with high risk of complications. However, the procedure is on rare occasion the most prudent option as when, for example, anatomical (e.g., large fibroids obstructing the cervical canal), medical (e.g., eclamptic shock or maternal acute major organ failure), or traumatic (uterine injury) conditions compel immediate delivery, surgical repair, or both [27]. Taking into account the putative risk of rupture or hemorrhage resulting from induction-type terminations may also sway clinicians to recommend hysterotomy, especially when no D&E option is available. A recent series from a teaching hospital in India recorded 10 nonemergent hysterotomies in women electing second-trimester abortion combined with permanent sterilization. Indications were two prior cesareans (five women); placenta previa (three women); psychiatric illness (one woman); rheumatic heart disease (one woman); and epilepsy (one woman). This facility routinely provides second-trimester induction abortions using prostaglandins. The only complication was hemorrhage occurring in one patient who was treated medically without transfusion [28].

Misestimation and failure in induced abortion

Underestimation of gestational age

Underestimation of gestational age can result in preventable complications, particularly when the gestational age lies beyond the surgical skills of the provider or when cervical priming is omitted in a patient with a noncompliant cervix. Facilities providing abortion without ultrasonographic confirmation of gestational age should advise patients about this possibility during the informed consent process. Clinical dating using the patient's history and pelvic examination can sometimes be inaccurate, irrespective of clinician experience (Chapter 6). Patient anxiety, obesity, and uterine retroversion make gestational age assessment particularly challenging. As a result, providers typically obtain ultrasound confirmation when uterine size is uncertain or exceeds 12 weeks.

In a series of 15 cases of uterine perforation during D&E, the authors found underestimation of gestational age by 2 weeks or more in six patients [29]. Seven patients had not undergone preoperative ultrasonography. In three cases the surgeon unwisely proceeded with the abortion despite an assessment that cervical dilation was inadequate.

Telltale signs of underestimation during D&E include more amniotic fluid than anticipated and larger-than-expected fetal parts or umbilical cord diameter. When underestimation is suspected, the provider should stop the procedure and use ultrasonography to estimate gestational age. In the case of an early- or mid-second-trimester pregnancy with a compliant cervix, an experienced surgeon may be able to dilate the cervix safely using mechanical dilation. Usually, however, the safer strategy is to stop and prepare the cervix with osmotic dilators or prostaglandins before completing surgical evacuation. An alternative is to switch the procedure to a labor-induction abortion. Amended consents and prophylactic antibiotics are advisable in these circumstances.

Failed attempted abortion

Failed surgical abortion is rare. In a large prospective study conducted from 1975 to 1978, the proportion of failed first-trimester surgical abortions was 2.3 per 1,000 procedures [30]. According to voluntary self-reports by NAF member clinics, the frequency following first-trimester surgical abortion has remained constant during the last decade at about 0.5 per 1,000 cases; some underreporting is likely, however. Several factors increase the risk for this complication. Uterine anomalies, whether congenital (e.g., bicornuate or septate uterus) or acquired (e.g., fibroids, synechiae), are associated with a high risk of failed attempted abortion. In a study of 33,000 first-trimester abortions, the relative risk of failed abortion in women with uterine anomalies was 90 times that of women with normal anatomy; multiple prior pregnancies, early gestational age, and operator inexperience also conferred increased risk [30]. In another series, involving 25 failed vacuum abortions, four patients had septate uteri, three had rudimentary horns, and eight had tubal ectopics [31].

Recent reports have addressed the risk of failure with early surgical abortion. Using a protocol involving sensitive human chorionic gonadotropin (hCG) testing, intraoperative ultrasonography, and manual vacuum aspiration, a physician performed surgical abortions on 2,399 patients with gestations of less than 6 weeks. Only three (0.13%) required reaspirations for continuing pregnancies, which were discovered expeditiously. Three additional reaspirations were performed for hematometra [32]. Among 1,132 patients having vacuum abortions at less than 6 weeks' gestation by several experienced physicians at a large Planned Parenthood affiliate, the risk of failed abortion was 2% after rigorous follow-up [33].

Failed attempted abortion is usually recognized by immediate gross tissue examination with backlighting or the use of magnification when necessary. Clinic staff members can be trained to become proficient examiners of tissue specimens. Routine screening of tissue aspirates may on occasion uncover important ancillary findings including suspicion of hydatidiform mole, multiple gestation, or fetal deformity, disclosure of which may prove useful in genetic counseling [34].

Postoperative ultrasonography is usually diagnostic of failed attempted abortion, but formal ultrasound consultation is sometimes necessary. Collapsed sacs and small intact gestational sacs in bicornuate, septate, or large fibroid uteri, as well as cornual/interstitial implantations, can be challenging to visualize. A useful first-trimester evacuation technique with uterine duplication anomalies is to direct a malleable sound into the pregnant cavity under ultrasound guidance (Chapter 13).

In some instances, failed abortion is not recognized immediately. Patients who report persistent pregnancy symptoms after a week warrant evaluation for continuing pregnancy. However, not every woman with a failed abortion experiences or acknowledges pregnancy symptoms. Although current data do not support the need for a routine postabortion visit for all patients [35], scheduling follow-up for those with risk factors for failed abortion is prudent unless the provider unequivocally confirmed successful abortion at the time of the procedure. Low-sensitivity urine hCG assays offer a simple and inexpensive means of screening patients after surgical abortion. A positive latex-agglutination hCG slide test (sensitivity of about 1,500 to 2,000 mIU/ml) 2 weeks after surgical abortion warrants assessment for retained placenta, ongoing pregnancy, or gestational trophoblastic disease. When failed abortion is diagnosed, most patients choose to undergo repeat uterine evacuation, as did all patients in the aforementioned series by Kaunitz [30] and Valle [31].

Failed attempted abortion may or may not adversely affect obstetrical outcomes in women who continue their pregnancies. Data are limited to small case series. A recent US single-institution report described 18 failed attempted vacuum abortions, 11 (60%) of which occurred at 7 weeks' gestation or less. By 6 weeks after the procedure, only 12 failures (67%) had been discovered. Seven patients elected to continue their pregnancies, and another four exceeded the upper-gestational-age limit for an abortion. Among these 11 continuing pregnancies, seven (77%) had complications: growth restriction occurred in two; preterm labor in two, and premature membrane rupture in three. In all, eight of 11 newborns survived. Two mothers had postpartum depression and seven expressed guilt, underscoring the potential emotional burden of experiencing traumatic obstetrical outcomes after a reversal of the initial decision to abort [36].

Retained tissue

Incomplete abortion

Retained products of conception is one of the more common complications of surgical abortion. Worldwide, the frequency of reaspiration after first-trimester surgical abortion varies from 0.29 to 1.96% and in the second trimester, from 0.40 to 2.70% (Table 15.2).

Women with retained products commonly present with lower abdominal pain and bleeding. Although symptoms usually arise within the first week, patients with subtle symptoms may not seek immediate attention. Infection occurs infrequently provided the operators are well trained, use sterile technique, and the uterus has not been injured. The uterus may feel enlarged and soft, and ultrasonography reveals a heterogeneous echo complex in the cavity. However, gray-scale ultrasonography and bimanual uterine examination cannot distinguish between retained products of conception and hematometra unless placental tissue protrudes from the cervical os or fetal bone is seen on ultrasonography [37]. Also, intrauterine collections of varying echogenicity represent normal ultrasound findings after surgical abortion and do not usually warrant intervention in asymptomatic women [38,39].

The pathology report after reaspiration may also be unhelpful or misleading. In a pilot study with a convenience sample of 200 women undergoing first- and second-trimester surgical abortions by a single experienced operator, a pathologist identified scattered villi microscopically in 32% of specimens obtained by repeat vacuum curettage for 30 seconds immediately after clinically complete evacuation (Christensen D, 1995, unpublished observations). Thus, the presence of villi on pathology slides after successful surgical abortion is an expected finding and is not diagnostic of retained tissue.

After surgical abortion, small amounts of retained products may pass spontaneously, avoiding the need for further intervention. If large amounts of tissue are left, the patient is at risk for bleeding and infection. Endometritis following untreated incomplete abortion can evolve into salpingitis and, occasionally, sepsis [53]. Therefore, prompt vacuum reaspiration or prostaglandin therapy (e.g., misoprostol 800 μg vaginally) is the treatment in symptomatic cases; sharp metal curettage should not be used as the primary means of evacuation. Aspiration is preferred over expectant or medical management if signs of infection, hemorrhage, severe pain, or serious anemia are present. Antibiotic treatment after reevacuation is optional unless the provider suspects infection.

Thoroughness is the key in reducing the risk of retained products after surgical abortion. Proper surgical technique includes positioning the vacuum cannula well into the endometrial cavity and suctioning until tissue is no longer forthcoming; a gritty sensation is often detectable as the cannula moves against the emptied uterine cavity (Chapter 10). Intraoperative ultrasonography may be helpful in difficult cases. Although some clinicians perform a sharp curette check at the end of the procedure, no data exist concerning the advisability of this practice and it may carry some risk.

Hematometra

Hematometra refers to accumulation of blood in the uterine cavity. This gynecological term is preferable to obsolete

Table 15.2 Frequency of reaspiration[a] after induced abortion

Study	Study Period	Facility	Gestational Age (weeks LMP)	Total Patients	Comments	Frequency of Re-aspiration (%)
Grimes et al [40]	1971–1975	Multicenter, mostly inpatient (USA)	13–24	11,254	Induction with $PGF_{2\alpha}$ ($n = 1{,}241$) Induction with saline ($n = 10{,}013$)	36.10 28.27
Peterson et al [41]	1972–1981	One hospital clinic (USA)	13–22	11,720	Surgeon experience related. Some acute and some remote in time	0.30
Hakim-Elahi et al [5]	1971–1987	Freestanding clinics (USA)	≤14	170,000	Repeat suction on day of surgery: 0.18% (88% = hematometra) Repeat suction subsequently: 0.17%	0.35
Hodgson & Portmann [42]	1972–1973	Freestanding clinic (USA)	≤12	10,453	Retained tissue	0.43
Wulff & Freiman [43]	1973–1976	Freestanding clinic (USA)	≤14	16,410	Failed and incomplete abortion	0.54
Wadhera [44]	1975–1980	Hospitals (Canada)	≤13 (84% of cases)	351,879	Retained products of conception	1.96
Hill & MacKenzie [45]	1976–1987	Hospital (Great Britain)	14–19 (88% of cases) Induction, PGE_2	2,308	Readmission for surgical evaluation	1.40
Hern [46]	1977–1982	Freestanding clinic (USA)	17–25 (D&E plus urea)	1,000	Repeat aspiration, acute or remote	2.70
Altman et al [47]	1979–1980	Hospital (USA)	13–18 (83% of cases) Evacuation primarily by vacuum aspiration	1,392	Repeat aspiration	0.36
Jacot et al [48]	1986–1990	Hospital–attached clinic (Canada)	≤14 (vacuum) 15–20 (D&E)	3,225 547	Incomplete abortion Incomplete abortion	0.90 0.40
NAF [49]	1992–1995	Freestanding clinics (USA)	≤13 (87% of cases)	1,024,428	Repeat procedures (voluntary self-reporting)	0.29
Hern [50]	1990–1999	Freestanding clinic (USA)	18–34 Oxytocin induction	1,677	Reaspiration	1.60
Pridmore & Chambers [51]	1992–1998	Public ambulatory surgery center (Australia)	4–13	11,982	Need for repeat aspiration	1.65
Choudhary et al [28]	1997–2001	Teaching hospital (India)	≤12	961	Failed plus incomplete abortions	1.46
Patel et al [52]	2002–2003	19 affiliated outpatient clinics (USA)	12–23 6/7	2,218	One case only (associated with a perforation)	0.05
Kapp et al [16]	2006	13 maternity hospitals (Tashkent, Uzbekistan)	14–24 Induction MSP or saline/PGF	108 saline/PGF 120 MSP	Curettage for retained placenta (routinely performed after saline inductions by some physicians in this study)	64.8 1.7

[a] The terms repeat aspiration, reaspiration, and repeat suctioning are those of the investigators and are synonymous.
NAF = National Abortion Federation; MSP = misoprostol; PGF = prostaglandin $F_{2\alpha}$

descriptions such as "postabortal syndrome," "redo syndrome," "postabortal pain syndrome," and retained clot. The frequency of this complication after suction curettage is about 2 per 1,000 [5,54]. In one study of 170,000 vacuum abortions, 88% of patients requiring remote aspiration (n = 285) had hematometra rather than retained products of conception [5]. Studies comparing general anesthesia with local anesthesia have not shown differences in the frequency of hematometra [5].

The volume of liquid and clotted blood varies, as does the timing of presentation. For example, accumulation of 250 to 1500 ml of blood causes low midline pelvic pressure and cramping within 15 minutes and up to several hours after the procedure. When large volumes of blood are sequestered in the uterus, hypotension may occur. Alternatively, patients may have vasovagal reactions from the pain of uterine distension. Accumulations of less than 100 ml are more common and can remain asymptomatic, even for a few weeks. Patients may have sudden expulsion of clots, pelvic pressure, and mild fever. Typically, pelvic examination reveals an enlarged, firm, and tender uterus; ultrasonography shows an intrauterine heterogeneous echo complex (Fig. 15.1). The process is often self-limiting and responds immediately to repeat suctioning. Reaspiration can be accomplished with an electric suction machine, manual vacuum aspirator, or even wall suction in an emergency department. Mild temperature elevations are usually not indicative of infection; these usually resolve rapidly with reevacuation, regardless of antibiotic coverage.

Prophylactic uterotonic agents may reduce the risk of postabortal hematometra, although data are sparse. Approaches include oral ergot derivatives, such as ergonovine 0.1 mg intramuscularly or intracervically, or low-dose locally administered vasopressin [55,56]. Small intrauterine accumulations of blood visible on ultrasonography after surgical abortion are normal, may take several days to dissolve or expel, and should be regarded as a natural physiologic event that seldom requires intervention [38,39,57].

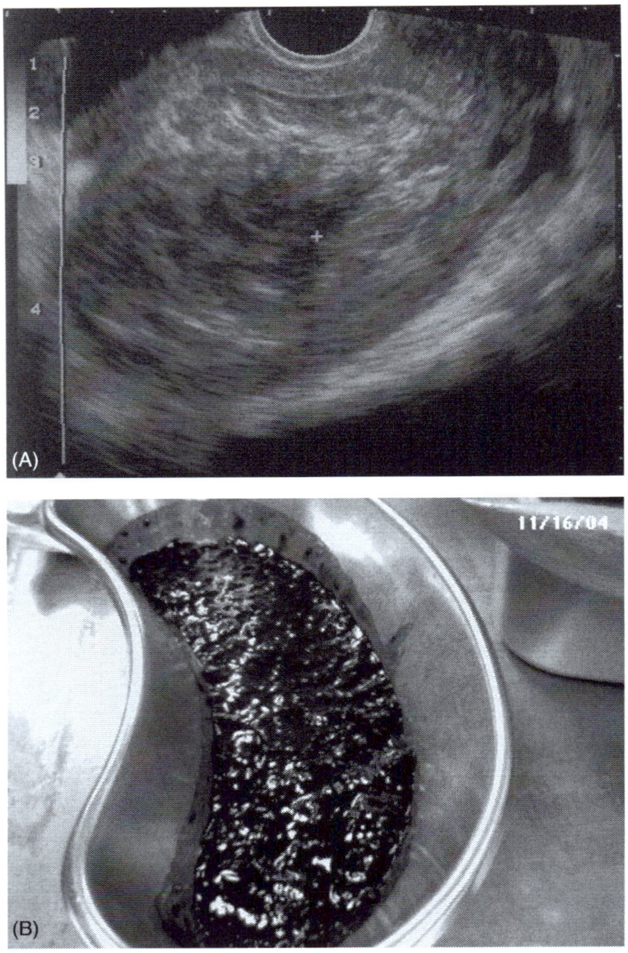

Figure 15.1 (A) Transvaginal ultrasound image showing intracavitary heterogeneous echoes in a patient with hematometra diagnosed 4 days after aspiration abortion at 12 weeks' gestation. (B) Uterine reaspiration yielded approximately 150 cc of blood clots and serum only.

Hemorrhage

Uterine hemorrhage associated with abortion can result from cervical laceration, perforation, retained tissue, uterine atony or rupture, uterine scar-related problems, arteriovenous malformations, placental abnormalities (accreta, increta and percreta), or coagulopathy. Because of the poor validity of estimates of blood loss and varying definitions of hemorrhage, sound comparisons of incidence are elusive. Over time, however, incidence rates in North America have trended downward, possibly reflecting greater surgical experience and more skill in the use of uterotonic agents (Table 15.3). The rare frequency of blood transfusion provides a better measure of serious blood loss.

Surgical inexperience and gestations beyond 10 weeks are associated with increased risk of uterine hemorrhage. Other risk factors include advanced maternal age and parity [62], prior cesarean delivery, number of uterine scars, uterine fibroids, and history of excessive postabortal or postpartum bleeding. By reducing uterine tone, halogenated anesthetic gases may also increase the risk of blood loss.

Several measures may reduce blood loss with abortion. Administration of vasopressin 4 units with paracervical anesthesia reduces bleeding with second-trimester D&E, and the effect increases with gestational age [63]. Peterson et al reported a decrease in the incidence of blood loss exceeding 500 ml from 9 per 1,000 D&Es to 2 per 1,000 in a large (n = 12,000) single-institution series after 1 ml of vasopressin was added to the local cervical anesthetic [41]. Pridmore and Chambers found similar improvement when 5 μg/ml of epinephrine was added to the intracervical block (n = 5,700 patients) [51]. Another study reported that local vasopressin produced a 50% reduction in blood loss at all gestations before 13 weeks [64].

Table 15.3 Single-institution reports of hemorrhage rates with induced abortion.

Study	Study Period	Facility	Abortion Method	Gestational Age (weeks LMP)	Total Patients	Blood Loss >250 ml/1,000 Cases	Comments
Hakim-Elahi et al [5]	1971–1987	Freestanding clinics (USA)	Vacuum aspiration	≤14	170,000	0.07[a]	No difference in morbidity between local (75%) and general (25%) anesthesia
Hodgson & Portmann [42]	1972–1973	Freestanding clinic (USA)	Vacuum aspiration	≤12	10,453	None	93% of patients <10 weeks LMP
Bozorgi [58]	1973–1974	Freestanding clinic (USA)	Vacuum aspiration	≤14	10,890	1.5	72% of patients <11 weeks LMP; 28% of patients 11–14 weeks LMP Increased incidence if surgeon less experienced
Wulff & Freiman [43]	1973–1976	Freestanding clinic (USA)	Vacuum aspiration	≤14	16,400	0.7	64% of patients <11 weeks LMP; 36% of patients 11–14 weeks LMP
Hodari et al [59]	1974–1976	Hospital (USA)	Vacuum aspiration	13–15	2,500	12.0[b]	97% of patients 13–15 weeks LMP No osmotic dilators used General anesthesia used in all cases, but agent(s) unspecified Oxytocin 10 units IV after operation completed Mean operating time 13 minutes
Pahl & Lundy [60]	1975–1977	Hospital (USA)	Saline, $PGF_{2\alpha}$, or both	13–25	1,839	20.0[c]	
Peterson et al [41]	1972–1981	One hospital clinic (USA)	D&E	13–22	11,720	0.9[d]	Incidence fell to 0.2% after 1 ml of vasopressin was added to the cervical anesthetic
Hill & MacKenzie [45]	1976–1987	Hospital (Great Britain)	Induction, PGE_2	14–19 (88% of cases)	2,308	5.6[b]	
Hern [46]	1977–1982	Freestanding clinic (USA)	D&E plus urea	17–25	1,000	21.0[d]	
Altman et al [47]	1979–1980	Hospital (USA)	Vacuum aspiration	13–18 (83% of cases)	1,392	8.6[c]	
Hern [50]	1990–1999	Freestanding clinic (USA)	Induction with oxytocin; digoxin or urea to cause fetal demise	18–34	1,677	38.0[d]	Only 3/27 required transfusion, 2 of whom had DIC
Choudhary et al [28]	1997–2001	Teaching hospital (India)	Vacuum aspiration	≤12	961	0.3	All were treated medically
Castleman et al [61]	1999–2002	Teaching hospital (Hanoi, Vietnam)	D&E	12–18	439	2.3	The only case had a large fibroid uterus
Patel et al [52]	2002–2003	19 affiliated outpatient clinics (USA)	D&E	12–23 6/7	2,218	4.1[d]	4 of 10 were associated with uterine perforation

[a] Enumerates only patients who required hospitalizations.
[b] Enumerates only patients who required transfusion.
[c] Blood loss >500 ml or patient required transfusion.
[d] Blood loss >500 ml.
DIC = disseminated intravascular coagulopathy.

Uterine atony

Uterine atony is a potentially serious complication of induced abortion. Clinicians should consider it whenever excessive blood loss occurs during or after an abortion.

Depending on the severity of bleeding, treatment may proceed sequentially or concomitantly. Treatment options include manual uterine massage, dilute intravenous oxytocin, intramuscular ergot derivatives, and low-dose cervical vasopressin injections (e.g., 4 to 6 pressor units injected in the paracervical tissue as part of cervical anesthesia). Intraoperative use of the four classes of uterotonic agents (oxytocin, ergot, vasopressin, and prostaglandins) reduces surgical blood loss in abortion, particularly after the first trimester. Elaborated at separate gene sites, they probably work synergistically to control bleeding.

For treating atony, rectal misoprostol has largely replaced intramuscular carboprost (250 μg, repeated every 15 minutes up to eight doses) in many centers as the initial high-intensity option. Five tablets per rectum (1000 μg) usually stop bleeding within a few minutes [65] and this regimen is both less expensive and potentially less noxious (vomiting, diarrhea, transient fever) than carboprost. Higher-dose vasopressin (10 units) in 20 ml of crystalloid, administered transcervically into the myometrium at multiple sites, produces rapid vasoconstriction that may last for up to 45 minutes.

Intrauterine tamponade with plain gauze [66] or with vasopressin- or thrombin-soaked [67] gauze packing can be an effective temporizing or therapeutic measure; so can balloon catheters [68]. Foley catheters with 30- to 75-ml balloons are standard equipment in many operative settings and have been inflated safely beyond their stated capacity in emergencies [68,69] with good clinical outcomes. For uterine cavities capable of greater distension, a larger intrauterine catheter [70] can inflate to volumes of 250 ml.

Surgical measures include encircling sutures around the uterus, hypogastric [71] or uterine artery ligation [72], and hysterectomy. B-Lynch [73] described a single suture surrounding the uterine wall. Of the simplified versions published since then [74,75], the modification by Pereira [76] is the only one that avoids entry into the uterus. A single-institution series of 28 postpartum cases using primarily the B-Lynch technique reported success in 82%. Among seven of these patients who underwent subsequent repeat cesareans, grooves or mild adhesions of the uterine serosa were observed in four cases [77]. Data are too limited to evaluate any effect on future fertility. Effective use of a Bakri balloon (Appendix, Fig. A-14) together with a B-Lynch compression suture has been reported [78].

Angiographic embolization is another treatment option for refractory atony [79,80]. Borgatta summarized 11 unpublished and seven published cases of embolization use in women undergoing spontaneous or induced abortions; three cases had atony as a contributing diagnosis. Seventeen of 18 women had successful treatment, including all 11 women with pregnancies beyond 14 weeks' gestation [79]. Angiographic embolization has clinical limitations; it takes about 1 hour to set up after the radiology team is assembled. It may be inadequate to treat multiple vessel injuries accompanying a large uterine laceration, and its success with placenta accreta/increta/percreta is mixed [79,80]. Occasionally, cases refractory to occlusion of the uterine artery alone will then respond when the utero-ovarian vessels are supplementally injected with occlusive agents [79]. On occasion, radiopaque dye alone may occlude a single damaged arteriole responsible for uncontrolled hemorrhage after D&E abortion [81].

Placental abnormalities

In ultrasonography studies, the reported prevalence of second-trimester placenta previa ranges from 2 to 6%; rates are higher if low-lying placentas are included [82]. Placenta previa itself (without placenta accreta) does not complicate abortion, including D&E [83,84]. Likewise, vasa previa has not been associated with abortion-related complications [85]. In terms of the pathophysiology of benign previas, serial ultrasonography of the progressing pregnancy illustrates an upward migration of the placenta toward the fundus as the placenta seeks the more fulsome blood supply available in the fundus, resulting in the relative atrophy of the portion overlying the less well-perfused lower segment and cervix [85]. As a result, unless placenta previa actually overlies a uterine scar (usually entailing a complete or wraparound previa), risk of abnormal placental adherence is low. Laminaria insertion is safe in the presence of benign placenta previa [86]. Even when an accreta is present, *insertion* of osmotic dilators does not usually trigger uncontrollable bleeding, but their removal may. Hence, the provider must be equipped to deal immediately with life-threatening hemorrhage at the start of any procedure in which placenta accreta is known or suspected. In a case-control study, Johnson et al [87] found that repeated sharp curettage procedures (OR 2.9, 95% CI 1.0, 8.5 for $\geq$3 abortions), but not multiple vacuum aspirations (OR 1.4, 95% CI 0.6, 3.1 for $\geq$3 abortions), were associated with risk of subsequent placenta previa. This finding carries stark implications for regions where sharp curettage is still commonly practiced for induced abortion or management of spontaneous abortion.

Placenta accreta carries the risk of torrential bleeding during uterine evacuation, and its frequency may be increasing as cesarean delivery becomes more common [88]. In a large series of D&E abortions, the estimated prevalence of placenta accreta was about 0.4 per 1,000 operations. All seven patients had at least one prior cesarean delivery, and all required hysterectomy for management of hemorrhage [89]. The most recent information on the relationship between cesarean delivery and placenta accreta comes from the Maternal-Fetal Medicine Units Network [90,91]. In these obstetrical populations the risk of placenta accreta,

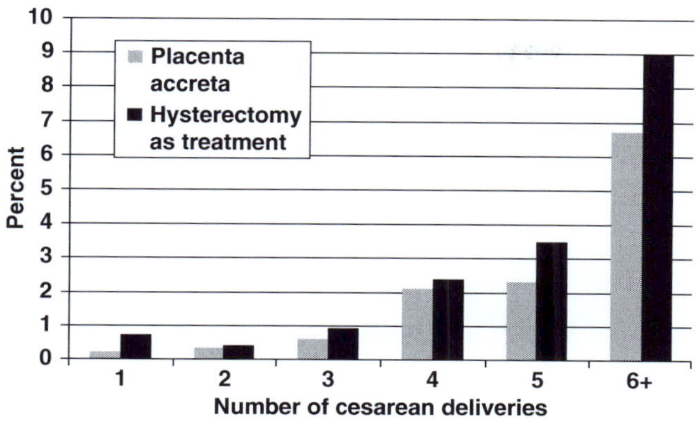

Figure 15.2 The relationship between number of cesarean deliveries and the risk of placenta accreta and hysterectomy for treatment (Data from Silver et al [90].)

and hysterectomy as its treatment, increased exponentially with the number of previous cesarean deliveries women had (Fig. 15.2).

Placenta accreta is rare in first-trimester abortion [92–94]. Second-trimester abortion patients with complete placenta previa and a history of cesarean delivery are at serious risk for placenta accreta. Placental localization for second-trimester patients with prior uterine incision may be helpful, with referral of suspicious cases to a skilled ultrasonographer. Color Doppler ultrasonography, computer-assisted tomography (CT) scanning, or magnetic resonance imaging (MRI) have varying diagnostic accuracy [95,96] (Fig. 15.3). The combination of initial color Doppler scanning (sensitivity 0.77, specificity 0.96) plus confirmatory MRI for equivocal cases (sensitivity 0.88, specificity 1.0) has been effective [97].

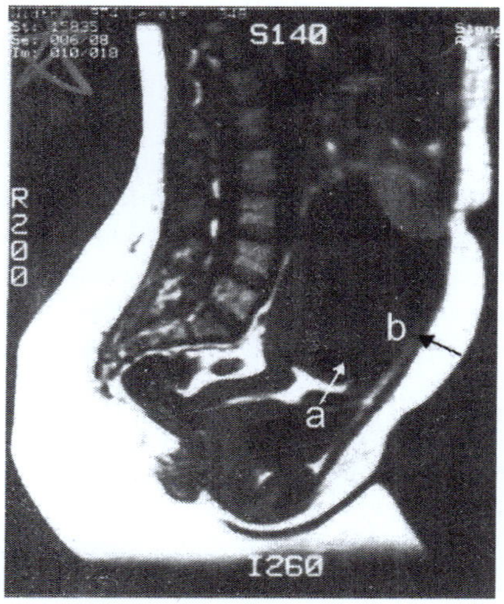

Figure 15.3 Magnetic resonance imaging (MRI) ruled out placenta accreta in a woman 23 weeks pregnant with placenta previa and a history of three prior cesarean deliveries. Sagittal T2-weighted image through the placenta previa. Normal placenta (a) remains dark and does not invade the anterior scar tissue (b), which remains lucid throughout.

Angiographic embolization has been used with mixed results to treat unremitting hemorrhage from placenta accreta following D&E. Borgatta [79] reported four successful preoperative embolizations among eight patients with high radiological suspicion of placenta accreta. These women underwent surgical abortion at or after 12 weeks' gestation. Steinauer and colleagues [80] reported successful uterine artery embolization in 38 of 42 patients. The four treatment failures had histologic confirmation of placenta accreta (increta or percreta) after hysterectomy. Eight women with cervical lacerations or perforations had successful embolizations.

When placenta accreta is suspected, performing the D&E in a hospital with full blood-bank capabilities is prudent. Second-trimester labor induction is contraindicated. The preoperative treatment plan should include extensive family counseling and mobilization of staff and supplies necessary to perform emergency hysterectomy with massive blood and clotting-factor replacement. Preoperative placement of an angiographic port is advisable in high-risk cases, especially those that suggest bladder involvement (placenta percreta). Prophylactic stenting of the ureter(s) deserves consideration as well. For select cases, allowing the adherent placenta to remain *in situ* is an option [98], sometimes in conjunction with administration of methotrexate to promote its reabsorption. Because these measures entail some risk of remote bleeding as well as infection [98] and no studies are available to gauge their overall benefit versus risk, expert consultation is advisable when contemplating their use.

Arteriovenous malformation

Uterine arteriovenous malformation (AVM) of the endometrium, a rare but life-threatening condition, can be congenital or acquired. Operations, trauma, infection, or neoplasm (e.g., gestational trophoblastic disease or carcinoma) can lead to abnormal communication between arteries and veins. With color Doppler ultrasound, CT scan, MRI, or angiography, an AVM appears as a loosely arrayed bundle of inchoate vessels resembling the findings seen at the site of a placenta accreta; hence they are sometimes misdiagnosed, one for the other [94].

An AVM can produce massive bleeding unresponsive to standard uterotonic therapy. In other instances, heavy or moderate persistent bleeding can occur hours, days, or months later. Hemorrhage associated with AVM has occurred spontaneously [99] and following spontaneous abortion [100], early medical abortion [101], and surgical abortion in the first [102] and second trimesters [103]. Conservative management has been successful for milder presentations [101], but serious bleeding warrants angiographic embolization, which has often been therapeutic, with anecdotal reports of subsequent successful delivery in five cases [104].

Disseminated intravascular coagulopathy

Disseminated intravascular coagulopathy (DIC) is an infrequent but dangerous complication. First-trimester frequency ranges from 0.0 to 0.08% [48,105] (Lichtenberg ES, 1995, unpublished observations) and in the second trimester, 0.0 to 0.5% [40,49,106]. The risk of DIC increases with advanced gestational age, prolonged fetal death, abruptio placentae, placenta previa or accreta, amniotic fluid embolism, and massive blood loss. DIC can follow an uncomplicated D&E in a patient without preexisting conditions (idiopathic DIC). In dedicated pregnancy termination facilities with experienced surgeons, idiopathic DIC is the most common clinical presentation of this condition. Intravascular infusion of amniotic fluid during the operation has long been hypothesized to trigger the clotting cascade, with the coagulopathy first becoming evident in the recovery room. In reality, fetal cells are invariably present in the maternal circulation beginning in early pregnancy, and no compelling evidence has explained why most pregnancies avoid this complication despite the obvious admixing of maternal and fetal elements in the maternal circulation.

In abortion practice, recognition of DIC is complicated by its infrequency, mimicry, and insidious onset. What begins as normal or absent bleeding may evolve into accumulation of intrauterine clot resembling postabortal hematometra before ultimately manifesting as DIC. The transformation from clotted bleeding to serosanguineous flow may take from 30 minutes to 6 hours or more. Differential diagnoses include uterine atony and operative trauma. Aggressive uterotonic therapy, reaspiration, and thorough digital examination of the uterus help to exclude these other conditions.

A coagulation panel is useful but not essential. Drops in fibrinogen level and platelet count and increased fibrinogen degradation products (fibrin split monomer) or D-dimer (molecules resulting from fibrinolysis of thrombi) are the most sensitive indices. Clinicians can diagnose DIC early in its course with a simple bedside test: failure of 10 cc of whole blood to produce a retracted, stable clot in a plain glass tube within 5 to 10 minutes indicates impaired clotting. Conversely, the presence of a solid clot excludes DIC from the differential diagnosis at that time.

Once the diagnosis of DIC is made, therapy consists of clotting factors and volume replacement and, if needed, red cell transfusions. Rapid treatment may forestall progression of DIC. Therefore, one or two large (16 to 18 gauge) intravenous ports should be established for rapid infusion. True blood loss may substantially exceed measured blood loss, because DIC is a systemic process involving small vessels throughout the body. When administered early in DIC, as little as 2 to 4 units of fresh frozen plasma (FFP) usually restore clotting function; occasionally, 5 to 8 units or more are needed. Each standard unit of FFP (200 to 250 ml) raises fibrinogen levels about 25 mg/dl. Although FFP derived from AB-negative donors is usual, specimens from AB-positive donors can be utilized safely if the patient receives full dose Rh-immune globulin.

Cryoprecipitate is another important acceptable clotting factor replacement. It is the cold precipitable fraction of FFP suspended in a minimal plasma volume and refrozen. Cryoprecipitate contains only fibrinogen (200–300 mg), factor VIII:C (80–120 units), von Willebrand factor, fibronectin, and factor XIII. Like FFP, cryoprecipitate is type-specific, has a shelf life of 1 year, and can be thawed rapidly by microwave. About 14 units are required to raise fibrinogen 100 mg/dl. The selection and number of units of products can be coordinated with blood bank personnel and guided by the severity of the coagulopathy; it has the advantage of equal effect at lower replacement volume but is more expensive.

Recombinant activated factor VII (rFVIIa) is a powerful, costly (US$9,000 to $18,000) synthetic procoagulant therapy [107]. Where available, it can serve as a last resort for unremitting hemorrhage because of tissue injury or coagulopathy [108]. Onset of action typically occurs 10 to 30 minutes after infusion. Thrombosis is a rare complication, mostly among patients extensively immobilized during convalescence.

Transfusion with packed red blood cells deserves consideration when orthostasis, confusion, or oliguria persist after volume replacement with crystalloid or plasma expanders. In a normal adult, blood volume comprises 8% of body weight (5,600 ml in a 70-kg [154-lb] adult). Young, healthy women with continuing acute blood loss below a hematocrit range of 15 to 19% may require transfusion [109,110]. Earlier transfusion may be indicated in women with cardiovascular or respiratory disease. Because the hematocrit does not equilibrate for several hours after acute blood loss, treatment is guided by a combination of blood pressure, pulse, urine output, and clinical judgment, and not solely by serial hematocrit levels. Attentive monitoring is the rule and should include periodic orthostatic vital signs, vaginal pad counts, measurement of urine output (>25–30 ml/hour), inspection for cutaneous bleeding sites, evaluation of patient consciousness, and serial hematocrit determinations and clotting indices. Cessation of vaginal bleeding is often the first sign of successful therapy. Once uncomplicated DIC is reversed, it rarely recurs.

Infection

Endoparametritis

Worldwide, the frequency of infection after first-trimester surgical abortion varies widely from 0.1 to 4.7% (Table 15.4). This disparity reflects differences in method of ascertainment, definition of infection, and inclusion of outpatient cases. In the second trimester, infection rates with both medical and surgical abortion methods have remained within the narrow range of 0.4 to 2% in North America and Great Britain, except during the 1970s when instillation regimens

Table 15.4 Frequency of infection following first-trimester vacuum aspiration abortion.

Study	Study Period	Facility	Gestational Age (Weeks LMP)	Total Patients	Antibiotic Prevention	Criteria for Diagnosis of Infection	Frequency of Infection (%)
Hakim-Elahi et al [5]	1971–1987	Freestanding clinics (USA)	≤14	170,000	None	Fever was not a requisite criterion Any pelvic tenderness Suspicious history	0.46
Hodgson & Portmann [42]	1972–1973	Freestanding clinic (USA)	≤12	10,453	Infrequently	Pain, fever, bleeding	0.28
Wulff & Freiman [43]	1973–1976	Freestanding clinic (USA)	≤14	16,400	Yes	Temp. ≥38°C ≥1 day	0.10
Wadhera [44]	1975–1980	Hospitals (Canada)	≤13	351,879	Variable	Not specified	0.18
Heisterberg & Kringelbach [111]	1980–1985	Hospital (Denmark)	≤12	5,851	None	Temp. ≥38°C Antibiotic therapy	2.40 3.20
Fried et al [112]	1987	Hospital (Sweden)	≤15	1,000	Preoperative doxycycline if chlamydia culture was positive	Not specified	4.70
Choudhary et al [28]	1997–2001	Teaching hospital (India)	≤12	961	Two oral antibiotics for each patient	Excessive discharge plus lower abdominal or adnexal tenderness; all were treated orally	1.8

of induction abortion were still being refined (Table 15.5). Higher rates reported in Scandinavia could in part reflect the larger number of providers, each of whom do a small number of cases annually, as well as more sensitive clinical triggers for invoking the diagnosis.

Typically, signs and symptoms of postabortal endometritis arise within the first few days. Some combination of reported pain, fever, pelvic tenderness, and white count elevation is usually, but not invariably, present. The cervix should be tested for sexually transmitted pathogens; blood or uterine cultures are rarely informative. Because untreated infection can result in chronic pelvic pain, dyspareunia, infertility, and, on occasion, sepsis, a high index of suspicion and expedient treatment are warranted.

Established risk factors for postabortal infection include age less than 20 years; previous pelvic inflammatory disease (PID); and the presence of sexually transmitted pathogens in the cervix at the time of abortion, particularly chlamydia [114–116] or gonorrhea. Studies of prophylactic treatment of bacterial vaginosis are of limited quality and thus inconclusive [117] (Chapter 7). Most postabortal infections occur in women without these risk factors.

Two randomized trials have addressed the efficacy of vaginal cleansing to prevent postabortal infection before surgical abortion. Chlorhexidine digluconate was not found superior to sterile saline washing or no vaginal preparation. Prophylactic antibiotics were not used in either study [118,119].

Administration of prophylactic antibiotics reduces the risk of infection following surgical abortion by about 40%[120]. This protective effect was evident not only in women with antecedent risk factors (history of PID, positive preoperative chlamydia culture, or preoperative bacterial vaginosis), but also in low-risk groups. Two recent US prevalence studies [121,122] showed that carriage rates of chlamydia and gonorrhea are highest among Black women and lowest among White women by a factor of two to four times, with higher rates found among females age 14 to 19 years and highest rates among those with a history of gonorrhea or chlamydia in the previous 12 months. At a large public hospital pregnancy termination clinic in the USA, 11.4 and 2.6% of women tested positive during 2006 for chlamydia and gonorrhea, respectively [123]. Knowing prevalence data in a specific demographic population seeking abortion may influence strategies for postabortal infection prevention (e.g., screen-and-treat versus routine coverage). Routine perioperative antibiotic coverage may prevent up to half of all postabortal infections in the USA and is highly cost-effective.

The optimum drug regimen for routine antibiotic prevention remains unclear. Most studies have used tetracyclines or nitroimidazoles (e.g., metronidazole or tinidazole). Penicillins, erythromycin, and ofloxacin are superior to placebo but were used in only one study each [120]. No randomized trial has compared routine preoperative versus postoperative antibiotic treatment in preventing postabortal infection. In the UK, the Royal College of Obstetricians and Gynaecologists (RCOG) recommends a more aggressive approach: presumptive therapy of chlamydia with doxycycline or azithromycin plus anaerobic bacteria coverage with rectal metronidazole, rather than short-course prophylaxis. However, the RCOG guidance also acknowledges that "other regimens may be equally appropriate"[124].

Ascending genital tract infections are typically polymicrobial, and patients who present with serious postabortal infection should receive a full course of broad-spectrum antibiotic therapy. Retained tissue evident clinically or radiographically warrants prompt reaspiration after an initial loading dose of antibiotics. Oral antibiotic treatment with one or more antibiotics is acceptable in a compliant patient who can tolerate the medications and has a favorable prognosis for cure in that she is not immunocompromised, severely ill, or suspected to have a tubo-ovarian abscess. A US multicenter trial has demonstrated effective outpatient treatment of mild-to-moderate PID in this favorable-prognosis group, including long-term follow-up of fertility preservation, using a single 2-gm injection of cefoxitin plus a single dose of 1 gm of probenecid orally followed by 100 mg of oral doxycycline twice daily for 14 days [125]. If patients fail to improve after 2 to 3 days of oral medication, parenteral therapy is warranted. For the period 1991 to 2001 in California, PID hospitalization rates declined by 62% and those for tubo-ovarian abscess decreased by 33%, possibly representing a shift to more outpatient therapy of PID [126].

Toxic shock syndromes

Toxic shock syndromes, heralded by shortness of breath, malaise, tachycardia, hypotension, and major organ system failure, are serious infections resulting from elaboration of bacterial cytotoxins that systemically attack integral cellular functions affecting vascular permeability, such as mitochondrial homeostasis [127]. These infections usually result in rapid multisystem deterioration and death. Sutkin and colleagues [128] reported acute onset of these symptoms 8 hours after insertion of a second set of laminaria prior to D&E abortion. Broad-spectrum antibiotics successfully treated amnionitis resulting from heavy growth of *Staphylococcus aureus* with staphylococcal enterotoxin C expression, permitting surgery to go forward. Mourton and Rich [129] have reported survival of a patient with classic findings of toxic shock syndrome 12 hours after endometrial biopsy. Her blood cultures grew Group A β-hemolytic *Streptococcus*. After fluid resuscitation and broad-spectrum antibiotics, she underwent total abdominal hysterectomy and bilateral salpingo-oophorectomy. The operative specimen was not tested for the presence of cytotoxins.

In addition to some strains of *Staphylococcus aureus* and group A *Streptococcus*, certain clostridial strains can also elaborate cytotoxins. *Clostridium perfringens* (formerly *welchii*) is the most common clostridial organism; like all clostridial

Table 15.5 Frequency of infection following second-trimester abortion.

Study	Study Period	Facility	Abortion Method	Gestational Age (Weeks LMP)	Total Patients	Antibiotic Prevention	Criteria for Diagnosis of Infection	Rate of Infection (%)
Grimes et al [113]	1971–1975	Multicenter, mostly inpatient (USA)	D&E	13–20	6,213	Unknown	Temp. ≥38°C for ≥1 day	1.34
							Endometritis	0.85
Hodari et al [59]	1974–1976	Hospital (USA)	D&E	13–18	2,500	13.4%	Temp. >38°C for ≥3 days and/or hospitalized for ≥2 days	0.40
Peterson et al [41]	1972–1981	One hospital clinic (USA)	D&E	13–22	11,720	100%	Temp. >38°C for ≥2 days after the first 24 hours	From 1.0 to 0.5 (p <0.004) after tetracycline routinized
Hill & MacKenzie [45]	1976–1987	Hospital (Great Britain)	Induction, PGE_2	14–19 (88% of cases)	2,308	1.9%	Two proven and six suspected cases	0.40
Hern [46]	1977–1982	Freestanding clinic (USA)	D&E plus urea	17–25	1,000	98.0%	Uterine tenderness responsive to outpatient antibiotics or brief temp. ≥38°C	0.60
Jacot et al [48]	1986–1990	Hospital-attached clinic (Quebec, Canada)	D&E	15–20	547	≥17 weeks LMP or history of PID	Any	2.00
							Three or more criteria (abdominal pain, uterine or adnexal tenderness, temp. ≥38°C for one day, elevated WBC or ESR, positive findings with laparoscopy)	0.70
							Hospitalization	0.40
Hern [50]	1990–1999	Freestanding clinic (USA)	Oxytocin induction; digoxin or urea to cause fetal demise	18–34	1,677	100%	All cases associated with PROM	0.30
Patel et al [52]	2002–2003	19 affiliated outpatient clinics (USA)	D&E	12–23 6/7	2,218	Not stated	One case only (sepsis/DIC/death)	0.05

WBC = white blood cells; ESR = erythrocyte sedimentation rate; LMP = last menstrual period; PID = pelvic inflammatory disease; PROM = premature membrane rupture; DIC = disseminated intravascular coagulopathy.

species, it is a spore-forming, rod-shaped, gram-positive anaerobe found predominantly in soil and contaminated water, and thereby in the intestines of grazing animals and humans. Experts theorize that anal-vaginal contamination results in vaginal carriage and that in some individuals these bacteria ascend the genital tract postpartum and after spontaneous or induced abortion [130]. *Clostridium sordellii* is a rare clostridial species found in about 1% of clostridial cultures. As of April 2008, seven deaths have occurred from clostridial infection in North American women undergoing first-trimester medical abortion. Six women used the evidence-based protocol of 200-mg mifepristone followed in 1 to 3 days by 800 μg of vaginal misoprostol, and one woman used mifepristone with buccal misoprostol. All exhibited a toxic shock-like presentation with absent or low fever, insidious onset, hemoconcentration, multiorgan failure and rapid demise. *Clostridium sordellii* was identified in six of these seven infections by a gene probe specific to this organism; the other case was identified as *Clostridium perfringens*. One case was reported from Quebec Province, Canada [131]; four cases, all from California, were reported by the CDC where bacteriologic subtyping identified each as associated with *Clostridium sordellii* [132]. Comparison by the CDC of the medication lot numbers eliminated pill contamination as a cause of infection [132].

Although reports have identified prolonged asymptomatic vaginal carriage of *C. sordellii* in 0.5 to 10% of healthy women, the precise etiology of this cluster of cases involving primarily an uncommon species of *Clostridium* remains unknown. From the time of its approval by the US Food and Drug Administration in 2000 until mid-2008, more than 840,000 doses of mifepristone have been sold in the USA (it is not commercially available in Canada), making the case-fatality rate from the six reported US deaths less than 1.0 per 100,000. All US *sordellii* mortalities have occurred in coastal states of the Western USA. The fatal *perfringens* case occurred in a noncoastal Western state. This distribution suggests a geographic predilection of clostridial species for certain geologic or climatic regions, and investigators are designing a large prevalence study to test this hypothesis. No reported *C. sordellii* or *perfringens* infections or toxic shock deaths have been reported among 2 million European women users of mifepristone.

Serious and often fatal clostridial infections have been reported during pregnancy unrelated to abortion and in women undergoing gynecologic procedures both in North America and Europe [130,133,134] (Zane SB, 2008, unpublished observations). One patient who had a spontaneous abortion at 18 weeks' gestation was treated after presentation with five antibiotics, dopamine, and fluid resuscitation. She is the sole surviving patient in the world literature among childbearing women infected with *C. sordellii* [130]. CDC laboratory testing confirmed that this strain of *C. sordellii* produced no lethal toxin.

In contrast to these disheartening outcomes, clinicians have achieved success by rapidly treating culture-proven clostridial endometritis following D&E abortion using peri-abortal oral doxycycline or standard broad-spectrum parenteral antibiotics, provided that the offending strain of clostridium does not produce endotoxin [135].

Pelvic abscess

Pelvic abscess is uncommon after second-trimester induced abortion and rarely occurs in the first trimester. Fifty per cent of patients with tubo-ovarian abscesses have a prior history of pelvic infection [136]. Increased susceptibility to abscess also exists in women with compromised immunity, as in those with human immunodeficiency virus/acquired immunodeficiency syndrome (HIV/AIDS) infection and high viral titers, or those debilitated and nutritionally deprived from substance abuse. Especially susceptible are women with poor nutrition and transport whose abortions are performed by untrained personnel. When these women develop infection resulting from natural occurrence, uterine injury, retained tissue, or unhygienic practices, they often experience long delays in obtaining trained medical evaluation and treatment, setting the stage for advanced infectious morbidity and mortality.

Most patients with untreated pelvic abscesses become acutely ill over time with severe abdominal or pelvic discomfort, high fevers, abdominal rebound tenderness, and exquisite adnexal pain on one or both sides. In acute, rapid-developing cases, leukocytosis is dramatic, ranging from 17,500/μl to more than 30,000/μl. Subtler and more slowly evolving cases can occur in patients with mature, walled-off abscesses or extensive adhesions from prior infection. Patients with life-threatening multiorgan involvement may present with mild or absent subjective, clinical, and laboratory findings other than severe malaise and toxic appearance because of failure of their immune system to mount an aggressive defense. Persistent low-grade fever, lack of energy, adnexal tenderness, and imaging studies point the way to diagnosis of this sometimes perplexing condition. In experienced hands, ultrasound has both high sensitivity (93%) and specificity (99%) in identifying abscesses [137].

Of the two widely used broad-spectrum intravenous antibiotic therapies, the beta-lactam-containing combination of doxycycline with cefoxitin or cefotetan has no advantage over the regimen of clindamycin plus an aminoglycoside [138]. Overall, 75% of patients with pelvic abscesses respond to medical therapy. Therapeutic surgical intervention is indicated in patients with progressive clinical deterioration and in those whose fever and pelvic pain remain unabated after 48 to 72 hours of medical therapy. Failure occurs more frequently in patients with recurrent infection; large (more than 8 cm), bilateral, or complex abscesses; compromised immunity; and chronic processes. Drainage of abscesses by ultrasound-guided needle aspiration can be highly effective in selected cases, avoiding laparotomy. Given the current array of assisted reproductive technologies, preservation of the uterus and at least one ovary is highly desirable in women with pelvic abscesses who desire future childbearing. When unilateral adnexectomy is elected for well-confined disease, risk of recurrent abscess during a woman's fertile years remains high because of residual scarring and, possibly, dormant pathogens.

Patients with sepsis require supportive care with large volumes of intravenous fluids to restore normal perfusion; pressor agents (dopamine and dobutamine) may be needed. Acute respiratory distress syndrome, DIC, and renal failure can develop rapidly. Patients who do not respond to initial measures may require hysterectomy and bilateral salpingectomy as a life-saving measure [53,139].

Postabortal endocarditis

Postabortal endocarditis is rare, difficult to diagnose, and often resistant to aggressive broad-spectrum antibiotic therapy [140]. Up to 75% of patients who develop postsurgical endocarditis have preexisting abnormalities of the heart [141] that are often asymptomatic. Predisposing conditions include prior endocarditis, whether recognized or not (rheumatic fever); existing prosthetic valve or surgical shunts; intravenous exposure through illicit drug use, injection therapy, or recent tattoos; immunocompromise (e.g., HIV/AIDS); and poor dentition with caries or chronic periodontal disease. Few affected patients have reported these conditions owing to their subtle nature or to privacy concerns. Usually a single heart valve is affected with reports of tricuspid, aortic, and pulmonic involvement, but multivalvular vegetation has also been reported [142]. Group B *Streptococcus* is the most common culprit and is uniformly sensitive to penicillin G, but absence of initial symptoms referent to the heart often results in late discovery, when the condition is far advanced. Clinical recovery, ultrasound evidence of shrinking of valvular vegetations, and improved cardiac flow gradients are encouraging signs. Refractory or pernicious cases frequently require valve replacement.

Although providers may differ in their approach to women with high-risk conditions, the American College of Obstetricians and Gynecologists does not recommend endocarditis prophylaxis for dilation and curettage, abortion, sterilization, or insertion or removal of intrauterine devices, irrespective of patient cardiac risk status [141].

Uterine injury

Low cervical tears

Lacerations of the anterior lip of the cervical portio occur most commonly when the tenaculum releases under traction. A less common type of injury can occur when a large fetal part, typically the calvarium, is pulled or expelled through the cervix. This type of tear occasionally extends several centimeters into the body of the cervix and often requires suturing, but it rarely affects large enough branches of the uterine artery to require extensive dissection.

Using atraumatic tenacula and applying traction steadily can avoid some tears. A number of techniques are available to gain a secure purchase on the cervix. These techniques include grasping a generous bite of cervical tissue; placing a tenaculum on the cervix vertically with one tooth inside the cervical canal; or using tandem tenacula, one at the 3 o'clock and the other at the 9 o'clock position of the cervicovaginal folds. In addition, use of osmotic dilators significantly reduces the risk of cervical injury during abortion [143]. Peterson reported a decrease in serious cervical trauma in early midtrimester D&E (from 0.8 to 0.4%) and later D&E (from 5.2 to 1.5%) when laminaria replaced dilation solely with graduated rigid dilators [41].

Treatment options include observation alone; clamp compression for 5 to 10 minutes; the application of silver nitrate or other styptic solutions, such as ferric subsulfate solution (Monsel's solution), and finally suturing. Surgical repair is best accomplished using absorbable suture in a running, locking stitch. Occasionally the bladder flap requires dissection and retraction to provide exposure for repair of extensive tears of the anterior cervix. Better lighting, lateral retractors, and surgical assistants are often needed to repair severe cervical injuries properly; hence, an operating room may be necessary.

High cervical tears

High cervical tears (cervical fractures) result from stretch-induced injury to the internal cervical os. The injury may be partial- or full-thickness, the latter creating a passage into the paracervical space. These lacerations can occur during labor induction [45] as well as during surgical abortion. Development of cervicovaginal fistulas can occur during labor-induction abortions; the posterior cervix bulges into the vagina, then ruptures, with delivery through the fistula. These injuries were more common with abortions induced with intra-amniotic prostaglandin $F_{2\alpha}$ [144].

Tears of the distal endocervix can traumatize lower cervical branches of the uterine artery and vein, which lie in the retroperitoneum (Fig. 15.4). In these instances, a hematoma may form, and vaginal bleeding is often light. Large hematomas can develop, leading to hypovolemia. Because of tamponade within the retroperitoneum and arteriolar spasm, blood loss may be slowly progressing and laterally sequestered, avoiding the development of rebound tenderness and resulting in delayed diagnosis.

Tears of the proximal portion of the internal os can disrupt upper cervical branches of the uterine artery and vein, which generally lie above the peritoneal reflection (Fig. 15.4). No retroperitoneal envelope is available to provide tamponade in these cases, and life-threatening hemoperitoneum can develop rapidly.

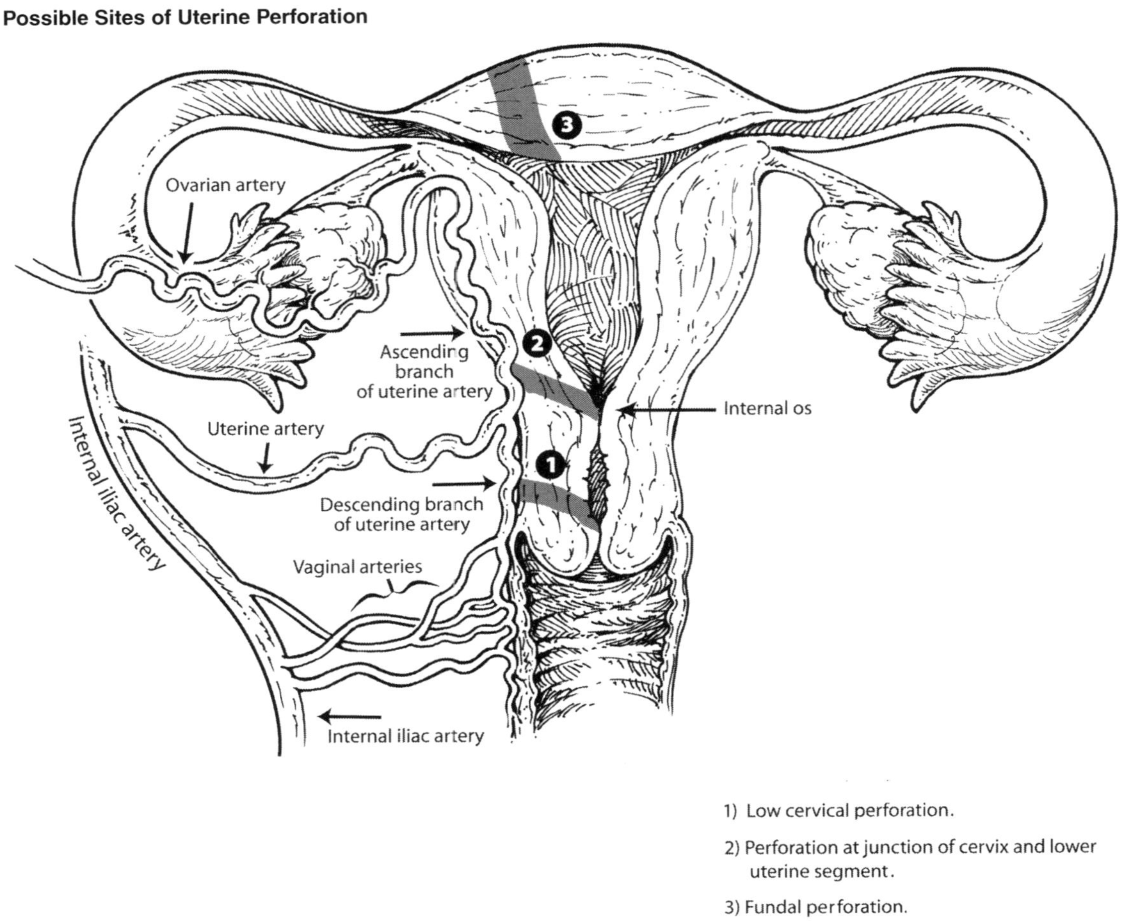

Figure 15.4 Possible sites of uterine perforation. (1) Low cervical lacerations can injure descending branches of uterine artery; (2) lacerations at the internal os (often related to overstretching of the sphincteric junction of cervix and lower uterine segment) can injure ascending branches of uterine artery; (3) fundal perforation. Regions lateral to the fundus and corpus are more vascular than in the midline.

The lateral aspects of the cervix are most vulnerable to stretch-induced injury, placing parametrial arterioles at risk. Spasm of these injured vessels results in episodic bleeding and can mislead the clinician in the belief that the injury has resolved spontaneously. Sudden massive internal and external bleeding has occurred with such tears up to 4 weeks after the original trauma.

Clinicians should suspect endocervical injury whenever postoperative bleeding persists despite a well-contracted uterus or when patients exhibit unexplained postoperative orthostatic hypotension unresponsive to fluid resuscitation. As fluid shifts occur and red cells are mobilized by means of demargination, serial hematocrit levels may show little or no drop for several hours, depending on the extent of the bleeding. Digital palpation of the endocervical barrel may reveal the defect. Bleeding from small non-perforating lacerations may stop permanently with application of Monsel's solution. Bleeding that stops temporarily when ring forceps are placed circumferentially at the level of the internal os, but resumes upon their removal, indicates a need for further therapy. Hysteroscopy can be diagnostic and therapeutic (cautery) when bleeding is light enough to permit endoscopic visualization [145]. Nonpenetrating injuries may respond to balloon tamponade after first-trimester [146] and D&E abortions [68]. Large or full-thickness penetrating lacerations usually require angiographic treatment or surgical repair using a vaginal or abdominal approach. Balloon tamponade or uterine packing (with vasopressin) can at times be curative and nearly always will temporarily slow bleeding enough to allow time for angiographic or surgical treatment.

A slowly developing pelvic hematoma may be insidious, with only mild tenderness, rectal pressure, and modest abnormalities of laboratory tests. Pelvic hematomas may be difficult to palpate if they are lateral or high, and rectal examination can be especially helpful in these circumstances. When palpated, fresh hematomas are uniformly tender. Pelvic ultrasound, CT scan, and MRI are sensitive, but sometimes nonspecific, diagnostic tests for hematomas.

Some hematomas can be managed with observation only. Repetitive hematocrit determinations and serial imaging measurements indicate when the hematoma has stabilized. Broad-spectrum antibiotic therapy may be prudent, given the communication with the vaginal flora. Large hematomas (more than 500–800 ml or 8–10 cm in diameter), failure of the hematoma to stabilize, or the appearance of infection should prompt intervention. Treatment options include ultrasonography- or CT-guided needle aspiration, angiographic embolization, and vaginal or abdominal surgical repair. When a hematoma resolves without intervening infection and without invasive therapy that breaches the peritoneum, adhesion formation within the pelvis is uncommon. Under these circumstances, fertility is not impaired, in contrast with the aftermath of most pelvic abscesses.

High cervical tears cannot entirely be prevented. However, avoiding forceful mechanical dilation and making appropriate use of osmotic dilators or cervical priming agents may lessen somewhat the risk of this complication.

Perforation

Perforation is an uncommon but potentially serious complication. The risk is highest with inexperienced providers and with advanced patient parity or gestational age [147]. Early reports of increased risk of perforation with general anesthesia were not confirmed in a subsequent study by the same investigators [148]. In a more recent large first-trimester study in which 51,000 of 170,000 patients underwent general anesthesia with intravenous methohexital, uterine perforation occurred in only 0.09 per 1,000 cases [5] (Table 15.6). However, some perforations are probably unsuspected and undetected. For example, only two of 14 uterine wall perforations were recognized in a series of 706 patients undergoing concurrent first-trimester vacuum abortion and laparoscopic sterilization [149]. On the other hand, Choudhary et al [28] more recently reported a single-institution series of 288 women undergoing simultaneous vacuum abortion and laparoscopic sterilization in which the one perforation visualized laparoscopically was in fact noted by the vaginal surgeon at the time of the uterine aspiration.

Suspicion of perforation is raised when instruments pass farther than expected, often without discernible resistance; when excessive bleeding occurs; or when contact with the gritty surface of the endometrium is lost during aspiration or curettage. Awake patients may exhibit sudden or unexpected pain, although this finding is nonspecific. Signs can include hypotension and occasionally detection of bowel or omentum in the cannula or cervix. Confirming all major fetal parts during or after D&E is advisable; failure to identify all major pregnancy elements raises suspicion of retained tissue or perforation with tissue in the peritoneal cavity [155]. Delayed recognition of these complications, especially bowel injury, can be life-threatening [156,157]. In general, any woman with protracted abdominal pain after abortion, especially if lateralized or accompanied by abdominal rebound tenderness, requires evaluation to exclude perforation, rupture, or dehiscence.

The most frequent site of perforation is the relatively avascular anterior or posterior midline surface (Fig. 15.4). In a series of 30 perforations in women undergoing vacuum abortion combined with laparoscopic sterilization [158], 60% occurred in the fundus, 30% in the midline of the corpus, and 10% on the side. Most penetrating injuries in the first trimester resolve without treatment or sequelae. Perforations likely to be more problematic are situated laterally, are larger than 1.2 cm in diameter, occur after the first trimester, result in acute pain or symptomatic blood loss, or involve bowel. Perioperative ultrasound may be useful in documenting whether a perforation has occurred and in monitoring the cul-de-sac for accumulation of blood [159]. Although laparoscopy is more expensive and inconvenient, it is a better diagnostic tool. Culdocentesis is an inexpensive and safe technique to assess blood in the cul-de-sac as well. Blood in the cul-de-sac may result from uterine injury, or from rupture of an ectopic pregnancy or ovarian cyst.

Experienced operators have safely completed first-trimester abortion immediately after known or suspected small midline perforations. Intraoperative ultrasound can guide completion of the procedure in such cases. Alternatively, the abortion can be deferred for a week or more to allow healing in patients with an intact sac who remain stable after an uncomplicated perforation. Preventative antibiotics are advised during the waiting period.

In the absence of heavy vaginal bleeding (i.e., more than 200 ml or suspected injury to abdominal contents), patients with small perforations can be observed closely in an outpatient setting for pain, orthostasis, declining hematocrit, and abdominal rebound tenderness. In most cases, patients who are clinically stable 2 to 4 hours after surgery can be discharged safely with a responsible chaperone. Oral antibiotics are advisable, and patients should receive explicit instructions and warnings, 24-hour emergency phone contact information, and a timely follow-up appointment. This conservative protocol for women with known or suspected low-risk perforations has been advocated by a variety of authors [149–151,153].

Unstable patients and those with other injuries require surgical intervention. Laparoscopy may fail to detect subtle but consequential injury to bowel. Whereas some surgeons can inspect the full length of the bowel with laparoscopy, others feel more comfortable performing this evaluation by laparotomy.

Small bowel is the most common viscera injured with uterine perforation because of its central pelvic location and length [156,160]. In a case series of surgical abortion-related bowel injuries referred to a large academic medical center in India [157], large bowel injuries (often the sigmoid colon)

Table 15.6 Frequency of uterine perforation with intrauterine instrumentation.

Study	Study Period	Surgical Site	Instrumentation	Total Patients	Comments	Perforation Frequency (per 1,000 cases)
White et al [150]	1974–1976	Hospital (USA)	Uterine sounding during sterilization	635	Teaching service	30.40
Chi & Feldblum [151]	1974–1976	Hospitals (international)	Uterine sounding during sterilization	20,757	18 medical centers in 11 countries surveyed	1.80 (laparoscopic tubal ligation), 1.20 (mini-lap tubal ligation)
Hakim-Elahi et al [5]	1971–1987	Freestanding clinics (USA)	Vacuum abortion ≤14 weeks LMP	170,000	No difference in rates between local (75%) and general (25%) anesthesia	0.09
Hodgson & Portmann [42]	1972–1973	Freestanding clinic (USA)	Vacuum abortion ≤12 weeks LMP	10,453		0.90
Freiman & Wulff [152]	1973 –1976	Freestanding clinic (USA)	Vacuum abortion, first trimester	20,000	Rate in last 8,000 cases = 0.75	1.40
Bozorgi [58]	1973–1974	Freestanding clinic (USA)	Vacuum abortion ≤14 weeks LMP	10,890		0.20
Wadhera [44]	1975–1980	Hospitals (Canada)	Vacuum abortion or induction to 20+ weeks LMP	351,879	84% of cases ≤13 weeks LMP	1.30
Peterson et al [41]	1972–1981	One hospital clinic (USA)	D&E, 13–22 weeks LMP	17,720	Laminaria introduced in 1977. One surgeon did most cases >18 weeks LMP	2.00 (Excludes cases managed expectantly)
Lindell & Flam [153]	1982–1992	Hospitals (Sweden)	Vacuum abortion, first trimester	84,850	Records reviewed at six public hospitals in greater Stockholm	1.70
Kaali et al [149]	1986–1987	Freestanding clinic (USA)	Vacuum abortion, first trimester	6,408	Abortion alone	1.30
			Concurrent sterilization and vacuum abortion, first trimester	706	Concurrent laparoscopic tubal ligation and first-trimester vacuum abortion	2.80 (suspected), 15.60 (actual)
Pridmore & Chambers [51]	1992–1998	Public ambulatory surgery center (Australia)	Vacuum 4–12 weeks LMP	12,040		0.50
			D&E 13–20 weeks LMP	1,925	More osmotic dilator treatments for scarred cervices or uteri improved outcomes	3.10
Hern [50]	1990–1999	Freestanding clinic (USA)	Oxytocin induction; digoxin or urea to cause fetal demise; 18–34 weeks LMP	1,677	One case of cervical laceration (2,500 ml estimated blood loss)	0.60
Choudhary et al [28]	1997–2001	Teaching hospital (India)	Vacuum at ≤12 weeks LMP	961	30% had concurrent laparoscopic sterilization	1.00
Castleman et al [61]	1999–2002	Teaching hospital (Hanoi, Vietnam)	12–18 weeks LMP	439	Misoprostol only for cervical ripening	4.60
Patel et al [52]	2002–2003	19 affiliated outpatient clinics (USA)	12–23 6/7 weeks LMP	2,218	Buccal misoprostol (100%) + laminaria (43%) for ripening	0.45
De La Vega et al [154]	1998–2006	Hospital (USA)	D&E, 13–26 weeks LMP	2,291	Risk factors: advanced maternal age and gestation >20 weeks	2.60

were often associated with posterior uterine wall perforations, whereas anterior wall or fundal perforations more often resulted in small bowel injury. Reporting a series of small-bore bowel injuries associated with gynecologic laparoscopic procedures, Soderstrom [160] noted that free air was seen in only one-third of injured patients using flat plate radiographs, but most patients became symptomatic (pain, distension, fever, and anorexia) within 72 hours. Large bowel injuries became symptomatic earlier than damaged small bowel because of fecal content [160]. In another series, laparoscopically associated injuries to large bowel led to greater likelihood of developing intra-abdominal abscess and pleural effusion than those to small bowel [161]. During abortion, other adjacent pelvic organs, such as the bladder or ureter [27], can sustain injury as well.

Identifying the cause of the perforation can be difficult. In a Swedish study involving 145 first-trimester perforations, 47% were discovered during aspiration, and 21% were noted during dilation [153]. Many clinicians use a sharp curette or small forceps to confirm that the uterine cavity is empty; 31% of perforations were discovered during this phase, reflecting that this "security check" carries some risk.

Because of the rarity of perforation, randomized controlled trials cannot evaluate the potential benefit of intraoperative ultrasonography. A before-after study from one hospital found that use of intraoperative ultrasound guidance lowered the risk of perforation during D&E and shortened operating time [162]. In a large prospective study of risk factors for uterine perforation in first- and second-trimester abortions, use of osmotic dilators had a protective effect [147]. Use of a sound to measure the depth of the fundus has been associated with perforation during diagnostic dilation and curettage [150], and this practice may entail risk in the abortion setting as well. In a 13-year retrospective review from China of uterine perforations that occurred during first-trimester surgical abortion, the sound was the perforating instrument in 23% of cases [163].

Atraumatic dehiscence (complete separation of myometrium with preservation of overlying abdominal or bladder peritoneum) has been described in D&E abortion [164]. Second-trimester rupture or dehiscence may be slow to develop and initially confused with uterine atony, retained tissue, or pelvic infection.

Asherman syndrome

Asherman syndrome includes scarring either in the endometrial cavity or in the cervical canal [165]. Although they may coexist, the two lesions are usually seen separately. Reported consequences of this condition include amenorrhea, secondary infertility, spontaneous abortion, and preterm delivery, but failed attempted abortion can occur as well [166].

Asherman syndrome after surgical abortion is uncommon and is usually readily correctable. In a large, single-institution report of surgical abortions, the frequency of documented Asherman syndrome was about 16 per 100,000 cases [5]. Most reported cases have involved cervical agglutination without evidence of synechiae in the cavity. In an early case series, nine of 12 cases involved cervical stenosis, while three involved intracavitary adhesions [167]. Chapman and Chapman [168] reported seven cases associated with induced abortion, six of which had cervical agglutination; all were corrected by cervical dilation alone. In a report of the cervical agglutination form of Asherman syndrome attributable to induced abortion, all 10 women achieved normal periods after therapy. Three of the patients had abortions by sharp curettage rather than vacuum aspiration, and the average time to diagnosis for all subjects was 11 months (range: 5–18 months)[169]. No case of Asherman syndrome has been reported after medical abortion using any of the common regimens.

Asherman syndrome typically presents as diminished or no uterine bleeding. Further, the patient may have a history of cyclical cramping if the os is occluded; hematometra is uncommon [165]. Dilating the cervix to a diameter of 7 to 8 mm using paracervical anesthesia can be both diagnostic and therapeutic.

Although still widely used for diagnosis, hysterosalpingography has false-positive rates as high as 30%; three-dimensional (3-D) ultrasound is much more accurate, especially in identifying and categorizing cervical agglutination in the presence or absence of cavitary scarring [170]. Hysteroscopy offers the most precise diagnosis, a vantage for lysis of adhesions under direct vision, and a vehicle for the identification and removal of the conceptus during elective abortion [166]. Milder forms of Asherman syndrome have uniformly optimistic prospects [171]. Although feasible in an office setting, hysteroscopy requires additional expense and skill and is not without complications. In the series cited earlier using 3-D ultrasound as a screening tool [170], two of 18 patients who underwent simultaneous hysteroscopy and laparoscopy experienced uterine perforations. Efficacy of widely practiced nonsurgical therapies such as sequential hormone replacement therapy (e.g., 2 mg oral conjugated estrogen twice daily for 10–14 days), intrauterine stenting (catheter balloons such as the Cook balloon uterine tent or intrauterine contraceptive devices for several weeks), or antibiotics (e.g., oral doxycycline 100 mg twice daily for 10–14 days) is unproven.

The epidemiology of uterine adhesions remains unclear. Sharp curettage appears related to Asherman syndrome [169], providing yet another reason to abandon an archaic tool that dates back to the 1800s. Whether other variations in abortion technique (e.g., preoperative cervical priming with osmotic dilators or prostaglandins, size and type of instrument used as a cervical dilator, use of sharp "check" curettage, or administration of perioperative antibiotics) influence the risk is unknown.

Thrombosis and embolism

Deep vein thrombosis

Deep vein thrombosis (DVT) is infrequently reported in association with abortion. It leads to pulmonary embolism in approximately 20% of cases. Heritable thrombophilias, such as Factor V Leiden deficiency, are strong risk factors, as are obesity, diabetes, age greater than 40 years, trauma, immobilization, and malignancy [172]. Pain, swelling, point tenderness, and inflammation vary greatly depending on the size and progression of the thrombus. Onset of DVT may be gradual, and the physiologic swelling associated with pregnancy may confound recognition of its symptoms. Noninvasive testing with plethysmography and ultrasound are imperfect screening techniques; venography is the definitive diagnostic tool.

Heparin is the mainstay of treatment; low-molecular-weight heparin (enoxaparin) is now widely used for both prophylaxis and the acute phase of treatment. Patients without risk factors who are undergoing short outpatient operations require no prophylactic measures. Those with risk factors may benefit from pneumatic compression devices, enoxaparin, or subcutaneous unfractionated heparin, particularly if a multiple-day hospitalization is contemplated (e.g., labor-induction abortion).

Pulmonary embolism

Pulmonary embolism is an important cause of abortion mortality [173]. The CDC described 10 cases of fatal pulmonary embolism from 1972 to 1975. These deaths occurred 2 to 50 days after abortion [174]. In addition to pregnancy, most patients had at least one other risk factor, including obesity, hypertension, cancer, family history of embolism, contraindicated recent use of oral contraceptives, or discontinuation of heparin therapy for DVT because of side effects. The authors estimated the overall incidence of fatal and non-fatal pulmonary embolism as 10 to 20 cases per 100,000 induced abortions [174].

Detection of pulmonary embolism is not always straightforward. Symptoms may be nonspecific and of variable severity. Classic signs include rapid or difficult breathing; pleuritic chest pain; and in about half of patients, anxiety, cough, and râles. Arterial hypoxemia occurs in most patients. Only a minority (approximately 5%) of pregnant women suspected of having pulmonary embolism will have the diagnosis radiographically validated after evaluation. Chest radiograph is required to rule out other causes and to interpret ventilation-perfusion scans. More recently, spiral computed tomography has supplanted ventilation-perfusion scans (60% indeterminate) on the grounds of both clinical benefit and cost-effectiveness [175]. Pulmonary angiography is the diagnostic gold standard but is expensive, invasive, and more risky than alternative tests. Anticoagulation with heparin initially, followed by warfarin therapy, is the mainstay of treatment. Treatment reduces mortality from approximately 15% to less than 1%.

Amniotic fluid embolism

Although rare, occurring in 1:10,000 to 1:80,000 pregnancies [176], amniotic fluid embolism has emerged as an important cause of death associated with second-trimester abortion, with a mortality rate as high as 80% [173]. This catastrophe is usually unforeseeable and often fatal. DIC complicates 40 to 60% of cases that survive beyond the initial insult. The risk of amniotic fluid embolism increases with advancing gestational age, as well as with older labor-induction methods and hysterotomy [177]. The most frequent presentation of amniotic fluid embolism is cardiorespiratory collapse. Sometimes a brief instance of dyspnea or feeling of impending doom precedes cessation of breathing, oxygen desaturation, cardiac electromechanical dissociation, and profound hypotension.

Although its etiology remains unclear, progress in identifying the presence and origin of this condition is ongoing. A number of studies have routinely identified trophoblasts and squamous cells of presumed fetal origin in the circulation of healthy gravidas after the first trimester [178–180]. Large volumes of homologous amniotic fluid are harmless in primate models. Because human maternal exposure to fetal elements is therefore a common occurrence, Clark [181] has posited that uniquely susceptible maternal-fetal pairs are necessary to produce amniotic fluid embolism. In such pairs, disturbance of the pregnancy may inoculate the pregnant woman with fetally derived antigen, which causes an anaphylactoid reaction. Gei and Hankins [182] have speculated that fetal particles in the maternal circulation may cause pulmonary microemboli that trigger release of arachidonic acid metabolites, stimulating an anaphylactoid response. These mediators may exist in the plasma, leukocytes, and fetal gut.

Pathological verification can be arduous and elusive. A diligent search should include central venous blood (for fetal squames, vernix, or eosinophilic leukocytic granules), sputum (for fetal squames), and bronchoalveolar lavage (for stained epithelial cells). Examiners should analyze maternal peripheral blood for the presence of fetally derived cells and debris and also test the blood with an array of highly specialized enzymatic markers (ZnCP-1, monoclonal antibody to TKH-2, and STN) before ruling out the diagnosis.

Treatment is supportive including endotracheal intubation, intracardiac epinephrine, and cardioversion. If the patient survives the primary event in an outpatient setting, she should be transferred promptly to a hospital for intensive care. Management may include replacement of clotting factors for DIC and intravenous dopamine plus prolonged ventilatory assistance for adult respiratory distress syndrome. Survival has been reported with an artificial membrane lung, and in another case, full-scale cardiopulmonary bypass.

Other conditions

Anaphylaxis

Anaphylaxis requires prior sensitization. It results from IgE-mediated antigen stimulation on the surface of basophils and mast cells, causing release of an array of dermatologic, vasoactive, and bronchospastic proteins. Most manifestations are mild, causing flushing or urticaria. In severe forms, acute bronchospasm, increased alveolar-capillary permeability, and profound hypotension may lead to airway obstruction, hypotensive shock, and extensive bilateral pulmonary edema.

Once the suspected antigen is withdrawn, treatment consists of airway access, ventilation, cardiac support, and fluid maintenance. Initial drug therapy includes epinephrine (0.3–0.5 ml of 1:1,000 solution subcutaneously or 3–5 ml of 1:10,000 intravenously or via endotracheal tube, repeated periodically as needed) and diphenhydramine (0.5–1.0 mg/kg intravenously). Steroids can be added if the patient requires more intensive therapy (hydrocortisone, 250–1000 mg intravenously, or methylprednisolone, 1–2 g intravenously). Inhaled beta-agonists (metaproterenol 0.3 ml or albuterol 0.5 ml in 2.5 ml normal saline) and aminophylline (0.25–0.5 gm intravenously) are used to treat resistant bronchospasm. In an emergency department study of 103 cases, 19% had recurrences at a mean interval of 10 hours (range, 2–38 hours). These recurrences were variably associated with initial symptom onset at least 30 minutes after exposure, inadequate epinephrine dosing, and underuse of steroids [183].

Vasovagal syncope

In abortion practice, a vasovagal reaction can occur in association with paracervical anesthesia, cervical dilation, or venipuncture. Although its etiology is unknown, vasovagal reaction is associated with stressful conditions such as pain, emotional upset, and prolonged standing. Upon standing upright, healthy individuals normally experience a drop in intrathoracic pressure of approximately 15%, a reduction of stroke volume of about 20%, and a corresponding decline in arterial pressure [184]. During a vasovagal reaction, the patient's skin is cold and clammy, and she often reports light-headedness, nausea, or visual changes. Moderate hypotension and bradycardia in the range of 30 to 50 beats per minute are common. Transient seizure-like muscular activity can occur. Brief disorientation may follow momentary unconsciousness, but true postictal states are rare.

Resting in a horizontal position or with the legs elevated is all that most patients require. Most episodes resolve in a few minutes without treatment. Severe or prolonged incidents can be treated with atropine, 0.4 to 1.0 mg intravenously, antiemetics, hydration and, rarely, airway support.

Asthmatic reactions

Eight per cent of patients seeking abortion report current use of at least intermittent asthma medication. Patients with asthma who merit special concern during presurgical screening are those with (1) symptoms requiring continuous antiinflammatory or steroid therapy; (2) frequent exacerbations or nocturnal dyspnea (more than one to two episodes per week); (3) a recent attack requiring medical therapy; and/or (4) current acute symptoms. In an observational cohort study of pregnant asthmatic women at 16 US health centers for the period 1994 to 1999, obesity (BMI ≥ 30) was significantly associated with asthma exacerbations (cough, dyspnea, or wheezing, OR 1.3, 95% CI 1.1–1.7, $p = 0.01$) after controlling for smoking and race, but not with hospitalizations for asthma, need for steroid treatment, or worsening asthma pattern overall [185].

Although acute asthmatic attacks in well-prepared abortion patients are rare, facilities must be prepared to treat severe asthmatic complications. Mild dyspnea usually responds to two puffs of nebulized beta$_2$-adrenergic agonist (albuterol, salmeterol) using self-administration or mask. Puffer dosing can be repeated every 20 to 30 minutes for up to three doses. A calm nursing presence is therapeutic. Second-level therapy involves parenteral sympathomimetic agents (subcutaneous epinephrine, 0.3 to 0.5 ml of 1:1,000 solution every 20 minutes up to three doses, or subcutaneous terbutaline, 250 μg every 15 minutes up to three doses).

A third level of treatment consists of methylxanthine therapy. Aminophylline is the only agent available for parenteral dosing and is highly effective in conjunction with nebulized beta adrenergics, parenteral sympathomimetics, or inspired anesthetic gases. The aminophylline loading dose is 5 mg/kg/30 minutes intravenously, and the maintenance dose is 0.5 to 1.0 mg/kg/hour.

A fourth level of therapy as a final recourse for refractory bronchospasm is the use of inspired halogenated gases such as desflurane or sevoflurane. These agents, where available, are extremely effective in opposing severe bronchoconstriction. Because they act as tocolytic agents upon smooth muscle, however, they carry risk of inciting uterine hemorrhage, possibly requiring intensive uterotonic therapy as a countermeasure.

Hydration is a key feature of treatment in all cases. Pulse oximetry is pivotal in early detection of airway compromise and valuable in gauging therapeutic success. The goal is to maintain oxygen saturation at 95% or better. Failure over time to raise oxygen saturation to 90% calls into question the need for intubation. Prolonged desaturation after intensive outpatient therapy requires hospitalization.

Seizures

Although grand mal, petit mal, toxic drug-induced, and idiopathic seizures can be distinguished clinically, acute treatment of these conditions is the same. This treatment consists of chin thrust (to dislodge the tongue from the oropharynx), mask oxygen, and parenteral anticonvulsants. Most seizures encountered in abortion settings are self-resolving solely with supportive measures and do not recur acutely. Anxiety, *nil per os* (NPO) status, or physical discomfort may contribute to their causation. Repetitive or prolonged seizure episodes warrant referral for expert treatment and evaluation.

Parenteral benzodiazepines (diazepam 5–10 mg or midazolam 2.5–5 mg) usually stop seizures for a period of 30 to 45 minutes, while lorazepam 1 to 2 mg is usually effective for 2 to 3 hours. Short-acting barbiturates represent an alternative first-line therapy. Intravenous thiopental (75–150 mg), propofol (50–100 mg), and methohexital (50–100 mg) are highly effective in temporarily controlling seizure activity. Although these doses do not abolish the gag reflex in most patients, it is prudent to administer these drugs in a setting with an experienced airway manager, pulse oximetry, intubation equipment, and nursing staff assignable to continuous monitoring. Complete loading and daily dosages of anticonvulsive therapy are considerably higher than those used during acute treatment and are best left to clinicians who will undertake the long-term monitoring of the patient.

Conclusion

Legal-induced abortion is one of the safest and most thoroughly studied procedures in medicine. Although surgical abortion complications are not completely avoidable, the following practices can minimize their occurrence:

- Accurate determination of gestational age before abortion;
- Limiting procedures to those in which the surgeon is skilled and experienced;
- Appropriate emergency consultation and hospital referral when necessary;
- Simple regimens of anesthesia and evacuation of the uterus;
- Routine periabortal antibiotics or presumptive treatment of sexually transmitted infections;
- Use of only sterile instruments inside the uterus ("no-touch" technique);
- Judicious use of osmotic dilators or prostaglandins to soften and open the cervix, particularly after 14 gestational weeks;
- Adequate cervical dilation;
- Gentle and thorough uterine evacuation;
- Avoiding sharp curettage;
- Prompt use of uterotonic drugs to treat atony;
- Maintaining a high index of suspicion for occult injury and insidious medical complications;
- Careful tissue examination to confirm successful abortion;
- Assiduous monitoring during and after surgery; and
- 24-hour telephone access to a clinician knowledgeable about postabortal complications.

References

1 Cates W Jr, Grimes DA, Schulz KF. The public health impact of legal abortion: 30 years later. *Perspect Sex Reprod Health* 2003; **35**: 25–28.

2 Grimes DA. Estimation of pregnancy-related mortality risk by pregnancy outcome, United States, 1991 to 1999. *Am J Obstet Gynecol* 2006; **194**: 92–94.

3 Bartlett LA, Berg CJ, Shulman HB et al. Risk factors for legal induced abortion-related mortality in the United States. *Obstet Gynecol* 2004; **103**: 729–737.

4 Chang J, Elam-Evans LD, Berg CJ et al. Pregnancy-related mortality surveillance–United States, 1991–1999. *MMWR Surveill Summ* 2003; **52**: 1–8.

5 Hakim-Elahi E, Tovell HM, Burnhill MS. Complications of first-trimester abortion: a report of 170,000 cases. *Obstet Gynecol* 1990; **76**: 129–135.

6 Henshaw SK. (1999) Unintended pregnancy and abortion: a public health perspective. In: Paul M, Lichtenberg ES, Borgatta L, Grimes DA, Stubblefield PG, eds. *A Clinician's Guide to Medical and Surgical Abortion*. Churchill Livingstone, New York, 1999, 11–22.

7 Boonstra H, Gold RB, Richards CL, Finer LB. *Abortion in Women's Lives*. Guttmacher Institute, New York, 2006.

8 Reece EA. Perspectives on obesity, pregnancy, and birth outcomes in the United States: the scope of the problem. *Am J Obstet Gynecol* 2008; **198**: 23–27.

9 Dark AC, Miller L, Kothenbeutel RL, Mandel L. Obesity and second-trimester abortion by dilation and evacuation. *J Reprod Med* 2002; **47**: 226–230.

10 Marchiano DA, Thomas AG, Lapinski R, Balwan K, Patel J. Intraoperative blood loss and gestational age at pregnancy termination. *Prim Care Update Ob Gyns* 1998; **5**: 204–205.

11 O'Connell K, Jones HE, Lichtenberg ES, Paul M. Second-trimester surgical abortion practices: a survey of National Abortion Federation members. *Contraception* 2008; **78**: 492–499.

12 Grimes DA, Schulz KF. Morbidity and mortality from second-trimester abortions. *J Reprod Med* 1985; **30**: 505–514.

13 Lawson HW, Frye A, Atrash HK, Smith JC, Shulman HB, Ramick M. Abortion mortality, United States, 1972 through 1987. *Am J Obstet Gynecol* 1994; **171**: 1365–1372.

14 Autry AM, Hayes EC, Jacobson GF, Kirby RS. A comparison of medical induction and dilation and evacuation for second-trimester abortion. *Am J Obstet Gynecol* 2002; **187**: 393–397.

15 Turok DK, Gurtcheff SE, Esplin MS et al. Second trimester termination of pregnancy: a review by site and procedure type. *Contraception* 2008; **77**: 155–161.

16 Kapp N, Todd CS, Yadgarova KT et al. A randomized comparison of misoprostol to intrauterine instillation of hypertonic saline plus a prostaglandin $F_{2\alpha}$ analogue for second-trimester induction termination in Uzbekistan. *Contraception* 2007; **76**: 461–466.

17 Goh SE, Thong KJ. Induction of second trimester abortion (12–20 weeks) with mifepristone and misoprostol: a review of 386 consecutive cases. *Contraception* 2006; **73**: 516–519.

18 Green J, Borgatta L, Sia M et al. Intervention rates for placental removal following induction abortion with misoprostol. *Contraception* 2007; **76**: 310–313.

19 Burgoine GA, Van Kirk SD, Romm J, Edelman AB, Jacobson S-L, Jensen JT. Comparison of perinatal grief after dilation and evacuation or labor induction in second trimester terminations for fetal anomalies. *Am J Obstet Gynecol* 2005; **192**: 1928–1932.

20 Virk J, Zhang J, Olsen J. Medical abortion and risk of subsequent adverse pregnancy outcome. *N Engl J Med* 2007; **357**: 648–653.

21 Kalish RB, Chasen ST, Rosenzweig LB, Rashbaum WK, Chervenak FA. Impact of midtrimester dilation and evacuation on subsequent pregnancy outcome. *Am J Obstet Gynecol* 2002; **187**: 882–885.

22 Chasen ST, Kalish RB, Gupta M, Kaufman J, Chervenak FA. Obstetrical outcomes after surgical abortion at > or = 20 weeks' gestation. *Am J Obstet Gynecol* 2005; **193**: 1161–1164.

23 Jackson JE, Grobman WA, Haney E, Casele H. Mid-trimester dilation and evacuation with laminaria does not increase the risk for severe subsequent pregnancy complications. *Int J Gynaecol Obstet* 2007; **96**: 12–15.

24 Woo J, Fine P, Goetzl L. Abortion disclosure and the association with domestic violence. *Obstet Gynecol* 2005; **105**: 1329–1334.

25 Meirik O, Bergström R. Outcome of delivery subsequent to vacuum-aspiration abortion in nulliparous women. *Acta Scand Gynecol Obstet* 1983; **62**: 499–509.

26 Zhou W, Sorenson HT, Olsen J. Induced abortion and subsequent pregnancy duration. *Obstet Gynecol* 1999; **94**: 948–953.

27 Meyer NL, Addis IB, Lipscomb GH. Ureteral avulsion during uterine dilatation and evacuation: a case report. *J Reprod Med* 2006; **51**: 581–583.

28 Choudhary N, Saha SC, Gopalan S. Abortion procedures in a tertiary care institution in India. *Int J Gynaecol Obstet* 2005; **91**: 81–86.

29 Darney PD, Atkinson E, Hirabayashi K. Uterine perforation during second-trimester abortion by cervical dilation and instrumental extraction: a review of 15 cases. *Obstet Gynecol* 1990; **75**: 441–444.

30 Kaunitz AM, Rovira EZ, Grimes DA, Schulz KF. Abortions that fail. *Obstet Gynecol* 1985; **66**: 533–537.

31 Valle RF, Sabbagha RE. Management of first trimester pregnancy termination failures. *Obstet Gynecol* 1980; **55**: 625–629.

32 Edwards J, Carson SA. New technologies permit safe abortion at less than six weeks' gestation and provide timely detection of ectopic gestation. *Am J Obstet Gynecol* 1997; **176**: 1101–1106.

33 Paul ME, Mitchell CM, Rogers AJ, Fox MC, Lackie EG. Early surgical abortion: efficacy and safety. *Am J Obstet Gynecol* 2002; **187**: 407–411.

34 Fulcheri E, di Capua E, Ragni N. Histologic examination of products of conception at the time of pregnancy termination. *Int J Gynaecol Obstet* 2003; **80**: 315–316.

35 Grossman D, Ellertson C, Grimes DA, Walker D. Routine follow-up visits after first-trimester induced abortion. *Obstet Gynecol* 2004; **103**: 738–745.

36 Roshan D. Pregnancy outcomes after failed abortion. *Obstet Gynecol* 2006; **107**(Abstract), 97S.

37 Kurtz AB, Shlansky-Goldberg RD, Choi HY, Needleman L, Wapner RJ, Goldberg BB. Detection of retained products of conception following spontaneous abortion in the first trimester. *J Ultrasound Med* 1991; **10**: 387–395.

38 Bar-Hava I, Aschkenazi S, Orvieto R et al. Spectrum of normal intrauterine cavity sonographic findings after first-trimester abortion. *J Ultrasound Med* 2001; **20**: 1277–1281.

39 Debby A, Golan A, Sadan O, Rotmensch S, Malinger G. Sonographic characteristics of the uterine cavity following first-trimester uterine evacuation. *Ultrasound Obstet Gynecol* 2008; **31**: 555–559.

40 Grimes DA, Schulz KF, Cates W Jr, Tyler CW Jr. Midtrimester abortion by intraamniotic prostaglandin $F_{2\alpha}$. Safer than saline? *Obstet Gynecol* 1977; **49**: 612–616.

41 Peterson WF, Berry FN, Grace MR, Gulbranson CL. Second-trimester abortion by dilatation and evacuation: an analysis of 11,747 cases. *Obstet Gynecol* 1983; **62**: 185–190.

42 Hodgson JE, Portmann KC. Complications of 10,453 consecutive first-trimester abortions: a prospective study. *Am J Obstet Gynecol* 1974; **120**: 802–807.

43 Wulff GJ Jr, Freiman SM. Elective abortion. Complications seen in a freestanding clinic. *Obstet Gynecol* 1977; **49**: 351–357.

44 Wadhera S. Early complication risks of legal abortions, Canada, 1975–1980. *Can J Public Health* 1982; **73**: 396–400.

45 Hill NC, MacKenzie IZ. 2308 second trimester terminations using extra-amniotic fluid or intra-amniotic prostaglandin E_2: an analysis of efficacy and complications. *Br J Obstet Gynaecol* 1989; **96**: 1424–1431.

46 Hern WM. Serial multiple laminaria and adjunctive urea in late outpatient dilation and evacuation abortion. *Obstet Gynecol* 1984; **63**: 543–549.

47 Altman AM, Stubblefield PG, Schlam JF, Loberfeld R, Osathanodh R. Midtrimester abortion with Laminaria and vacuum evacuation on a teaching service. *J Reprod Med* 1985; **30**: 601–606.

48 Jacot FR, Poulin C, Bilodeau AP et al. A five-year experience with second-trimester induced abortions: no increase in complication rate as compared to the first trimester. *Am J Obstet Gynecol* 1993; **168**: 633–637.

49 National Abortion Federation. Summary of abortion statistics. National Abortion Federation, Washington (DC), 1996.

50 Hern WM. Laminaria, induced fetal demise, and misoprostol in late abortion. *Int J Gynaecol Obstet* 2001; **75**: 279–286.

51 Pridmore BR, Chambers DG. Uterine perforation during surgical abortion: a review of diagnosis, management, and prevention. *Aust N Z J Obstet Gynaecol* 1999; **39**: 349–353.

52 Patel A, Talmont E, Morfesis J et al. The Planned Parenthood Federation of America Buccal Misoprostol Waiver Group. Adequacy and safety of buccal misoprostol for cervical preparation prior to termination of second-trimester pregnancy. *Contraception* 2006; **73**: 420–430.

53 Stubblefield PG, Grimes DA. Septic abortion. *N Engl J Med* 1994; **331**: 310–314.

54 Nathanson BN. The postabortal pain syndrome: a new entity. *Obstet Gynecol* 1973; **41**: 739–740.

55 Sands RX, Burnhill MS, Hakim-Elahi E. Postabortal uterine atony. *Obstet Gynecol* 1974; **43**: 595–598.

56 Dean CL, Chez RA. Using vasopressin in paracervical block. *Contemp OB/GYN* 1993; **38**: 42–44.

57 Haddad S, Ruach M, Ohel G. Sonographic demonstration of endometrial fluid collection following termination of pregnancy. *Obstet Gynecol* 1992; **79**: 703–704.

58 Bozorgi N. Statistical analysis of first-trimester pregnancy terminations in an ambulatory surgical center. *Am J Obstet Gynecol* 1977; **127**: 763–768.

59 Hodari AA, Peralta J, Quiroga PJ, Gerbi EB. Dilatation and curettage for second-trimester abortions. *Am J Obstet Gynecol* 1977; **127**: 850–854.

60 Pahl IR, Lundy LE. Experience with midtrimester abortion. *Obstet Gynecol* 1979; **53**: 587–591.

61 Castleman LD, Oanh KT, Hyman AG, Thuy le T, Blumenthal PD. Introduction of the dilation and evacuation procedure for second-trimester abortion in Vietnam using manual vacuum aspiration and buccal misoprostol. *Contraception* 2006; **74**: 272–276.

62 Grimes DA, Kafrissen ME, O'Reilly KR, Binkin NJ. Fatal hemorrhage from legal abortion in the United States. *Surg Gynecol Obstet* 1983; **157**: 461–466.

63 Schulz KF, Grimes DA, Christensen DD. Vasopressin reduces blood loss from second-trimester dilatation and evacuation abortion. *Lancet* 1985; **2**: 353–356.

64 Higier J, Krajewski J, Turowski J, Symonowicz N. The influence of ornithine 8-vasopressin preparation upon blood loss after induced abortions performed under local analgesia. *Ginekol Pol* 1970; **41**: 731–734.

65 O'Brien P, El-Refaey H, Gordon A, Geary M, Rodeck CH. Rectally administered misoprostol for the treatment of postpartum hemorrhage unresponsive to oxytocin and ergometrine: a descriptive study. *Obstet Gynecol* 1998; **92**: 212–214.

66 Hendsch SA, Cohn GM. The safety and efficacy of uterine packing in postpartum hemorrhage: A retrospective study. *Obstet Gynecol* 2002; **99** (Abstract), 86S.

67 Bobrowski RA, Jones TB. A thrombogenic uterine pack for postpartum hemorrhage. *Obstet Gynecol* 1995; **85**: 836–837.

68 Kauff ND, Chelmow D, Kawada CY. Intractable bleeding managed with Foley catheter tamponade after dilation and evacuation. *Am J Obstet Gynecol* 1995; **173**: 957–958.

69 Marcovici I, Scoccia B. Postpartum hemorrhage and intrauterine balloon tamponade. A report of three cases. *J Reprod Med* 1999; **44**: 122–126.

70 Bakri YN, Amri A, Abdul Jabbar F. Tamponade-balloon for obstetrical bleeding. *Int J Gynaecol Obstet* 2001; **74**: 139–142.

71 Papp Z, Tóth-Pál E, Papp C et al. Hypogastric artery ligation for intractable pelvic hemorrhage. *Int J Gynaecol Obstet* 2006; **92**: 27–31.

72 Philippe HJ, d'Oreye D, Lewin D. Vaginal ligature of uterine arteries during postpartum hemorrhage. *Int J Gynaecol Obstet* 1997; **56**: 267–270.

73 B-Lynch C, Coker A, Lawal AH, Abu J, Cohen MJ. The B-Lynch surgical technique for the control of massive postpartum hemorrhage: an alternative to hysterectomy? *Br J Obstet Gynaecol* 1997; **104**: 372–375.

74 Cho JH, Jun HS, Lee CN. Hemostatic suturing technique for uterine bleeding during cesarean delivery. *Obstet Gynecol* 2000; **96**: 129–131.

75 Hayman RG, Arulkumaran S, Steer PJ. Uterine compression sutures: surgical management of postpartum hemorrhage. *Obstet Gynecol* 2002; **99**: 502–506.

76 Pereira A, Nunes F, Pedroso S, Saraiva J, Retto H, Meirinho M. Compressive uterine sutures to treat postpartum bleeding secondary to uterine atony. *Obstet Gynecol* 2005; **106**: 569–572.

77 Baskett TF. Uterine compression sutures for postpartum hemorrhage: efficacy, morbidity, and subsequent pregnancy. *Obstet Gynecol* 2007; **110**: 68–71.

78 Nelson WL, O'Brien JM. The uterine sandwich for persistent uterine atony: combining the B-Lynch compression suture with an intrauterine Bakri balloon. *Am J Obstet Gynecol* 2007; **196**: e9–10.

79 Borgatta L, Chen AY, Reid SK, Stubblefield PG, Christensen DD, Rashbaum WK. Pelvic embolization for treatment of hemorrhage related to spontaneous and induced abortion. *Am J Obstet Gynecol* 2001; **185**: 530–536.

80 Steinauer JE, Diedrich JT, Wilson MW, Darney PD, Vargas JE, Drey EA. Uterine artery embolization in postabortion hemorrhage. *Obstet Gynecol* 2008; **111**: 881–889.

81 Lichtenberg ES. Angiography as treatment for a high cervical tear. A case report. *J Reprod Med* 2003; **48**: 287–289.

82 Taipale P, Hiilesmaa V, Ylöstalo P. Diagnosis of placenta previa by transvaginal sonographic screening at 12–16 weeks in a nonselected population. *Obstet Gynecol* 1997; **83**: 364–367.

83 Thomas AG, Alvarez M, Friedman F Jr, Brodman ML, Kim J, Lockwood C. The effect of placenta previa on blood loss in second-trimester pregnancy termination. *Obstet Gynecol* 1994; **84**: 58–60.

84 Halperin R, Vaknin Z, Langer R, Bukovsky I, Schneider D. Late midtrimester pregnancy termination in the presence of placenta previa. *J Reprod Med* 2003; **48**: 175–178.

85 Oyelese Y, Smulian JC. Placenta previa, placenta accreta, and vasa previa. *Obstet Gynecol* 2006; **107**: 927–941.

86 Nakayama D, Masuzaki H, Miura K, Hiraki K, Yoshimura S, Ishimaru T. Effect of placenta previa on blood loss in second-trimester abortion by labor induction using gemeprost. *Contraception* 2007; **75**: 238–240.

87 Johnson LG, Mueller BA, Daling JR. The relationship of placenta previa and history of induced abortion. *Int J Gynaecol Obstet* 2003; **81**: 191–198.

88 Wu S, Kocherginsky M, Hibbard JU. Abnormal placentation: twenty-year analysis. *Am J Obstet Gynecol* 2005; **192**: 1458–1461.

89 Rashbaum WK, Gates EJ, Jones J, Goldman B, Morris A, Lyman WD. Placenta accreta encountered during dilation and evacuation in the second trimester. *Obstet Gynecol* 1995; **85**: 701–703.

90 Silver RM, Landon MB, Rouse DJ et al. Maternal morbidity associated with multiple repeat cesarean deliveries. *Obstet Gynecol* 2006; **107**: 1226–1232.

91 Grobman WA, Gersnoviez R, Landon MB. Pregnancy outcomes for women with placenta previa in relation to the number of prior cesarean deliveries. *Obstet Gynecol* 2007; **110**: 1249–1255.

92 Höpker M, Fleckenstein G, Heyl W, Sattler B, Emons G. Placenta percreta in week 10 of pregnancy with consecutive hysterectomy: case report. *Hum Reprod* 2002; **17**: 817–820.

93 Balkanli-Kaplan P, Gucer F, Oz-Puyan F, Yuce MA, Kutlu K. Placenta percreta diagnosed after first-trimester pregnancy termination: a case report. *J Reprod Med* 2006; **51**: 662–664.

94 Walter AJ, McCullough AE, Patel MD, Cornella JL. Placenta increta presenting as a delayed postabortal hemorrhage. *Obstet Gynecol* 1999; **93**: 846.

95 Lerner JP, Deane S, Timor-Tritsch IE. Characterization of placenta accreta using transvaginal sonography and color Doppler imaging. *Ultrasound Obstet Gynecol* 1995; **5**: 198–201.

96 Ludmir J, Holland GA, Bader T et al. The value of magnetic resonance imaging in the evaluation of patients at risk for placenta accreta. SPO abstracts. *Am J Obstet Gynecol* 1993; **168** (Abstract): 429.

97 Warshak CR, Eskander R, Hull AD et al. Accuracy of ultrasonography and magnetic resonance imaging in the diagnosis of placenta accreta. *Obstet Gynecol* 2006; **108**: 573–581.

98 Kayem G, Davy C, Goffinet F, Thomas C, Clément D, Cabrol D. Conservative versus extirpative management in cases of placenta accreta. *Obstet Gynecol* 2004; **104**: 531–536.

99 Morikawa M, Yamada T, Yamada H, Minakami H. Effect of gonadotropin-releasing hormone agonist on a uterine arteriovenous malformation. *Obstet Gynecol* 2006; **108**: 751–753.

100 Hoffman MK, Meilstrup JW, Shackelford DP, Kaminski PF. Arteriovenous malformations of the uterus: an uncommon cause of vaginal bleeding. *Obstet Gynecol Surv* 1997; **52**: 736–740.

101 Wiebe ER, Switzer P. Arteriovenous malformations of the uterus associated with medical abortion. *Int J Gynaecol Obstet* 2000; **71**: 155–158.

102 Halperin R, Schneider D, Maymon R, Peer A, Pansky M, Herman Arteriovenous malformation after uterine curettage: a report of 3 cases. *J Reprod Med* 2007; **52**: 445–449.

103 Goldberg RP, Flynn MK. Pregnancy after medical management of a uterine arteriovenous malformation. A case report. *J Reprod Med* 2000; **45**: 961–963.

104 Poppe W, Van Assche FA, Wilms G, Favril A, Baert A. Pregnancy after transcatheter embolization of a uterine arteriovenous malformation. *Am J Obstet Gynecol* 1987; **156**: 1179–1180.

105 Kafrissen ME, Barke MW, Workman P, Schulz KF, Grimes DA. Coagulopathy and induced abortion methods: rates and relative risks. *Am J Obstet Gynecol* 1983; **147**: 344–345.

106 Hern WM. Laminaria versus Dilapan osmotic cervical dilators for outpatient dilation and evacuation abortion: randomized cohort comparison of 1,001 patients. *Am J Obstet Gynecol* 1994; **171**: 1324–1328.

107 Alfirevic Z, Elbourne D, Pavord S et al. Use of recombinant activated factor VII in primary postpartum hemorrhage: the Northern European Registry 2000–2004. *Obstet Gynecol* 2007; **110**: 1270–1278.

108 Pepas LP, Arif-Adib M, Kadir RA. Factor VIIa in puerperal hemorrhage with disseminated intravascular coagulation. *Obstet Gynecol* 2006; **108**: 757–761.

109 Weiskopf RB, Viele MK, Feiner J et al. Human cardiovascular and metabolic response to acute, severe isovolemic anemia. *JAMA* 1998; **279**: 217–221.

110 Viele MK, Weiskopf RB. What can we learn about the need for transfusion from patients who refuse blood? The experience with Jehovah's Witnesses. *Transfusion* 1994; **34**: 396–401.

111 Heisterberg L, Kringelbach M. Early complications after induced first-trimester abortion. *Acta Obstet Gynecol Scand* 1987; **66**: 201–204.

112 Fried G, Östlund E, Ullberg C, Bygdeman M. Somatic complications and contraceptive techniques following legal abortion. *Acta Obstet Gynecol Scand* 1989; **68**: 515–521.

113 Grimes DA, Schulz KF, Cates W Jr, Tyler CW Jr. Mid-trimester abortion by dilation and evacuation: a safe and practical alternative. *N Engl J Med* 1977; **296**: 1141–1145.

114 Barbacci MB, Spence MR, Kappus EW, Burkman RC, Rao L, Quinn TC. Postabortal endometritis and isolation of *Chlamydia trachomatis*. *Obstet Gynecol* 1986; **68**: 686–690.

115 Wein P, Kloss M, Garland SM. Postabortal pelvic sepsis in association with *Chlamydia trachomatis*. *Aust N Z J Obstet Gynaecol* 1990; **30**: 347–350.

116 Blackwell AL, Thomas PD, Wareham K, Emery SJ. Health gains from screening for infection of the lower genital tract in women attending for termination of pregnancy. *Lancet* 1993; **342**: 206–210.

117 Larsson PG, Bergman B, Forsum U, Platz-Christensen JJ, Påhlson C. Mobiluncus and clue cells as predictors of PID

after first-trimester abortion. *Acta Obstet Gynecol Scand* 1989; **68**: 217–220.

118 Lundh C, Meirik O, Nygren K-G. Vaginal cleansing at vacuum abortion does not reduce risk of postoperative infection. *Acta Obstet Gynecol Scand* 1983; **62**: 275–277.

119 Varli IH, Lindelius A, Bergström A. Is preoperative vaginal cleansing necessary for control of infection after first trimester vacuum curettage? *Acta Obstet Gynecol Scand* 2005; **84**: 650–653.

120 Sawaya GF, Grady D, Kerlikowske K, Grimes DA. Antibiotics at the time of induced abortion: the case for universal prophylaxis based on a meta-analysis. *Obstet Gynecol* 1996; **87**: 884–890.

121 Miller WC, Ford CA, Morris M et al. Prevalence of chlamydial and gonococcal infections among young adults in the United States. *JAMA* 2004; **291**: 2229–2236.

122 Datta SD, Sternberg M, Johnson RE. Gonorrhea and chlamydia in the United States among persons 14 to 39 years of age, 1999 to 2002. *Ann Intern Med* 2007; **147**: 89–96.

123 Patel AA. Prevalence of chlamydia and gonorrhea in a public pregnancy termination clinic. *Contraception* 2007; **76**(Abstract): 166.

124 Royal College of Obstetricians and Gynaecologists. *The Care of Women Requesting Induced Abortion*. Evidence-based clinical guideline number 7. RCOG Press, London, 2004.

125 Ness RB, Trautmann G, Richter HE. Effectiveness of treatment strategies in some women with pelvic inflammatory disease: a randomized trial. *Obstet Gynecol* 2005; **106**: 573–580.

126 Paik CK, Waetjen LE, Xing G, Sweet RL. Epidemiology of pelvic inflammatory disease and tubo-ovarian abscess, 1991–2001. *Obstet Gynecol* 2005; **105**(Abstract): 23S.

127 Petit P, Bréard J, Montalescot V et al. Lethal toxin from *Clostridium sordellii* induces cell apoptotic death by disruption of mitochondrial homeostasis in HL-60 cells. *Cell Microbiol* 2003; **5**: 761–777.

128 Sutkin G, Capelle SD, Schlievert PM, Creinin MD. Toxic shock syndrome after laminaria insertion. *Obstet Gynecol* 2001; **98**: 959–961.

129 Mourton S, Rich W. Group A streptococcal toxic shock syndrome after an office endometrial biopsy: a case report. *J Reprod Med* 2006; **51**: 665–668.

130 Cohen AL, Bhatnagar J, Reagan S. Toxic shock associated with *Clostridium sordellii* and *Clostridium perfringens* after medical and spontaneous abortion. *Obstet Gynecol* 2007; **110**: 1027–1033.

131 Sinave C, Le Templier G, Blouin D et al. Toxic shock syndrome due to *Clostridium sordellii*: a dramatic postpartum and postabortion disease. *Clin Infect Dis* 2002; **35**: 1441–1443.

132 Fischer M, Bhatnagar J, Guarner J et al. Fatal toxic shock syndrome associated with *Clostridium sordellii* after medical abortion. *N Engl J Med* 2005; **353**: 2352–2360.

133 Rørbye C, Petersen IS, Nilas L. Postpartum *Clostridium sordellii* infection associated with fatal toxic shock syndrome. *Acta Obstet Gynecol Scand* 2000; **79**: 1134–1135.

134 Aldape MJ, Bryant AE, Stevens DL. *Clostridium sordellii* infection: epidemiology, clinical findings, and current perspectives on diagnosis and treatment. *Clin Infect Dis* 2006; **43**: 1436–1446.

135 Lichtenberg ES, Henning C. Conservative management of clostridial endometritis. *Am J Obstet Gynecol* 2004; **191**: 266–270.

136 Walker CK, Landers DV. Pelvic abscesses: new trends in management. *Obstet Gynecol Surv* 1991; **46**: 615–624.

137 Taylor KJ, Wasson JR, DeGraaff C, Rosenfield AT, Andriole VT. Accuracy of grey-scale ultrasound diagnosis of abdominal and pelvic abscesses in 220 patients. *Lancet* 1978; **1**: 83–84.

138 Reed SD, Landers DV, Sweet RL. Antibiotic treatment of tubo-ovarian abscess: comparison of broad-spectrum beta-lactam agents versus clindamycin-containing regimens. *Am J Obstet Gynecol* 1991; **164**: 1556–1562.

139 Stubblefield PG, Borgatta L. Complications of induced abortion. In: Pearlman MD, Tintinali JE, Dyne PL, eds. *Obstetric and Gynecologic Emergencies: Diagnosis and Management*. McGraw-Hill, New York, 2004.

140 Palys EE, Li J, Gaut PL, Hardy WD. Tricuspid valve endocarditis with Group B Streptococcus after an elective abortion: the need for new data. *Infect Dis Obstet Gynecol* 2006; 43253.

141 American College of Obstetricians and Gynecologists. Antibiotic prophylaxis for gynecologic procedures. ACOG Practice Bulletin No. 74. *Obstet Gynecol* 2006; **108**: 225–234.

142 Jeppson PC, Park A, Chen CCG. Multivalvular bacterial endocarditis after suction curettage abortion. *Obstet Gynecol* 2008; **112**: 452–455.

143 Schulz KF, Grimes DA, Cates W Jr. Measures to prevent cervical injury during suction curettage abortion. *Lancet* 1983; **1**: 1182–1185.

144 Lowensohn R, Ballard C. Cervicovaginal fistula: an apparent increased incidence with prostaglandin F2 alpha. *Am J Obstet Gynecol* 1974; **119**: 1057–1061.

145 Townsend DE, Barbis SD, Mathews RD. Vasopressin and operative hysteroscopy in the management of delayed postabortion and postpartum bleeding. *Am J Obstet Gynecol* 1991; **165**: 616–618.

146 Goldrath MH. Uterine tamponade for the control of acute uterine bleeding. *Am J Obstet Gynecol* 1983; **147**: 869–872.

147 Grimes DA, Schulz KF, Cates W Jr. Prevention of uterine perforation during curettage abortion. *JAMA* 1984; **251**: 2108–2111.

148 MacKay HT, Schulz KF, Grimes DA. Safety of local versus general anesthesia for second-trimester dilatation and evacuation abortion. *Obstet Gynecol* 1985; **66**: 661–665.

149 Kaali SG, Szigetvari IA, Bartfai GS. The frequency and management of uterine perforations during first-trimester abortions. *Am J Obstet Gynecol* 1989; **161**: 406–408.

150 White MK, Ory HW, Goldenberg LA. A case-control study of uterine perforations documented at laparoscopy. *Am J Obstet Gynecol* 1977; **129**: 623–625.

151 Chi I, Feldblum P. Uterine perforation during sterilization by laparoscopy and minilaparotomy. *Am J Obstet Gynecol* 1981; **139**: 735–736.

152 Freiman SM, Wulff GJ Jr. Management of uterine perforation following elective abortion. *Obstet Gynecol* 1977; **50**: 647–650.

153 Lindell G, Flam F. Management of uterine perforations in connection with legal abortions. *Acta Obstet Gynecol Scand* 1995; **74**: 373–375.

154 De La Vega GA, Nemiroff R, Debbs R. Complications of second-trimester dilation and evacuation. *Obstet Gynecol* 2007; **109** (Abstract): 21S.

155 Givens VM, Lipscomb GH. Retained fetal parts after elective second-trimester dilation and evacuation. *Obstet Gynecol* 2007; **109**: 526–527.

156 Imoedemhe DA, Ezimokhai M, Okpere EE, Aboh IF. Intestinal injuries following induced abortion. *Int J Gynaecol Obstet* 1984; **22**: 303–306.

157 Jhobta RS, Attri AK, Jhobta A. Bowel injury following induced abortion. *Int J Gynaecol Obstet* 2007; **96**: 24–27.

158 Sharma JB, Malhotra M, Pundir P. Laparoscopic oxidized cellulose (Surgicel) application for small uterine perforations. *Int J Gynaecol Obstet* 2003; **83**: 271–275.

159 Lajinian S, Margono F, Mroueh J. Sonographic appearance of suspected iatrogenic uterine perforation: A case report. *J Reprod Med* 1994; **39**: 911–912.

160 Soderstrom RM. Bowel injury litigation after laparoscopy. *J Am Assoc Gynecol Laparosc* 1993; **1**: 74–77.

161 Baggish MS. One-hundred and thirty small and large-bowel injuries associated with gynecologic laparoscopic operations. *J Gynecol Surg* 2007; **23**: 83–95.

162 Darney PD, Sweet RL. Routine intraoperative ultrasonography for second trimester abortion reduces incidence of uterine perforation. *J Ultrasound Med* 1989; **8**: 71–75.

163 Chen LH, Lai SF, Lee WH, Leong NK. Uterine perforation during elective first trimester abortions: a 13-year review. *Singapore Med J* 1995; **36**: 63–67.

164 Lichtenberg ES, Frederiksen MC. Cesarean scar dehiscence as a cause of hemorrhage after second-trimester abortion by dilation and evacuation. *Contraception* 2004; **70**: 61–64.

165 Lo ST, Ramsay P, Pierson R, Manconi F, Munro MG, Fraser IS. Endometrial thickness measured by ultrasound scan in women with uterine outlet obstruction due to intrauterine or upper cervical adhesions. *Hum Reprod* 2008; **23**: 306–309.

166 Luk J, Allen RA, Schantz-Dunn J, Goldberg AB. Intrauterine adhesions as a risk factor for failed first-trimester pregnancy termination. *Contraception* 2007; **76**: 331–333.

167 Hakim-Elahi E. Postabortal amenorrhea due to cervical stenosis. *Obstet Gynecol* 1976; **48**: 723–724.

168 Chapman K, Chapman R. Asherman's syndrome: a review of the literature, and a husband and wife's 20-year worldwide experience. *J R Soc Med* 1990; **83**: 576–580.

169 March CM, Israel R. Intrauterine adhesions secondary to elective abortion. Hyseteroscopic diagnosis and management. *Obstet Gynecol* 1976; **48**: 422–424.

170 Knopman J, Copperman AB. Value of 3D ultrasound in the management of suspected Asherman's syndrome. *J Reprod Med* 2007; **52**: 1016–1022.

171 Valle RF, Sciarra JJ. Intrauterine adhesions: hysteroscopic diagnosis, classification, treatment, and reproductive outcome. *Am J Obstet Gynecol* 1988; **158**: 1459–1470.

172 Krivak TC, Zorn KK. Venous thromboembolism in obstetrics and gynecology. *Obstet Gynecol* 2007; **109**: 761–777.

173 Lawson HW, Atrash JK, Franks AL. Fatal pulmonary embolism during legal induced abortion in the United States from 1972 to 1985. *Am J Obstet Gynecol* 1990; **162**: 986–990.

174 Kimball AM, Hallum AV, Cates W Jr. Deaths caused by pulmonary thromboembolism after legally induced abortion. *Am J Obstet Gynecol* 1978; **132**: 169–174.

175 Doyle NM, Ramirez MM, Mastrobattista JM, Monga M, Wagner LK, Gardner MO. Diagnosis of pulmonary embolism: a cost-effectiveness analysis. *Am J Obstet Gynecol* 2004; **191**: 1019–1023.

176 Clark SL, Hankins GDV, Dudley DA, Didly GA, Porter TF. Amniotic fluid embolism: analysis of the national registry. *Am J Obstet Gynecol* 1995; **172**: 1158–1169.

177 Guidotti RJ, Grimes DA, Cates W Jr. Fatal amniotic fluid embolism during legally induced abortion, United States, 1972 to 1978. *Am J Obstet Gynecol* 1981; **141**: 257–261.

178 Hawes CS, Suskin HA, Petropoulos A, Latham SE, Mueller UW. A morphologic study of trophoblast isolated from peripheral blood of pregnant women. *Am J Obstet Gynecol* 1994; **170**: 1297–1300.

179 Clark SL, Pavlova Z, Greenspoon J, Horensten J, Phelan JP. Squamous cells in the maternal pulmonary circulation. *Am J Obstet Gynecol* 1986; **154**: 104–106.

180 Lee W, Ginsburg KA, Cotton DB, Kaufman RH. Squamous and trophoblastic cells in the maternal pulmonary circulation identified by invasive hemodynamic monitoring during the peripartum period. *Am J Obstet Gynecol* 1986; **155**: 999–1001.

181 Clark SL. New concepts of amniotic fluid embolism: a review. *Obstet Gynecol Surv* 1990; **45**: 360–368.

182 Gei A, Hankins GDV. Amniotic fluid embolism: An update. *Contemp OB/GYN* 2000; **45**: 53–66.

183 Ellis AK, Day JH. Incidence and characteristics of biphasic anaphylaxis: a prospective evaluation of 103 patients. *Ann Allergy Asthma Immunol* 2007; **98**: 64–69.

184 Grubb BP. Neurocardiogenic syncope and related disorders of orthostatic intolerance. *Circulation* 2005; **111**: 2997–3006.

185 Hendler I, Schatz M, Momirova V et al. Association of obesity with pulmonary and nonpulmonary complications of pregnancy in asthmatic women. *Obstet Gynecol* 2006; **108**: 77–82.

16

CHAPTER 16
Answering questions about long-term outcomes

Carol J. Rowland Hogue PhD, MPH, Lori A. Boardman MD, ScM, and Nada Stotland MD, MPH

LEARNING POINTS

- Studying potential long-term outcomes of abortion is challenging because of limitations in study design and data quality.
- First-trimester induced abortion is not associated with adverse pregnancy outcomes in the future.
- Abortion has no association with an increased risk of cancer, and some studies suggest a small decrease in the risk of endometrial and ovarian cancers.
- The most common emotional response to abortion is a sense of relief.
- No credible evidence supports a syndrome of lasting psychological trauma after abortion.

Introduction

Women seeking abortion are generally young and healthy. Therefore, considerable attention has been given to potential long-term health effects of induced abortion, particularly in regards to future fertility, cancer of the breast, and psychological outcomes. Fortunately, substantial evidence indicates that abortion is a safe procedure with few late sequelae. Patients may have concerns and questions about the long-term safety of abortion, however, because they either lack information or have received misinformation. Using a series of commonly asked questions, this chapter reviews the evidence regarding long-term outcomes and provides information that clinicians can use when counseling patients.

Abortion and future reproductive health

"My letter to the President focused on psychological effects of abortion because we had long since concluded that the physical sequelae of abortion were no different than those found in women who carried pregnancy to term or who had never been pregnant. I had nothing further to add to that subject in my letter to the President (Surgeon General Everett Koop [1])."

Management of Unintended and Abnormal Pregnancy, 1st edition. By M Paul, ES Lichtenberg, L Borgatta, DA Grimes, PG Stubblefield, MD Creinin

Why worry about the reproductive sequelae of induced abortion?

Surgeon General Everett Koop, in his testimony to a Congressional Subcommittee in 1989 excerpted in the previous paragraph, reflects a consensus that induced abortion does not pose a risk for subsequent reproductive health. Nevertheless, concerns among women arise, and they need to know the facts. Recent claims that induced abortion increases the risk of preterm delivery and mood disorders [2] have contributed to these concerns.

Many women seeking termination of their current pregnancy may choose to bear children in the future. Some will try to become pregnant again, only to experience secondary infertility. Others (perhaps one in three) will experience a clinical or subclinical early pregnancy loss. At least 1 in 20 subsequent births will be premature or of low birth weight. On occasion, women will have serious pregnancy complications, including ectopic pregnancy or fetal demise. When complications do occur, women naturally seek causes and explanations. Providers need to inform women about whether an abortion may affect future reproductive health.

Does having one abortion imperil the woman's future reproductive health?

A comprehensive review of this question was published in 1982 [3] and subsequently updated [4]. The authors concluded that the answer depends on the type of abortion procedure and the gestational age at the time of abortion.

Studies that do not separate induced from spontaneous abortion shed no light on the question; whereas induced abortion is usually performed on healthy women, spontaneous abortion is a reproductive complication that may be associated with medical conditions and other adverse reproductive outcomes. Unsafe, illegal abortions and those performed by dilation and sharp curettage (D&C), particularly when performed under general anesthesia, may increase the risk of preterm delivery.

Secondary infertility is not increased after induced abortion [4,5]. Other reproductive outcomes extensively studied are ectopic pregnancy and preterm delivery.

Ectopic pregnancy

Ectopic pregnancy following one or more abortions has been studied extensively [6–13]. Carefully controlled studies of the effect of one or more surgical induced abortions on ectopic pregnancy find no measurable increased risk. These studies illustrate some of the methodological challenges inherent in epidemiologic studies of the late effects of induced abortion.

Control group comparability

Competing reproductive factors and events make choosing the right comparison group difficult. Women using contraception effectively are less likely to have unintended pregnancies, and thus they have less need for induced abortion. Women who have never been pregnant or who are pregnant for the first time have, by definition, not been exposed to a prior induced abortion. Women giving birth are, on average, less likely to have experienced a previous induced abortion than a randomly selected group of nonpregnant women or a group of pregnant women chosen to represent all pregnancy outcomes (i.e., induced abortion of this pregnancy as well as delivery)[14]. In a case-control study of ectopic pregnancy in Italy, for example, the odds ratio (OR) associated with one prior abortion was 2.1 when compared with women giving birth, but 1.2 when compared with women hospitalized for nonobstetric reasons. Results for the effect of multiple induced abortions in this study were similarly biased [15].

Regardless of how investigators chose to control for the potential impact of prior induced abortions, the results were similar. For women with one prior abortion, adjusted ORs for ectopic pregnancy ranged from 0.9 to 1.4, and none was significantly elevated. Samples were large enough in four studies to rule out a twofold excess risk. For women with two or more prior abortions, adjusted ORs varied more broadly, from 0.2 to 2.6. This range reflects the smaller sample sizes and wider confidence limits, but none of the results was statistically significant.

Selective recall

Like many studies of the reproductive health effects of induced abortion, the studies of ectopic pregnancy are case-control investigations. Researchers asked women with an ectopic pregnancy (cases) about their previous abortions and then compared their responses with those of controls. Study results depend on the accurate recall of past abortion history; however, the highly charged emotional environment surrounding abortion makes women reluctant to reveal a past abortion history. This reluctance results in selective recall, that is, women who have a poor pregnancy outcome are more likely to mention their abortion history to the interviewer than are women in the control group [16,17]. Such selective recall biases the results of case-control studies toward finding a spurious excess risk, perhaps by as much as 20 to 50% over the true risk. Selective recall could explain the small (but nonsignificant) increased ORs found for pregnancies following one induced abortion in three of the studies of ectopic pregnancy [6–8].

Prospective studies that begin with the woman's abortion experience do not suffer from selective recall bias, but such expensive and time-consuming investigations are less common than the more economical case-control studies. In one Norwegian study [18], the adjusted incidence density ratio (number of incident cases divided by the length of follow-up among subjects) for ectopic pregnancy was 1.2 (95% CI 0.5, 3.1) for women with two or more induced abortions compared with those with one abortion.

Competing risk factors

Even when the control group is appropriate, the study must control adequately for competing risk factors. Women who terminate a pregnancy differ from those who do not in ways that affect reproductive health. For example, they are more likely to smoke [3] and to be exposed to sexually transmitted infections (STIs) through a greater number of sexual partners, earlier age at first sex, preexisting pelvic inflammatory disease, and less reliance on condoms for protection from STIs.

Studies that fail to control for competing risk factors will overestimate the impact of induced abortions on poor reproductive functioning. Examples of such studies include ectopic pregnancy (OR of 1.87 [95% CI 0.84, 4.16])[19]; placenta previa (adjusted OR of 1.28 [95% CI 1.00, 1.63] for one or more induced abortions)[18]; neonatal sepsis (adjusted OR of 2.20 [95% CI 1.73, 2.29])[20]; and secondary infertility (adjusted OR of 2.1 [95% CI 1.1, 4.0] for one induced abortion and 2.3 [95% CI 1.0, 5.3] for more than one induced abortion)[21]. When the lower limit of the 95% confidence interval is greater than 1.0, the effect is said to be statistically significant (i.e., the probability of a difference of this size resulting from chance is less than 5%). Thus, with the exception of the ectopic pregnancy study, these more flawed studies concluded that induced abortion slightly increased the risk of adverse outcomes (odds ratios ranging from 1.28 to 2.3).

Preterm delivery

Well-conducted, prospective studies uniformly find that one vacuum aspiration in the first trimester does not increase the risk of preterm delivery. However, many flawed studies of induced abortion have been published; some conclude that induced abortion increases preterm delivery risk, whereas others do not find an elevated risk. Common and pervasive flaws include relying on the woman's recall to document abortion [22], failing to control for major confounding (a mixing or blurring of effects), using incorrect comparison groups [23,24], and imprecision about the abortion method. Flaws introduce biases away from the null hypothesis. For example, a review of literature that did not take these flaws into consideration [2] disputed earlier conclusions regarding preterm delivery, although other investigators [25–27] concur that one surgical abortion does not increase the risk of preterm delivery in the next pregnancy.

The only studies free from selective recall are cohort designs that document the induced abortion through abortion records. Several such large, population-based studies show no effect of induced abortion on early or late preterm delivery or low birth weight [23,24,26]. Such studies have more scientific credibility.

Studies that control more effectively for confounding find no effect of induced abortion on preterm delivery [28], even among teenagers with repeat pregnancies [29,30], although Reime did report a significant association between history of abortion and very low birth weight among primiparous teenagers. Case-control studies that report elevated risk of very early preterm delivery associated with history of abortion, such as the EPIPAGE study in France [22], point to infectious causes of preterm delivery. This finding suggests that undiagnosed infectious complications of previous abortions may increase risk of preterm delivery in subsequent pregnancies.

Because first-born infants are at increased risk of preterm delivery, comparing second-born to first-born infants introduces bias. Incorrect comparison groups include gravida 2, para 1 (i.e., two pregnancies, one birth) compared with gravida 2, induced abortion 1, para 0. An excellent illustration of this bias is in the study by Zhou [23,24]. Although often cited as positive evidence of an abortion effect, this study shows no effect of previous induced abortion on first-born infants' risk of low birth weight [24] and minimal, crude effect for preterm delivery [23]. This crude effect would likely have disappeared if the authors conducted a proper multivariate analysis for para 0 women.

Does medical abortion have an impact on subsequent reproduction?

Emerging evidence suggests no elevated risk to subsequent pregnancies associated with prior medical abortion using mifepristone regimens. Although one population-based, case-control study of ectopic pregnancy reported an OR of 2.8 for previous medical abortion [13], only 24 women in this study reported having had a medical abortion (13 cases and 11 controls). A much larger, prospective study [27] found no association between medical abortion and subsequent ectopic pregnancy, when compared with women who had surgical abortion in the previous study. Results for low birth weight and preterm birth were similar in another large, multicenter study in China [31].

Do other abortion procedures increase reproductive risks?

With respect to other types of procedures, study findings are not as definitive:

- Abortion performed by D&C, particularly if performed under general anesthesia, may result in uterine synechiae (uterine scarring) that increase the risk of subsequent midtrimester spontaneous abortions and low-birth-weight deliveries.
- Second-trimester procedures have not been studied as extensively as have first-trimester procedures, but there is no evidence from the published literature that labor-induction abortion methods are associated with significantly increased risk of adverse pregnancy outcomes [4,32].
- Dilation and evacuation (D&E) procedures may pose some risk, especially if cervical dilation is not carried out gradually with osmotic dilators [4,33]. A recent small cohort study found no important differences in adverse pregnancy outcomes after standard D&E[1] versus intact D&E [34].

If one abortion does not harm reproductive health, are multiple abortions also safe?

Earlier studies suggested little or no increased risk of more than one abortion compared with one abortion [4,35]. However, the evidence is mixed in more recent studies. Retrospective recall of two or more vacuum aspiration procedures was associated with vaginal bleeding during the first two trimesters of pregnancy in North Carolina [36] and with very early preterm births in the large EUROPOP study conducted in 16 countries [37]. Although some investigators [25] accept this finding as evidence that multiple abortions do increase preterm delivery risk, the association may not be causal.

A likely explanation for any observed "dose-response" effect of multiple abortions on infection-associated, early preterm loss is unmeasured confounding. In a study in

[1] While the authors here adopt the term "standard D&E" as the US Supreme Court used it in *Gonzalez V. Carhart*, 127 S.C&. 1610 (2007), to refer to non-intact d&Es, the term is not medical, and the authors in no way suggest that any one variant of D&E is more or less standard than another.

Finland of 26,976 pregnancies occurring from 1989 to 2001 in which abortion history was obtained at 20 weeks' gestation, the sample size was large enough for precise estimates of effect for fetal distress (various measures) and admission to neonatal intensive care (adjusted odds ratio [AOR] = 1.29 [95%. CI 0.90, 1.85]) as well as low birth weight (AOR = 1.26 [95% CI 0.79, 2.00]), intrauterine growth restriction (AOR = 0.99 [95% CI 0.70, 1.40]), preterm delivery (AOR = 1.35 [95% CI 0.91, 2.02]), cesarean delivery (AOR = 1.15 [95% CI 0.85, 1.55]), but not perinatal death (AOR = 0.52, [95% CI 0.07, 3.75])[26].

What can the provider do to assist the woman in preserving her reproductive health?

Four measures may help:

- Provide prophylactic antibiotics. Postabortal infection or preexisting and nontreated STIs are risk factors for subsequent secondary infertility, ectopic pregnancy, and fetal loss. Prophylactic antibiotics at the time of the abortion procedure protect against pelvic infection [38].
- Counsel the woman regarding her reproductive health risk factors. The abortion visit is an opportunity to provide contraceptives and contraceptive counseling, as well as education about the risks of STIs and smoking.
- Provide appropriate informed consent, including the potential risks of the abortion procedure.
- Encourage the woman to report her abortion history when she seeks reproductive health care in the future. In rare instances, an unrecognized complication of the abortion procedure can be the cause of a subsequent problem. To rule out such complications, her provider needs to know about her past experience with induced abortion.

Abortion and cancer

Numerous studies have addressed the possible relationship between induced abortion and the subsequent development of cancer, particularly that of the breast. Most of the initial evidence was derived from case-control studies in which researchers frequently relied on interviews to gather information regarding pregnancy history. As noted earlier, this method of ascertainment is prone to numerous biases, including underreporting of both induced and spontaneous abortions, particularly among the control women in whom the disease had not developed [17,39–42]. Published abortion rates in such studies range widely, from less than 2% to more than 30%, which may in part reflect these differences in reporting. Whether women with cancer are more likely to report a risk factor than women who serve as controls, however, remains debatable [17,41,43].

Does induced abortion increase a woman's risk of nongynecological malignancies?

Numerous investigators have evaluated induced abortion as a potential risk factor for carcinoma of the thyroid. In a pooled analysis of 14 case-control studies, a history of induced abortion did not appear to correlate with an increased risk of thyroid cancer [44]. On the other hand, findings from prospective cohort studies range from protective effects associated with spontaneous abortion [45] to increased risks of papillary or follicular thyroid carcinoma among women with histories of either spontaneous abortions (OR 1.4 [95% CI 0.9, 2.1]) or voluntary terminations (OR 3.1 [95% CI 1.5, 6.2]). The study authors caution, however, that the elevated risk seen in women with a history of induced abortion may reflect surveillance bias [46].

With regard to cancers of the gastrointestinal tract, Kvale and Heuch [47] conducted a cohort study assessing the relationship between colorectal cancer and various reproductive risk factors in 63,000 women enrolled in a breast cancer screening program in Norway. Following adjustment for potential confounders, they found a significantly increased risk (OR 1.72 [95% CI 1.14, 2.62]) of rectal cancer in women who had had two or more abortions, but they did not stratify between spontaneous and induced abortions. On the other hand, La Vecchia [48] found a decreased risk of colon carcinoma among women with a history of two or more induced abortions (RR 0.4, $p < 0.05$). In case-control studies of both gastric cancer [49] and pancreatic cancer [50], no association was demonstrated among women with a history of either spontaneous or induced abortion. As for cancers of renal and hematologic sites, little has been written and the findings are inconclusive [48]. None of these cancers has a plausible link to abortion.

Does induced abortion increase a woman's risk of gynecological malignancies?

The majority of the literature regarding cancers of the pelvic organs focuses on ovarian carcinoma. Negri [51] reviewed 16 case-control studies that provided data on abortion history: nine demonstrated no association between abortion and subsequent development of ovarian cancer, six showed an inverse relationship, and one reported a nonsignificant association. However, many of these investigations included not only spontaneous and induced abortions, but also stillbirths. Three of these studies examined induced abortions independently and found a protective effect of induced abortion on ovarian cancer risk, particularly for those women undergoing two or more pregnancy terminations [52]. Mori et al [53] had similar results, as did Greggi [54]. In a prospective cohort study, Jacobson [55] documented improved survival in ovarian cancer patients who had two or more abortions (RR 0.5 [95% CI 0.3, 0.9]), although these results have not been confirmed in subsequent published literature [56].

Methodological problems plague many of the studies on cervical and endometrial cancers. In an ecological study based on official abortion statistics and regional cancer rates in the former Soviet Union, Remennick [57] reported a significant association between cervical cancer and a history of two or more abortions. However, because of the limitations of this study design, the author was unable to control for confounding risk factors, such as sexual behavior. When risk factors including age, education, number of sexual partners, smoking, and early age at first coitus and first birth were placed into a multivariate logistic regression model, Parazzini [58] found no association between number of induced abortions and invasive squamous cell carcinoma of the cervix. However, Parazzini [59], in a separate case-control study, did demonstrate an increased risk of adenocarcinoma of the cervix in women with a history of induced abortion (OR 3.7, 95% CI 1.6, 8.2). These results conflict with those of Brinton [60].

As for endometrial cancer, evidence largely points to either no association or an inverse relationship [61,62]. Of note, two studies have shown a positive association between induced abortion and endometrial cancer [63,64]. In the Brinton study, multiple terminations did not affect the risk estimate, raising questions, as the authors note, about the biologic credibility of the association. Instead, reporting bias, uncontrolled confounding, or chance may in part explain the observed relationship.

Does induced abortion increase a woman's risk of breast cancer?

Studies examining the relationship between induced abortion and breast cancer are far more numerous. Many of these studies are of case-control design and show inconsistent findings. However, multiple large prospective cohort studies have now been published, the results of which provide the most appropriate information to use when counseling women concerned about this issue.

In 1996, Brind published a review and meta-analysis on breast cancer and abortion, including 23 studies that distinguished between spontaneous and induced abortion [65]. Of these studies, 12 showed no association between induced abortion and breast cancer; four reported nearly significant associations, and seven reported significant elevations in risks of breast cancer in women who had induced abortions. Five of these studies were published after 1989 and were among the works most commonly cited as showing a link between induced abortion and breast cancer [66–70].

The evidence addressing the association between breast cancer and abortion does not meet a number of the criteria for causality [71] (Table 16.1). First, the initial rationale for biological plausibility (i.e., pregnancy interruption negates the protection from mammary tumorigenesis associated with full-term pregnancy) described by Russo and Russo in 1980 [72] has been supplanted with evidence to the contrary. An incomplete pregnancy of short duration may in fact impart the benefits of a full-term pregnancy with respect to the development of breast cancer [73]. The mechanism by which this protective effect is postulated to occur involves placental human chorionic gonadotropin (hCG), an important regulator of cellular differentiation, proliferation, and apoptosis. Placental hCG, which rises rapidly in the first trimester and peaks at roughly 8 to 10 weeks of gestation, also induces the production of inhibin, a tumor-suppressor factor, in the mammary epithelium, thus protecting the breast against carcinogenic initiation [74]. Supporting the protective effect of short-term exposure to hCG is evidence of a reduced risk of breast cancer among women receiving hCG injections as part of a weight loss regimen or infertility treatment [75].

Second, as Rosenberg [76] points out, a typical difference in risk of 50% (OR of 1.5) is a weak effect and could easily result from bias in observational studies. In our examination of the research on induced abortion and breast cancer, the strength of association, where one exists, is consistently small with relative risks and odds ratios rarely exceeding 1.4.

Consistency of results is also lacking. For example, subsequent authors have failed to confirm Daling's [69] finding

Table 16.1 Some criteria for judging causality (Adapted from Hill [71]).

1. Strength of the association. The greater the relative risk (for cohort studies) or odds ratio (for case-control studies), the more likely the association is causal.
2. Consistency. The association has been observed in a variety of populations under a variety of circumstances.
3. Specificity. The exposure causes a specific effect.
4. Temporality. The cause precedes the effect in time.
5. Dose-response relationship. The greater the exposure, the greater the magnitude of effect.
6. Biological plausibility. There is a rational biological explanation for the association.
7. Coherence. The association is in accord with existing knowledge of the natural history and biology of the disease.
8. Experimental evidence. Laboratory data support the human findings.
9. Analogy. Similar exposures are associated with similar effects.

of an association between induced abortion and breast cancer [77–80]. Disparate results have also been reported for certain subgroups of women, such as young women, nulliparae, multiparae, or women undergoing abortions before their first birth [39,77]. Examination of these studies reveals no clear, reproducible subset of women for whom induced abortion increases the risk of development of breast cancer.

A preferable way to examine the relationship between breast cancer and abortion is to start with a population of women who had abortions and then follow them for the development of breast cancer (i.e., a cohort study). Melbye et al [78], in a cohort of 1.5 million Danish women, demonstrated that induced abortions had no overall effect on the risk of breast cancer. Although the authors found a statistically significant increase in risk among women who had undergone second-trimester abortions after 18 weeks' gestation, this increase did not affect the overall result, because most abortions occurred in the first trimester. On the other hand, abortion at less than 7 weeks' gestation was associated with a statistically insignificant decrease in risk of subsequent development of breast cancer. Caution is warranted because of the small number of women with breast cancer who underwent very early abortions, and only 14 of the 10,246 women (0.14%) with breast cancer had a history of induced abortion after 18 weeks.

Other more recent, large cohort studies confirm the findings of Melbye [73,81]. For example, using data from 59,000 women recruited into the Black Women's Health Study, Palmer et al [81] found that among nulliparous women, the incidence rate ratio (following adjustment for multiple factors) for any induced abortion relative to none was 0.9 (95% CI 0.5, 1.4).

In summary, what can providers tell patients about the impact of induced abortion on the future development of cancer?

Regarding sites other than the breast, the literature is sparse and conclusions are difficult to draw. However, limited evidence to date suggests that induced abortion is not a risk factor for future cancers and may be protective for endometrial and ovarian carcinomas. As for breast cancer, the picture has become clear. Although findings from the case-control studies are inconsistent, more credible cohort studies convincingly point to a lack of association between induced abortion and the subsequent development of breast cancer. In fact, the American College of Obstetricians and Gynecologists [82], the National Cancer Institute [83], the American Cancer Society [84], and the World Health Organization [85] have all concluded that no evidence supports a causal relationship between breast cancer and induced abortion. At present, patients may be reassured that induced abortions performed in the first and early second trimesters of pregnancy have little, if any, impact on their baseline risk of breast cancer.

Psychological sequelae

No convincing evidence suggests that induced abortion causes important negative psychiatric sequelae. As noted earlier for other outcomes, the study of the psychiatric consequences of abortion is fraught with misleading allegations and methodological difficulties. For example, normal feelings, such as sadness, are confused with psychiatric illnesses, such as depression [86].

After months or years, distinguishing the possible impact of an induced abortion from other life events may be impossible. Subsequent life events and circumstances influence a woman's memory of and attitude toward past life events and decisions. Moreover, an unplanned or unwanted pregnancy can itself be a powerfully stressful life event. Prospective assessment is thus better than retrospective recall. However, few studies prospectively assess the effects of abortion over women's lifetime [87]. Prospective assessment is difficult because women who have abortions prefer to put the experience behind them. Requiring long-term follow-up, especially in the absence of substantive evidence of psychological harm, would impose an undue burden.

Studies of psychological aspects of abortion often lack a control group, especially studies claiming to detect negative sequelae. For a woman contemplating abortion, the only real alternative is to deliver and then either care for the child or place the child for adoption. Although using women who chose to continue their pregnancies as controls might seem reasonable, these women are not comparable. Women who choose to continue their pregnancies differ from those who elect abortion in cogent psychosocial baseline variables (financial and relational status, caretaking responsibilities, domestic violence, preparedness, and desire to assume the responsibilities of motherhood); indeed, these are the very factors that influence women to continue or terminate pregnancies [88,89]. Neither is it possible to assign pregnant women randomly to abortion or continued pregnancy/delivery.

Despite the methodological problems, if serious psychiatric sequelae resulted from a procedure performed over a million times a year in the USA, and many more worldwide, those sequelae would have become apparent by now. Tens of millions of abortions have been provided in the USA, and no such sequelae have emerged [90,91].

Do factors other than the abortion per se influence a woman's psychological responses to the abortion experience?

The psychological outcome of an abortion is most directly related to the psychological condition of the woman before her abortion [92]. Many factors can influence the patient's response to her abortion experience (Chapter 3), and only a few will be discussed briefly here.

Social burdens

Women living in poverty, abusive relationships, chaotic social conditions, or caring for dependents with inadequate social support often have difficulty obtaining contraceptives and refusing unprotected intercourse [93,94]. These social circumstances also have a negative effect on women's mood and mental functioning before and after abortion [95,96].

Personal relationships

Women often elect abortion because of failed relationships with the men who impregnated them. Pregnancy itself can precipitate a man's flight. The woman, who might have wanted the pregnancy, may decide that raising a child is now untenable. Although the decision to have an abortion is hers, she must cope emotionally with two losses: her lover and her pregnancy. If the threat of abandonment occurs in a relationship that already includes children, such an ultimatum may jeopardize the family's well-being. A woman may feel that she has no choice but to terminate the pregnancy in order to protect her relationship and her children [97].

Religious conflicts

Many of the same religious denominations that forbid abortion also forbid or frown upon extramarital intercourse and contraceptives. Women who belong to these faiths may feel more comfortable engaging in sexual activity when "swept away" by romantic feelings rather than planning to have intercourse and making contraceptive arrangements. If pregnancy ensues, however, they may find the prospect of having a child out of wedlock unacceptable. Women who choose abortion in these circumstances face a religious dilemma: to eschew their faith and the social network that goes with it; to decide that the precepts of their religious leaders regarding sex and abortion are unrealistic and can therefore be ignored; to confess to their religious leaders and congregation and risk ostracism in hopes of understanding and forgiveness; or to keep the abortion secret and bear their guilt alone [98,99]. Each of these choices carries a psychological burden.

Youth

In the USA, the proliferation of state laws mandating parental involvement in the abortion decisions of minors reflects an assumption that young women lack the capacity to make decisions about pregnancy. Despite the fact that adolescents are on average less psychologically mature than adults, research demonstrates that they are as capable as adults of making informed, rational decisions concerning their pregnancies [100]. In addition, no evidence suggests that adolescents experience poorer outcomes than adults [101–104].

Rape

A woman pregnant by rape carries within her a pregnancy that combines her genetic heritage with that of a man who has committed a horrendous assault on her. Some women in these circumstances choose to carry to term, whereas others seek abortion services. Among the latter group may be some women who, absent the rape, would not want to abort even an unintended pregnancy. For such women, as for sexual assault survivors in general, either option (continuing the pregnancy or ending it) may entail great psychological stress.

Incest

Pregnancy conceived by incest is still more psychologically complex. The perpetrator may be someone on whom the pregnant woman (often a minor) depends for support such as a family member, and he may make sexual activity a condition of love and care. Family members to whom she turns for support may nevertheless blame her, abandon her, and/or abjure her to silence.

Antiabortion activism

In the USA, abortion has been legal nationwide only since 1973, and it has become increasingly legally constrained since that time (Chapter 4). To undergo a procedure that was recently illegal and that vociferous groups would like to make illegal again carries a very different emotional valence than to have an abortion in a culture, like Japan's or Russia's, where abortion is more accepted [105,106].

Antiabortion demonstrators may attempt to deter patients from entering clinics. They often carry placards bearing gory photographs and plead with women not to "kill their babies." They sometimes attack abortion providers and vandalize and bomb abortion clinics. Even when not overtly violent, these demonstrations evoke anxiety and fear among women and their companions [107,108].

Recently, the allegation that abortion damages women psychologically has become the central, avowed strategy of antiabortion activists [109]. Despite the testimony of scientific experts, assertions to this effect are enshrined in state laws and even in a US Supreme Court decision (Chapter 4). Most people trust government entities to provide accurate information. They are not aware that national and state legislatures and courts can assert, and make binding decisions on the basis of, claims clearly contrary to the scientific evidence [110]. Being convinced that a procedure is psychologically damaging is a risk factor for psychological damage in those who contemplate or undergo that procedure [111].

What is the most common emotional response following abortion?

The most common emotional response following abortion is relief [112]. Women invest substantial emotional energy and deliberation in the decision to have an abortion, and carrying out the decision resolves the stressful situation. Some women, as well as their partners, report that this decision-making was the first time in their lives that they had thought ahead to their futures and taken responsibility and control.

Some women experience guilt after having an abortion. They may feel that they have placed their well-being over the potential life of the embryo or fetus, or that their emotional and physical resources were not sufficient to support another life [113]. Many women feel a sense of sadness about the loss of a pregnancy. Feelings of guilt and loss resolve spontaneously within days or weeks in most cases, do not impair women's ability to function, and do not constitute a psychological disorder or psychiatric illness [102,114].

Very few data are available comparing psychological responses in women having early medical versus surgical abortions. One recent prospective investigation found no significant differences in postabortal anxiety, depression, or low self-esteem among women randomized to medical abortion using mifepristone-prostaglandin or vacuum aspiration [115–117].

Does abortion increase a woman's risk for future psychiatric illness?

Until 1973, most studies of the psychological sequelae of abortion in the USA involved women who either underwent illegal operations or managed to gain access to legal abortion on the grounds of mental or general health impairment. Women seeking abortion on these grounds often had to obtain supporting opinions from several physicians or convince a panel of physicians of the validity of their need for the procedure. Some women claimed suicidal intent or feigned mental illnesses in order to obtain permission for abortion. Psychoanalytic theories before 1973 attributed abortion to unconscious psychological conflict, but this hypothesis has never been confirmed in scientific studies.

In contrast to the USA and many other countries, European countries generally permit abortions and provide abortion services as part of national health plans accessible to women of all socioeconomic strata. Most of the studies of psychological sequelae have necessarily been performed in these countries. Much of the literature is decades old, probably because those studies were so reassuring that further research was unlikely to be useful. Recent reviews of the literature, including one by the American Psychological Association, confirm that the most rigorous studies show no association between induced abortion and major psychiatric sequelae [118–120]. Using psychiatric hospitalization as a marker for significant psychiatric illness, postpartum women are over 10 times as likely to require psychiatric hospitalization as women who have had induced abortions.

What are the specific risk factors for psychiatric illness following abortion?

Women who have psychiatric illness before an abortion are likely to continue to have psychiatric illness following an abortion [91,120]. The stressful circumstances leading to the abortion may contribute to an exacerbation or recurrence of preexisting disease. Preexisting psychiatric illnesses can also compromise a woman's ability to protect herself against unwanted or unprotected intercourse and pregnancy and make her vulnerable to antiabortion groups eager to use her distress as an example of the moral evil and health dangers of abortion.

Women who decide to terminate pregnancies on genetic or medical grounds would otherwise have preferred to carry their pregnancies. These women and their partners tend to be older than the average pregnant couple, and many have delayed childbearing; therefore these pregnancies may be especially wanted and valued. Abortion under these circumstances entails not only ambivalence over the loss of a wanted pregnancy, but also the perceived failure to conceive or maintain a normal pregnancy [121,122]. These circumstances may also threaten the relationship.

What is the evidence for an "abortion trauma syndrome"?

A growing body of scientific and popular publications claims evidence for a so-called "abortion trauma syndrome" or "postabortion depression and psychosis [123,124]." These studies suffer from the aforementioned methodological shortcomings [119]. Some use databases not originally compiled to address the impact of abortion and without information on either the preabortion mental state of the subjects or the psychosocial circumstances under which the abortion occurred. Some reports are anecdotal, involving self-selected populations of women who are often linked to a religious denomination strongly opposed to abortion or who have been treated by clinicians with similar negative beliefs [125]. A Public Broadcasting System program available on the Internet, "Postabortion Politics," depicts the arguments and meetings of groups that assert these misconceptions [126]. The program and these studies portray women racked by guilt, sadness, and preoccupation with the aborted "child," causing interference with their current relationships and functional capacities; these effects are attributed to abortions that the women underwent years or decades before. Notably, no one syndrome, or constellation of signs and symptoms, has been described; moreover, no such "abortion trauma syndrome" is included in the *Diagnostic and Statistical Manual of Mental Disorders*, 4th Edition [127].

What can the provider do to assist women in coping with a problem pregnancy and abortion?

No evidence suggests that therapeutic counseling is more necessary for the woman considering abortion than for the woman deciding to have a baby or an operation. The resources most important for healthy coping with a problem pregnancy and abortion include information about pregnancy options, access to services needed to carry out a woman's decision, and the respect and support of loved ones and health professionals regardless of the choice a woman makes. Some patients appreciate the opportunity to discuss the nature of their social supports and resources for maximizing them.

Providers should inform patients that a wide range of emotional responses is normal after abortion. These emotions should resolve spontaneously within days or weeks and should not interfere with a woman's ability to carry out her usual activities. Women with persistent symptoms or symptoms that interfere with normal activities warrant referral for mental health care. Likewise, women who attribute psychological suffering or symptoms to abortions may benefit from counseling by a nonjudgmental, supportive therapist. Providers also should seek specialty consultation for women who are unable to give informed consent, who cannot arrive at a decision because of paralyzing ambivalence, or who have psychiatric illness that requires treatment. Patients who are in abusive relationships should be referred to appropriate resources.

Conclusion

In conclusion, the most common emotional response to induced abortion is relief. Few women suffer emotional complications of abortion. The psychological sequelae of abortion must always be viewed in the context of the alternative for the pregnant woman: childbirth followed by childrearing or adoption. These outcomes all carry greater emotional risks.

References

1 Koop, Surgeon General Everett, C. Medical and psychological impact of abortion. In: *Hearing Before the Human Resources and Intergovernmental Relations Subcommittee of the Committee on Government Operations, House of Representatives, One Hundred First Congress – First Session*. US Government Printing Office, Washington (DC), 1989.

2 Thorp JM Jr, Hartmann KE, Shadigian E. Long-term physical and psychological health consequences of induced abortion: review of the evidence. *Obstet Gynecol Surv* 2003; **58**: 67–79.

3 Hogue C, Cates W Jr, Tietze C. The effects of induced abortion on subsequent reproduction. *Epidemiol Rev* 1982; **4**: 66–94.

4 Atrash HK, Hogue CJ. The effect of pregnancy termination on future reproduction. *Baillieres Clin Obstet Gynaecol* 1990; **4**: 391–405.

5 Frank P, McNamee R, Hannaford PC, Kay CR, Hirsch S. The effect of induced abortion on subsequent fertility. *Br J Obstet Gynaecol* 1993; **100**: 575–580.

6 Levin AA, Schoenbaum SC, Stubblefield PG, Zimicki S, Monson RR, Ryan KJ. Ectopic pregnancy and prior induced abortion. *Am J Public Health* 1982; **72**: 253–256.

7 Daling JR, Chow WH, Weiss NS, Metch BJ, Soderstrom R. Ectopic pregnancy in relation to previous induced abortion. *JAMA* 1985; **253**: 1005–1008.

8 Skjeldestad FE, Atrash HK. Evaluation of induced abortion as a risk factor for ectopic pregnancy; a case-control study. *Acta Obstet Gynecol Scand* 1997; **76**: 151–158.

9 Skjeldestad FE, Gargiullo PM, Kendrick JS. Multiple induced abortions as risk factor for ectopic pregnancy; a prospective study. *Acta Obstet Gynecol Scand* 1997; **76**: 691–696.

10 Atrash HK, Strauss LT, Kendrick JS, Skjeldestad FE, Ahn YW. The relation between induced abortion and ectopic pregnancy. *Obstet Gynecol* 1997; **89**: 512–518.

11 Burkman RT, Mason KJ, Gold EB. Ectopic pregnancy and prior induced abortion. *Contraception* 1988; **37**: 21–27.

12 Holt VL, Daling JR, Voigt LF et al. Induced abortion and the risk of subsequent ectopic pregnancy. *Am J Public Health* 1989; **79**: 1234–1238.

13 Bouyer J, Coste J, Shojaei T et al. Risk factors for ectopic pregnancy: a comprehensive analysis based on a large case-control, population-based study in France. *Am J Epidemiol* 2003; **157**: 185–194.

14 Weiss NS, Daling JR, Chow WH. Control definition in case-control studies of ectopic pregnancy. *Am J Public Health* 1985; **75**: 67–68.

15 Parazzini F, Ferraroni M, Tozzi L, Ricci E, Mezzopane R, La Vecchia C. Induced abortions and risk of ectopic pregnancy. *Hum Reprod* 1995; **10**: 1841–1844.

16 Hogue CJ. Low birth weight subsequent to induced abortion: a historical prospective study of 948 women in Skopje, Yugoslavia. *Am J Obstet Gynecol* 1975; **123**: 675–681.

17 Lindefors-Harris BM, Eklund G, Adami HO, Meirik O. Response bias in a case-control study: analysis utilizing comparative data concerning legal abortions from two independent Swedish studies. *Am J Epidemiol* 1991; **134**: 1003–1008.

18 Taylor VM, Kramer MD, Vaughan TL, Peacock S. Placenta previa in relation to induced and spontaneous abortion: a population-based study. *Obstet Gynecol* 1993; **82**: 88–91.

19 Kalandidi A, Doulgerakis M, Tzonou A, Hsieh CC, Aravandinos D, Trichopoulos D. Induced abortions, contraceptive practices, and tobacco smoking as risk factors for ectopic pregnancy in Athens, Greece. *Br J Obstet Gynaecol* 1991; **98**: 207–213.

20 Germain M, Krohn MA, Daling JR. Reproductive history and the risk of neonatal sepsis. *Paediatr Perinat Epidemiol* 1995; **9**: 48–58.

21 Tzonou A, Hsieh CC, Trichopoulos D et al. Induced abortions, miscarriages, and tobacco smoking as risk factors for secondary infertility. *J Epidemiol Community Health* 1993; **47**: 36–39.

22 Moreau C, Kaminski M, Ancel PY et al. Previous induced abortions and the risk of very preterm delivery: results of the EPIPAGE study. *BJOG* 2005; **112**: 430–437.

23 Zhou W, Sorensen HT, Olsen J. Induced abortion and subsequent pregnancy duration. *Obstet Gynecol* 1999; **94**: 948–953.

24 Zhou W, Sørensen HT, Olsen J. Induced abortion and low birthweight in the following pregnancy. *Int J Epidemiol* 2000; **29**: 100–106.

25 Papiernik E. Is the high rate of preterm birth in the United States linked to previous induced abortions? *Pediatrics* 2006; **118**: 795–796.

26 Raatikainen K, Heiskanen N, Heinonen S. Induced abortion: not an independent risk factor for pregnancy outcome, but a challenge for health counseling. *Ann Epidemiol* 2006; **16**: 587–592.

27 Virk J, Zhang J, Olsen J. Medical abortion and the risk of subsequent adverse pregnancy outcomes. *N Engl J Med* 2007; **357**: 648–653.

28 Henriet L, Kaminski M. Impact of induced abortions on subsequent pregnancy outcome: the 1995 French national perinatal survey. *BJOG* 2001; **108**: 1036–1042.

29 Lao TT, Ho LF. Induced abortion is not a cause of subsequent preterm delivery in teenage pregnancies. *Hum Reprod* 1998; **13**: 758–761.

30 Reime B, Schücking BA, Wenzlaff P. Reproductive outcomes in adolescents who had a previous birth or an induced abortion compared to adolescents' first pregnancies. *BMC Pregnancy Childbirth* 2008; **8**: 4.

31 Chen A, Yuan W, Meirik L et al. Mifepristone-induced early abortion and outcome of subsequent wanted pregnancy. *Am J Epidemiol* 2004; **160**: 110–117.

32 Lurie S, Levy R, Katz Z, Appelman Z, Insler V. The influence of midtrimester termination of pregnancy on subsequent fertility: four to five years follow-up. *Contraception* 1994; **50**: 239–241.

33 Schneider D, Halperin R, Langer R, Caspi E, Bukovsky I. Abortion at 18–22 weeks by laminaria dilation and evacuation. *Obstet Gynecol* 1996; **88**: 412–414.

34 Chasen ST, Kalish RB, Gupta M, Kaufman J, Chervenak FA. Obstetric outcomes after surgical abortion at > or = 20 weeks' gestation. *Am J Obstet Gynecol* 2005; **193**: 1161–1164.

35 Infante-Rivard C, Gauthier R. Induced abortion as a risk factor for subsequent fetal loss. *Epidemiol* 1996; **7**: 540–542.

36 Yang J, Savitz DA, Dole N et al. Predictors of vaginal bleeding during the first two trimesters of pregnancy. *Paediatr Perinat Epidemiol* 2005; **19**: 276–283.

37 Ancel PY, Lelong N, Papiernik E, Saurel-Cubizolles MJ, Kaminski M. History of induced abortion as a risk factor for preterm birth in European countries: results of the EUROPOP survey. *Hum Reprod* 2004; **19**: 734–740.

38 Sawaya GF, Grady D, Kerlikowske K, Grimes DA. Antibiotics at the time of induced abortion: the case for universal prophylaxis based on a meta-analysis. *Obstet Gynecol* 1996; **87**: 884–890.

39 Kelsey JL, Gammon MD, John EM. Reproductive factors and breast cancer. *Epidemiol Rev* 1993; **15**: 36–47.

40 Lehrer S. Pregnancy termination and risk of breast cancer. *JAMA* 1996; **276**: 31–32.

41 Tang MT, Weiss NS, Daling JR, Malone KE. Case-control differences in the reliability of reporting a history of induced abortion. *Am J Epidemiol* 2000; **151**: 1139–1143.

42 Rookus MA. Reporting bias in case-control studies on induced abortion and breast cancer. *Am J Epidemiol* 2000; **151**: 1144–1147.

43 Hartge P. Abortion, breast cancer, and epidemiology. *N Engl J Med* 1997; **336**: 127–128.

44 Negri E, Dal Maso L, Ron E et al. A pooled analysis of case-control studies of thyroid cancer. II. Menstrual and reproductive factors. *Cancer Causes Control* 1999; **10**: 143–155.

45 Memon A, Darif M, Al-Saleh K, Suresh A. Epidemiology of reproductive and hormonal factors in thyroid cancer: evidence from a case-control study in the Middle East. *Int J Cancer* 2002 ; **97**: 82–89.

46 Truong T, Orsi L, Dubourdieu D, Rougier Y, Hémon D, Guénel P. Role of goiter and of menstrual and reproductive factors in thyroid cancer: a population-based case-control study in New Caledonia (South Pacific), a very high incidence area. *Am J Epidemiol* 2005; **161**: 1056–1065.

47 Kvåle G, Heuch I. Is the incidence of colorectal cancer related to reproduction? A prospective study of 63,000 women. *Int J Cancer* 1991; **47**: 390–395.

48 La Vecchia C, Negri E, Franceschi S, Parazzini F. Long-term impact of reproductive factors on cancer risk. *Int J Cancer* 1993; **53**: 215–219.

49 La Vecchia C, D'Avanzo B, Franceschi S, Negri E, Parazzini F, Decarli A. Menstrual and reproductive factors and gastric-cancer risk in women. *Int J Cancer* 1994; **59**: 761–764.

50 Fernandez E, La Vecchia C, D'Avanzo B, Negri E. Menstrual and reproductive factors and pancreatic cancer risk in women. *Int J Cancer* 1995; **62**: 11–14.

51 Negri E, Franceschi S, La Vecchia C, Parazzini F. Incomplete pregnancies and ovarian cancer risk. *Gynecol Oncol* 1992; **47**: 234–238.

52 Negri E, Franceschi S, Tzonou A et al. Pooled analysis of 3 European case-control studies: I. Reproductive factors and risk of epithelial ovarian cancer. *Int J Cancer* 1991; **49**: 50–56.

53 Mori M, Harabuchi I, Miyake H, Casagrande JT, Henderson BE, Ross RK. Reproductive, genetic, and dietary risk factors for ovarian cancer. *Am J Epidemiol* 1988; **128**: 771–777.

54 Greggi S, Parazzini F, Paratore MP et al. Risk factors for ovarian cancer in central Italy. *Gynecol Oncol* 2000; **79**: 50–54.

55 Jacobson JS, Neugut AI, Garbowski GC et al. Reproductive risk factors for colorectal adenomatous polyps (New York City, NY, United States). *Cancer Causes Control* 1995; **6**: 513–518.

56 Nagle CM, Bain CJ, Green AC, Webb PM. The influence of reproductive and hormonal factors on ovarian cancer survival. *Int J Gynecol Cancer* 2008; **18**: 407–413.

57 Remennick LI. Induced abortion as cancer risk factor: a review of epidemiological evidence. *J Epidemiol Community Health* 1990; **44**: 259–264.

58 Parazzini F, La Vecchia C, Negri E, Cecchetti G, Fedele L. Reproductive factors and the risk of invasive and intraepithelial cervical neoplasia. *Br J Cancer* 1989; **59**: 805–809.

59 Parazzini F, La Vecchia C, Negri E, Fasoli M, Cecchetti G. Risk factors for adenocarcinoma of the cervix: a case-control study. *Br J Cancer* 1988; **57**: 201–204.

60 Brinton LA, Tashima KT, Lehman HF et al. Epidemiology of cervical cancer by cell type. *Cancer Res* 1987; **47**: 1706–1711.

61 Parslov M, Lidegaard O, Klintorp S et al. Risk factors among young women with endometrial cancer: a Danish case-control study. *Am J Obstet Gynecol* 2000; **182**: 23–29.

62 Xu WH, Xiang YB, Ruan ZX et al. Menstrual and reproductive factors and endometrial cancer risk: results from a population-based case-control study in urban Shanghai. *Int J Cancer* 2004; **108**: 613–619.

63 McPherson CP, Sellers TA, Potter JD et al. Reproductive factors and risk of endometrial cancer. The Iowa Women's Study. *Am J Epidemiol* 1996; **143**: 1195–1202.

64 Brinton LA, Sakoda LC, Lissowska J et al. Reproductive risk factors for endometrial cancer among Polish women. *Br J Cancer* 2007; **96**: 1450–1456.

65 Brind J, Chinchilli VM, Severs WB, Summie-Long J. Induced abortion as an independent risk factor for breast cancer: a comprehensive review and meta-analysis. *J Epidemiol Community Health* 1996; **50**: 481–496.

66 Howe HL, Senie RT, Bzduch H, Herzfeld P. Early abortion and breast cancer risk among women under age 40. *Int J Epidemiol* 1989; **18**: 300–304.

67 Daling JR, Malone KE, Voigt LF, White E, Weiss NS. Risk of breast cancer among young women: relationship to induced abortion. *J Natl Cancer Inst* 1994; **86**: 1584–1592.

68 White E, Malone KE, Weiss NS, Daling JR. Breast cancer among young US women in relation to oral contraceptive use. *J Natl Cancer Inst* 1994; **86**: 505–514.

69 Daling JR, Brinton LA, Voigt LF et al. Risk of breast cancer among white women following induced abortion. *Am J Epidemiol* 1996; **144**: 373–380.

70 Newcomb PA, Storer BE, Longnecker MP, Mittendorf R, Greenberg ER, Willett WC. Pregnancy termination in relation to risk of breast cancer. *JAMA* 1996; **275**: 283–287.

71 Hill AB. The environment and disease: association or causation? *Proc R Soc Med* 1965; **58**: 295–300.

72 Russo J, Russo IH. Susceptibility of the mammary gland to carcinogenesis, II. Pregnancy interruption as a risk factor in tumor incidence. *Am J Pathol* 1980; **100**: 497–512.

73 Michels KB, Xue F, Colditz GA, Willet WC. Induced and spontaneous abortion and incidence of breast cancer among young women: a prospective cohort study. *Arch Intern Med* 2007; **167**: 814–820.

74 Russo IH, Russo J. Primary prevention of breast cancer by hormone-induced differentiation. *Recent Results Cancer Res* 2007; **174**: 111–130.

75 Bernstein L, Hanisch R, Sullivan-Halley J, Ross RK. Treatment with human chorionic gonadotropin and risk of breast cancer. *Cancer Epidemiol Biomarkers Prev* 1995; **4**: 437–440.

76 Rosenberg L, Palmer JR, Kaufman DW, Strom BL, Schottenfeld D, Shapiro S. Breast cancer in relation to the occurrence and time of elective and spontaneous abortion. *Am J Epidemiol* 1988; **127**: 981–989.

77 Tavani A, La Vecchia C, Franceschi S, Negri E, D'Avanzo B, Decarli A. Abortion and breast cancer risk. *Int J Cancer* 1996; **65**: 401–405.

78 Melbye M, Wohlfahrt J, Olsen JH et al. Induced abortion and the risk of breast cancer. *N Engl J Med* 1997; **336**: 81–85.

79 Beral V, Bull D, Doll R, Reeves G. Collaborative Group on Hormonal Factors in Breast Cancer. Breast cancer and abortion: collaborative reanalysis of data from 53 epidemiological studies, including 83,000 women with breast cancer from 16 countries. *Lancet* 2004; **363**: 1007–1016.

80 Brewster DH, Stockton DL, Dobbie R, Bull D, Beral V. Risk of breast cancer after miscarriage or induced abortion: a Scottish record linkage case-control study. *J Epidemiol Community Health* 2005; **59**: 283–287.

81 Palmer JR, Wise LA, Adams-Campbell LL, Rosenberg L. A prospective study of induced abortion and breast cancer in African-American women. *Cancer Causes Control* 2004; **15**: 105–111.

82 American College of Obstetricians and Gynecologists. Induced abortion and breast cancer risk. ACOG Committee Opinion Number 285, August 2003. *Int J Gynaecol Obstet* 2003; **83**: 233–235.

83 National Cancer Institute. (2003) Summary report: early reproductive events and breast cancer workshop [Online]. Bethesda (MD): National Cancer Institute. 25 Mar 2003 [cited 2009 Jan 9]. Available from: URL:http://www.nci.nih.gov/cancerinfo/ere-workshop-report

84 American Cancer Society. Can having an abortion cause or contribute to breast cancer? [Online]. 11 Aug 2008 [cited 2009 Jan 9]. Available from: URL:http://www.cancer.org/docroot/CRI/content/CRI_2_6x_Can_Having_an_Abortion_Cause_or_Contribute_to_Breast_Cancer.asp

85 World Health Organization. Induced abortion does not increase breast cancer risk. Fact Sheet #240. [Online]. 2000 Jun [cited 2008 Jul 8]. Available from: URL: http://www.who.int/mediacentre/factsheets/fs240/en/index.html

86 Cohen SA. Abortion and mental health: myths and realities. *Guttmacher Policy Review* 2006; **9**: 8–11.

87 Schmiege S, Russo NF. Depression and unwanted first pregnancy: longitudinal cohort study. *BMJ* 2005; **331**: 1303.

88 Broen AN, Moum T, Bødtker AS, Ekeberg O. The course of mental health after miscarriage and induced abortion: a longitudinal, five-year follow-up study. *BMC Med* 2005; **3**: 18.

89 Evins G, Chescheir N. Prevalence of domestic violence among women seeking abortion services. *Womens Health Issues* 1996; **6**: 204–210.

90 Adler NE, David HP, Major BN, Roth SH, Russo NF, Wyatt GE. Psychological responses after abortion. *Science* 1990; **248**: 41–44.

91 Gilchrist AC, Hannaford PC, Frank P, Kay CR. Termination of pregnancy and psychiatric morbidity. *Br J Psychiatry* 1995; **167**: 243–248.

92 Broen AN, Moum T, Bodtker AS, Ekeberg O. Predictors of anxiety and depression following pregnancy termination: a longitudinal five-year follow-up study. *Acta Obstet Gynecol Scand* 2006; **85**: 317–323.

93 Boyer D, Fine D. Sexual abuse as a factor in adolescent pregnancy and child maltreatment. *Fam Plann Perspect* 1992; **24**: 4–11, 19.

94 Kaye DK, Mirembe F, Bantebya G, Johansson A, Ekstrom AM. Domestic violence as risk factor for unwanted pregnancy and induced abortion in Mulago Hospital, Kampala, Uganda. *Trop Med Int Health* 2006; **11**: 90–101.

95 Golding JM. Intimate partner violence as a risk factor for mental disorders: A meta-analysis. *J Family Violence* 1999; **14**: 99–132.

96 Major B, Cozzarelli C. Psychosocial predictors of adjustment to abortion. *J Soc Issues* 1992; **48**: 121–142.

97 Major B, Cozzarelli C, Testa M, Mueller P. Male partners' appraisals of undesired pregnancy and abortion: implications for women's adjustment to abortion. *J Appl Soc Psychol* 1992; **22**: 599–614.

98 Hoffman JP, Johnson SM. Attitudes towards abortion among religious traditions in the United States: change or continuity? *Sociol Relig* 2005; **66**: 161–182.

99 Tamburrino MB, Franco KN, Campbell NB, Pentz JE, Evans CL, Jurs SG. Postabortion dysphoria and religion. *South Med J* 1990; **83**: 736–738.

100 Ambuel B, Rappaport J. Developmental trends in adolescents' psychological and legal competence to consent to abortion. *Law Hum Behav* 1992; **16**: 129–154.

101 Felton GM, Parsons MA, Hassell JS. Health behavior and related factors in adolescents with a history of abortion and never-pregnant adolescents. *Health Care Women Int* 1998; **19**: 37–47.

102 Fergusson DM, Horwood LJ, Ridder EM. Abortion in young women and subsequent mental health. *J Child Psychol Psychiatry* 2006; **47**: 16–24.

103 Pope LM, Adler NE, Tschann JM. Postabortion psychological adjustment: are minors at increased risk? *J Adolesc Health* 2001; **29**: 2–11.

104 Quinton WJ, Major B, Richards C. Adolescents and adjustment to abortion: are minors at greater risk? *Psychol Public Policy Law* 2001; **7**: 491–514.

105 Major B, Gramzow RH. Abortion as stigma: cognitive and emotional implications of concealment. *J Pers Soc Psychol* 1999; **77**: 735–745.

106 Major B, O'Brien LT. The social psychology of stigma. *Annu Rev Psychol* 2005; **56**: 393–421.

107 Cozzarelli C, Major B. The effects of anti-abortion demonstrators and pro-choice escorts on women's psychological responses to abortion. *J Social Clin Psychol* 1994; **13**: 404–427.

108 Cozzarelli C, Major B, Karrasch A, Fuegen K. Women's experiences of and reactions to antiabortion picketing. *Basic and Applied Social Psychology* 2000; **22**: 265–275.

109 Reardon D. *Making Abortion Rare: A Healing Strategy for a Divided Nation*. Acorn Books, Springfield (IL), 1996.

110 Richardson CT, Nash R. Misinformed consent: the medical accuracy of state-developed abortion counseling materials. *Guttmacher Policy Review* 2006; **9**: 6–11.

111 Major B, Mueller PM, Hildebrandt K. Attributions, expectations, and coping with abortion. *J Pers Soc Psychol* 1985; **48**: 585–599.

112 Major B, Cozzarelli C, Cooper ML et al. Psychological responses of women after first-trimester abortion. *Arch Gen Psychiatry* 2000; **57**: 777–784.

113 Conklin MP, O'Connor BP. Beliefs about the fetus as a moderator of post-abortion psychological well-being. *J Soc Clin Psychol* 1995; **14**: 76–95.

114 Broen AN, Moum T, Bodtker AS, Ekeberg O. Reasons for induced abortion and their relation to women's emotional distress: a prospective, two-year follow-up study. *Gen Hosp Psychiatry* 2005; **27**: 36–43.

115 Ashok PW, Hamoda H, Flett GM, Kidd A, Fitzmaurice A, Templeton A. Psychological sequelae of medical and surgical abortion at 10–13 weeks gestation. *Acta Obstet Gynecol Scand* 2005; **84**: 761–766.

116 Lowenstein L, Deutsch M, Gruberg R et al. Psychological distress symptoms in women undergoing medical vs. surgical termination of pregnancy. *Gen Hosp Psychiatry* 2006; **28**: 43–47.

117 Sit D, Rothschild AJ, Creinin MD, Hanusa BH, Wisner KL. Psychiatric outcomes following medical and surgical abortion. *Hum Reprod* 2007; **22**: 878–884.

118 Boonstra H, Gold R, Richards C, Finer L. *Abortion in Women's Lives*. Guttmacher Institute, New York, 2006.

119 Charles VE, Polis CB, Sridhara SK, Blum RW. Abortion and long-term mental health outcomes: a systematic review of the evidence. Contraception 2008; **78**: 436–450.

120 American Psychological Association. Report of the APA Task Force on Mental Health and Abortion. [Online]. 2008 [cited 2009 Jan 9]. Available from:URL:http://www.apa.org/releases/abortion-report.pdf

121 Salvesen KA, Oyen L, Schmidt N, Malt UF, Eik-Nes SH. Comparison of long-term psychological responses of women after pregnancy termination due to fetal anomalies and after perinatal loss. *Ultrasound Obstet Gynecol* 1997; **9**: 80–85.

122 Kersting A, Dorsch M, Kreulich C et al. Trauma and grief 2–7 years after termination of pregnancy because of fetal anomalies–a pilot study. *J Psychosom Obstet Gynaecol* 2005; **26**: 9–14.

123 Bazelon E. Is there a post-abortion syndrome? *New York Times Magazine*, 40–47, 62, 66, 70, 21 January 2007. Available from URL:http://www.nytimes.com/2007/01/21/magazine/21abortion.t.html?scp=1&sq=January%2021%202007%20and%20post%20abortion%20syndrome&st=cse

124 Coleman PK, Reardon DC, Strahan T, Cougle JR. The psychology of abortion: a review and suggestions for future research. *Psychology and Health* 2005; **20**: 237–271.

125 Reardon D. *Aborted Women: Silent No More*. Loyola University Press, Chicago, 1987.

126 Public Broadcasting System Post-abortion politics. [Online] 2007 July 20 [cited 2008 Aug 15] Available from: URL:http://www. pbs.org/now/shows/329/

127 American Psychiatric Association. *Diagnostic and Statistical Manual of Mental Disorders*, 4th edition. American Psychiatric Press Inc., Washington (DC), 1995.

17

CHAPTER 17

Pregnancy loss

Alisa B. Goldberg MD, MPH, Daniela Carusi MD, MSc, and Carolyn Westhoff MD

LEARNING POINTS

- Failed early pregnancy can be managed expectantly, with misoprostol, or by suction curettage.
- Compared to suction curettage, expectant management of failed early pregnancy is less effective at causing complete abortion; it is associated with more bleeding and unscheduled curettages, but no increased risk of infection.
- Misoprostol, 800 μg administered vaginally and allowed 1 week to work, is approximately 80 to 85% effective at causing expulsion of an anembryonic pregnancy or early embryonic demise.
- In cases of incomplete abortion, expectant management is highly effective. Misoprostol, 600 to 800 μg given vaginally or orally, may speed completion.
- Management options for second-trimester pregnancy loss include dilation and evacuation or labor induction with misoprostol. Modern evidence comparing these techniques is limited.

Introduction

Pregnancy loss in the first or second trimester can result from failure of an embryo to develop, embryonic or fetal death, or spontaneous expulsion of a pregnancy. Much of the literature on pregnancy loss suffers from lack of uniform terminology and definitions. For purposes of national vital statistics reporting in the USA, researchers commonly define *spontaneous abortion* as pregnancy loss prior to 20 weeks' gestation. *Fetal death* is defined as intrauterine fetal demise (IUFD) at 20 weeks' gestation or greater, and a late fetal death is an IUFD after 28 weeks' gestation [1,2]. As early as 1903, Williams stated that the term "miscarriage" was used by laypeople and that clinicians preferred "spontaneous abortion [3]." Application of ultrasonography in contemporary medical practice has allowed for earlier and more precise diagnosis. The term *early pregnancy failure* (EPF) refers to first-trimester pregnancy loss categorized sonographically into two types. A pregnancy that develops without any fetal pole is called an *anembryonic gestation*. The presence of a gestational sac that contains an embryo (at least 5 mm in length) or fetus without evidence of cardiac motion is termed an *embryonic or fetal demise*. Among women with easy access to care, many spontaneous abortions are now identified with minimal or absent symptoms because of the widespread use of sonography.

Of the approximate 205 million pregnancies that occur worldwide each year, 133 million result in live birth, 42 million are terminated by induced abortion, and 30 million end in spontaneous pregnancy loss [4]. In the USA alone, spontaneous abortions exceed 900,000 reported cases annually [1], and many additional cases go unreported [5]. Because pregnancy loss is a frequent occurrence, women's health practitioners must be prepared to diagnose and treat this condition appropriately. After providing some background information on the epidemiology of pregnancy loss, this chapter describes approaches to the diagnosis and modern management of first-trimester pregnancy loss in general and second-trimester pregnancy loss resulting from IUFD. Pregnancy loss in the second trimester also can result from obstetric complications, such as placental abruption, chorioamnionitis, preterm premature rupture of membranes, and advanced cervical dilation with or without bulging membranes. Reviewing the pathophysiology, diagnosis, and management of obstetric complications is beyond the scope of this chapter, but physicians generally use or adapt dilation and evacuation (D&E) or induction techniques (Chapters 11 and 12) to treat such cases of pregnancy loss.

Management of Unintended and Abnormal Pregnancy, 1st edition. By M Paul, ES Lichtenberg, L Borgatta, DA Grimes, PG Stubblefield, MD Creinin
 ISBN: 9781405176965.

Epidemiology

Frequency estimates

Spontaneous abortion occurs in 8 to 20% of clinically recognized pregnancies. In the 2002 US National Survey of Family Growth, US women reported that 17% of pregnancies in the previous 5 years resulted in spontaneous abortion; correcting the estimate for the underreporting of induced abortion decreased the proportion to 15% [3]. Although social stigma is unlikely to lead to underreporting of spontaneous abortion, multiple sources agree that these events are underreported. Most studies do not include spontaneous abortion occurring before 5 completed menstrual weeks. The reported frequency of spontaneous abortion depends on the health care system, the source of the information, and the age distribution of the population.

Routine surveillance by the US Centers for Disease Control and Prevention (CDC) tracks births, fetal deaths, and induced abortions, but not pregnancy losses prior to 20 weeks' gestation. In 1999 the CDC estimated the number of clinically recognized pregnancies occurring between 1981 and 1991 to provide denominators for rates of pregnancy-related outcomes. Of all pregnancies that occurred during the study period, 62.5% resulted in live births, 21.9% ended in induced abortion, 13.8% were spontaneous abortions, 1.3% were ectopic, and 0.5% ended with fetal death after 20 weeks' gestation [1]. Applying these percentages to national birth data for the USA between 1991 and 1999, Grimes estimated that approximately 7,882,974 spontaneous abortions and 285,615 fetal deaths occurred during this interval [6]. Assuming consistent rates during this 8-year interval produces estimates of 985,372 spontaneous abortions and 35,702 fetal deaths per year.

The frequency of spontaneous abortion is greatest in the early or mid first trimester and progressively decreases throughout the second trimester. Older estimates suggest that 87% of spontaneous abortions occur before 13 weeks' gestation, 9% at 13 to 15 weeks' gestation, and 4% at 16 to 19 weeks' gestation [7]. A recent study indicates that the subsequent loss rate of pregnancies with fetal heart tones between 10 and 13 weeks' gestation is extremely low. In a large multicenter study of spontaneous pregnancy loss after amniocentesis, the control group included more than 31,000 women who had singleton pregnancies at 10 to 13 weeks' gestation with fetal heart tones and who did not have invasive prenatal diagnostic procedures; the spontaneous loss rate before 24 weeks' gestation was 0.94% [8]. Although infrequent, the rate of loss after documented heart tones increases with maternal age [8].

Risk factors

Many studies agree that the strongest risk factor for spontaneous abortion is advancing maternal age. Both trisomic and chromosomally normal spontaneous abortions increase with age. Monosomy is not associated with increasing maternal age, but all known trisomies are. A Danish study of all pregnancies from 1978 to 1992 with a hospital-based outcome included 101,851 spontaneous abortions [9]. Among women aged 20 to 24, 8.9% of all recorded pregnancies ended in spontaneous abortion compared to 74.7% of pregnancies among women aged 45 or older. In the Jerusalem Perinatal Cohort Study, which included 1,506 women with spontaneous abortions [10], women over age 35 had a markedly increased risk of spontaneous abortion (adjusted odds ratio 8.3, 95% CI 6.7, 10.3) compared to women aged 20 to 24. The risk for spontaneous abortion increased 16% with each additional year of maternal age. That study also showed that the risk increases with advancing paternal age (after adjustment for maternal age), but the effect is not as strong (odds ratio 1.9, 95% CI 1.6, 2.3 for men aged 35 to 39 compared to men aged 25 to 29). The highest risk for spontaneous abortion occurs with advanced age of both the woman and the man.

Other factors that have been consistently associated with spontaneous abortion include a short interpregnancy interval (generally less than 3 to 6 months) [11], a history of previous spontaneous abortion, and maternal diabetes [10]. Studies are inconsistent regarding previous induced abortion, but a large case-control study found no association [12]. Research examining this issue is limited by underreporting of induced abortions and the methodological difficulties of identifying a suitable control group (Chapter 16).

Smoking is the main clearly defined, modifiable risk factor for spontaneous abortion. Maternal smoking during pregnancy increases the risk of spontaneous abortion in a dose-dependent fashion; however, prepregnancy smoking is unrelated [13,14]. Heavy paternal smoking is also associated with spontaneous abortion [15]. Alcohol consumption and high levels of caffeine intake may be weakly associated with spontaneous abortion [16]. Occupational exposures have been the subject of many studies, but associations are not well defined. In contrast, factors weakly associated with a reduced risk of spontaneous abortion include higher parity, higher maternal or paternal education, and higher social class [10]. Occurrence of spontaneous abortion in the USA does not vary by race; according to national statistics, however, Black race is associated with an increased risk of fetal death at 20 weeks' gestation and beyond [2].

In comparison to first-trimester anembryonic pregnancies, fetal death after 13 weeks' gestation is weakly associated with aneuploidies and more strongly related to thrombophilias [17,18]. Later losses are also related to maternal infections, genetic syndromes, and structural abnormalities.

Morbidity and mortality

Since 1979 the CDC has conducted surveillance of deaths in the USA from all pregnancy outcomes, including spontaneous abortions at less than 20 weeks' gestation. From

1981 to 1991, the overall case-fatality rate was 0.7 per 100,000 spontaneous abortions. The risk of death was higher among non-White women, those over aged 35, and those beyond 12 weeks' gestation [7]. Reported causes of spontaneous abortion-related deaths included infection 59%, hemorrhage 18%, embolism 13%, anesthesia-related complications 5%, and other causes 5%. Disseminated intravascular coagulopathy (DIC) was associated with half of the cases where it was not listed as the primary cause of death [7].

Pregnancies complicated by IUFD may be associated with an increased risk of maternal death, but data are conflicting. A single-institution retrospective analysis found no increased risk of maternal morbidity or mortality associated with IUFD compared to delivery of a viable fetus at a similar gestational age [19]. However, a recent estimation of maternal death rate by pregnancy outcome based on US national statistics suggests that the risk of maternal death is greater with IUFD than with live birth, spontaneous abortion, or legal induced abortion [6]. These data include second- and third-trimester IUFDs and do not report on underlying diagnoses or etiologies of the fetal demise.

Diagnosis

Spontaneous abortion is diagnosed by history of bleeding and pain, physical examination, and by ultrasound examination when available. Serial serum quantitative human chorionic gonadotropin (hCG) monitoring helps in some cases. Because routine, early first-trimester prenatal sonogram for dating or for first-trimester screening is highly prevalent in the USA and many other countries, women often receive the diagnosis of EPF prior to the development of any symptoms.

Sonography

Sonographic findings diagnostic of EPF include either an embryo 5 mm or greater in size without cardiac activity or a mean gestational sac diameter 13 mm or greater with absent yolk sac. A recent report using 5 to 6 mHz transducers found that 100% specificity was not reached until a cutoff of 16 mm (Chapter 6). With or without symptoms, these findings indicate EPF. Because both pregnancy dating and sonography are imperfect, diagnosis of spontaneous abortion in a woman with a wanted pregnancy may require two sonographic assessments to differentiate an EPF from a misdated pregnancy. When no yolk sac is visible, the clinician must also consider the diagnosis of ectopic pregnancy. In addition to ultrasound, serial hCG levels performed approximately 2 days apart can help distinguish normal from abnormal pregnancies. When a yolk sac is not clearly visible on ultrasound and serial hCG levels are not rising normally, uterine evacuation with inspection of tissue for the presence of villi can definitively distinguish between ectopic pregnancy and EPF (Chapter 18).

Early pregnancy failures have been further classified sonographically as anembryonic gestations or embryonic or fetal demises. In the large, multicenter Management of Early Pregnancy Failure (MEPF) trial, US researchers defined anembryonic pregnancy as an empty gestational sac with a mean diameter of at least 16 mm or insufficient growth of the sac over at least 5 days. If the gestational sac contained a yolk sac but hCG levels increased less than 15% over a 2-day period, then EPF was confirmed. Embryonic or fetal demise was diagnosed in the absence of fetal heart motion with an embryonic pole or crown-rump length of at least 5 mm, or the absence of growth over time of a smaller embryo [20].

Clinical diagnosis

The clinical stage of the spontaneous abortion process is described according to the presence or absence of symptoms at the time of presentation, the degree of cervical dilation, and the amount of tissue already passed [21] (Fig. 17.1). Mild bleeding with a closed cervix is prevalent in early pregnancy. In a woman with a positive pregnancy test, this clinical picture is often called *threatened abortion* in the absence of sonographic findings.

If history, examination, or sonogram indicates that the patient has passed tissue, then the diagnosis is either *incomplete abortion* or *complete abortion* depending on the amount of residual tissue in the uterus. No single objective standard differentiates these two entities, and the decision to intervene on clinical grounds often results in a patient receiving a diagnosis of incomplete abortion regardless of whether retained products of conception are present. If the cervix is dilated, contractions are in progress, and no tissue has yet passed, then the clinical diagnosis is imminent or *inevitable abortion*.

The distinctions among these diagnostic subgroups may guide treatment options, and they are generally needed for the purposes of coding and reimbursement in the USA. For instance, the term *missed abortion* is clinically outdated, but it may be the best diagnosis code for an asymptomatic woman with an anembryonic pregnancy or embryonic demise by sonogram. No data indicate that these clinical diagnostic distinctions are useful to ascribe etiology.

The time of diagnosis tends to occur later in women whose early pregnancy loss is diagnosed only with the advent of pain and bleeding; it occurs sooner in women who undergo a routine, early first-trimester sonogram, whether for dating or for first-trimester screening.

Management of early pregnancy loss

Spontaneous loss of a desired pregnancy is emotionally distressing for the woman and her partner. Health care personnel can help these patients and their families by showing empathy and support at all times. Women carrying undesired pregnancies may feel relieved that the loss occurred

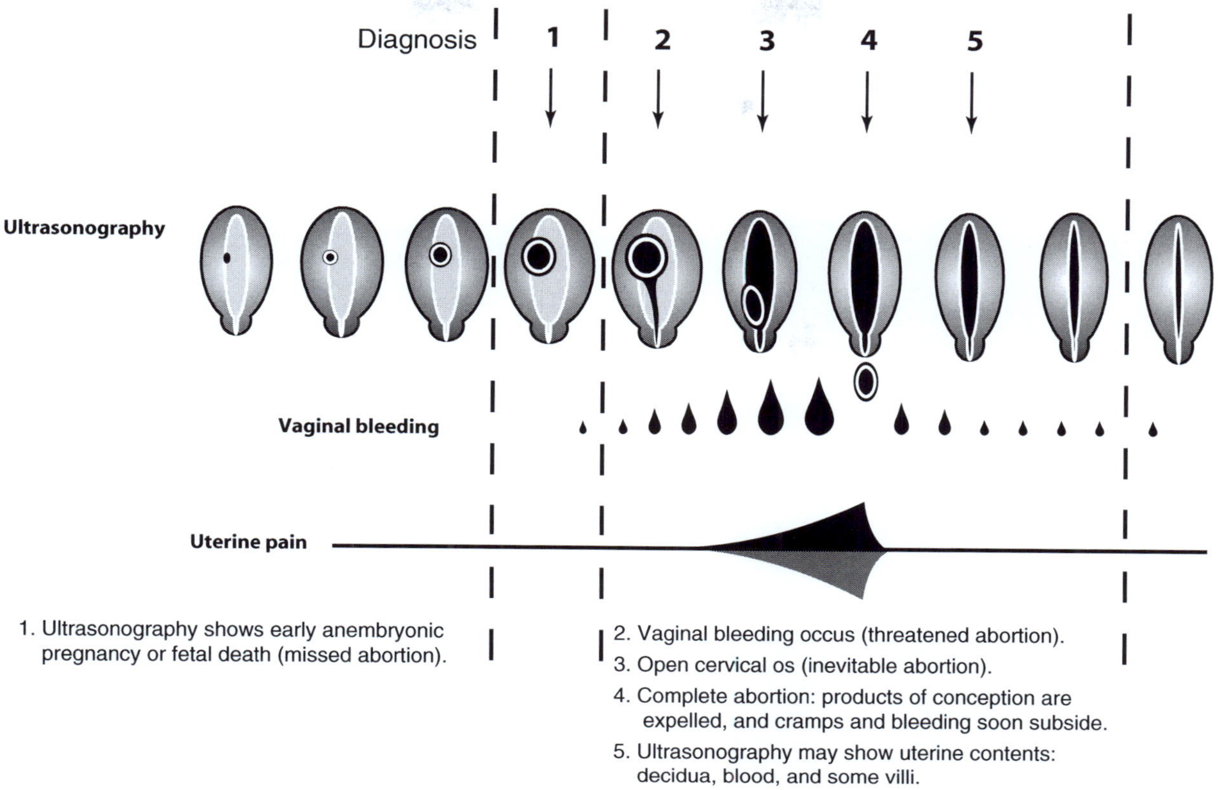

Figure 17.1 Natural course of spontaneous abortion (miscarriage) with opportunities for intervention. (Adapted and reprinted with permission from Ankum et al [21].)

spontaneously, avoiding the need for an induced abortion. Alternatively, some women make the decision to terminate their pregnancy, present for an induced abortion, and are diagnosed with a pregnancy loss incidentally on ultrasound. The provider should inform such patients of the diagnosis, as it may alter their preference for management and their insurance coverage for the procedure. Likewise, equivocal findings should be explained. Anecdotally, most women choose to proceed with the induced abortion as originally planned without a definitive diagnosis, but some women prefer to obtain a follow-up ultrasound for confirmation.

Once the diagnosis of pregnancy loss is established, the clinician should discuss management options with the patient. Options include expectant, medical, and surgical management. A patient in the first or second trimester who is clinically stable with no evidence of hemorrhage or infection does not require immediate uterine evacuation and should be given adequate time to consider her options. When faced with a pregnancy loss, some women request immediate uterine evacuation and others prefer to wait until they feel emotionally ready or can obtain another medical opinion. Patient preference deserves strong consideration when selecting a management option. A study of quality-of-life outcomes found that women managed according to their preference had the best outcomes [22]. The effectiveness of treatment plans, medication-dosing regimens, surgical techniques, and risk of complications vary by gestation. Women who are Rh(D) negative and have had any bleeding during the current pregnancy should receive anti-D immune globulin at the time of their initial assessment. Rh(D)-negative women with no bleeding should receive anti-D immune globulin when they initiate treatment.

Management of first-trimester pregnancy loss

For more than 60 years in the USA, dilation and curettage (D&C) with either a sharp or vacuum curette has been the treatment of choice for early pregnancy loss [23]. As is still the case in some countries with restrictive abortion laws, universal D&C was adopted in the USA to prevent hemorrhage and sepsis in an era when abortion was illegal; antibiotics, synthetic prostaglandins, and ultrasound were unavailable; and a large proportion of women presenting with presumed complications of spontaneous pregnancy loss actually had undergone clandestine and unsafe induced abortions. Despite liberalization of abortion laws and numerous medical advances, routine curettage remains standard treatment for pregnancy loss in many places. Today in countries where abortion is legal, spontaneous abortions usually are truly spontaneous, and they are often diagnosed with ultrasound in asymptomatic women. Moreover, safer vacuum aspiration methods and prostaglandin analogs such as misoprostol are increasingly available worldwide. In light of these changes, the ideal management of spontaneous pregnancy loss needs to be revisited.

Surgical management

Vacuum aspiration to evacuate a failed pregnancy in the first trimester is performed in a fashion similar to first-trimester pregnancy termination (Chapter 10). Clinicians can use either an electric vacuum source or a handheld manual vacuum aspirator (MVA). The procedure can readily be accomplished using local anesthesia or moderate sedation in an outpatient facility [24] except in certain cases of severe maternal disease or serious pregnancy-related complications (Chapter 7). Surgical management of EPF is the treatment of choice for women who present with heavy vaginal bleeding or signs of infection with possible retained tissue and for those in whom the diagnosis of ectopic pregnancy cannot be excluded. If ultrasound fails to confirm an intrauterine pregnancy prior to uterine evacuation, villi are not identified after uterine aspiration, and serial hCG levels are not falling appropriately, the patient warrants treatment for ectopic pregnancy (Chapter 18).

Although 95% of induced abortions in the USA occur in freestanding clinics or physicians' offices [25], studies from Europe and North America suggest that spontaneous abortions are commonly managed in hospitals with suction curettage in an operating room [26–28]. Data have confirmed the safety of induced abortions performed in nonhospital settings [29], and no evidence suggests that different scenarios are medically necessary for the two conditions [26]. Moreover, one study found that MVA in an outpatient setting using local anesthesia or moderate sedation saved a significant amount of time and money compared to suction curettage in a hospital operating room [30]. A recent study evaluated the treatment preferences and satisfaction of women with EPF who chose between suction curettage in an office or operating room setting. Many women expressed strong preferences, and the priorities of the women differed. Women who preferred the office setting regarded privacy and a desire to avoid drugs and remain awake as highly important. Satisfaction was high in both groups, although underestimating the amount of discomfort of procedures performed without intravenous sedation or general anesthesia was associated with lower levels of satisfaction in the office group. Women in the operating room group were four times more likely to have hemorrhage-related complications, which the authors attributed to use of halogenated gases for general anesthesia [31].

Expectant management

Although suction curettage for first-trimester pregnancy loss is an extremely safe procedure, it may not be necessary in all cases. In a large observational study, 686 women with a failed early pregnancy or incomplete abortion chose between expectant management and suction curettage under general anesthesia. The 478 (70%) women who chose expectant management were followed for 4 weeks, or longer if they requested extended observation, to determine if they completely expelled the products of conception without requiring curettage. Women who initially presented with an incomplete abortion were the most likely to have complete expulsion. Regardless of initial diagnosis, success rates improved the longer women waited before intervention [32] (Table 17.1). Because spontaneous abortion is a physiologic process that often begins with abnormal embryonic development or demise and then progresses with cervical softening, bleeding, uterine contractions, and expulsion, it makes sense that complete abortion rates are higher among those diagnosed later in the process and those given more time (Fig. 17.1).

Several randomized clinical trials have compared expectant management to suction curettage [33–37]. These studies demonstrated a wide range of efficacy of expectant management. Efficacy is influenced by the type of pregnancy failure at the time of initial diagnosis, the interval allowed

Table 17.1 Types of miscarriage and outcome in patients who chose expectant management. Values are numbers (percentages). (Reprinted with permission from Luise et al [32].)

		Complete miscarriage[a]		
Group classification at diagnosis	Patients	By day 7	By day 14	Successful outcome by day 46
Incomplete miscarriage	221 (49)	117 (53)	185 (84)	201 (91)
Missed miscarriage	138 (31)	41 (30)	81 (59)	105 (76)
Anembryonic pregnancy	92 (20)	23 (25)	48 (52)	61 (66)
Total	451 (100)	181 (40)	314 (70)	367 (81)

[a] No suction curettage performed.

> **Summary: Expectant Management of Early Pregnancy Loss**
> Based on the evidence to date, it appears that 7 to 14 days of expectant management can enable approximately 75 to 85% of women with an incomplete abortion and 30 to 60% of those with an embryonic demise to avoid suction curettage and its small surgical and anesthetic risks [32,39]. Expectant management is associated with more unscheduled curettages and more bleeding, but no increased risk of infection.

before intervention, and the criteria used for intervention. Specifically, many studies of expectant management routinely performed suction curettage for all women who were noted to have an endometrial thickness on ultrasound greater than 15 mm after a given time interval, including those who were asymptomatic. This practice has likely inflated the published failure rates of expectant management. Nonetheless, these studies consistently showed that expectant management is less effective at achieving complete emptying of the uterus than suction curettage, but most did not observe an increase in complications. A Cochrane review, which included randomized trials conducted through 2005 enrolling a total of 689 women, concluded that expectant management is associated with an increased risk of incomplete abortion (RR 5.37; 95% CI 2.57, 11.22), more unscheduled curettages (RR 4.78; 95% CI 1.99, 11.48), and more bleeding than surgical management, but a decreased risk of infection (RR 0.29; 95% CI 0.09, 0.87) [38]. Most of the trials of expectant management either made no mention of prophylactic antibiotics or reported that they were not used. The Miscarriage Treatment (MIST) trial, a recent randomized trial designed specifically to compare rates of infection among 1,200 women allocated to expectant, medical, or surgical management, found no difference in infection rates among the three groups. No prophylactic antibiotics were used in this study. Significantly more women in the expectant management group required transfusions ($n = 7$, 2%) compared to those in the surgical management group ($n = 0$). Transfusion rates in the medical and surgical management groups did not differ significantly [39].

Medical management

Although expectant management of first-trimester pregnancy loss expands women's treatment options, some women may find the uncertainty about the timing and completeness of pregnancy passage undesirable. Active management with medications gives women more control over the process and may help to avoid surgical intervention.

Mifepristone, an anti-progesterone, and misoprostol, a prostaglandin E1 analog, have been studied extensively for use in early medical abortion. When used in combination, these drugs are highly effective at terminating a pregnancy up to 63 days' gestation (Chapter 9). These same drugs have been studied for treatment of first-trimester pregnancy loss, as has the combination of methotrexate and misoprostol. However, the US Food and Drug Administration (FDA) has not evaluated these medications for this purpose.

Researchers have evaluated mifepristone on its own as treatment for first-trimester pregnancy failure. In a randomized trial, a single 600-mg oral dose led to complete tissue passage for 77% of subjects within 5 days, performing significantly better than the placebo [40]. Medication abortion studies using mifepristone and misoprostol have demonstrated no change in efficacy when mifepristone doses are reduced from 600 to 200 mg [41]. This finding appears to apply to spontaneous abortions as well [42].

Because medical management of spontaneous abortion relies more on uterine expulsion than interruption of an ongoing pregnancy, the mifepristone dose may not be necessary at all. A nonrandomized trial compared the combination of mifepristone and vaginal misoprostol with the same misoprostol dose used alone. The two groups had similar success rates (71 to 74%) [43]. A recent randomized trial comparing misoprostol alone to mifepristone plus misoprostol for EPF also found no difference in success rates with the addition of mifepristone [44]. Similarly, misoprostol combined with methotrexate is no better than misoprostol alone in managing a failed early pregnancy [45]. Whereas adding mifepristone improves the efficacy of medical abortion with misoprostol (Chapter 9), the limited evidence to date suggests that adding mifepristone or methotrexate does not improve the efficacy of misoprostol alone when used for spontaneous abortion. For unclear reasons, success rates for the medical management of EPF remain substantially lower than those reported for medical abortion, regardless of regimen used.

Misoprostol compared to suction curettage

A number of trials have compared misoprostol to suction curettage for the management of failed early pregnancy. These trials have shown success rates of 50 to 90% for women treated medically and 91 to 100% for those treated with electric or manual vacuum aspiration (i.e., no unplanned, repeat procedures) [20,39,46–53]. Although fewer subjects receiving misoprostol achieved success with initial therapy, most were ultimately able to avoid a surgical intervention.

Numerous factors may account for the wide range of success rates with misoprostol, including dose, route of administration, type of spontaneous abortion, definitions of success, indications for suction curettage, and duration of follow-up before surgical intervention. Studies have shown that 800 μg of vaginal misoprostol is more effective than 600 μg given by the same route [54] or 400 μg given orally [55]. Two studies comparing the 800-μg vaginal dose to the same dose given orally showed no difference in effectiveness, with the vaginal route producing more vomiting [56] and the oral dose producing more diarrhea [57]. Adequate duration of follow-up before surgical intervention may be more important than misoprostol dose. Completion rates were 50 to 60% when researchers offered surgical management 1 to 3 days after treatment [47,52,53] versus 70 to 90% when researchers waited 1 to 2 weeks before considering suction curettage [20,39,46,48,49].

Criteria for surgical intervention also matter. Some researchers intervened when endometrial thickness by ultrasound passed a set cutoff value, whereas others did so only if the gestational sac had failed to pass. One trial using a 15-mm endometrial thickness cutoff found a success rate of only 28% after one misoprostol dose, and 53% after two doses [52]. Alternatively, the MEPF trial, which used a 30-mm endometrial cutoff and 8 days of follow-up, achieved an 84% success rate [20]. In that study, endometrial thickness was a poor predictor of the need for curettage [58]. Medical abortion studies have similarly shown that the only important criterion for determining success of the procedure is passage of the gestational sac (Chapter 9). Although women who ultimately require curettage have a thicker endometrial stripe on average than those who do not, endometrial thickness on ultrasound is a poor predictor of the need for curettage [59].

Efficacy also may vary with type of pregnancy failure. The MEPF trial analyzed success rates by diagnosis and found significantly lower success rates with anembryonic gestations (81%) than with embryonic/fetal deaths or incomplete abortions (88 and 93%, respectively) [20]. Incomplete abortions, which begin spontaneously and are near completion, may have the highest success rates with medical management. Trials specifically looking at the medical management of incomplete abortions show success rates of 80 to 96% [39,46,48,49]. Reported success rates are lower if women with incomplete abortions are allowed only 1 to 3 days to pass retained tissue before surgical intervention (50 to 71%) [39,47]. Other predictors of success with medical management of early pregnancy failure include spontaneous vaginal bleeding within the 24 hours preceding misoprostol use and parity less than two [60].

Most studies found increased bleeding [39,46–49,61] or a larger drop in hemoglobin concentration [53,61] with misoprostol than with surgical therapy, but the clinical significance of this difference has been questioned. In the MEPF study, the average drop in hemoglobin was only 0.5 g/dl greater for those in the medical group than the surgical group; however, more medically treated women dropped their hemoglobin by more than 3 g/dl or reached a nadir more than 10 g/dl from their baseline. Additionally, more women in the misoprostol group found their bleeding unacceptable (12% vs. 5% in the surgical group) [61]. The MEPF and the MIST trials as well as others found that women treated with misoprostol had more days of bleeding than those treated surgically [39,46].

The MEPF and MIST trials found no significant difference in infection rates when comparing misoprostol to surgical management [20,39]. Other studies have found higher rates of antibiotic use and infection in the subjects randomized to surgical therapy [47,48].

Studies have shown variable results regarding pain. Some studies found that subjects in the misoprostol groups required more analgesia than those in the surgical groups [20,47,52], whereas others have shown the opposite [48,49]. The choice of analgesia used during the surgical procedure likely influences these results.

Misoprostol can produce gastrointestinal side effects, such as nausea and diarrhea. These side effects occur more frequently with oral or sublingual misoprostol than with vaginal administration [57,62,63]. When compared to surgical management, trials have shown higher rates of gastrointestinal side effects in women using oral or vaginal misoprostol [47,49]. The MEPF trial found that, compared to those having surgery, significantly more subjects receiving vaginal misoprostol experienced nausea (53% vs. 29%), vomiting (20% vs. 7%), and diarrhea (24% vs. 10%) [20].

Misoprostol compared to expectant management

A number of trials have compared misoprostol to expectant management for first-trimester pregnancy loss. In cases of early demise or anembryonic gestation, all trials showed that misoprostol was superior to no therapy or placebo, with success rates of 72 to 83% at 1 to 2 days of follow-up for the misoprostol groups versus 12 to 17% with placebo [64–66]. A longer, 7-day follow-up period increased success rates to 87% for misoprostol and 29% for placebo [67]. In contrast, several studies specifically looking at incomplete abortion did not show an advantage to misoprostol over expectant management. The 70 to 100% success rates for the misoprostol groups did not differ significantly from the 75 to 86% success with 7 to 14 days of expectant management [39,67,68]. However, a meta-analysis comparing the efficacy of expectant, medical, and surgical management of first-trimester spontaneous abortion suggests that medical management is more effective than expectant management for incomplete abortion [69]. Additionally, an expert panel suggests that medical management is a reasonable option for women with an incomplete abortion who prefer immediate treatment and wish to avoid surgery [70].

Most studies found no differences in bleeding between misoprostol treatment and expectant management [39,54,66,67]. In the MIST study, seven transfusions occurred in the expectant group, three in the medical group, and none in the surgical group. This difference was only statistically significant when comparing expectant to surgical management [39]. Two small studies found more fever or infection with misoprostol use than with expectant management [54,68]; whereas the MIST study, designed to look at

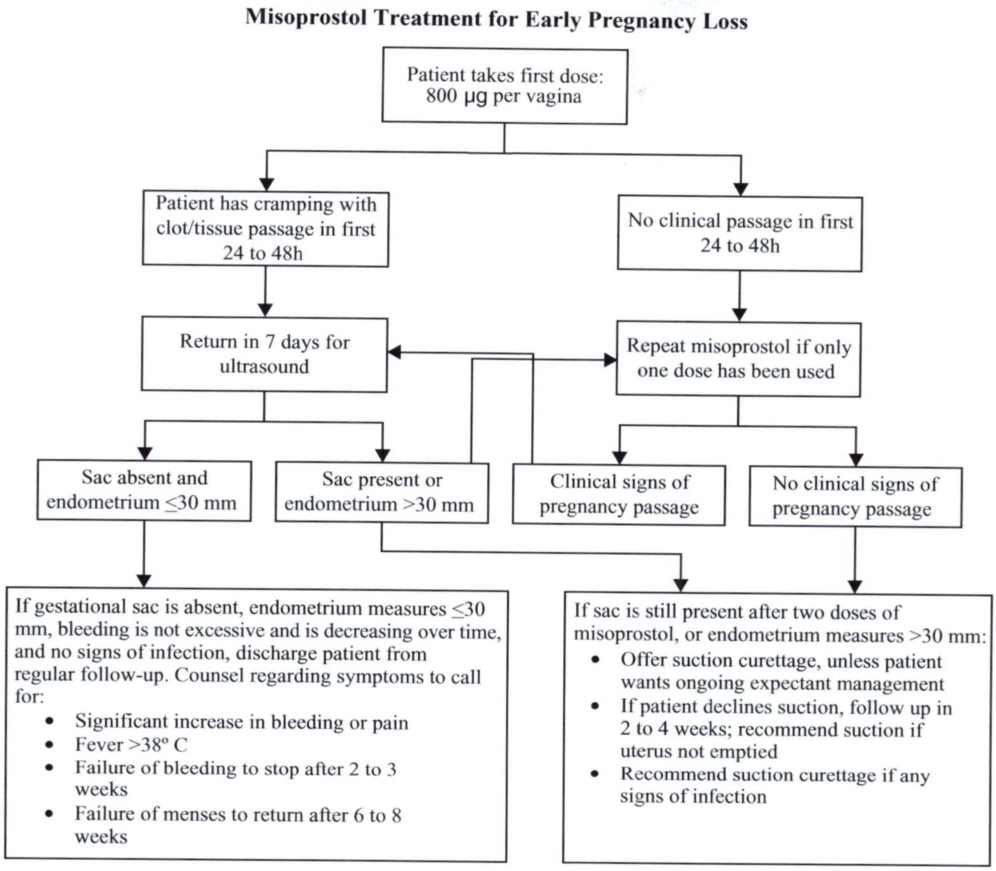

Figure 17.2 Algorithm for the use of misoprostol for management of early pregnancy loss.

infectious complications, found no difference with medical, surgical, or expectant management [39].

Management of second-trimester pregnancy loss because of fetal demise

Most patients diagnosed with a fetal death in the second trimester prefer active management because carrying a demised fetus, especially late in gestation, is stressful [17]. However, in a hemodynamically stable patient with no evidence of infection, uterine evacuation is not urgent. Patients with fetal demise should be given adequate time to process the diagnosis and consider their management options.

A study from the early 1960s suggested that 80 to 90% of women with fetal death spontaneously labored within 2 weeks of the fetal demise [71]; however, a recent expert opinion suggests that the interval may be considerably longer [17]. We could not identify any recent studies specifically evaluating expectant management of fetal demise in the second trimester. Potential risks of expectant management include delivery outside of a clinical setting, hemorrhage from maternal coagulopathy, and infection.

Summary: Medical Management of Early Pregnancy Loss

Available data indicate that 60 to 90% of patients who prefer to avoid surgical management may be able to do so with misoprostol. Based on studies in a large number of subjects, the best dose to maximize effectiveness and minimize side effects among women with an anembryonic pregnancy or embryonic demise is 800 μg per vagina, with the possibility of repeating the dose in 24 hours (Fig. 17.2). For women with an incomplete abortion and no evidence of infection, expectant management is a highly effective and reasonable option. Women with an incomplete abortion who prefer active management can receive an 800-μg vaginal dose or a 600-μg oral dose of misoprostol [70]. Success is further optimized by allowing at least 1 week before diagnosing a treatment failure and avoiding surgical intervention as long as the gestational sac has passed. In the absence of a gestational sac, decisions for surgical intervention should be made on clinical grounds (e.g., heavy or persistent bleeding or clinical infection with concern for retained products of conception). Although misoprostol therapy is consistently superior to expectant management in the case of early fetal/embryonic death or anembryonic gestation, it offers less benefit in cases of incomplete abortion where expectant management is highly effective.

Older studies reported a 25% rate of coagulopathy among women with fetal demise for more than 4 weeks [17]. More recently, of 238 women with IUFD, most were delivered within 1 week of the demise and 3% of women with no co-existing obstetric disease had coagulation abnormalities. Pregnancy-related conditions, especially abruption and uterine perforation, were associated with an increased risk of coagulation abnormalities [72]. Whether uterine evacuation of a recently demised fetus carries an increased risk of hemorrhage and DIC compared to induced abortion at a similar gestational age is unknown. In cases of fetal demise, some providers recommend preprocedure laboratory evaluation for coagulation defects (platelet count, prothrombin time [PT], partial thromboplastin time [PTT], and international normalized ratio [INR]).

Women desiring active management of an IUFD in the second trimester are generally managed either with D&E in locations where providers with the requisite skills are available or by induction of labor, often with misoprostol.

Surgical management

D&E for the indication of fetal demise is performed in the same way as D&E for second-trimester pregnancy termination (Chapter 11). Long-standing demise may make fetal tissue softer and easier to remove. Complications include hemorrhage, infection, retained tissue requiring reevacuation, cervical laceration, and uterine perforation (Chapter 15). Similar to cases of second-trimester induced abortion, the risk of serious complications is low but increases with advancing gestational age.

No epidemiologic evidence suggests that amniotic fluid embolism (AFE) is more likely to occur with uterine evacuation of a demised fetus than with induced abortion at a comparable gestational age. This extremely rare complication was primarily associated with older uterine instillation methods for abortion [73], but a few cases of AFE have been reported in women having second-trimester D&Es for fetal demise [74, 75]. The incidence of AFE in the second trimester is unknown but is likely lower than in the third trimester. A population-based study of singleton births in California from 1994 to 1995 reported an incidence of AFE of 1 in 20,646 with a 26% maternal mortality [76].

A variety of infections can cause fetal death. However, aside from cases of septic abortion, we could find no evidence suggesting that D&E performed for IUFD is associated with any higher risk of endometritis or sepsis than D&E performed for induced abortion. Similarly, no data have compared the infection rates associated with modern methods of labor induction and those associated with D&E when used for the management of IUFD.

The possible increased risks of hemorrhage, DIC, and maternal death with late second-trimester fetal demise warrant consideration as to the ideal location for managing these patients. Women faced with fetal demise often have an option for hospital-based care that patients having induced abortions may not. However, many hospitals have no provider of D&E services, leaving only the option of induction of labor. Because the absolute risks of major complications using modern D&E or induction techniques for fetal demise are not known, evidence to guide recommendations is lacking. Providers should consider the facility's capacity to manage complications and the proximity to emergency referral resources when making decisions about the appropriate setting.

Medical management

Many women with fetal demise undergo labor induction rather than surgery. Labor-induction procedures commonly take place in hospital settings, where patients can be monitored for heavy bleeding or fever, receive analgesics and antiemetics as needed, and undergo surgical removal of the placenta if required. As with other labor inductions, medication choices include oxytocin, PGE_2 (dinoprostone or sulprostone), or misoprostol, although higher doses are often required in the second trimester compared to later in gestation.

Regimens are well defined for second-trimester medical abortion (Chapter 12). The FDA has approved use of dinoprostone vaginal suppositories for second-trimester labor induction. Among patients undergoing induced abortion or treatment of fetal demise, a 20-mg dose of PGE_2 was no more effective than 10 mg followed by high-dose oxytocin. Patients receiving the higher dose experienced more fever and vomiting, and one case of hypotension and two cases of refractory fever occurred in this group [77]. Dinoprostone is a relatively expensive drug that requires refrigeration, limiting its practicality for this indication.

Numerous studies have confirmed the safety and efficacy of misoprostol for labor induction, although FDA labeling for misoprostol does not include this indication. Misoprostol's low cost and stability at room temperature make it a popular option for this purpose. When compared to oxytocin regimens, misoprostol resulted in faster delivery times and higher rates of complete abortion within 24 hours (>90% success vs. 62 to 85%). These studies included patients with both ongoing pregnancies and demised fetuses, and they used 400 μg of misoprostol orally every 4 hours [78] or a 600-μg vaginal loading dose followed by 400 μg vaginally every 4 hours [79]. When given at a lower dose less frequently, 200 μg every 12 hours, misoprostol was inferior to high-dose oxytocin [80].

Misoprostol appears equivalent to dinoprostone when using doses of 600 μg vaginally every 12 hours or a 600-μg vaginal dose followed by 400 μg orally every 12 hours [81]. Equivalence to PGE_2 has been demonstrated with misoprostol doses as low as 100 to 200 μg vaginally every 12 hours [82], with the advantage of producing less severe pain, fever, and vomiting [83]. Using 100 μg of misoprostol vaginally every 4 hours may be more effective than PGE_2, although in one study this regimen was associated with more bleeding and incomplete expulsion [84].

These trials combined women undergoing induced abortion and those with fetal demise. However, studies comparing these two groups have consistently shown faster induction to delivery times in cases of fetal demise. Both PGE_2 [83,85,86] and misoprostol demonstrate mean delivery times of 10 to 13 hours with fetal demise [83,87–90]. Other studies have shown that the misoprostol dose can be lowered in cases of fetal demise. For induced abortions, a dose of 400 μg per vagina every 6 hours is more effective than 200 μg by the same route every 6 or 12 hours [87,91], or 400 μg given orally every 6 hours [92]. In cases of fetal demise a dose of 200 μg vaginally every 6 hours appears as effective as the 400-μg dose [87,91].

Dosing interval may be important in accelerating uterine evacuation. Studies of labor induction for fetal demise that used 100 to 200 μg of misoprostol every 12 hours showed a wide range of 24-hour completion rates, with some studies reporting rates under 80% [82,91,93] and others 92 to 94% [94,95]. Studies that compared twice-daily to more frequent dosing found higher 24-hour completion rates when doses were given every 4 to 6 hours, but similar completion rates at 48 hours [91,93].

As with first-trimester misoprostol studies, research protocols for second-trimester induction are heterogenous. In some studies, researchers place laminaria tents within the cervix prior to administering the study drugs [79,80]. However, one trial showed that placing laminaria at the time of the first vaginal dose of misoprostol added no benefit [96], while another found slower induction to delivery times [97]. Outside of the USA, mifepristone is used extensively in combination with misoprostol for second-trimester induction abortion, resulting in higher efficacy and shortened induction-to-abortion intervals compared to using misoprostol alone (Chapter 12). A small trial that included women with fetal demise compared mifepristone to laminaria given 1 day before second-trimester induction of labor with misoprostol. This study found a shorter induction-to-delivery time with mifepristone [98]. Studies vary in terms of giving oxytocin routinely [81,83], and many studies combine second- and third-trimester inductions [82,93,94]. Despite this heterogeneity, most trials of misoprostol for labor induction for fetal demise show mean induction-to-delivery intervals of 10 to 16 hours [82,83,86–88,90,93,99,100], and completion rates of 80 to 100% within 24 hours [86,88,90,91,93,100,101].

The American College of Obstetricians and Gynecologists (ACOG) discourages use of misoprostol when a patient has a scarred uterus and a viable fetus [102]. Studies of second-trimester induction of labor with misoprostol have included women with a uterine scar, as the smaller uterus is likely to confer less risk of rupture. Although a few case reports have described uterine rupture with second-trimester use of misoprostol [82,91], uterine rupture can occur with oxytocin as well [103,104]. Dickinson retrospectively reviewed 101 cases of second-trimester misoprostol use in women with prior cesarean sections. No cases of uterine rupture occurred, and the frequency of major complications or blood loss was not increased when compared to women with an unscarred uterus [105].

Summary: Medical Management of Fetal Demise

Based on the evidence to date, a recent expert panel recommends using 200 μg of misoprostol vaginally every 6 hours for women with IUFD at 13 to 17 weeks' gestation (maximum daily dose 1600 μg), 100 μg of misoprostol vaginally every 6 hours for women with IUFD at 18 to 26 weeks' gestation (maximum daily dose 800 μg) and 25 to 50 μg of misoprostol every 4 hours for women with IUFD from 27 to 43 weeks' gestation (maximum daily dose 600 μg). If the first dose does not induce regular contractions, the next dose may be doubled. Women with previous cesarean sections should receive lower range doses of misoprostol, and doses should not be doubled [106]. Pretreatment with mifepristone appears beneficial. Patients who have uterine scars should be counseled about the rare risk of uterine rupture, which could potentially occur with any medical induction method.

D&E compared to induction of labor for fetal demise

We could identify no studies that specifically compared the relative safety of induction of labor using misoprostol with D&E in cases of fetal demise. One recent observational study found a higher rate of retained placenta with misoprostol induction abortions than D&E techniques [107]. In this study, which included women with IUFD, patients undergoing labor induction were at increased risk of induction failure or retained tissue requiring curettage. The authors found no significant increased risk of transfusion, intravenous antibiotics, cervical laceration, organ damage, or hospital readmission. However, the only two cases of major organ damage requiring repair occurred among women with failed medical inductions: one woman with a prior cesarean scar experienced uterine rupture, and another had a uterine perforation on rescue D&E.

Evaluation of second-trimester fetal loss

For patients who desire future pregnancy, a single second-trimester fetal death should prompt a fetal karyotype analysis, inspection of the fetus for abnormalities, and placental pathologic analysis [108]. Confirmation of a chromosomal problem may reduce the need for other testing. Obtaining a full karyotype of the pregnancy requires recovery and culture of embryonic tissue or chorionic villi. The cells will grow in culture only if sent as a fresh specimen (not in formalin); even fresh specimens will fail to grow in culture approximately 5% of the time [109]. If cells fail to grow in culture, then the florescence *in situ* hybridization (FISH) test can be performed. With FISH testing, probes for select chromosomes enable identification of the number of those chromosomes per cell. The test does not screen for all chromosomal abnormalities; however, by selecting the chromosomes most commonly associated with pregnancy loss, approximately 80% of aneuploid pregnancies can be identified [110]. No studies have specifically compared the success of cell culture with specimens obtained surgically versus those passed spontaneously. Fresher specimens, cultured soon after removal or expulsion from the uterus, may yield better cell growth.

Autopsy of medically delivered intact fetuses has been shown to alter the final diagnosis and patient counseling in 27% of cases with normal chromosomes [111]. Induction of labor and often intact D&E (Chapters 11 and 20) enable removal of an intact fetus for inspection and grieving purposes. Evidence of placental infarction may warrant maternal thrombophilia and antiphospholipid antibody screening. Infectious and toxicology screening may depend on maternal clinical status and fetal and placental pathology [17].

Septic abortion

Women having a spontaneous abortion who are hemodynamically unstable or have signs of sepsis, including high fever and white blood cell count, altered mental status, hypovolemia, hypotension, or tachycardia, should receive broad-spectrum intravenous antibiotic therapy and undergo prompt uterine evacuation. Patients who fail to respond to these measures or those with an acute abdomen may require laparotomy and possible hysterectomy. In these severe cases, the diagnosis of clostridial sepsis should be considered. Cases of *Clostridium sordellii* sepsis have been reported after both spontaneous and medically induced abortions [112]. Management of clostridial sepsis is similar to management of septic abortion from other pathogens, although patients may have a greater need for hysterectomy and a worse prognosis (Chapter 15).

Women presenting with spontaneous abortion without sepsis but with signs of infection including abdominal pain, fever, uterine tenderness, and/or abnormal bleeding should receive broad-spectrum antibiotics. In addition, uterine evacuation is warranted for women with suspected retained products of conception. It also should be considered when sonography suggests no retained products but the patient fails to respond quickly to broad-spectrum antibiotics alone [113]. Parenteral antibiotic regimens recommended by the CDC for the treatment of pelvic inflammatory disease are appropriate [114].

Although two randomized trials comparing doxycycline to placebo for prophylaxis prior to suction curettage for incomplete abortion showed no reduction in infection with doxycycline, multiple trials and a meta-analysis indicate that universal antibiotic prophylaxis reduces the risk of postabortal infection after surgical abortion (Chapters 14 and 15). No evidence to date supports the routine use of prophylactic antibiotics in cases of expectant or medical management of pregnancy loss.

Counseling, education, and consent for patients with pregnancy loss

Counseling patients with pregnancy loss includes focusing on their emotional needs, treatment options, and their desire for future pregnancies. The loss of a wanted pregnancy often exacts a high emotional toll. In such cases, providers can acknowledge the sadness of the loss, the prospects of attempting another pregnancy, and the improbability that the woman's own behavior caused the loss. The counselor should obtain a pregnancy history, as prior live births or losses may affect the patient's perspective as well as her odds of complications in the future.

In order to give informed consent, patients must understand the risks and benefits of each treatment alternative and have ample opportunity to ask and receive answers to their questions (Chapter 5). Given that the risks of suction curettage are similar when performed for pregnancy loss or induced abortion, many providers use similar consent forms for surgical management regardless of diagnosis. Unlike for induced abortion in the USA, no state mandates special consent forms for management of fetal demise; however, procedures and consent for disposal of the products of conception may differ by state.

For medical management of spontaneous abortion, important risks to discuss include bleeding, infection, incomplete uterine evacuation, and failure of the treatment requiring vacuum aspiration. With up to two vaginal doses of 800-μg misoprostol, failure rates after first-trimester medical management are approximately 15% if patients wait at least 1 week to pass the pregnancy [20,56,67]. With second-trimester misoprostol treatment, at least 85% of patients will pass the pregnancy within 24 hours [91,99,101], and 90 to 100% will do so within 48 hours [82,90,93].

Other factors may also influence the choice of management options. In the first trimester, medical management allows a patient to complete expulsion in the privacy of her own home, usually avoiding surgical risks. However, she must be prepared to bleed more heavily than she might with surgical management [47,61] and to self-treat any pain or cramping. Patients using home medical management must have access to a telephone and transportation, if needed for emergency care.

In the second trimester, available medical resources may limit a woman's options. Many hospital facilities do not have skilled surgical abortion providers on-site, so labor induction is the only alternative. Medical treatment may be preferred by patients who desire comprehensive fetopsy as part of the evaluation for fetal demise or who simply prefer to deliver an intact fetus. Furthermore, some patients may wish to see or hold their fetus for grieving purposes. Intact D&E (Chapter 11) also may have these advantages. Because intact D&E depends on achieving adequate cervical dilation, however, not all procedures result in an intact fetus even in the most experienced hands. Counselors need to explain these benefits and limitations before the patient decides on a treatment method.

Follow-up

Some evidence suggests that routine follow-up is not necessary for many women after uncomplicated first-trimester induced abortion [115], but the same may not hold true for women experiencing loss of a desired pregnancy. Studies suggest that after a spontaneous abortion, many women appreciate the opportunity to follow up with their care provider to have their loss acknowledged and their grief legitimized and to have the opportunity to discuss possible underlying etiologies and the risk of recurrence [116,117].

Conclusion

Pregnancy loss is a common condition that requires adept management by practitioners of women's health care. Diagnosis can be made clinically or more precisely using ultrasonography. Early pregnancy failures can be managed expectantly, with medication, or surgically. Expectant management is a safe option for clinically stable women with incomplete abortions. Medical management with misoprostol allows most women with early pregnancy failure to complete their abortion and avoid surgery. Vacuum aspiration remains the most effective and efficient way to ensure complete uterine evacuation, and it can be accomplished easily in the outpatient setting using manual or electric suction devices. Management options for second-trimester fetal demise include labor induction or D&E where clinicians with the requisite skills are available. Patients experiencing loss of a desired pregnancy benefit from a follow-up visit to acknowledge the loss and discuss its implications. Those desiring pregnancy and experiencing multiple early losses or a second-trimester loss may benefit from referral to counselors or specialists to address their complex needs.

References

1 Saraiya M, Berg CJ, Shulman H, Green CA, Atrash HK. Estimates of the annual number of clinically recognized pregnancies in the United States, 1981–1991. *Am J Epidemiol* 1999; **149**: 1025–1029.

2 National Center for Health Statistics and Centers for Disease Control and Prevention [Online]. Hyattsville (MD): National Center for Health Statistics. Health, United States, 2007 with Chartbook on Trends in the Health of Americans: Appendix II – Definitions and Methods. 2008 [cited 2009 Jan 11]. Available from: URL: http://www.CDC.gov/nchs/data/hus/hus07.pdf

3 Williams J. *Obstetrics: A Text-Book for the Use of Students and Practitioners*. D. Appleton & Co., New York, 1903.

4 Sedgh G, Henshaw S, Singh S, Åhman E, Shah IH. Induced abortion: estimated rates and trends worldwide. *Lancet* 2007; **370**: 1338–1345.

5 Jones RK, Kost K. Underreporting of induced and spontaneous abortion in the United States: an analysis of the 2002 National Survey of Family Growth. *Stud Fam Plann* 2007; **38**: 187–197.

6 Grimes DA. Estimation of pregnancy-related mortality risk by pregnancy outcome, United States, 1991 to 1999. *Am J Obstet Gynecol* 2006; **194**: 92–94.

7 Saraiya M, Green CA, Berg CJ, Hopkins FW, Koonin LM, Atrash HK. Spontaneous abortion-related deaths among women in the United States—1981–1991. *Obstet Gynecol* 1999; **94**: 172–176.

8 Eddleman KA, Malone FD, Sullivan L et al. Pregnancy loss rates after midtrimester amniocentesis. *Obstet Gynecol* 2006; **108**: 1067–1072.

9 Nybo Andersen AM, Wohlfahrt J, Christens P, Olsen J, Melbye M. Maternal age and fetal loss: population based register linkage study. *BMJ* 2000; **320**: 1708–1712.

10 Kleinhaus K, Perrin M, Friedlander Y, Paltiel O, Malaspina D, Harlap S. Paternal age and spontaneous abortion. *Obstet Gynecol* 2006; **108**: 369–377.

11 Buss L, Tolstrup J, Munk C et al. Spontaneous abortion: a prospective cohort study of younger women from the general population in Denmark. Validation, occurrence, and risk determinants. *Acta Obstet Gynecol Scand* 2006; **85**: 467–475.

12 Parazzini F, Chatenoud L, Tozzi L, Di Cintio E, Benzi G, Fedele L. Induced abortion in the first trimester of pregnancy and risk of miscarriage. *Br J Obstet Gynaecol* 1998; **105**: 418–421.

13 Chatenoud L, Parazzini F, di Cintio E et al. Paternal and maternal smoking habits before conception and during the first trimester: relation to spontaneous abortion. *Ann Epidemiol* 1998; **8**: 520–526.

14 Nielsen A, Hannibal CG, Lindekilde BE et al. Maternal smoking predicts the risk of spontaneous abortion. *Acta Obstet Gynecol Scand* 2006; **85**: 1057–1065.

15 Venners SA, Wang X, Chen C et al. Paternal smoking and pregnancy loss: a prospective study using a biomarker of pregnancy. *Am J Epidemiol* 2004; **159**: 993–1001.

16 Rasch V. Cigarette, alcohol, caffeine consumption: risk factors for spontaneous abortion. *Acta Obstet Gynecol Scand* 2003; **82**: 182–188.

17 Silver RM. Fetal death. *Obstet Gynecol* 2007; **109**: 153–167.

18 Stephenson M, Kutteh W. Evaluation and management of recurrent early pregnancy loss. *Clin Obstet Gynecol* 2007; **50**: 132–145.

19 Magann EF, Chauhan SP, Bofill JA, Waddell D, Rust OA, Morrison JC. Maternal morbidity and mortality associated with

intrauterine fetal demise: five-year experience in a tertiary referral hospital. *South Med J* 2001; **94**: 493–495.

20 Zhang J, Gilles JM, Barnhart K et al. A comparison of medical management with misoprostol and surgical management for early pregnancy failure. *N Engl J Med* 2005; **353**: 761–769.

21 Ankum WM, Wieringa-De Waard M, Bindels PJ. Management of spontaneous miscarriage in the first trimester: an example of putting informed shared decision making into practice. *BMJ* 2001; **322**: 1343–1346.

22 Wieringa-De Waard M, Hartman EE, Ankum WM, Reitsma JB, Bindels PJ, Bonsel GJ. Expectant management versus surgical evacuation in first trimester miscarriage: health-related quality of life in randomized and non-randomized patients. *Hum Reprod* 2002; **17**: 1638–1642.

23 Creinin MD, Schwartz JL, Guido RS, Pymar HC. Early pregnancy failure–current management concepts. *Obstet Gynecol Surv* 2001; **56**: 105–113.

24 Castadot RG. Pregnancy termination: techniques, risks, and complications and their management. *Fertil Steril* 1986: **45**: 5–17.

25 Finer LB, Henshaw SK. Abortion incidence and services in the United States in 2000. *Perspect Sex Reprod Health* 2003; **35**: 6–15.

26 Harris LH, Dalton VK, Johnson TR. Surgical management of early pregnancy failure: history, politics, and safe, cost-effective care. *Am J Obstet Gynecol* 2007; **196**: 445 e1–5.

27 Hemminki E. Treatment of miscarriage: current practice and rationale. *Obstet Gynecol* 1998; **91**: 247–253.

28 Wiebe E, Janssen P. Management of spontaneous abortion in family practices and hospitals. *Fam Med* 1998; **30**: 293–296.

29 Grimes DA, Cates W Jr, Tyler CW Jr. Comparative risk of death from legally induced abortion in hospital and nonhospital facilities. *Obstet Gynecol* 1978; **51**: 323–326.

30 Blumenthal PD, Remsburg RE. A time and cost analysis of the management of incomplete abortion with manual vacuum aspiration. *Int J Gynaecol Obstet* 1994; **45**: 261–267.

31 Dalton VK, Harris L, Weisman CS, Guire K, Castleman L, Lebovic D. Patient preferences, satisfaction, and resource use in office evacuation of early pregnancy failure. *Obstet Gynecol* 2006; **108**: 103–110.

32 Luise C, Jermy K, May C, Costello G, Collins WP, Bourne TH. Outcome of expectant management of spontaneous first trimester miscarriage: observational study. *BMJ* 2002; **324**: 873–875.

33 Nielsen S, Hahlin M. Expectant management of first-trimester spontaneous abortion. *Lancet* 1995; **345**: 84–86.

34 Hurd WW, Whitfield RR, Randolph JF Jr, Kercher ML. Expectant management versus elective curettage for the treatment of spontaneous abortion. *Fertil Steril* 1997; **68**: 601–606.

35 Jurkovic D, Ross JA, Nicolaides KH. Expectant management of missed miscarriage. *Br J Obstet Gynaecol* 1998; **105**: 670–671.

36 Chipchase J, James D. Randomised trial of expectant versus surgical management of spontaneous miscarriage. *Br J Obstet Gynaecol* 1997; **104**: 840–841.

37 Wieringa-de Waard M, Vos J, Bonsel GJ, Bindels PJ, Ankum WM. Management of miscarriage: a randomized controlled trial of expectant management versus surgical evacuation. *Hum Reprod* 2002; **17**: 2445–2450.

38 Nanda K, Peloggia A, Grimes D, Lopez L, Nanda G. Expectant care versus surgical treatment for miscarriage. *Cochrane Database Syst Rev* 2006; **2**: CD003518.

39 Trinder J, Brocklehurst P, Porter R, Read M, Vyas S, Smith L. Management of miscarriage: expectant, medical, or surgical? Results of randomised controlled trial (miscarriage treatment [MIST] trial). *BMJ* 2006; **332**: 1235–1240.

40 Lelaidier C, Baton-Saint-Mleux C, Fernandez H, Bourget P, Frydman R. Mifepristone (RU 486) induces embryo expulsion in first trimester non-developing pregnancies: a prospective randomized trial. *Hum Reprod* 1993; **8**: 492–495.

41 Anonymous. Comparison of two doses of mifepristone in combination with misoprostol for early medical abortion: a randomised trial. World Health Organisation Task Force on Post-ovulatory Methods of Fertility Regulation. *BJOG* 2000; **107**: 524–530.

42 Coughlin LB, Roberts D, Haddad NG, Long A. Medical management of first trimester miscarriage (blighted ovum and missed abortion): is it effective? *J Obstet Gynaecol* 2004; **24**: 69–71.

43 Grønlund A, Grønlund L, Clevin L, Andersen B, Palmgren N, Lidegaard Ø. Management of missed abortion: comparison of medical treatment with either mifepristone + misoprostol or misoprostol alone with surgical evacuation. A multi-center trial in Copenhagen County, Denmark. *Acta Obstet Gynecol Scand* 2002; **81**: 1060–1065.

44 Stockheim D, Machtinger R, Wiser A et al. A randomized prospective study of misoprostol or mifepristone followed by misoprostol when needed for the treatment of women with early pregnancy failure. *Fertil Steril* 2006; **86**: 956–960.

45 Autry A, Jacobson G, Sandhu R, Isbill K. Medical management of non-viable early first trimester pregnancy. *Int J Gynaecol Obstet* 1999; **67**: 9–13.

46 Moodliar S, Bagratee JS, Moodley J. Medical vs. surgical evacuation of first-trimester spontaneous abortion. *Int J Gynaecol Obstet* 2005; **91**: 21–26.

47 Chung TK, Lee DT, Cheung LP, Haines CJ, Chang AM. Spontaneous abortion: a randomized, controlled trial comparing surgical evacuation with conservative management using misoprostol. *Fertil Steril* 1999; **71**: 1054–1059.

48 Weeks A, Alia G, Blum J et al. A randomized trial of misoprostol compared with manual vacuum aspiration for incomplete abortion. *Obstet Gynecol* 2005; **106**: 540–547.

49 Bique C, Ustá M, Debora B, Chong E, Westheimer E, Winikoff B. Comparison of misoprostol and manual vacuum aspiration for the treatment of incomplete abortion. *Int J Gynaecol Obstet* 2007; **98**: 222–226.

50 de Jonge ET, Makin JD, Manefeldt E, De Wet GH, Pattinson RC. Randomised clinical trial of medical evacuation and

surgical curettage for incomplete miscarriage. *BMJ* 1995; **311**: 662.

51 Demetroulis C, Saridogan E, Kunde D, Naftalin AA. A prospective randomized control trial comparing medical and surgical treatment for early pregnancy failure. *Hum Reprod* 2001; **16**: 365–369.

52 Graziosi GC, Mol BW, Reuwer PJ, Drogtrop A, Bruinse HW. Misoprostol versus curettage in women with early pregnancy failure after initial expectant management: a randomized trial. *Hum Reprod* 2004; **19**: 1894–1899.

53 Muffley PE, Stitely ML, Gherman RB. Early intrauterine pregnancy failure: a randomized trial of medical versus surgical treatment. *Am J Obstet Gynecol* 2002; **187**: 321–325; discussion 325–326.

54 Kovavisarach E., Jamnansiri C. Intravaginal misoprostol 600 microg and 800 microg for the treatment of early pregnancy failure. *Int J Gynaecol Obstet* 2005; **90**: 208–212.

55 Creinin MD, Moyer R, Guido R. Misoprostol for medical evacuation of early pregnancy failure. *Obstet Gynecol* 1997; **89**: 768–772.

56 Ngoc NT, Blum J, Westheimer E, Quan TT, Winikoff B. Medical treatment of missed abortion using misoprostol. *Int J Gynaecol Obstet* 2004; **87**: 138–142.

57 Pang MW, Lee TS, Chung TK. Incomplete miscarriage: a randomized controlled trial comparing oral with vaginal misoprostol for medical evacuation. *Hum Reprod* 2001; **16**: 2283–2287.

58 Reeves MF, Lohr PA, Harwood BJ, Creinin MD. Ultrasonographic endometrial thickness after medical and surgical management of early pregnancy failure. *Obstet Gynecol* 2008; **111**: 106–112.

59 Cowett AA, Cohen LS, Lichtenberg ES, Stika CS. Ultrasound evaluation of the endometrium after medical termination of pregnancy. *Obstel Gynecol* 2004; **103**: 871–875.

60 Creinin MD, Huang X, Westhoff C, Barnhart K, Gilles JM, Zhang J. Factors related to successful misoprostol treatment for early pregnancy failure. *Obstet Gynecol* 2006; **107**: 901–907.

61 Davis AR, Hendlish SK, Westhoff C et al. Bleeding patterns after misoprostol vs. surgical treatment of early pregnancy failure: results from a randomized trial. *Am J Obstet Gynecol* 2007; **196**: 31 e1–7.

62 Tang OS, Lau WN, Ng EH, Lee SW, Ho PC. A prospective randomized study to compare the use of repeated doses of vaginal with sublingual misoprostol in the management of first trimester silent miscarriages. *Hum Reprod* 2003; **18**: 176–181.

63 Tang OS, Ho PC. Pilot study on the use of sublingual misoprostol for medical abortion. *Contraception* 2001; **64**, 315–317.

64 Herabutya Y, O-Prasertsawat P. Misoprostol in the management of missed abortion. *Int J Gynaecol Obstet* 1997; **56**: 263–266.

65 Lister MS, Shaffer LE, Bell JG, Lutter KQ, Moorma KH. Randomized, double-blind, placebo-controlled trial of vaginal misoprostol for management of early pregnancy failures. *Am J Obstet Gynecol* 2005; **193**: 1338–1343.

66 Wood SL, Brain PH. Medical management of missed abortion: a randomized clinical trial. *Obstet Gynecol* 2002; **99**: 563–566.

67 Bagratee JS, Khullar V, Regan L, Moodley J, Kagoro H. A randomized controlled trial comparing medical and expectant management of first trimester miscarriage. *Hum Reprod* 2004; **19**: 266–271.

68 Shelley JM, Healy D, Grover S. A randomised trial of surgical, medical, and expectant management of first trimester spontaneous miscarriage. *Aust N Z J Obstet Gynaecol* 2005; **45**: 122–127.

69 Sotiriadis A, Makrydimas G, Papatheodorou S, Ioannidis JP. Expectant, medical, or surgical management of first-trimester miscarriage: a meta-analysis. *Obstet Gynecol* 2005; **105**: 1104–1113.

70 Blum J, Winikoff B, Gemzell-Danielsson K, Ho PC, Schiavon R, Weeks A. Treatment of incomplete abortion and miscarriage with misoprostol. *Int J Gynaecol Obstet* 2007; **99**: S186–189.

71 Goldstein DP, Johnson JP, Reid DE. Management of intrauterine fetal death. *Obstet Gynecol* 1963; **21**: 523–529.

72 Maslow AD, Breen TW, Sarna MC, Soni AK, Watkins J, Oriol NE. Prevalence of coagulation abnormalities associated with intrauterine fetal death. Can J Anaesth 1996; **43**: 1237–1243.

73 Guidotti RJ, Grimes DA, Cates W Jr. Fatal amniotic fluid embolism during legally induced abortion, United States, 1972 to 1978. *Am J Obstet Gynecol* 1981; **141**: 257–261.

74 Ray BK, Vallejo MC, Creinin MD et al. Amniotic fluid embolism with second trimester pregnancy termination: a case report. *Can J Anaesth* 2004; **51**: 139–144.

75 Mainprize TC, Maltby JR. Amniotic fluid embolism: a report of four probable cases. *Can Anaesth Soc J* 1986; **33**: 382–387.

76 Gilbert WM, Danielsen B. Amniotic fluid embolism: decreased mortality in a population-based study. *Obstet Gynecol* 1999; **93**: 973–977.

77 Owen J, Hauth JC. Concentrated oxytocin plus low-dose prostaglandin E2 compared with prostaglandin E2 vaginal suppositories for second-trimester pregnancy termination. *Obstet Gynecol* 1996; **88**: 110–113.

78 Ramin KD, Ogburn PL, Danilenko DR, Ramsey PS. High-dose oral misoprostol for mid-trimester pregnancy interruption. *Gynecol Obstet Invest* 2002; **54**: 176–179.

79 Ramsey PS, Savage K, Lincoln T, Owen J. Vaginal misoprostol versus concentrated oxytocin and vaginal PGE2 for second-trimester labor induction. *Obstet Gynecol* 2004; **104**: 138–145.

80 Owen J, Hauth JC. Vaginal misoprostol vs. concentrated oxytocin plus low-dose prostaglandin E2 for second trimester pregnancy termination. *J Matern Fetal Med* 1999; **8**: 48–50.

81 Mendilcioglu I, Simsek M, Seker PE, Erbay O, Zorlu CG, Trak B. Misoprostol in second and early third trimester for termination of pregnancies with fetal anomalies.*Int J Gynaecol Obstet* 2002; **79**: 131–135.

82 De Heus R, Graziosi GC, Christiaens GC, Bruinse HW, Mol BW. Medical management for termination of second and third

trimester pregnancies: a comparison of strategies. *Eur J Obstet Gynecol Reprod Biol* 2004; **116**: 16–21.

83 Jain JK, Mishell DR Jr. A comparison of intravaginal misoprostol with prostaglandin E2 for termination of second-trimester pregnancy. *N Engl J Med* 1994; **331**: 290–293.

84 Makhlouf AM, Al-Hussaini TK, Habib DM, Makarem MH. Second-trimester pregnancy termination: comparison of three different methods. *J Obstet Gynaecol* 2003; **23**: 407–411.

85 Debby A, Sagiv R, Girtler O, Sadan O, Glezerman M, Golan A. Extra-amniotic prostaglandin E2 for midtrimester termination of pregnancy in live fetuses vs. fetal demise. *Arch Gynecol Obstet* 2003; **268**: 301–303.

86 Dickinson JE, Godfrey M, Evans SF. Efficacy of intravaginal misoprostol in second-trimester pregnancy termination: a randomized controlled trial. *J Matern Fetal Med* 1998; **7**: 115–119.

87 Dickinson JE, Evans SF. The optimization of intravaginal misoprostol dosing schedules in second-trimester pregnancy termination. *Am J Obstet Gynecol* 2002; **186**: 470–474.

88 Jain JK, Kuo J, Mishell DR Jr. A comparison of two dosing regimens of intravaginal misoprostol for second-trimester pregnancy termination. *Obstet Gynecol* 1999; **93**: 571–575.

89 Niromanesh S, Hashemi-Fesharaki M, Mosavi-Jarrahi A. Second trimester abortion using intravaginal misoprostol. *Int J Gynaecol Obstet* 2005; **89**: 276–277.

90 Srisomboon J, Pongpisuttinun S. Efficacy of intracervicovaginal misoprostol in second-trimester pregnancy termination: a comparison between live and dead fetuses. *J Obstet Gynaecol Res* 1998; **24**: 1–5.

91 Edwards RK, Sims SM. Outcomes of second-trimester pregnancy terminations with misoprostol: comparing 2 regimens. *Am J Obstet Gynecol* 2005; **193**: 544–548.

92 Dickinson JE, Evans SF. A comparison of oral misoprostol with vaginal misoprostol administration in second-trimester pregnancy termination for fetal abnormality. *Obstet Gynecol* 2003; **101**: 1294–1299.

93 Chittacharoen A, Herabutya Y, Punyavachira P. A randomized trial of oral and vaginal misoprostol to manage delivery in cases of fetal death. *Obstet Gynecol* 2003; **101**: 70–73.

94 Bugalho A, Bique C, Machungo F, Faáundes A. Induction of labor with intravaginal misoprostol in intrauterine fetal death. *Am J Obstet Gynecol* 1994; **171**: 538–541.

95 Fadalla FA, Mirghani OA, Adam I. Oral misoprostol vs. vaginal misoprostol for termination of pregnancy with intrauterine fetal demise in the second-trimester. *Int J Gynaecol Obstet* 2004; **86**: 52–53.

96 Jain JK, Mishell DR Jr. A comparison of misoprostol with and without laminaria tents for induction of second-trimester abortion. *Am J Obstet Gynecol* 1996; **175**: 173–177.

97 Borgatta L, Chen AY, Vragovic O, Stubblefield PG, Magloire CA. A randomized clinical trial of the addition of laminaria to misoprostol and hypertonic saline for second-trimester induction abortion. *Contraception* 2005; **72**: 358–361.

98 Prairie BA, Lauria MR, Kapp N, Mackenzie T, Baker ER, George KE. Mifepristone versus laminaria: a randomized controlled trial of cervical ripening in midtrimester termination. *Contraception* 2007; **76**: 383–388.

99 Merrell DA, Koch MA. Induction of labour with intravaginal misoprostol in the second and third trimesters of pregnancy. *S Afr Med J* 1995; **85**: 1088–1090.

100 Pongsatha S, Tongsong T. Therapeutic termination of second trimester pregnancies with intrauterine fetal death with 400 micrograms of oral misoprostol. *J Obstet Gynaecol Res* 2004; **30**: 217–220.

101 Eng NS, Guan AC. Comparative study of intravaginal misoprostol with gemeprost as an abortifacient in second trimester missed abortion. *Aust N Z J Obstet Gynaecol* 1997; **37**: 331–334.

102 American College of Obstetricians and Gynecologists, Committee on Obstetric Practice. ACOG Committee Opinion No. 228: Induction of labor with misoprostol. Washington (DC): American College of Obstetricians and Gynecologists, November 1999, reaffirmed 2008.

103 Dickinson JE, Newnham JP, Roberts RV, Reid SE. Oxytocin induced second trimester uterine rupture. *Aust N Z J Obstet Gynaecol* 1986; **26**: 251–252.

104 Yapar EG, Senöz S, Urkütür M, Batioglu S, Gökmen O. Second trimester pregnancy termination including fetal death: comparison of five different methods. *Eur J Obstet Gynecol Reprod Biol* 1996; **69**: 97–102.

105 Dickinson JE. Misoprostol for second-trimester pregnancy termination in women with a prior cesarean delivery. *Obstet Gynecol* 2005; **105**: 352–356.

106 Gómez Ponce de León R, Wing D, Fiala C. Misoprostol for intrauterine fetal death. *Int J Gynaecol Obstet* 2007; **99**: S190–1903.

107 Autry AM, Hayes EC, Jacobson GF, Kirby RS. A comparison of medical induction and dilation and evacuation for second-trimester abortion. *Am J Obstet Gynecol* 2002; **187**: 393–397.

108 American College of Obstetrics and Gynecology, Committee on Genetics. ACOG Committee Opinion No. 383: Evaluation of stillbirths and neonatal deaths. *Obstet Gynecol* 2007; **110**: 963–966.

109 Hogge WA, Bymes AL, Lanasa MC, Surti U. The clinical use of karyotyping spontaneous abortions. *Am J Obstet Gynecol* 2003; **189**: 397–400.

110 Jobanputra V, Sobrino A, Kinney A, Kline J, Warburton D. Multiplex interphase FISH as a screen for common aneuploidies in spontaneous abortions. *Hum Reprod* 202; **17**: 1166–1170.

111 Boyd PA, Tondi F, Hicks NR, Chamberlain PF. Autopsy after termination of pregnancy for fetal anomaly: retrospective cohort study. *BMJ* 2004; **328**: 137.

112 Cohen AL, Bhatnagar J, Reagan S et al. Toxic shock associated with *Clostridium sordellii* and *Clostridium perfringens* after medical and spontaneous abortion. *Obstet Gynecol* 2007; **110**: 1027–1033.

113 Stubblefield PG, Grimes DA. Septic abortion. *N Engl J Med* 1994; **331**: 310–314.

114 Centers for Disease Control and Prevention, Workowski KA, Berman SM. Sexually transmitted diseases treatment guidelines, 2006. *MMWR Recomm Rep* 2006; **55**: 1–94.

115 Grossman D, Ellertson C, Grimes DA, Walker D. Routine follow-up visits after first-trimester induced abortion. *Obstet Gynecol* 2004; **103**: 738–745.

116 Brier N. Understanding and managing the emotional reactions to a miscarriage. *Obstet Gynecol* 1999; **93**: 151–155.

117 Griebel CP, Halvorsen J, Golemon TB, Day AA. Management of spontaneous abortion. *Am Fam Physician* 2005; **72**: 1243–1250.

18

CHAPTER 18
Ectopic pregnancy

Jennifer L. Kulp MD and Kurt T. Barnhart MD, MSCE

> **LEARNING POINTS**
> - The majority (more than 95%) of cases of ectopic pregnancy occur in the fallopian tube, with most implanting in the ampulla.
> - Patient factors conferring the greatest risk of ectopic pregnancy include a history of a previous ectopic pregnancy, known tubal damage or previous tubal surgery, failure of a progestin-only contraceptive, and a history of transabdominal tubal sterilization.
> - Patients with an ectopic pregnancy can present in early pregnancy with amenorrhea, abdominal pain, or vaginal bleeding.
> - Diagnosis of ectopic pregnancy may require serial high-resolution ultrasounds and serum quantitative human chorionic gonadotropin (hCG) assays.
> - Medical treatment of ectopic pregnancy with methotrexate allows properly selected patients to avoid surgery.

Introduction

Ectopic pregnancy occurs when a fertilized ovum implants outside the endometrial cavity, most commonly in the fallopian tube [1]. The exact incidence of ectopic pregnancy is difficult to determine. Traditional methods of measuring rates of ectopic pregnancy, such as the use of hospital records, are no longer accurate due to the increasing numbers of ectopic pregnancies managed in outpatient settings. Using US national survey data on inpatient admissions and visits to hospital emergency and outpatient departments, the Centers for Disease Control and Prevention (CDC) estimated that ectopic pregnancy accounted for 2% of all pregnancies (19.7 per 1,000 reported pregnancies) in the USA in 1992. Because this analysis did not include patients managed exclusively in physicians' offices, the true incidence of ectopic pregnancy is undoubtedly greater. Although the number of US women hospitalized for ectopic pregnancy has decreased over time, data suggest that the incidence of ectopic pregnancy increased sixfold from 1970 to 1992 [2]. For unclear reasons, studies have consistently reported lower rates of ectopic pregnancy (less than 1%) in women presenting for induced abortion [3,4].

Ectopic pregnancy remains an important cause of mortality and morbidity in women of reproductive age. In the 1990s, ectopic pregnancy accounted for 6% of all pregnancy-related deaths in the USA [5]. Although the mortality rate from ectopic pregnancy declined from 84.2 deaths per 100,000 ectopic pregnancies in 1979 to 1980 to about 32 per 100,000 during 1991 to 1999 [6], ectopic pregnancy remains the leading cause of maternal death in the first trimester. Most deaths occur due to rupture of the fallopian tube and massive hemorrhage. The cost of treating ectopic pregnancy is considerable, totaling approximately 1.1 billion US dollars in 1992 [7]. Based on a systematic review of the distribution of causes of maternal death worldwide, the World Health Organization found that reported deaths from ectopic pregnancy accounted for nearly 5% of maternal mortality in developed countries and less than 1% in developing countries [8]. Although ectopic pregnancy remains an important public health problem in developing countries where limited resources and poor access to care often lead to late diagnosis, the relative contribution of ectopic pregnancy to maternal mortality is low compared to hemorrhage, infection, hypertensive disorders, and unsafe abortion [8].

Because more than 60% of US women seek abortion care during the first 8 weeks of pregnancy [9], abortion providers have an opportunity to decrease morbidity from ectopic pregnancy by diagnosing and treating the condition early. This chapter assists this process by describing risk factors and diagnostic algorithms for ectopic pregnancy, as well as

Management of Unintended and Abnormal Pregnancy, 1st edition. By M Paul, ES Lichtenberg, L Borgatta, DA Grimes, PG Stubblefield, MD Creinin
 ISBN: 9781405176965.

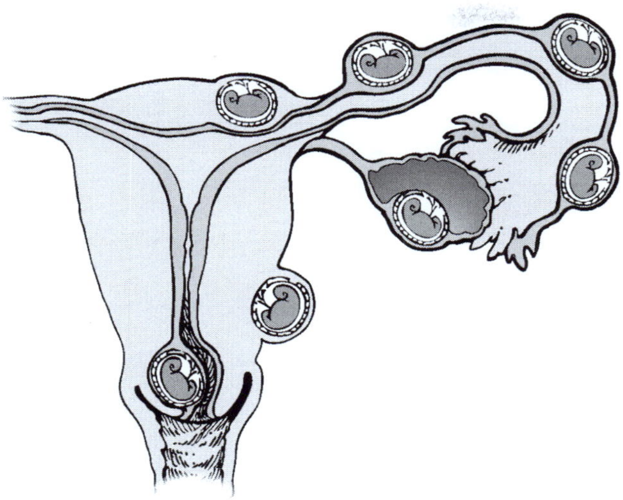

Figure 18.1 Possible sites of ectopic pregnancy. Although most ectopic pregnancies implant in the fallopian tube, extratubal locations may occur.

approaches to medical and surgical management of the condition. Most of the chapter pertains to ectopic pregnancies located in the fallopian tube because they are the most common type; less frequent types of extrauterine pregnancies are described at the end of the chapter.

Table 18.1 Risk factors for ectopic pregnancy. (Adapted from Seeber et al [16], Ankum et al [17], and Bouyer et al [18].)

Risk Factor	Odds Ratio
High Risk	
Previous tubal surgery	6.0–21.0
Tubal sterilization[a]	3.0–9.3
Previous ectopic pregnancy	8.3–47.0
In utero exposure to DES	2.4–13.0
Current use of IUD	1.1–45.0
Tubal pathology	3.5–25.0
Moderate Risk	
Infertility	1.1–28.0
Previous genital infections	2.5–3.7
Multiple sexual partners	1.4–4.8
Low Risk	
Previous pelvic infection	0.9–3.8
Cigarette smoking	2.3–3.9
Vaginal douching	1.1–3.1
First intercourse < age 18	1.1–2.5

[a] Tubal sterilization refers to sterilization procedures performed transabdominally. The risk of ectopic pregnancy after transcervical sterilization is not known.

Background

Pathogenesis

Most (more than 95%) cases of ectopic pregnancy occur in the fallopian tube. Tubal ectopic pregnancies implant most frequently in the ampulla (70%), followed by the isthmus (12%), the fimbria (11.1%), and the cornua (2.4%) [1]. Rare locations for ectopic pregnancies are the ovary, the abdominal cavity, and the cervix (Fig. 18.1). As cesarean section rates increase, reports of implantation at the site of the scar (cesarean scar ectopic pregnancies) are becoming more frequent.

Ectopic pregnancy occurs in the fallopian tube when proliferating trophoblasts invade the tubal wall. The ampullary portion of the fallopian tube is more distensible than other areas of the tube. Ectopic gestations implanting at this site are often found within the tubal lumen and may result in tubal abortion rather than tubal rupture. In contrast, ectopic pregnancies that implant in the narrow isthmus portion of the fallopian tube are more prone to rupture [10].

The etiology of tubal ectopic pregnancy may be due to slowed migration of the blastocyst as it travels through the fallopian tube, resulting in implantation before it reaches the uterine cavity. Impaired movement in the fallopian tube can be secondary to tubal damage from underlying disease, inflammation, or hormonal factors that affect tubal mobility [11]. Intrinsic factors of the blastocyst do not appear to play a role in the etiology of ectopic implantation. Studies analyzing the karyotypes of ectopic embryos have not found greater than expected rates of chromosomal abnormalities [12,13]. However, abnormalities in molecular signaling surrounding the event of implantation may be important [11].

Risk factors

Many factors have been associated with an increased risk of ectopic pregnancy [14–18] (Table 18.1). Factors conferring the greatest risk include a history of a previous ectopic pregnancy and damage to the fallopian tube, either from prior tubal surgery or from tubal pathology such as salpingitis. Women with ectopic pregnancies are three times more likely to have had one prior ectopic pregnancy, and 16 times more likely to have had two prior ectopic pregnancies compared to those with intrauterine pregnancies [14]. A patient with an ectopic pregnancy has up to a 10 to 15% chance of recurrence; this risk varies by treatment method of the original ectopic pregnancy, with salpingostomy having the greatest risk of recurrence [15]. Women who have had reconstructive tubal surgeries are also at high risk. Most likely, the condition requiring the surgery (e.g., salpingitis, adhesive disease, or ectopic pregnancy) is the causative factor for future ectopic pregnancies rather than the procedure itself.

Salpingitis is another important risk factor for ectopic pregnancy. One study found salpingitis isthmica nodosa, a condition that results in anatomic thickening of the proximal portion of the fallopian tubes with multiple luminal diverticula, in approximately 14% of the fallopian tubes containing an ectopic pregnancy versus none of the controls [19]. Genital infections associated with salpingitis, such as chlamydia, gonorrhea, and pelvic inflammatory disease, increase the risk for ectopic pregnancy [17]. One retrospective study found odds ratios for ectopic pregnancy of 2.1 in women who had a history of two prior chlamydial infections and 4.5 in women with three or more prior chlamydial infections [20].

Women exposed to diethylstilbestrol (DES) *in utero* may develop reproductive tract anomalies, including a T-shaped uterus and foreshortened fallopian tubes with small tubal ostia and minimal fimbrial tissue [21]. *In utero* DES exposure carries a ninefold increased risk of ectopic pregnancy [22]. Women who become pregnant after tubal sterilization or while using intrauterine contraception or progestin-only methods are at greater risk for ectopic pregnancy. Patients who conceive following transabdominal tubal sterilization have a ninefold increased risk of ectopic pregnancy [23]. The 10-year cumulative probability of ectopic pregnancy after such procedures is approximately 0.07% [24]. Tubal sterilization using bipolar coagulation carries a greater risk than other transabdominal methods, such as postpartum bilateral salpingectomy [25]. Rates of ectopic pregnancy after transcervical sterilization are unknown. As many as half of pregnancies occurring in women with a levonorgestrel intrauterine system in place may be ectopic, whereas the rate is 1 in 16 pregnancies in women using a copper intrauterine device [24]. Women who conceive while using a progestin-only method of contraception, such as oral contraceptives or implants, have a slightly greater risk of ectopic pregnancy compared to those who become pregnant while not using any type of contraception [24]. More importantly, because contraception decreases a woman's overall chance of becoming pregnant the absolute risk of developing an ectopic pregnancy is still lower.

Assisted reproductive technologies (ART) also increase the risk of ectopic pregnancy. In 2004, the frequency of ectopic pregnancy following *in vitro* fertilization was 2%, which represents a decrease from the 3% rate reported in 1999. The risk of ectopic pregnancy is greatest in couples with tubal factor infertility [26], most likely due to damaged fallopian tubes in this population. Patients with hydrosalpinges undergoing ART have greater rates of ectopic pregnancy [27,28]. Furthermore, exogenous hormones administered for ovulation induction can alter tubal motility [29–31]. The method of embryo transfer may influence the risk as well, with embryos placed at deep fundal locations having a greater risk for implanting in the fallopian tube than those placed in midfundal locations [32].

For reasons that remain unclear, smoking is also a risk factor for ectopic pregnancy [18,33]. Smoking may lead to impaired immunity, which places women at increased risk for developing genital infections, or smoking may alter fallopian tube mobility, thereby increasing the risk of a tubal implantation.

Clinical assessment

Signs and symptoms

The signs and symptoms of ectopic pregnancy are neither sensitive nor specific. Patients with an ectopic pregnancy may present in the first trimester of pregnancy with amenorrhea, abdominal pain, or vaginal bleeding. However, these symptoms also occur commonly in patients with threatened or spontaneous abortion, making the conditions difficult to differentiate based on clinical assessment alone. In one series, women with ectopic pregnancy presented with complaints of pain in 64 to 80% of cases and with vaginal bleeding in 67 to 83% of cases. In most patients, the vaginal bleeding was mild [34]. Abdominal pain described as moderate to severe or sharp increases the risk of ectopic pregnancy [35]. The minority of patients who present with tubal rupture can exhibit syncope, light-headedness, tachycardia, or hypovolemic shock.

Signs present on physical examination that increase the likelihood of ectopic pregnancy include unilateral or bilateral abdominal tenderness, peritoneal signs such as rebound or guarding, or cervical motion tenderness. A tender adnexal mass is evident in a minority of patients. Women with a uterine size greater than 8 weeks are less likely to have an ectopic pregnancy [35]. The examination in a patient with an ectopic pregnancy also may be nonfocal [36].

Diagnosis

History and physical examination alone will not usually confirm a diagnosis of ectopic pregnancy. Differentiating an ectopic pregnancy from an early intrauterine pregnancy (IUP) or spontaneous abortion usually requires a combination of serum quantitative human chorionic gonadotropin (hCG) measurements, pelvic ultrasound and, in some cases, dilation and curettage [37] (Fig. 18.2). With a normal IUP, specific landmarks using transvaginal ultrasonography typically appear during the following gestational weeks [38]:

- Gestational sac — 4.5 weeks
- Yolk sac — 5 weeks
- Embryonic cardiac activity — 6 weeks.

Sometimes ultrasonography allows for an immediate diagnosis of ectopic pregnancy. In units with skilled ultrasonographers, 70 to 90% of women ultimately diagnosed with an ectopic pregnancy had a mass or gestational sac seen in the adnexa by transvaginal ultrasound [39,40]. However, in other settings the majority of initial ultrasounds in women ultimately diagnosed with an ectopic pregnancy are nondiagnostic [41]. The ultrasound finding of an extraovarian, noncystic adnexal mass in a woman with no intrauterine pregnancy and a positive hCG assay has a sensitivity of 84 to

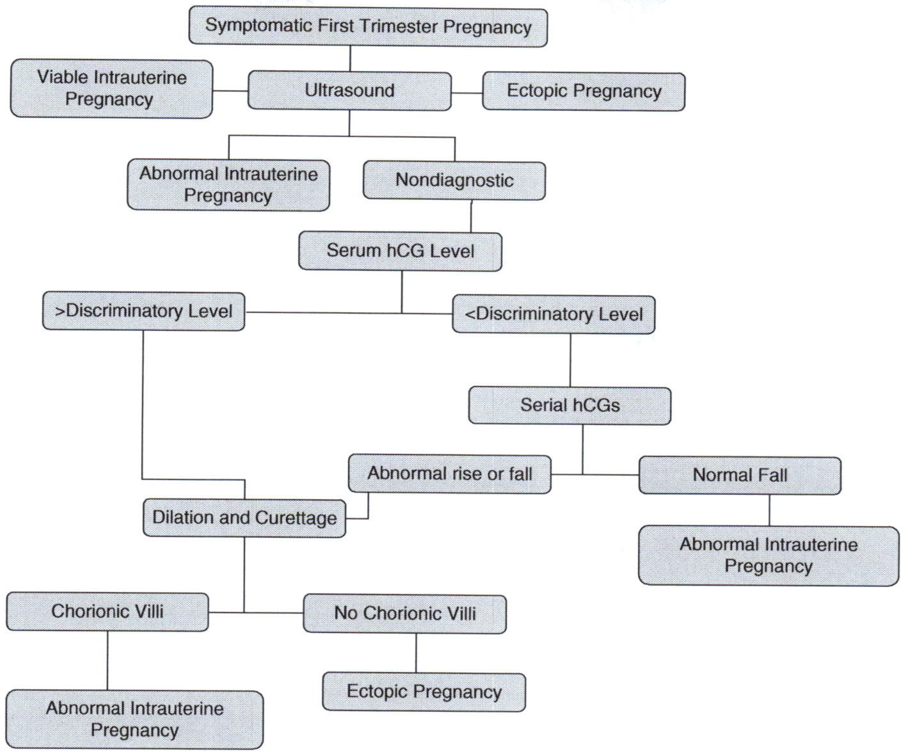

Figure 18.2 Diagnostic algorithm for ectopic pregnancy (Adapted with permission from Seeber et al [37].)

90% and a specificity of 94 to 99% for the diagnosis of ectopic pregnancy [40,42,43]. When ectopic pregnancies are visualized on ultrasound, they most frequently appear as a homogeneous mass (58%); less often, they appear as a mass with a hyperechoic ring around a gestational sac (20%) or as a gestational sac with an embryonic pole, with or without gestational cardiac activity (13%) [40].

Other ultrasound findings can be seen in patients with ectopic pregnancies. A pseudogestational sac is a fluid collection in the endometrial cavity that represents bleeding from decidualized endometrial tissue (Fig. 18.3). Unlike a true gestational sac, it is centrally located in the endometrial cavity. Patients with an ectopic pregnancy may also have a corpus luteum cyst that is located on the same side as the ectopic gestation in 70 to 85% of cases [40,44,45]. Blood in the pelvis is evident on ultrasound in 30% of ectopic pregnancy cases and may represent tubal rupture or blood leaking from the fallopian tube [40].

The serum hCG level at which an intrauterine pregnancy should be seen on ultrasound is called the "discriminatory level" (Chapter 6). Depending on the equipment and skills of the personnel at a particular institution, the discriminatory level for transvaginal ultrasonography usually ranges from about 1,500 to 2,500 mIU/ml. A lower discriminatory level is less likely to delay the diagnosis of an ectopic pregnancy, whereas a higher cutoff decreases the risk of missing or dis-

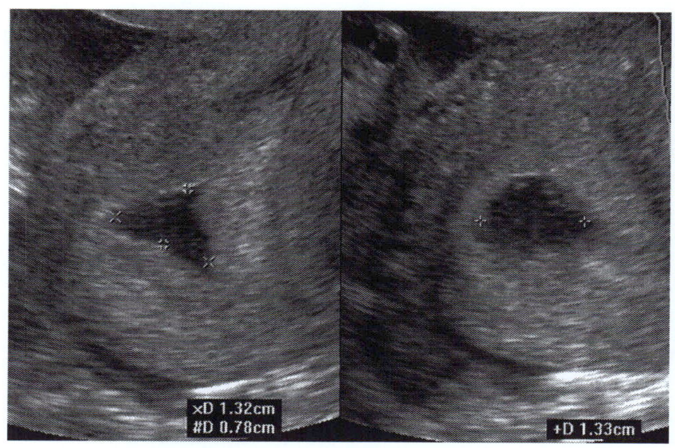

Figure 18.3 Two transvaginal ultrasound images of a pseudogestational sac in a woman with an ectopic pregnancy. The pseudosac is composed of decidualized endometrium (the echogenic rim) and fluid within the endometrial cavity (the anechoic central area outlined by calipers). This fluid is usually either blood or secretions from the hypersecretory endometrium. True early gestational sacs are usually round or elliptical in shape, located eccentrically in the uterine corpus, and surrounded by two bright echogenic rings (so-called choriodecidual reaction or "double-decidual sign"). In contrast, this pseudogestational sac is irregular in shape, centrally located in the uterine cavity, and lacks a double-decidual sign. Often, the pseudogestational sac will come to a point that points toward the cervix, as is the case in this example. (Courtesy of Dr. Matthew Reeves.)

rupting a viable intrauterine pregnancy. If the serum hCG level is above the discriminatory cutoff and transvaginal ultrasonography does not identify an intrauterine pregnancy, then the diagnosis of an abnormal pregnancy is confirmed; however, distinguishing a spontaneous abortion from an ectopic pregnancy remains critical. If the hCG level is below the discriminatory cutoff at the time of presentation, then the patient may have an early intrauterine pregnancy, a failed pregnancy, or an ectopic pregnancy. Serial hCG levels are required to make the diagnosis.

Using quantitative radioimmunoassay, hCG can be detected at levels as low as 1 mIU/ml in the serum and 20 mIU/ml in the urine (Chapter 6). Its appearance in serum and urine coincides with implantation, which occurs approximately 6 to 12 days after ovulation [46]. In viable intrauterine pregnancies with starting hCG levels less than 10,000 mIU/ml, the minimum expected rise in hCG over 48 hours is 53% based on a 99% confidence interval. In rare viable intrauterine pregnancies, the rise in hCG levels may be as low as 35% [47,48]. However, 20% of ectopic gestations can produce an initial hCG pattern identical to that of an intrauterine pregnancy, so an important part of the diagnostic algorithm includes performing an ultrasound once the hCG level reaches the discriminatory cutoff [49]. A decreasing hCG level indicates an abnormal pregnancy. A rapid decline in hCG of 21 to 35% over 48 hours is most indicative of a spontaneous abortion [48], but some ectopic pregnancies have a fast decline in hCG levels as well. Therefore, continuing to obtain serial hCG levels until they fall to undetectable levels is important.

In the majority of cases (70%) of ectopic pregnancy, the rise in hCG levels is slower than that expected for a viable intrauterine pregnancy, or the decline is slower than that expected for a spontaneous abortion [37]. If a woman has a nondiagnostic ultrasound, an initial hCG level above the discriminatory cutoff, and hCG levels that are rising or falling abnormally, performing uterine aspiration can then aid in determining the final diagnosis (Fig. 18.2). Identification of chorionic villi in the tissue aspirate confirms the diagnosis of an abnormal intrauterine pregnancy, and no further therapy is necessary. Absence of chorionic villi establishes the diagnosis of ectopic pregnancy, and further treatment is warranted.

Sometimes histological examination is not readily available or accurate. In this situation, a serum quantitative hCG level can be obtained prior to aspiration and 12 to 24 hours later. Data from the medical abortion literature shows that after expulsion of a viable IUP, a drop in the hCG level of at least 50% (average 66%) can be expected at 24 hours [50]. Another study assessing the use of misoprostol for the expulsion of nonviable pregnancies found an expected hCG decline of 80% at approximately 24 hours after misoprostol administration [51]. Within 24 hours after surgical evacuation of an abnormal intrauterine pregnancy, the expected decrease in hCG from preoperative levels is at least 21 to 35%, and is often greater. More information is needed to set a precise minimum expected hCG percent fall after suction curettage. By setting a lower expected minimum decrease in hCG levels postoperatively, fewer patients will be treated incorrectly for an assumed ectopic pregnancy. Performing suction curettage instead of empiric treatment with methotrexate for a presumed ectopic pregnancy does not increase the complication rate [52].

Serum progesterone measurements are not frequently used in diagnostic algorithms for ectopic pregnancy. Serum progesterone levels are greater in viable intrauterine pregnancies than in abnormal pregnancies, and a progesterone level less than 5 ng/ml can accurately rule out a viable IUP. However, a single progesterone level is not useful for diagnosing an ectopic pregnancy, as no definitive value distinguishes an ectopic pregnancy from other abnormal intrauterine pregnancies [53,54].

Up to 50% of women with ectopic pregnancies are asymptomatic and do not have known risk factors [55]. Ideally, screening could allow for early detection of ectopic pregnancy and prevent tubal rupture and the need for surgical management. However, screening for ectopic pregnancy is not recommended due to the low prevalence of the condition and the high false-positive rate of current screening tools [56,57].

Management of tubal pregnancy

Medical management

An ectopic pregnancy can be treated medically with methotrexate, allowing properly selected patients to avoid surgery. Methotrexate is a folic acid antagonist that binds competitively to dihydrofolate reductase and decreases production of folic acid. Because folic acid is needed for DNA synthesis, methotrexate inhibits the synthesis of purines and pyrimidines, and therefore mitosis. Methotrexate affects rapidly dividing cells, and cytotrophoblasts are particularly sensitive to the drug.

Patients eligible for methotrexate treatment of ectopic pregnancy are hemodynamically stable, reliable, and able to return for follow-up monitoring. Traditional relative contraindications to methotrexate treatment include an ectopic gestation greater than 3.5 cm in size as measured by ultrasound or the presence of gestational cardiac activity or an hCG level greater than 5,000 mIU/ml [58]. Although adhering to these guidelines may increase the success rate of methotrexate therapy, other studies suggest that methotrexate is effective in patients who do not fit these criteria [59,60]. Success rates of methotrexate therapy decrease with greater pretreatment hCG levels. In patients treated with the single-dose methotrexate protocol, success rates are significantly lower when pretreatment hCG levels exceed 5,000 mIU/ml [61]. Certain medical conditions are absolute

Table 18.2 Methotrexate protocols.

	Treatment Day								
	0	1	2	3	4	5	6	7	11
Single-dose	T&S, CBC, recent serum hCG, (may need LFTs, Cr)[a] MTX 50 mg/m^2				Serum hCG			Serum hCG, CBC, LFTs, Cr MTX if <15% decrease in serum hCG from day 4	
Two-dose	T&S, CBC, recent serum hCG, (may need LFTs, Cr)[a] MTX 1mg/kg				Serum hCG MTX			Serum hCG, CBC, LFTs, Cr MTX if <15% decrease in serum hCG from day 4	Serum hCG MTX if <15% decrease in serum hCG from day 7
Multi-dose[b]	T&S, CBC, recent serum hCG, (may need LFTs, Cr)[a] MTX 1mg/kg	LEU 0.1mg/kg	Serum hCG MTX	LEU	Serum hCG MTX	LEU	Serum hCG MTX	LEU	

CBC: complete blood count; LFTs: liver function tests; Cr: serum creatinine; T&S: type and screen; MTX: methotrexate; LEU: leucovorin
For all protocols: After initial decline in serum hCG level, check titers weekly until undetectable or in the multidose protocol until less than 15 mIU/ml.
[a] For otherwise healthy patients, the provider may choose not to draw pretreatment LFTs or creatinine.
[b]Continue methotrexate and leucovorin until 15% decrease in hCG levels between two consecutive titers.

contraindications to methotrexate: immunodeficiency, chronic liver disease or alcoholism, preexisting blood dyscrasias, active pulmonary disease, peptic ulcer disease, hematologic or renal dysfunction, breastfeeding, and known sensitivity to methotrexate [62].

Methotrexate is commonly used for the treatment of disorders such as arthritis and malignancies, but it was first used to treat ectopic pregnancies in the 1980s. Stovall et al [63] described the first protocol for outpatient treatment of ectopic pregnancy. In this "multidose" methotrexate protocol (Table 18.2), methotrexate is administered at a dose of 1 mg/kg intramuscularly on days 1, 3, 5, and 7. Leucovorin is given on days 2, 4, 6, and 8 at a dose of 0.1 mg/kg intramuscularly. Leucovorin is a folic acid analog that decreases the side effects resulting from multiple doses of methotrexate, such as mucositis or leukopenia. When leucovorin is used in this manner, it is called leucovorin "rescue." In this multidose protocol, up to four doses of methotrexate are given in the first week of treatment until serum hCG levels decrease by 15% on two consecutive titers. Weekly hCG levels are checked until the level declines to less than 15 mIU/ml. If hCG levels increase or plateau after the first week of treatment, then a second course of methotrexate can be administered. The multidose methotrexate protocol has a success rate of greater than 90% [63,64].

A "single-dose" methotrexate protocol (Table 18.2) was developed with the goal of enhancing patient compliance without decreasing the efficacy of the treatment. In this protocol, a single dose of methotrexate (50 mg/m^2 intramuscularly) is administered without leucovorin rescue (day 1). The patient receives a second dose of methotrexate if hCG titers do not decrease by 15% between days 4 and 7. The hCG levels are checked until they are undetectable. In this protocol, up to 20% of patients will require more than one dose of methotrexate [59]. The mean time to resolution of the ectopic pregnancy is 35 days, but it may take as long as 109 days. The success rate of the single-dose protocol ranges from 64 to 89%, making it less effective than the multidose protocol [65–67]. A meta-analysis comparing the two protocols found a 1.96 odds ratio for increased risk of tubal rupture when using the single-dose protocol. After controlling for pretreatment risk factors for treatment failure, including initial hCG level and the presence of gestational cardiac activity, the failure rate for the single-dose regimen was five times greater than that of the multidose protocol [67].

A "two-dose" methotrexate protocol (Table 18.2) has recently been developed with the goal of providing better efficacy than the single-dose protocol without increasing the complexity of the treatment or requiring more patient visits. Using this protocol, the patient receives two doses of methotrexate during the first week of treatment on days 1 and 4. An additional dose can be administered on day 7 or day 11 if hCG titers do not decrease by at least 15% between days 4 and 7. In a trial with 100 patients, the two-dose protocol was found to be safe and well tolerated [68].

When used in the protocols to treat ectopic pregnancy, methotrexate is generally well tolerated. Approximately 30% of patients treated with the single-dose protocol experienced side effects compared to 40% of those receiving the multidose protocol [67]. The most common side effects were gastrointestinal symptoms (nausea, vomiting) and stomatitis. Elevated liver transaminases usually occurred only with multidose regimens. Other side effects, such as alopecia or pneumonitis, rarely occurred in women receiving methotrexate for treatment of ectopic pregnancy.

Pretreatment blood work includes a complete blood count (CBC), liver transaminases, serum creatinine, a serum quantitative hCG level, and determination of Rh(D) antigen status. In healthy women, simplifying the required blood work to a pretreatment hemoglobin, Rh status, and a recent hCG level may be appropriate. In patients with a history of pulmonary disease, obtaining a chest x-ray is prudent due to the increased albeit small risk of interstitial pneumonitis.

Once a patient receives methotrexate, hCG levels are repeated according to the protocol being used (Fig. 18.2). Concentrations of hCG may increase between days 1 and 4 due to continuing production of hCG after methotrexate treatment. Serial ultrasound monitoring is unnecessary; the ectopic gestation may actually increase in size due to hematoma formation, and this finding is not predictive of treatment failure [69,70]. Tubal hematoma formation or tubal abortion may cause transient abdominal pain in patients undergoing methotrexate therapy. This pain usually occurs 3 to 7 days after the first dose of methotrexate, lasts 4 to 12 hours, and can often be managed conservatively [71].

A patient who requires surgery for her ectopic pregnancy after methotrexate therapy is considered a treatment failure. Abdominal pain lasting more than 12 hours or orthostatic hypotension may indicate tubal rupture, warranting surgical management. An increase or plateau of hCG levels after the first week of methotrexate therapy may also indicate treatment failure [58].

Surgical management

Surgical treatment of ectopic pregnancy is required when methotrexate is contraindicated or has failed and in cases of ruptured ectopic pregnancy or a coexisting wanted intrauterine pregnancy. Some patients choose surgical management over methotrexate therapy; benefits include treatment in one visit and fewer follow-up visits for monitoring. Although standard surgical treatment for ectopic pregnancy originally entailed laparotomy, laparoscopy has become the dominant approach in contemporary medical practice. In a study comparing laparoscopic salpingostomy to salpingostomy performed via laparotomy, the laparoscopic approach was associated with decreases in operating time, blood loss during the procedure, length of hospital stay, cost, and convalescence time [72]. No difference was found in future fertility or repeat ectopic pregnancy between the two approaches, although the rate of persistent ectopic pregnancy was greater after laparoscopy. Ultimately, the preferred approach will depend on several factors, including the surgeon's skill set and the hemodynamic stability of the patient. Laparotomy may allow for a faster entry into the abdominal cavity and better visualization in a patient with uncontrolled bleeding.

Surgical treatment of ectopic pregnancy includes salpingectomy (excision of the fallopian tube) or salpingostomy (removal of the ectopic pregnancy through an incision in the fallopian tube). Surgical management is often guided by surgeon preference, as available studies do not strongly favor one method over another. Some studies, but not all, have found a greater pregnancy rate after salpingostomy as compared to salpingectomy [15,73–77]. However, salpingostomy may carry a slightly greater risk of repeat ectopic pregnancy compared to salpingectomy [15,73]. The decision to perform a salpingostomy or salpingectomy is often made intraoperatively, and no strict criteria exist for recommending one versus the other. Expert opinion generally favors a salpingectomy in the following situations: uncontrolled bleeding, recurrent ectopic pregnancy in the same tube, ectopic gestation greater than 5 cm in size, or a damaged fallopian tube.

When performing a salpingostomy, injecting a solution of vasopressin (0.2 units/ml) into the fallopian tube at the site of the ectopic pregnancy may help to reduce blood loss. A longitudinal incision should be made using a unipolar needle on the antimesenteric border of the fallopian tube. The surgeon can then flush the products of conception from the fallopian tube using high-pressure irrigation. Any bleeding from the fallopian tube can be controlled with electrosurgical fulguration. The fallopian tube can heal by secondary intention or be sutured. One study found no significant difference in postoperative tubal patency rates, future fertility, or repeat ectopic pregnancy rates in patients who underwent salpingostomy with or without tubal suturing [73].

Persistent ectopic pregnancy occurs in 3 to 20% of patients after salpingostomy [15]. Detection of these cases requires weekly monitoring of serum hCG levels postoperatively. A plateau or rise in hCG levels signals a persistent ectopic pregnancy, which should be treated with a single dose of methotrexate. After treatment with methotrexate, hCG levels are followed until they are no longer detectable. In one study that assessed the predictive value of a postoperative day 1 serum hCG titer, the average decline in hCG level was 60%, and a drop of less than 50% was predictive of a persistent ectopic pregnancy [78]. Preoperative factors that increase the risk of persistent ectopic pregnancy include fewer than 42 days from onset of the patient's last menstrual period prior to treatment, an ectopic gestation less than 2 cm in diameter, or a rapidly increasing hCG level (greater than 40% per day) [79,80]. Administering prophylactic methotrexate at a dose of 1 mg/kg within 24 hours of surgery may decrease the risk of persistent ectopic pregnancy, but this approach remains controversial [81]. Side effects from this single dose of methotrexate are mild and occur in 5 to 8% of patients [72]. Some experts advocate prophylactic methotrexate only in certain circumstances, such as in patients at high risk for persistent ectopic pregnancy or when the surgeon is not certain of complete removal of the tubal gestation [82].

Studies comparing laparoscopic salpingostomy to multidose methotrexate therapy found no difference in treatment success rates. Patients receiving methotrexate had more side effects and a lower health-related quality of life compared to those treated surgically. Research also demonstrates similar success rates in women treated with single-dose methotrexate therapy or laparoscopic salpingostomy, although approximately 20% of medically treated patients received more than one dose of methotrexate. Rates of posttreatment tubal patency, future fertility, and repeat ectopic pregnancies did not significantly differ between the two groups [72].

Reproductive outcome

Although multiple studies have examined fertility after ectopic pregnancy, varying treatment modalities and rates of follow-up make this outcome difficult to measure. In one review, 57% of patients treated with conservative laparoscopic surgery for ectopic pregnancy had a subsequent intrauterine pregnancy, similar to 58 to 61% of patients treated with methotrexate [83]. Preexisting fallopian tube damage is likely a major factor in future reproductive success after an ectopic pregnancy. One study found that at 1 year posttreatment, 75% of women without tubal damage were pregnant compared to 55% of women with prior tubal damage [75]. Women with an ectopic pregnancy are at risk for recurrence; approximately 10% (range 5 to 28%) will have another ectopic pregnancy [75,83,84].

Rare types of ectopic pregnancy

Heterotopic pregnancy

A heterotopic pregnancy is the coexistence of an intrauterine and an ectopic gestation. In the majority of cases of heterotopic pregnancy, the ectopic gestation is found in the fallopian tube. Traditionally, heterotopic pregnancies occurred at a rate of 1 in 30,000 pregnancies but they are now more frequent, occurring in 1 of 3,900 pregnancies overall and 1.5 of 1,000 pregnancies conceived through assisted reproductive technologies [85–87]. The reassuring presence of an intrauterine pregnancy on ultrasound may delay the diagnosis of the ectopic gestation. Treatment of heterotopic pregnancies usually involves salpingectomy; methotrexate is contraindicated in a patient with a desired intrauterine pregnancy. In cases of undesired pregnancy, a possible treatment option could include uterine aspiration of the intrauterine pregnancy, followed by methotrexate treatment of the ectopic gestation in those patients meeting the criteria for medical management. Case reports describe successful treatment with local injection of potassium chloride [88–90]. In heterotopic pregnancies, the intrauterine pregnancy is more likely to end in a spontaneous or induced abortion when compared to singleton ART pregnancies. Perinatal outcomes are similar between the two groups [87].

Interstitial (cornual) pregnancy

Located at the junction of the fallopian tube and uterine cavity, interstitial (cornual) pregnancies comprise less than 3% of all ectopic gestations [1] (see Plate 18.1). Risk factors for interstitial ectopic pregnancies include a history of ipsilateral salpingectomy, previous ectopic pregnancy, and *in vitro* fertilization [91]. Interstitial ectopic pregnancies can be difficult to differentiate from intrauterine pregnancies and require an experienced ultrasonographer to make the diagnosis. Interstitial pregnancies are eccentrically located in the endometrial cavity with extremely thin surrounding myometrium, typically less than 5 mm. Their similarity to intrauterine pregnancies may delay the diagnosis. In one series, 14 of 32 interstitial pregnancies presented after rupture through the uterine wall [91]. Treatment traditionally consists of laparotomy with a corneal resection or a hysterectomy. Case reports describe treatment of these pregnancies with laparoscopic resection or a combined laparoscopic and hysteroscopic approach [92–95]. Treatment of nonruptured interstitial pregnancies with methotrexate also has been described [93,96].

Abdominal pregnancy

Abdominal pregnancies are rare types of ectopic pregnancies [1]. They occur in the peritoneal cavity and can be found on the omentum, pelvic sidewall, or abdominal organs. The etiology of abdominal ectopic pregnancies remains unclear. They may result from primary peritoneal implantation or secondary implantation of an aborted tubal pregnancy. Patients with abdominal ectopic pregnancies can present with a variety of signs and symptoms. Ultrasound is useful for initial diagnosis, but CT scan or MRI may be necessary for confirmation. Although diagnosis can occur at any gestational age, some abdominal ectopic pregnancies progress to the third trimester. Late diagnosis places patients at risk for life-threatening hemorrhage or hypovolemic shock if the placenta invades a large vessel [97].

The optimum management for abdominal ectopic pregnancy is not clear. Treatment in the first trimester usually consists of laparoscopic removal of the pregnancy [98]; methotrexate may not be efficacious [99]. Management of pregnancies that have progressed to the second and third trimesters is determined on a case-by-case basis but usually entails laparotomy. Prompt intervention is indicated due to the life-threatening risk of continuing to carry these pregnancies. A few case reports have described delivery of viable fetuses after diagnosis in the third trimester, but fetal morbidity is high [100,101]. Disposition of the placenta remains controversial; the surgeon may choose to leave it *in situ* if the placenta is attached to large blood vessels or organs. Patients with placentas left *in situ* warrant close monitoring, as they are at risk for sepsis, secondary hemorrhage, and other complications [97,102].

Ovarian pregnancy

Ovarian pregnancies account for approximately 3% of all ectopic pregnancies [1,103]. Patients may present with signs and symptoms similar to those seen in fallopian tube ectopic pregnancies, such as amenorrhea, abdominal pain, and vaginal bleeding. A large percentage of patients with ovarian pregnancies present after rupture has occurred [103]. On ultrasound examination, ovarian pregnancies can be difficult to distinguish from fallopian tube pregnancies. Intraoperatively, ovarian pregnancies are frequently mistaken for ruptured ovarian cysts or other ovarian pathologies [104], and the diagnosis is made at the time of histologic examination. Treatment of ovarian pregnancies consists of cystectomy, ovarian wedge resection, or oophorectomy, all of which may be accomplished laparoscopically [105].

Cervical pregnancy

A cervical pregnancy occurs when a fertilized oocyte implants within the endocervical canal. Cervical pregnancies account for less than 1% of ectopic pregnancies [1]. Risk factors for cervical pregnancies include prior dilation and sharp curettage (D&C), which may be reported in 50 to 68% of patients [106,107], prior cesarean delivery, or *in-vitro* fertilization treatment [106,108]. The main symptom of cervical pregnancy is painless vaginal bleeding.

Most case reports of cervical ectopic pregnancies have used ultrasound for diagnosis. Ultrasound criteria used to diagnose a cervical pregnancy include the following:

- A gestational sac in the cervix with peritrophoblastic flow (with or without an embryonic or fetal pole)
- An enlarged cervix with hourglass uterine shape
- Multiple echogenic areas within the cervix.

A closed internal cervical os or a pregnancy below the level of the uterine arteries helps to differentiate a cervical pregnancy from an isthmico-cervical pregnancy [106,109,110]. A cervical pregnancy can be mistaken for an intrauterine pregnancy implanted in the lower uterine segment or an early spontaneous abortion with the gestational sac located in the cervix. Serial ultrasound examinations are useful for diagnosis. The gestational sac in spontaneous abortions tends to change position in the cervix and become increasingly irregular. In cervical ectopic pregnancies, the gestational sac remains in the same position and retains its shape or grows larger. Moreover, gestational cardiac motion may be seen in cervical ectopic pregnancies, unlike in spontaneous abortions. MRI is another useful diagnostic modality [111]. Although more expensive and not as readily available as ultrasound, MRI may be helpful when ultrasound evaluation is indeterminate.

Historically, cervical ectopic pregnancies were diagnosed at the time of dilation and curettage, when massive hemorrhage occurred, often requiring hysterectomy. In contemporary practice, diagnosis of cervical pregnancy more commonly occurs before surgical intervention. In an attempt to preserve fertility, numerous treatment modalities have been used as adjuncts to suction curettage, including intracervical Foley catheter tamponade, uterine artery embolization, internal iliac artery ligation, cervical packing, cervical cerclage, and cervical amputation [112–114]. Case reports suggest that treatment with methotrexate, either systemically or via direct injection with or without potassium chloride, may have success rates exceeding 80% [106,112,114–117].

Cesarean section scar pregnancy

Cesarean section scar pregnancy is a rare type of ectopic gestation in which the pregnancy implants into a uterine scar from a prior cesarean section. The pregnancy is implanted in the muscle (intramural) and not connected to the endometrial cavity. Cesarean scar pregnancies occur in up to 1 in 1,800 pregnancies [118], and the incidence may be increasing due to heightened awareness by sonographers. Current data are limited to case reports, and diagnosis and treatment are not standardized. The most common symptom may be painless vaginal bleeding [118]. Ultrasound (transvaginal and Doppler) is useful in making the diagnosis. The sonographer may see a mass or gestational sac anterior to a previous cesarean section scar that appears to bulge outward toward the bladder. Abnormal vascularity in this area of the lower uterine segment may be visualized with the use of Doppler and helps differentiate a cesarean ectopic pregnancy from a spontaneous abortion.

Various treatments for cesarean scar ectopic pregnancy have been described, and include surgery via an abdominal approach or dilation and curettage, systemic or direct injection of methotrexate or direct injection of potassium chloride into the ectopic gestation, and expectant management [118–120]. In the first trimester, laparotomy or laparoscopy with local wedge resection or hysterectomy provides definitive management [119,120]. Dilation and curettage for cesarean scar pregnancy may result in excessive blood loss and the need for uterine tamponade with a Foley catheter [121]. One case series reported an approximate 70% success rate with local injection of methotrexate [121]. However, the risks with this type of management include uterine rupture or significant hemorrhage. Because the risk of hemorrhage or uterine rupture with expectant management of a cesarean scar pregnancy appears to be high, this approach is not recommended [118,121]. A second-trimester cesarean scar pregnancy requires surgical management. One small series reported a 5% risk of recurrent cesarean scar pregnancy in future pregnancies [122]. Viable full-term gestations following cesarean scar pregnancies have been reported [122].

Conclusion

Despite advances in diagnosis and management, ectopic pregnancy remains an important public health problem worldwide. In the USA, ectopic pregnancy is still the leading cause of maternal death in the first trimester. Ectopic pregnancies occur most frequently in the fallopian tube. Abortion providers can play an important role in decreasing morbidity from ectopic pregnancy by remaining vigilant for the diagnosis. Algorithms using ultrasonography and serum hCG assays facilitate early diagnosis. Many unruptured tubal pregnancies can be treated medically using methotrexate regimens.

References

1 Bouyer J, Coste J, Fernandez H, Pouly JL, Job-Spira N. Sites of ectopic pregnancy: a 10 year population-based study of 1800 cases. *Hum Reprod* 2002; **17**: 3224–3230.

2 Centers for Disease Control and Prevention. Ectopic pregnancy—United States, 1990–1992. *JAMA* 1995; **273**: 533.

3 Hakim-Elahi E, Tovell HM, Burnhill MS. Complications of first-trimester abortion: a report of 170,000 cases. *Obstet Gynecol* 1990; **76**: 129–135.

4 Edwards J, Carson SA. New technologies permit safe abortion at less than six weeks' gestation and provide timely detection of ectopic gestation. *Am J Obstet Gynecol* 1997; **176**: 1101–1106.

5 Chang J, Elam-Evans LD, Berg CJ et al. Pregnancy-related mortality surveillance—United States, 1991–1999. *MMWR Surveill Summ* 2003; **52**: 1–8.

6 Grimes DA. Estimation of pregnancy-related mortality risk by pregnancy outcome, United States, 1991 to 1999. *Am J Obstet Gynecol* 2006; **194**: 92–94.

7 Washington AE, Katz P. Ectopic pregnancy in the United States: economic consequences and payment source trends. *Obstet Gynecol* 1993; **81**: 287–292.

8 Khan KS, Wojdyla D, Say L, Gulmezoglu AM, Van Look PF. WHO analysis of causes of maternal death: a systematic review. *Lancet* 2006; **367**: 1066–1074.

9 Gamble SB, Strauss LT, Parker WY, Cook DA, Zane SB, Hamdan S. Abortion surveillance—United States, 2005. *MMWR Surveill Summ* 2008; **57**: SS–13.

10 Senterman M, Jibodh R, Tulandi T. Histopathologic study of ampullary and isthmic tubal ectopic pregnancy. *Am J Obstet Gynecol* 1988; **159**: 939–941.

11 Attar E. Endocrinology of ectopic pregnancy. *Obstet Gynecol Clin North Am* 2004; **34**: 779–794.

12 Goddijn M, van der Veen F, Schuring-Blom GH, Ankum WM, Leschot NJ. Cytogenetic characteristics of ectopic pregnancy. *Hum Reprod* 1996; **11**: 2769–2771.

13 Coste J, Fernandez H, Joyé N et al. Role of chromosome abnormalities in ectopic pregnancy. *Fertil Steril* 2000; **74**: 1259–1260.

14 Barnhart KT, Sammel MD, Gracia CR, Chittams J, Hummel AC, Shaunik A. Risk factors for ectopic pregnancy in women with symptomatic first-trimester pregnancies. *Fertil Steril* 2006; **86**: 36–43.

15 Yao M, Tulandi T. Current status of surgical and nonsurgical management of ectopic pregnancy. *Fertil Steril* 1997; **67**: 421–433.

16 Seeber B, Barnhart KT. In: Gibbs RS, Karlan BY, Haney AF, Nygaard IE, eds. *Danforth's Obstetrics and Gynecology*, 10th edn. Philadelphia: Lippincott, Williams & Wilkins, 2006.

17 Ankum WM, Mol BW, van der Veen F, Bossuyt PM. Risk factors for ectopic pregnancy: a meta-analysis. *Fertil Steril* 1996; **65**: 1093–1099.

18 Bouyer J, Coste J, Shojaei T et al. Risk factors for ectopic pregnancy: a comprehensive analysis based on a large case-control, population-based study in France. *Am J Epidemiol* 2003; **157**: 185–194.

19 Kutluay L, Vicdan K, Turan C, Batiolu S, Ouz S, Gökmen O. Tubal histopathology in ectopic pregnancies. *Eur J Obstet Gynecol Reprod Biol* 1994; **57**: 91–94.

20 Hillis SD, Owens LM, Marchbanks PA, Amsterdam LF, Mac Kenzie WR. Recurrent chlamydial infections increase the risks of hospitalization for ectopic pregnancy and pelvic inflammatory disease. *Am J Obstet Gynecol* 1997; **176**: 103–107.

21 DeCherney AH, Cholst I, Naftolin F. Structure and function of the fallopian tubes following exposure to diethylstilbestrol (DES) during gestation. *Fertil Steril* 1981; **36**: 741–745.

22 Goldberg JM, Falcone T. Effect of diethylstilbestrol on reproductive function. *Fertil Steril* 1999; **72**: 1–7.

23 Mol BW, Ankum WM, Bossuyt PM, van der Veen F. Contraception and the risk of ectopic pregnancy: a meta-analysis. *Contraception* 1995; **52**: 337–341.

24 Furlong LA. Ectopic pregnancy risk when contraception fails: a review. *J Reprod Med* 2002; **47**: 881–885.

25 Peterson HB, Xia Z, Hughes JM, Wilcox LS, Tylor LR, Trussell J. The risk of ectopic pregnancy after tubal sterilization. *N Engl J Med* 1997; **336**: 762–767.

26 Strandell A, Thorburn J, Hamberger L. Risk factors for ectopic pregnancy in assisted reproduction. *Fertil Steril* 1999; **71**: 282–286.

27 Barmat LI, Rauch E, Spandorfer S et al. The effect of hydrosalpinges on IVF-ET outcome. *J Assist Reprod Genet* 1999; **16**: 350–354.

28 Cohen MA, Lindheim SR, Sauer MV. Hydrosalpinges adversely affect implantation in donor oocyte cycles. *Hum Reprod* 1999; **14**: 1087–1089.

29 McBain JC, Evans JH, Pepperdell RJ, Robinson HP, Smith MA, Brown JP. An unexpectedly high rate of ectopic pregnancy following the induction of ovulation with human pituitary and chorionic gonadotrophin. *Br J Obstet Gynaecol* 1980; **87**: 5–9.

30 Gemzell C, Guillome J, Wang CF. Ectopic pregnancy following treatment with human gonadotropins. *Am J Obstet Gynecol* 1982; **143**: 761–765.

31 Cohen J, Mayaux MJ, Guihard-Moscato ML, Schwartz D. In-vitro fertilization and embryo transfer: a collaborative study of 1163 pregnancies on the incidence and risk factors of ectopic pregnancies. *Hum Reprod* 1986; **1**: 255–258.

32 Nazari A, Askari HA, Check JH, O'Shaughnessy A. Embryo transfer technique as a cause of ectopic pregnancy in in vitro fertilization. *Fertil Steril* 1993; **60**: 919–921.

33 Saraiya M, Berg CJ, Kendrick JS, Strauss LT, Atrash HK, Ahn YW. Cigarette smoking as a risk factor for ectopic pregnancy. *Am J Obstet Gynecol* 1998; **178**: 493–498.

34 Barnhart KT, Rinaudo P, Hummel A, Pena J, Sammel MD, Chittams J. Acute and chronic presentation of ectopic pregnancy may be two clinical entities. *Fertil Steril* 2003; **80**: 1345–1351.

35 Dart RG, Kaplan B, Varaklis K. Predictive value of history and physical examination in patients with suspected ectopic pregnancy. *Ann Emerg Med* 1999; **33**: 283–290.

36 Della-Giustina D, Denny M. Ectopic pregnancy. *Emerg Med Clin North Am* 2003; **21**: 565–584.

37 Seeber BE, Barnhart KT. Suspected ectopic pregnancy. *Obstet Gynecol* 2006; **107**: 399–413.

38 Laing F, Frates MC. Ultrasound evaluation during the first trimester of pregnancy. In: Callen PW, ed. *Ultrasonography in Obstetrics and Gynecology*, 4th edn. Philadelphia: WB Saunders, 2000.

39 Thoen LD, Creinin MD. Medical treatment of ectopic pregnancy with methotrexate. *Fertil Steril* 1997; **68**: 727–730.

40 Condous G, Okaro E, Khalid A et al. The accuracy of transvaginal ultrasonography for the diagnosis of ectopic pregnancy prior to surgery. *Hum Reprod* 2005; **20**: 1404–1409.

41 Barnhart KT, Katz I, Hummel A, Gracia CR. Presumed diagnosis of ectopic pregnancy. *Obstet Gynecol* 2002; **100**: 505–510.

42 Brown DL, Doubilet PM. Transvaginal sonography for diagnosing ectopic pregnancy: positivity criteria and performance characteristics. *J Ultrasound Med* 1994; **13**: 259–266.

43 Shalev E, Yarom I, Bustan M, Weiner E, Ben-Shlomo I. Transvaginal sonography as the ultimate diagnostic tool for the management of ectopic pregnancy: experience with 840 cases. *Fertil Steril* 1998; **69**: 62–65.

44 Walters MD, Eddy C, Pauerstein CJ. The contralateral corpus luteum and tubal pregnancy. *Obstet Gynecol* 1987; **70**: 823–826.

45 Jurkovic D, Bourne TM, Janiaux E, Campbell S, Collins WP. Transvaginal color Doppler study of blood flow in ectopic pregnancies. *Fertil Steril* 1992; **57**: 68–73.

46 Wilcox AJ, Baird DD, Weinberg CR. Time of implantation of the conceptus and loss of pregnancy. *N Engl J Med* 1999; **340**: 1796–1799.

47 Barnhart KT, Sammel MD, Rinaudo PF, Zhou L, Hummel AC, Guo W. Symptomatic patients with an early viable intrauterine pregnancy: HCG curves redefined. *Obstet Gynecol* 2004; **104**: 50–55.

48 Seeber BE, Sammel MD, Guo W, Zhou L, Hummel A, Barnhart KT. Application of redefined human chorionic gonadotropin curves for the diagnosis of women at risk for ectopic pregnancy. *Fertil Steril* 2006; **86**: 454–459.

49 Silva C, Sammel MD, Zhou L, Gracia C, Hummel AC, Barnhart K. Human chorionic gonadotropin profile for women with ectopic pregnancy. *Obstet Gynecol* 2006; **107**: 605–610.

50 Creinin MD. Change in serum beta-human chorionic gonadotropin after abortion with methotrexate and misoprostol. *Am J Obstet Gynecol* 1996; **174**: 776–778.

51 Barnhart KT, Bader T, Huang X, Frederick MM, Timbers KA, Zhang JJ. Hormone pattern after misoprostol administration for a nonviable first-trimester gestation. *Fertil Steril* 2004; **81**: 1099–1105.

52 Ailawadi M, Lorch SA, Barnhart KT. Cost-effectiveness of presumptively medically treating women at risk for ectopic pregnancy compared with first performing a dilatation and curettage. *Fertil Steril* 2005; **83**: 376–382.

53 McCord ML, Muram D, Buster JE, Arheart KL, Stovall TG, Carson SA. Single serum progesterone as a screen for ectopic pregnancy: exchanging specificity and sensitivity to obtain optimal test performance. *Fertil Steril* 1996; **66**: 513–516.

54 Mol BW, Lijmer JG, Ankum WM, van der Veen F, Bossuyt PM. The accuracy of single serum progesterone measurement in the diagnosis of ectopic pregnancy: a meta-analysis. *Hum Reprod* 1998; **13**: 3220–3227.

55 Stovall TG, Kellerman AL, Ling FW, Buster JE. Emergency department diagnosis of ectopic pregnancy. *Ann Emerg Med* 1990; **19**: 1098–1103.

56 Mol BW, Hajenius PJ, Ankum WM, Bossuyt PM, van der Veen F. Screening for ectopic pregnancy in symptom-free women at increased risk. *Obstet Gynecol* 1997; **89**: 704–707.

57 Mol BW, van der Veen F, Bossuyt PM. Symptom-free women at increased risk of ectopic pregnancy: should we screen? *Acta Obstet Gynecol Scand* 2002; **81**: 661–672.

58 American College of Obstetricians and Gynecologists. ACOG practice bulletin. Medical management of tubal pregnancy. No. 3, December 1998. Clinical management guidelines for obstetrician-gynecologists. *Int J Gynaecol Obstet* 1999; **65**: 97–103.

59 Lipscomb GH, Bran D, McCord ML, Portera JC, Ling FW. Analysis of three hundred fifteen ectopic pregnancies treated with single-dose methotrexate. *Am J Obstet Gynecol* 1998; **178**: 1354–1358.

60 Lipscomb GH, McCord ML, Stovall TG, Huff G, Portera SG, Ling FW. Predictors of success of methotrexate treatment in women with tubal ectopic pregnancies. *N Engl J Med* 1999; **341**: 1974–1978.

61 Menon S, Colins J, Barnhart KT. Establishing a human chorionic gonadotropin cutoff to guide methotrexate treatment of ectopic pregnancy: a systematic review. *Fertil Steril* 2007; **87**: 481–484.

62 American College of Obstetricians and Gynecologists. ACOG Practice Bulletin No. 94. Medical management of ectopic pregnancy. *Obstet Gynecol* 2008; **111**: 1479–1485.

63 Stovall TG, Ling FW, Buster JE. Outpatient chemotherapy of unruptured ectopic pregnancy. *Fertil Steril* 1989; **51**: 435–438.

64 Stovall TG, Ling FW, Gray LA, Carson SA, Buster JE. Methotrexate treatment of unruptured ectopic pregnancy: a report of 100 cases. *Obstet Gynecol* 1991; **77**: 749–753.

65 Stika CS, Anderson L, Frederiksen MC. Single-dose methotrexate for the treatment of ectopic pregnancy: Northwestern Memorial Hospital three-year experience. *Am J Obstet Gynecol* 1996; **174**: 1840–1846.

66 Lipscomb GH, Stovall TG, Ling FW. Nonsurgical treatment of ectopic pregnancy. *N Engl J Med* 2000; **343**: 1325–1329.

67 Barnhart KT, Gosman G, Ashby R, Sammel M. The medical management of ectopic pregnancy: a meta-analysis comparing "single dose" and "multidose" regimens. *Obstet Gynecol* 2003; **101**: 778–784.

68 Barnhart K, Hummel AC, Sammel MD, Menon S, Jain J, Chakhtoura N. Use of "2-dose" regimen of methotrexate to treat ectopic pregnancy. *Fertil Steril* 2007; **87**: 250–256.

69 Brown DL, Felker RE, Stovall TG, Emerson DS, Ling FW. Serial endovaginal sonography of ectopic pregnancies treated with methotrexate. *Obstet Gynecol* 1991; **77**: 406–409.

70 Atri M, Bret PM, Tulandi T, Senterman MK. Ectopic pregnancy: evolution after treatment with transvaginal methotrexate. *Radiology* 1992; **185**: 749–753.

71 Lipscomb GH, Puckett KJ, Bran D, Ling FW. Management of separation pain after single-dose methotrexate therapy for ectopic pregnancy. *Obstet Gynecol* 1999; **93**: 590–593.

72 Hajenius P, Mol JF, Mol BW, Bossuyt PM, Ankum WM, van der Veen F. Interventions for tubal ectopic pregnancy. *Cochrane Database Syst Rev* 2007; **1**: CD000324.

73 Tulandi T, Guralnick M. Treatment of tubal ectopic pregnancy by salpingotomy with or without tubal suturing and salpingectomy. *Fertil Steril* 1991; **55**: 53–55.

74 Silva PD, Schaper AM, Rooney B. Reproductive outcome after 143 laparoscopic procedures for ectopic pregnancy. *Obstet Gynecol* 1993; **81**: 710–715.

75 Job-Spira N, Bouyer J, Pouly JL et al. Fertility after ectopic pregnancy: first results of a population-based cohort study in France. *Hum Reprod* 1996; **11**: 99–104.

76 Mol BW, Matthijsse HC, Tinga DJ et al. Fertility after conservative and radical surgery for tubal pregnancy. *Hum Reprod* 1998; **13**: 1804–1809.

77 Bangsgaard N, Lund CO, Ottesen B, Nilas L. Improved fertility following conservative surgical treatment of ectopic pregnancy. *BJOG* 2003; **110**: 765–770.

78 Spandorfer SD, Sawin SW, Benjamin I, Barnhart KT. Postoperative day 1 serum human chorionic gonadotropin level as a predictor of persistent ectopic pregnancy after conservative surgical management. *Fertil Steril* 1997; **68**: 430–434.

79 Seifer DB, Gutmann JN, Doyle MB, Jones EE, Diamond MP, DeCherney AH. Persistent ectopic pregnancy following laparoscopic linear salpingostomy. *Obstet Gynecol* 1990; **76**: 1121–1125.

80 Kemmann E, Trout S, Garcia A. Can we predict patients at risk for persistent ectopic pregnancy after laparoscopic salpingotomy? *J Am Assoc Gynecol Laparosc* 1994; **1**: 122–126.

81 Graczykowski JW, Mishell DR Jr. Methotrexate prophylaxis for persistent ectopic pregnancy after conservative treatment by salpingostomy. *Obstet Gynecol* 1997; **89**: 118–122.

82 Gracia CR, Brown HA, Barnhart KT. Prophylactic methotrexate after linear salpingostomy: a decision analysis. *Fertil Steril* 2001; **76**: 1191–1195.

83 Pisarska MD, Carson SA, Buster JE. Ectopic pregnancy. *Lancet* 1998; **351**: 1115–1120.

84 Bernoux A, Job-Spira N, Germain E, Coste J, Bouyer J. Fertility outcome after ectopic pregnancy and use of an intrauterine device at the time of the index ectopic pregnancy. *Hum Reprod* 2000; **15**: 1173–1177.

85 Reece EA, Petrie RH, Sirmans MF, Finster M, Todd WD. Combined intrauterine and extrauterine gestations: a review. *Am J Obstet Gynecol* 1983; **146**: 323–330.

86 Tal J, Haddad S, Gordon N, Timor-Tritsch I. Heterotopic pregnancy after ovulation induction and assisted reproductive technologies: a literature review from 1971 to 1993. *Fertil Steril* 1996; **66**: 1–12.

87 Clayton HB, Schieve LA, Peterson HB, Jamieson DJ, Reynolds MA, Wright VC. A comparison of heterotopic and intrauterine-only pregnancy outcomes after assisted reproductive technologies in the United States from 1999 to 2002. *Fertil Steril* 2007; **87**: 303–309.

88 Fernandez H, Lelaidier C, Doumerc S, Fournet P, Olivennes F, Frydman R. Nonsurgical treatment of heterotopic pregnancy: a report of six cases. *Fertil Steril* 1993; **60**: 428–432.

89 Doubilet PM, Benson CB, Frates MC, Ginsburg E. Sonographically guided minimally invasive treatment of unusual ectopic pregnancies. *J Ultrasound Med* 2004; **23**: 359–370.

90 Goldstein JS, Ratts VS, Philpott T, Dahan MH. Risk of surgery after use of potassium chloride for treatment of tubal heterotopic pregnancy. *Obstet Gynecol* 2006; **107**: 506–508.

91 Tulandi T, Al-Jaroudi D. Interstitial pregnancy: results generated from the Society of Reproductive Surgeons Registry. *Obstet Gynecol* 2004; **103**: 47–50.

92 Meyer WR, Mitchell DE. Hysteroscopic removal of an interstitial ectopic gestation: a case report. *J Reprod Med* 1989; **34**: 928–929.

93 Lau S, Tulandi T. Conservative medical and surgical management of interstitial ectopic pregnancy. *Fertil Steril* 1999; **72**: 207–215.

94 Moon HS, Choi YJ, Park YH, Kim SG. New simple endoscopic operations for interstitial pregnancies. *Am J Obstet Gynecol* 2000; **182**: 114–121.

95 Katz DL, Barrett JP, Sanfilippo JS, Badway DM. Combined hysteroscopy and laparoscopy in the treatment of interstitial pregnancy. *Am J Obstet Gynecol* 2003; **188**: 1113–1114.

96 Fisch JD, Ortiz BH, Tazuke SI, Chitkara U, Giudice LC. Medical management of interstitial ectopic pregnancy: a case report and literature review. *Hum Reprod* 1998; **13**: 1981–1986.

97 Rahman MS, Al-Suleiman SA, Rahman J, Al-Sibai MH. Advanced abdominal pregnancy: observations in 10 cases. *Obstet Gynecol* 1982; **59**: 366–372.

98 Tsudo T, Harada T, Yoshioka H, Terakawa N. Laparoscopic management of early primary abdominal pregnancy. *Obstet Gynecol* 1997; **90**: 687–688.

99 Zinger M, Rosenfeld D. Failed treatment of abdominal pregnancy with methotrexate: a case report. *J Reprod Med* 2001; **46**: 392–394.

100 Ludwig M, Kaisi M, Bauer O, Diedrich K. The forgotten child: a case of heterotopic, intra-abdominal and intrauterine pregnancy carried to term. *Hum Reprod* 1999; **14**: 1372–1374.

101 Rahaman J, Berkowitz R, Mitty H, Gaddipati S, Brown B, Nezhat F. Minimally invasive management of an advanced abdominal pregnancy. *Obstet Gynecol* 2004; **103**: 1064–1068.

102 Attapattu JA, Menon S. Abdominal pregnancy. *Int J Gynaecol Obstet* 1993; **43**: 51–55.

103 Grimes HG, Nosal RA, Gallagher JC. Ovarian pregnancy: a series of 24 cases. *Obstet Gynecol* 1983; **61**: 174–180.

104 Hallatt JG. Primary ovarian pregnancy: a report of twenty-five cases. *Am J Obstet Gynecol* 1982; **143**: 55–60.

105 Hage PS, Arnouk IF, Zarou DM, Kim BH, Wehbeh HA. Laparoscopic management of ovarian ectopic pregnancy. *J Am Assoc Gynecol Laparosc* 1994; **1**: 283–285.

106 Ushakov FB, Elchalal U, Aceman PJ, Schenker JG. Cervical pregnancy: past and future. *Obstet Gynecol Surv* 1997; **52**: 45–59.

107 Vela G, Tulandi T. Cervical pregnancy: the importance of early diagnosis and treatment. *J Minim Invasive Gynecol* 2007; **14**: 481–484.

108 Karande VC, Flood JT, Heard N, Veeck L, Muasher SJ. Analysis of ectopic pregnancies resulting from in-vitro fertilization and embryo transfer. *Hum Reprod* 1991; **6**: 446–449.

109 Oyer R, Tarakjian D, Lev-Toaff A, Friedman A, Chatwani A. Treatment of cervical pregnancy with methotrexate. *Obstet Gynecol* 1988; **71**: 469–471.

110 Gun M, Mavrogiorgis M. Cervical ectopic pregnancy: a case report and literature review. *Ultrasound Obstet Gynecol* 2002; **19**: 297–301.

111 Jung SE, Byun JY, Lee JM, Choi BG, Hahn ST. Characteristic MR findings of cervical pregnancy. *J Magn Reson Imaging* 2001; **13**: 918–922.

112 Creinin MD, Feldstein VA. Conservative management options for cervical pregnancy: case reports and literature review. *Int J Fertil Menop Stud* 1995; **40**: 175–186.

113 Su TH, Wang YD, Chen CP, Lei SY. A conservative surgical treatment of cervical pregnancy with active bleeding: uterine artery ligation and cervicotomy. *Int J Gynaecol Obstet* 1992; **37**: 275–279.

114 Cosin JA, Bean M, Grow D, Wiczyk H. The use of methotrexate and arterial embolization to avoid surgery in a case of cervical pregnancy. *Fertil Steril* 1997; **67**: 1169–1171.

115 Kaplan BR, Brandt T, Javaheri G, Scommegna A. Nonsurgical treatment of a viable cervical pregnancy with intra-amniotic methotrexate. *Fertil Steril* 1990; **53**: 941–943.

116 Timor-Tritsch IE, Monteagudo A, Mandeville EO, Peisner DB, Anaya GP, Pirrone EC. Successful management of viable cervical pregnancy by local injection of methotrexate guided by transvaginal ultrasonography. *Am J Obstet Gynecol* 1994; **170**: 737–739.

117 Kung FT, Chang SY. Efficacy of methotrexate treatment in viable and nonviable cervical pregnancies. *Am J Obstet Gynecol* 1999; **181**: 1438–1444.

118 Rotas MA, Haberman S, Levgur M. Cesarean scar ectopic pregnancies: etiology, diagnosis, and management. *Obstet Gynecol* 2006; **107**: 1373–1381.

119 Valley MT, Pierce JG, Daniel TB, Kaunitz AM. Cesarean scar pregnancy: imaging and treatment with conservative surgery. *Obstet Gynecol* 1998; **91**: 838–840.

120 Lee CL, Wang CJ, Chao A, Yen CF, Soong YK. Laparoscopic management of an ectopic pregnancy in a previous Caesarean section scar. *Hum Reprod* 1999; **14**: 1234–1236.

121 Jurkovic D, Hillaby K, Woelfer B, Lawrence A, Salim R, Elson CJ. First-trimester diagnosis and management of pregnancies implanted into the lower uterine segment Cesarean section scar. *Ultrasound Obstet Gynecol* 2003; **21**: 220–227.

122 Ben Nagi J, Helmy S, Ofili-Yebovi D, Yazbek J, Sawyer E, Jurkovic D. Reproductive outcomes of women with a previous history of Caesarean scar ectopic pregnancies. *Hum Reprod* 2007; **22**: 2012–2015.

19

CHAPTER 19

Gestational trophoblastic disease

Neil J. Sebire MD and Michael J. Seckl MD, PhD

LEARNING POINTS

- Contemporary hydatidiform moles most commonly present as early pregnancy failure.
- Following a diagnosis of hydatidiform mole, patients require hCG follow-up to detect persistent trophoblastic neoplasia, which follows about 15% of complete hydatidiform moles and about 0.5% of partial hydatidiform moles.
- Most cases of persistent trophoblastic neoplasia can be treated successfully with relatively nontoxic chemotherapeutic regimens.
- Abnormal vaginal bleeding or other unusual symptoms following any type of pregnancy should raise suspicion for possible trophoblastic disease.

Introduction

Gestational trophoblastic disease refers to a range of defined entities including complete and partial hydatidiform mole, invasive mole, and the malignant tumors choriocarcinoma, placental site trophoblastic tumor, and its variants. In the context of abortion care, chief concerns are the reliable detection of hydatidiform mole and prevention of morbidity through identification of persistent gestational trophoblastic neoplasia (pGTN) [1]. Diagnosis of pGTN typically requires human chorionic gonadotropin (hCG) surveillance following uterine evacuation of hydatidiform moles; rising or plateauing hCG levels signal pGTN that may require chemotherapy. The aim of this chapter is not to review all aspects of gestational trophoblastic disease but rather to focus on early diagnosis of hydatidiform mole (HM) and its subsequent management, including screening after induced abortion or medical management of early pregnancy failure. Complications of GTN are best managed in specialist tertiary referral centers.

Epidemiology of hydatidiform mole

In the USA and Western Europe, hydatidiform mole occurs in approximately 1 in 500 to 1 in 1,200 pregnancies [2]. The incidence of both complete (CHM) and partial (PHM) hydatidiform mole varies by ethnicity, being greater in women of Asian origin. Incidence is also strongly associated with extremes of maternal age, with a small peak in relative risk in the early teens and a much larger peak occurring among women in their late forties [3]. All hydatidiform moles carry a risk of developing pGTN, which occurs following about 15% of CHM and 0.5% of PHM [4].

Management of Unintended and Abnormal Pregnancy, 1st edition. By M Paul, ES Lichtenberg, L Borgatta, DA Grimes, PG Stubblefield, MD Creinin
© 2009 Blackwell Publishing, ISBN: 9781405176965.

Genetics of hydatidiform moles

Hydatidiform moles represent a phenotype of abnormal placental development due to overexpression of paternally derived genes, and they are therefore abnormalities of imprinting. Complete and partial hydatidiform moles are genetically distinct. Complete moles are almost always diploid, with the genetic material exclusively of paternal origin. They derive from fertilization of an anucleate oocyte, either by a haploid sperm that undergoes duplication inside the oocyte or, more rarely, by two sperm. Partial moles are almost exclusively triploid, with one maternal and two paternal contributions to the genome. They usually arise from dispermic fertilization of an apparently normal oocyte (Fig. 19.1).

Presentation of moles and their early identification

According to classical dogma, PHM is associated with the presence of a fetus and coexistent patchy hydatidiform change of the placenta, whereas CHM lacks significant fetal development and demonstrates diffuse placental hydropic change. However, modern understanding of these pathologies negates such a simple distinction. Indeed, some cases of CHM show histologic evidence of early fetal-type

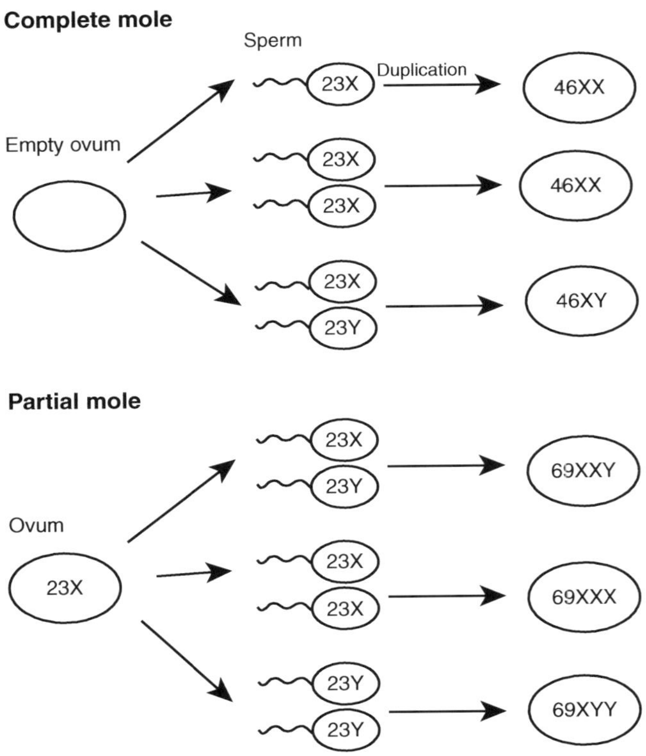

Figure 19.1 Cytogenetic origin of hydatidiform moles. Most complete moles are diploid (46 chromosomes) and androgenetic (i.e., the genetic material is exclusively of paternal origin). They arise from fertilization of an "empty" oocyte by either a haploid sperm that undergoes duplication or, rarely, by two haploid sperm. Partial moles are almost always triploid (69 chromosomes), and contain both maternal and paternal genetic contributions. Partial moles arise from fertilization of an apparently normal haploid ovum by two haploid sperm. (Reprinted with permission from Altieri A, Franceschi S, Ferlay J, Smith J, La Vecchia C. Epidemiology and aetiology of gestational trophoblastic diseases. Lancet Oncol 2003; 4:670–678.)

development [5], whereas most women with PHM present as early pregnancy failure without a clinically or sonographically identifiable fetus [6]. The changing clinical, sonographic, and histopathologic descriptions of these conditions require revised and updated criteria for their identification and diagnosis.

Pathology of hydatidiform moles

Molecular genetic analysis is the gold standard for the definitive diagnosis and subtyping of hydatidiform mole, although histopathologic examination remains the most common method of diagnosis for practical purposes. The diagnostic pathologic feature of molar pregnancy is abnormal proliferation of villus trophoblast. However, complete moles and partial moles each have distinctive histologic characteristics, even in the first trimester [7–9].

Classic second-trimester complete moles exhibit marked villus hydrops with extensive circumferential villus trophoblast hyperplasia and central "cistern" formation. However, most contemporary moles are evacuated in the first trimester when these features are not developed. The histopathologic diagnostic features at this early stage include a characteristic abnormal "budding" villus architecture with abnormally distributed villus trophoblast hyperplasia, a relative lack of villus hydrops, sheets of pleomorphic extravillus trophoblast, collapsed villus blood vessels, and marked stromal karyorrhectic debris, as well as abnormal extravillus trophoblastic invasion [8,9]. In addition, tests based on genetic characteristics of the HM subtypes may assist in the diagnosis of early CHM. The imprinted gene $p57^{KIP2}$ shows high levels of expression in cells with maternal nuclear DNA content, but it is repressed in cells that contain only paternal DNA. Therefore, normal placenta and PHM show nuclear positivity on immunostaining of villi with antibody to $p57^{KIP2}$, whereas androgenetic CHM does not [10,11].

Classic second-trimester partial moles exhibit a dual population of normal-sized and hydropic villi with focal trophoblast hyperplasia. In the first trimester, the changes are usually patchy and mild with limited villus hydrops and cistern formation, numerous vessels containing nucleated fetal red cells, patchy vascular "pseudoangiomatoid" change, abnormally shaped "scalloped" or "dentate" villi, and the presence of trophoblastic pseudoinclusions and villus stromal fibrosis. Trophoblast hyperplasia is patchy and in an abnormal distribution, often with a vacuolated appearance (Fig. 19.2).

In some cases, a definite diagnosis of early PHM may not be possible without the use of ancillary techniques such as assessment of ploidy using *in situ* hybridization or flow cytometry [12] or microsatellite polymorphism analysis (not available in routine practice) [13]. This requirement is especially true when limited material is submitted for examination. Furthermore, conceptions affected by other aneuploidies may appear histologically similar to PHM, although they lack the abnormal trophoblast hyperplasia of hydatidiform mole.

Changes in the clinical presentation of hydatidiform mole

In traditional obstetric and gynecologic teaching, patients with CHM presented with vaginal bleeding or passage of vesicles per vagina, uterine enlargement greater than expected for gestational age, and abnormally high levels of serum hCG. Potential medical complications included preeclampsia, hyperthyroidism, hyperemesis, anemia, or massive ovarian theca-lutein cysts [14].

However, with the increasing use of ultrasonography to assess uncomplicated pregnancies and those that present with vaginal bleeding, this classical presentation occurs rarely [15]. Most contemporary moles are evacuated before 12 weeks' gestation (around 10 weeks in the UK) [16,17]. This change in management has decreased dramatically the number of molar pregnancies presenting with the symptoms

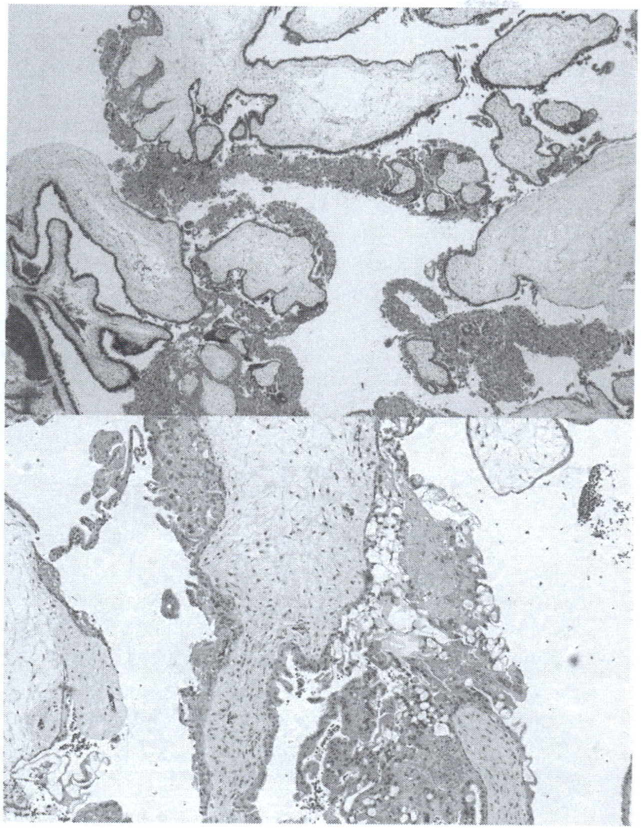

Figure 19.2 Photomicrographs of complete hydatidiform mole (top) and partial hydatidiform mole (bottom) demonstrating histopathologic features of abnormal budding architecture, cellular stroma with debris and abnormal trophoblast hyperplasia (complete mole), and abnormal irregularly shaped villi with trophoblastic pseudoinclusions and abnormal trophoblast proliferation (partial mole). H&E, original magnifications × 20.

and signs induced by overgrowth of trophoblast and excessive hCG secretion. In one study of women with confirmed CHM, 40% were entirely asymptomatic with the condition detected by routine sonography, whereas the remaining 60% presented with vaginal bleeding; only 2% reported symptoms such as hyperemesis, and no women reported any other systemic manifestations [18].

The role of ultrasonography in the diagnosis of hydatidiform mole

Although now seldom seen, the characteristic sonographic findings of second-trimester hydatidiform mole include a uterine cavity filled with a central heterogeneous mass with anechoic spaces of varying sizes and shapes (e.g., a "snowstorm" appearance) without associated fetal development (Chapter 6) [19]. In addition, theca-lutein ovarian cysts can occur secondary to high hCG levels, producing either a "soap bubble" or "spoke wheel" appearance of the enlarged ovaries. In the first trimester, hydatidiform changes on ultrasound examination are less readily apparent (Fig. 19.3).

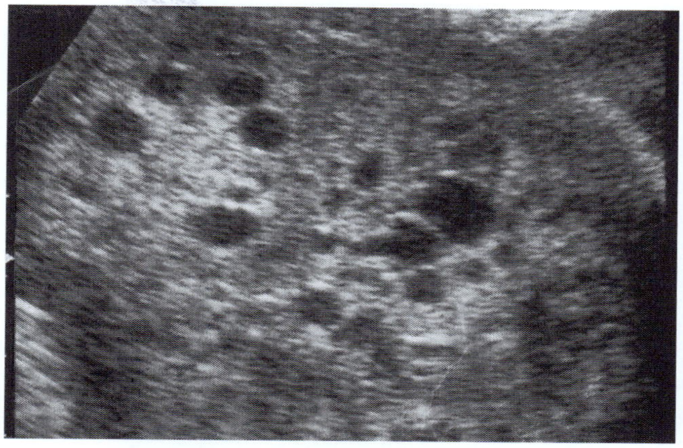

Figure 19.3 Early partial hydatidiform mole most commonly appears as an anembryonic pregnancy on ultrasonography. Occasionally, it manifests as multiple cystic spaces in the placenta, as shown in this ultrasound image.

Multiple studies have examined the ability of ultrasound to detect hydatidiform mole in early pregnancy, with initial reports suggesting detection rates of up to 80% for CHM. When PHM or CHM was not suspected prior to pathologic examination, the most common initial sonographic diagnosis was anembryonic pregnancy [20–24]. These early reports were based on small series from specialist centers.

Two recent larger studies found that in routine practice, preevacuation ultrasonography performed during the first or early second trimester correctly identified only 40 to 60% of molar pregnancies [16,25]. The largest study reviewed the preevacuation ultrasound findings in more than 1,000 consecutive patients referred to a UK regional trophoblastic disease unit for histologic review of possible or probable hydatidiform mole [16]. All cases of gestational trophoblastic disease suspected clinically, sonographically, or on the basis of histopathologic findings are registered at the center, allowing for the greatest possible ascertainment. The median gestational age at evacuation was 10 weeks (range 5 to 27 weeks). The final diagnosis was hydatidiform mole in 859 (82%) cases, including 253 (29%) CHM and 606 (71%) PHM.

Overall, only 40% of women with confirmed hydatidiform mole had a preevacuation ultrasound diagnosis suggesting molar pregnancy, including about 80% of CHM and 30% of PHM; the remaining cases appeared sonographically as anembryonic pregnancies. A nonsignificant trend occurred toward increasing ultrasound detection rate with advancing gestational age; sonographic features of hydatidiform mole were reported in 35% of cases before 14 weeks' gestation, compared to approximately 60% after this time. Of note, more than 10% of the cases identified as molar on ultrasound examination were in fact nonmolar hydropic abortions on histologic review. Based on this study, the sensitivity, specificity, and positive and negative predictive values for routine preevacuation ultrasound examination for hydatidiform mole are 44, 74, 88, and 23%, respectively. Because a proportion of early moles are simply not yet hydropic enough to be evident on ultrasound examination, current techniques will likely never result in 100% detection rates [9,26].

Occasionally, routine ultrasound examination demonstrates the presence of a morphologically normal fetus in association with apparent "molar" change of the placenta. These findings may represent a pregnancy with placental mosaicism for CHM [27] or a dichorionic twin pregnancy with a CHM and a normal co-twin. Partial mole is unlikely because triploid PHM rarely progresses, and the fetus is almost never structurally normal. In one large series of CHM/co-twin cases, the risk of pGTN was comparable to that reported following singleton CHM, and it did not differ between women who continued the pregnancy and those who had immediate uterine evacuation. However, pregnancy continuation was associated with several complications, including spontaneous abortion, later fetal demise, and preterm delivery [28]. Diffuse cystic sonographic "molar" changes of the placenta in association with an apparently normal fetus in the second or third trimester are usually due to placental mesenchymal dysplasia rather than hydatidiform mole [29].

Detection of hydatidiform mole in the abortion care setting

Most pregnancy terminations and pregnancy failures occur during the first trimester, and treatment options include aspiration or medical regimens. Appropriate management of these conditions will lessen the chance of missing an undiagnosed mole that may subsequently present with pGTN [30,31]. Data based on cases of pGTN following terminations of pregnancy suggest that delayed diagnosis results in poorer outcomes. Women presenting with clinical symptoms of pGTN have significantly more complications, morbidity, and requirements for radical surgery and combination chemotherapy than women identified by postevacuation hCG surveillance protocols [31].

Detecting early hydatidiform mole and its possible sequelae presents challenges, however. Tissue is not always available for histopathological examination. With home-based medical treatment regimens for induced abortion or early pregnancy failure, patients typically expel the products of conception outside of the clinical setting. Moreover, only 22% of North American abortion providers routinely submit tissue for pathological examination following surgical abortion [32]. Even when tissue is submitted, pathologists without special expertise in gestational trophoblastic disease may have problems identifying the subtle morphologic changes of early moles. Indeed, studies have shown poor interobserver correlation between pathologists, particularly in distinguishing partial moles from nonmolar hydropic abortions [33,34].

Because most early molar pregnancies are partial moles that present sonographically as anembryonic gestations [16], the most comprehensive approach would include universal ultrasound examination to identify any nonviable conceptions, followed by aspiration and formal histopathologic tissue analysis by specialists in placental pathology. However, such a policy is cost-prohibitive, especially because PHM rarely results in persistent disease. Moreover, this strategy excludes patients who prefer home-based medical methods of pregnancy termination.

Urine pregnancy testing postabortion can detect persistently elevated hCG levels that may signal complications including failed abortion, incomplete abortion, or the rare case of pGTN [31]. Following complete induced abortion, hCG levels decline rapidly at first and then more gradually; low-sensitivity urine pregnancy tests are usually negative by 2 to 3 weeks after surgical abortion, whereas sensitive tests may take 4 weeks or more (Chapter 6). A persistently positive test in the absence of other complications may signify pGTN. In this case, serum quantitative hCG levels should be followed every 1 to 2 weeks to assure that they return to normal or until pGTN is confirmed by persistently elevated hCG levels [35]. Because pGTN can occur after nonmolar gestations, hCG testing is advised for patients who have unexplained persistent abnormal bleeding 6 weeks following any pregnancy outcome [1,36].

For a variety of reasons, including that many women do not return for follow-up after induced or spontaneous abortion, some cases of HM will inevitably escape detection. A few cases of pGTN resulting from undiagnosed HM at the time of abortion have been reported [30,31]. Fortunately, given the rarity of molar pregnancy and the less than 1% risk that PHM will progress to pGTN, overall morbidity from undetected early HM is likely to be very low.

Management of hydatidiform mole

Uterine evacuation

Prompt uterine evacuation constitutes the initial management of hydatidiform mole. Use of suction rather than sharp curettage minimizes the risk of uterine perforation [37]. Evacuation of large moles is facilitated by adequate dilation using osmotic dilators and a large-bore cannula. To control bleeding following uterine aspiration, we recommend using a single dose of ergotamine to induce a sustained contraction. In general, clinicians should avoid repeated evacuations; they increase the risk of uterine perforation, and persistent molar tissue may be deeply invasive and likely to require chemotherapy [17]. Ultrasound examination, either B mode or combined with color Doppler flow assessment, may help confirm uterine evacuation or identify residual trophoblastic tissue [38–40]. Neither the American College of Obstetricians and Gynecologists (ACOG) nor the Royal College of Obstetricians and Gynaecologists (RCOG) supports medical methods of uterine evacuation for patients with suspected hydatidiform mole [1,36,41].

Follow-up hCG surveillance

All patients diagnosed with CHM or PHM require follow-up with serial hCG measurements for the early detection of pGTN. Serum monitoring provides the most accurate way of determining when the hCG falls to normal. The ACOG recommends measuring serum hCG within 2 days of evacuation, every 1 to 2 weeks while elevated, and then monthly for an additional 6 months [36]. The protocol followed at the trophoblastic disease center at Charing Cross Hospital, London, is as follows: hCG is measured in serum and urine every 2 weeks until normal and then in urine monthly until the end of the follow-up period. If the hCG becomes negative within 56 days (8 weeks), then we follow the patient for a total of 6 months from the time of molar evacuation. In contrast, follow-up is extended for a full 6 months of negative hCG values if hCG first normalizes more than 56 days after molar evacuation. We use the same periods of follow-up regardless of the type of hydatidiform mole [35]. Other centers in the world may vary this regimen; some use a shorter duration of follow-up, particularly for PHM [42]. Abbreviated follow-up may help overcome problems with patient compliance [43]; however, it also presents a small risk of missing pGTN with its rare but life-threatening complications, and therefore warrants further investigation.

Because cancer can produce multiple forms of hCG that are not all found in normal pregnancy, hCG assays used in cancer optimally would detect all forms of hCG. In addition to reported false-positive problems [44], most commercial assays are prone to false-negative results because they fail to detect variant forms of hCG [45]. Efforts are under way to develop a new generation of appropriate hCG assays for use in cancer.

Patients who have had a molar pregnancy are at increased risk for a subsequent hydatidiform mole and development of pGTN following any future pregnancy, even if nonmolar, due to reactivation of latent trophoblast [46]. Therefore, hCG surveillance is critical following any subsequent pregnancy, regardless of outcome. Reliable contraception is recommended during the initial follow-up period because a subsequent pregnancy complicates the interpretation of a rising hCG level, and the hormonal effects of pregnancy may reactivate latent trophoblastic disease. Use of the combined oral contraceptive pill (OCP) in this setting has been marked by controversy. Early experimental studies suggested that administration of exogenous hormones could stimulate GTN growth, and some observational studies reported an increased risk of pGTN in women using OCPs. However, a recent systematic review of the literature, including two randomized trials, failed to support this conclusion [47]. Moreover, the World Health Organization designates all hormonal contraceptive methods as Category 1 (no reason to deny) for women with benign or malignant gestational trophoblastic disease [48]. Nonetheless, some centers, including those in the UK, recommend avoiding hormonal contraception at least until hCG levels have returned to normal [17].

Persistent gestational trophoblastic neoplasia

Forms of pGTN

Persistent GTN complicates about 15% of CHM and about 0.5% of PHM [4,35]. The various forms of pGTN include noninvasive trophoblastic proliferation, invasive mole, choriocarcinoma, and placental site trophoblastic tumor.

Invasive mole occurs when villi from a CHM (or rarely PHM) penetrate into the myometrium or the uterine vasculature. Occasionally, villi penetrate through the full thickness of the myometrium (percreta), leading to uterine perforation or local pelvic extension. In contrast to choriocarcinoma, invasive mole contains distinct molar chorionic villi. The condition usually manifests clinically as pGTN following initial evacuation of a molar pregnancy, with persistent heavy vaginal bleeding and raised hCG levels. Sonography demonstrates focal areas of increased echogenicity within the myometrium [49] (Fig. 19.4). These findings mimic those of placental site trophoblastic tumor but they occur concurrently, or soon after, a proven molar gestation. Treatment usually involves standard chemotherapy

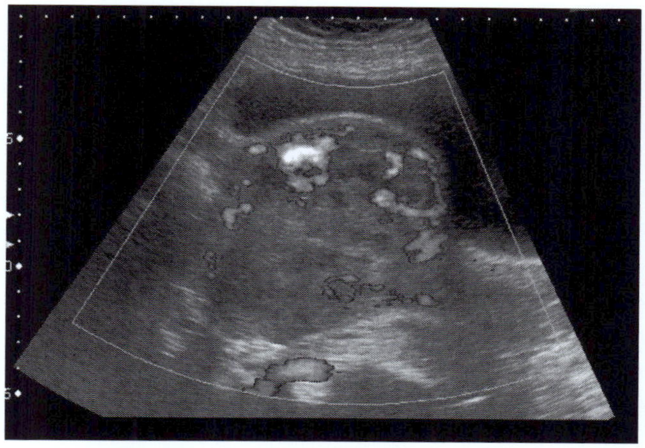

Figure 19.4 Ultrasonographic appearance of an invasive complete hydatidiform mole, showing a localized uterine mass with multiple echolucent cystic spaces and Doppler imaging demonstrating peripheral blood flow. See Plate 19.1.

protocols or surgery; adjunctive local ultrasound-guided injection of methotrexate also has been described [50].

Choriocarcinoma is a malignant neoplasm that exhibits differentiation toward villus cytotrophoblast and syncytiotrophoblast in the absence of chorionic villus structures. Choriocarcinoma occurs in approximately 1 in 20,000 pregnancies [36], and it can follow CHM, PHM, normal pregnancy, stillbirth, spontaneous abortion, or ectopic pregnancy. The incidence of choriocarcinoma after CHM is about a thousand-fold greater than that following a nonmolar pregnancy. Choriocarcinoma either presents as pGTN in patients on hCG surveillance or as clinically apparent, often metastatic, disease in other patients. Uterine choriocarcinoma appears as a hemorrhagic nodule, which metastasizes early to cervix, vagina, or distant sites. Unexplained intracerebral hemorrhage or acute cor pulmonale in a woman of childbearing age should always raise suspicion of choriocarcinoma.

Placental site trophoblastic tumor (PSTT) is distinct from choriocarcinoma both pathologically and clinically, growing more slowly and remaining localized often for several years. Placental site trophoblastic tumors tend to produce less hCG than choriocarcinoma. Spread is initially to adjacent structures and lymph nodes, although PSTT also can metastasize. Many PSTT will respond to aggressive chemotherapy regimens. The cure rate is high if the disease is detected within 4 years of the causative pregnancy, but patients presenting after this period almost universally succumb to the disease. Overall experience with PSTT is still limited [51].

Diagnosis and evaluation of pGTN

Persistent GTN typically presents as either plateauing or rising hCG concentrations during hCG surveillance (Fig. 19.5) or, uncommonly, with symptoms due to localized or metastatic disease. Although several staging systems have been suggested for pGTN, the FIGO 2000 Staging and Risk Factor Scoring System for GTN represents a unified worldwide system to allow comparison of outcome and treatment data across centers [52]. According to this system, any of the following criteria suffices for the diagnosis of postmolar pGTN:

- Plateauing hCG (±10%) for four measurements over a 3-week period or longer
- Rising hCG on three consecutive weekly measurements, over a period of 2 weeks or longer
- Histologic evidence of choriocarcinoma
- hCG exceeding 20,000 IU/L 4 weeks postuterine evacuation (because of the risk of uterine perforation)
- hCG level remaining elevated for 6 months or more postevacuation.

Identification of pGTN warrants further investigation to stage the disease. After a molar pregnancy, most women simply require a current serum hCG level, chest x-ray, and a pelvic Doppler ultrasound. Identification of a lesion on chest x-ray prompts further delineation by chest CT, as well as

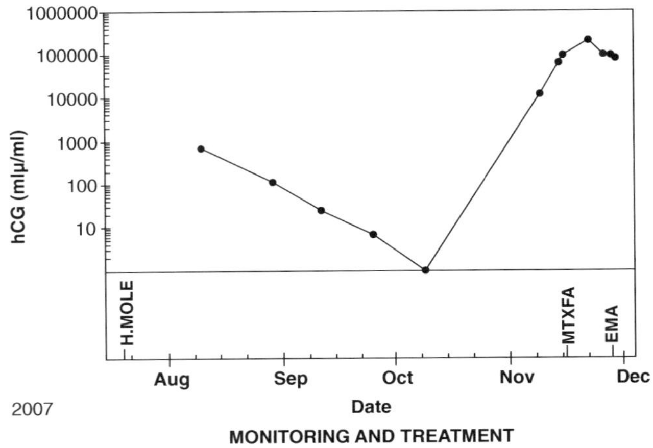

Figure 19.5 Plot of serum hCG concentrations following evacuation of an early complete hydatidiform mole, demonstrating a gradual fall in hCG levels followed by a marked increase, indicating persistent GTN requiring chemotherapy. H Mole = hydatidiform mole; MTXFA = methotrexate, folinic acid; EMA = etoposide, methotrexate, and actinomycin D.

brain MRI to help exclude CNS spread. If the brain MRI is normal, then a lumbar puncture to assess the cerebrospinal fluid serum hCG ratio helps exclude occult CNS disease. Specialists use the results of these studies to determine the stage and prognostic score to assign patients to high- or low-risk groups for developing disease that is resistant to single drug chemotherapy [53]. Other indications for treatment of pGTN include vaginal or intra-abdominal bleeding; metastases in the lung or vagina exceeding 2 cm; or metastases in the brain, gastrointestinal tract, or liver.

Treatment of low-risk patients

Most women who develop pGTN after a molar pregnancy will be low-risk, meaning that their disease has a low probability of becoming resistant to single-drug therapy with either methotrexate or actinomycin D. A variety of protocols exist [54–56] but no randomized trials have established the optimal agent or regimen [57].

Due to its favorable safety/side effect profile, methotrexate is used most commonly with or without folinic acid rescue. A nonrandomized study suggests that daily or alternate daily methotrexate treatment over a week is superior to weekly or less-frequent pulsed administrations [58]. At Charing Cross, we administer 50 mg of methotrexate intramuscularly on days 1, 3, 5, and 7 alternating with 15 mg of folinic acid orally 30 hours postmethotrexate on days 2, 4, 6, and 8, repeated every 2 weeks. Once the serum hCG has normalized, methotrexate treatment is continued for three further cycles (i.e., for 6 weeks of normal hCG levels). We estimate that 10^5 cancer cells may remain when hCG levels first become normal, so stopping therapy early increases relapse rates. The schedule is well tolerated with no alopecia. The incidence of mucositis, the most common toxicity, fell from 20% to less than 2% by increasing the folinic acid rescue from 7.5 to 15 mg [56]. Other less-frequent side effects include serositis and derangement in liver and renal function. Myelosuppression occurs rarely, and no second malignancies have yet been reported.

Several schedules also have been developed using actinomycin D. Daily administration for 5 days every 2 weeks is more efficacious and better tolerated than pulsed or biweekly single-dose regimens [58]. The short-term toxicity of actinomycin D exceeds that of methotrexate but, like methotrexate, it probably has no significant long-term sequelae [56].

The most sensitive indicator of methotrexate resistance is a plateau or rise in serum hCG levels over three or more values. The level of hCG at which resistance develops may guide the choice of salvage chemotherapy. At Charing Cross, we achieve high cure rates using single-agent actinomycin D if the hCG is less than 100 IU/L. If initial therapy was actinomycin D, a switch to methotrexate may be curative. Both actinomycin D failures and those patients developing methotrexate resistance with an hCG exceeding 100 IU/L can be cured with etoposide, methotrexate, and actinomycin D (EMA) combined with cyclophosphamide and vincristine (CO) [56].

Treatment of high-risk patients

Combination chemotherapy is the treatment of choice for high-risk patients. The most widely used regimen based on EMA/CO has remission rates of 80 to 95% [59,60]. EMA/CO chemotherapy is more toxic than single-agent therapy; short-term side effects include reversible alopecia, mucositis, myelosuppression, and peripheral neuropathy. Such high-risk treatment increases the risk of second tumors approximately 1.5-fold compared to the general population. A review of 275 high-risk patients at Charing Cross Hospital treated with EMA/CO chemotherapy showed a cumulative 5-year survival of 86%, with no deaths from GTN beyond 2 years after the initiation of chemotherapy. Presence of metastatic disease, especially combined liver and brain metastases, was associated with poor prognosis [59].

Patients with resistant GTN can still be salvaged after primary treatment failure, usually by a combination of further chemotherapy and surgical removal of resistant disease. As an adjunct to surgery or when surgery is not appropriate, we use a weekly alternating regimen of etoposide and cisplatin (EP) alternating with 1 day of EMA. This combination is toxic but effective, with salvage rates greater than 80% [61]. No other treatment regimens utilized thus far have proven as effective as EP/EMA.

Follow-up postchemotherapy

Following successful treatment, patients are followed up with regular serum and urine hCG measurements weekly for 6 weeks, biweekly for 3 months, and then with diminishing frequency until they require only biannual urine samples. In the UK, we continue follow-up indefinitely because we are uncertain when it is safe to stop. Current information indicates that the overall relapse rate is about 3%, with most relapses occurring within the first year of follow-up. We advise women not to conceive for 12 months, as pregnancy would mask early detection of relapsed disease and the preceding chemotherapy poses an increased risk of congenital anomalies.

Conclusion

With advances in technology and clinical practice over the last two decades, presentation of hydatidiform mole has moved from the second trimester to the earlier weeks of gestation. Because early moles lack the characteristic features of classic moles, this evolution is testing the limits of our current diagnostic modalities and opening up new avenues of clinical inquiry and research. By remaining clinically astute and aware of changes in the rapidly evolving field of gestational trophoblastic disease, abortion providers and other women's health practitioners can play an important role in decreasing morbidity from this rare but important set of disorders.

References

1 Royal College of Obstetricians and Gynaecologists. The management of gestational trophoblastic neoplasia. *RCOG Clinical Guideline No. 38.* Royal College of Obstetricians and Gynaecologists Press, London, 2004.

2 Smith HO. Gestational trophoblastic disease epidemiology and trends. *Clin Obstet Gynecol* 2003; **46**: 541–556.

3 Sebire NJ, Foskett M, Fisher RA, Rees H, Seckl M, Newlands ES. Risk of partial and complete hydatidiform molar pregnancy in relation to maternal age. *BJOG* 2002; **109**: 99–102.

4 Seckl MJ, Fisher RA, Salerno G et al. Choriocarcinoma and partial hydatidiform moles. *Lancet* 2000; **356**: 36–39.

5 Paradinas FJ, Fisher RA, Browne P, Newlands ES. Diploid hydatidiform moles with fetal red blood cells in molar villi: 1—pathology, incidence, and prognosis. *J Pathol* 1997; **181**: 183–188.

6 Sebire NJ, Rees H, Paradinas F, Seckl M, Newlands E. The diagnostic implications of routine ultrasound examination in histologically confirmed early molar pregnancies. *Ultrasound Obstet Gynecol* 2001; **18**: 662–665.

7 Sebire NJ, Rees H. Diagnosis of gestational trophoblastic neoplasia in early pregnancy. *Curr Diagn Pathol* 2003; **8**: 430–440.

8 Sebire NJ, Fisher RA, Rees HC. Histopathological diagnosis of partial and complete hydatidiform mole in the first trimester of pregnancy. *Pediatr Dev Pathol* 2003; **6**: 69–77.

9 Sebire NJ, Makrydimas G, Agnantis NJ, Zagorianakou N, Rees H, Fisher RA. Updated diagnostic criteria for partial and complete

hydatidiform moles in early pregnancy. *Anticancer Res* 2003; **23**: 1723–1728.

10 Castrillon DH, Sun D, Weremowicz S, Fisher RA, Crum CP, Genest DR. Discrimination of complete hydatidiform mole from its mimics by immunohistochemistry of the paternally imprinted gene product p57^{KIP2}. *Am J Surg Pathol* 2001; **25**: 1225–1230.

11 Fisher RA, Hodges MD, Rees HC et al. The maternally transcribed gene p57 (KIP2) (CDNK1C) is abnormally expressed in both androgenetic and biparental complete hydatidiform moles. *Hum Mol Genet* 2002; **11**: 3267–3272.

12 Berezowsky J, Zbieranowski I, Demers J, Murray D. DNA ploidy of hydatidiform moles and nonmolar conceptuses: a study using flow and tissue section image cytometry. *Mod Pathol* 1995; **8**: 775–781.

13 Fisher RA, Newlands ES. Gestational trophoblastic disease. Molecular and genetic studies. *J Reprod Med* 1998; **43**: 87–97.

14 Evans AC Jr, Soper JT, Hammond CB. Clinical features of molar pregnancies and gestational trophoblastic tumors. In: Hancock BW, Newlands ES, Berkowitz RS, Cole LA, eds. *Gestational Trophoblastic Neoplasia*, 2nd edn. [Online]. International Society for the Study of Trophoblastic Diseases; 2003 [cited 2008 Aug 7]. Available from: URL:http://www.isstd.org/gtd/08%20word%20for%20print.pdf

15 Paradinas FJ, Browne P, Fisher RA, Foskett M, Bagshawe KD, Newlands E. A clinical, histopathological and flow cytometric study of 149 complete moles, 146 partial moles and 107 nonmolar hydropic abortions. *Histopathol* 1996; **28**: 101–110.

16 Fowler DJ, Lindsay I, Seckl MJ, Sebire NJ. Routine preevacuation ultrasound diagnosis of hydatidiform mole: experience of more than 1000 cases from a regional referral center. *Ultrasound Obstet Gynecol* 2006; **27**: 76–80.

17 Berkowitz RS, Goldstein DP. Presentation and management of molar pregnancy. In: Hancock BW, Newlands ES, Berkowitz RS, Cole LA, eds. *Gestational Trophoblastic Neoplasia*, 2nd edn. [Online]. International Society for the Study of Trophoblastic Diseases; 2003 [cited 2008 Aug 7]. Available from: URL:http://www.isstd.org/gtd/09%20word%20for%20print.pdf

18 Gemer O, Segal S, Kopmar A, Sassoon E. The current clinical presentation of complete molar pregnancy. *Arch Gynecol Obstet* 2000; **264**: 33–34.

19 Santos-Ramos R, Forney JP, Schwarz BE. Sonographic findings and clinical correlations in molar pregnancy. *Obstet Gynecol* 1980; **56**: 186–192.

20 Fine C, Bundy AL, Berkowitz RS, Boswell SB, Berezin AF, Doubilet PM. Sonographic diagnosis of partial hydatidiform mole. *Obstet Gynecol* 1989: **73**: 414–418.

21 Sherer DM, Allen T, Woods J Jr. Transvaginal sonographic diagnosis of a hydatidiform mole occurring two weeks after curettage for an incomplete abortion. *J Clin Ultrasound* 1991; **19**: 224–226.

22 Lazarus E, Hulka C, Siewert B, Levine D. Sonographic appearance of early complete molar pregnancies. *J Ultrasound Med* 1999; **18**: 589–594.

23 Benson CB, Genest DR, Bernstein MR, Soto-Wright V, Goldstein DP, Berkowitz RS. Sonographic appearance of first trimester complete hydatidiform moles. *Ultrasound Obstet Gynecol* 2000; **16**: 188–191.

24 Lindholm H, Flam F. The diagnosis of molar pregnancy by sonography and gross morphology. *Acta Obstet Gynecol Scand* 1999; **78**: 6–9.

25 Johns J, Greenwold N, Buckley S, Jauniaux E. A prospective study of ultrasound screening for molar pregnancies in missed miscarriages. *Ultrasound Obstet Gynecol* 2005; **25**: 493–497.

26 Fowler DJ, Lindsay I, Seckl MJ, Sebire NJ. Histomorphometric features of hydatidiform moles in early pregnancy: relationship to detectability by ultrasound examination. *Ultrasound Obstet Gynecol* 2007; **29**: 76–80.

27 Makrydimas G, Sebire NJ, Thornton SE, Zagorianakou N, Lolis D, Fisher RA. Complete hydatidiform mole and normal live birth: a novel case of confined placental mosaicism: case report. *Hum Reprod* 2002; **17**: 2459–2463.

28 Sebire NJ, Foskett M, Paradinas FJ et al. Outcome of twin pregnancies with complete hydatidiform mole and healthy co-twin. *Lancet* 2002; **359**: 2165–2166.

29 Paradinas FJ, Sebire NJ, Fisher RA et al. Pseudo-partial moles: placental stem vessel hydrops and the association with Beckwith-Wiedemann syndrome and complete moles. *Histopathology* 2001; **39**: 447–454.

30 Lichtenberg ES. Gestational trophoblastic tumor after medical abortion. *Obstet Gynecol* 2003; **101**: 1137–1139.

31 Seckl MJ, Gillmore R, Foskett M, Sebire NJ, Rees H, Newlands ES. Routine terminations of pregnancy: should we screen for gestational trophoblastic neoplasia? *Lancet* 2004; **364**: 705–707.

32 O'Connell K, Jones HE, Simon M, Saporta V, Paul M, Lichtenberg S. First trimester surgical abortion practices: a survey of National Abortion Federation members. Contraception, in press.

33 Howat AJ, Beck S, Fox H, et al. Can histopathologists reliably diagnose molar pregnancy? *J Clin Pathol* 1993; **46**: 599–602.

34 Fukunaga M, Katabuchi H, Nagasaka T, Mikami Y, Minamiguchi S, Lage JM. Interobserver and intraobserver variability in the diagnosis of hydatidiform mole. *Am J Surg Pathol* 2005; **29**: 942–947.

35 Sebire NJ, Foskett M, Short D et al. Shortened duration of human chorionic gonadotropin surveillance following complete or partial hydatidiform mole: evidence for revised protocol of a UK regional trophoblastic disease unit. *BJOG* 2007; **114**: 760–762.

36 American College of Obstetricians and Gynecologists. Diagnosis and treatment of gestational trophoblastic disease. *ACOG Practice Bulletin No. 53*. American College of Obstetricians and Gynecologists, Washington, DC, 2004.

37 Seckl MJ, Newlands ES, Paradinas FJ. Gestational trophoblastic tumours. In: Souhami RL, Tannock I, Hohenberger P, Horlot JC, eds. *The Oxford Textbook of Oncology*, 2nd edn. Oxford University Press, Oxford, 2001.

38 Achiron R, Goldenberg M, Lipitz S, Mashiach S. Transvaginal duplex Doppler ultrasonography in bleeding patients suspected of having residual trophoblastic tissue. *Obstet Gynecol* 1993; **81**: 507–511.

39 Wolman I, Hartoov J, Pauzner D et al. Transvaginal sonohysterography for the early diagnosis of residual trophoblastic tissue. *J Ultrasound Med* 1997; **16**: 257–261.

40 Ben-Ami I, Schneider D, Maymon R, Vaknin Z, Herman A, Halperin R. Sonographic versus clinical evaluation as predictors of residual trophoblastic tissue. *Hum Reprod* 2005; **20**: 1107–1111.

41 Royal College of Obstetricians and Gynaecologists. The management of early pregnancy loss. *RCOG Clinical Guideline No. 25*. Royal College of Obstetricians and Gynaecologists Press, London, 2000.

42 Kerkmeijer L, Wielsma S, Bekkers R, Pyman J, Tan J, Quinn M. Guidelines following hydatidiform mole: a reappraisal. *Aust N Z J Obstet Gynaecol* 2006; **46**: 112–118.

43 Feltmate CM, Batorfi J, Fulop V, Goldstein DP, Doszpod J, Berkowitz RS. Human chorionic gonadotropin follow-up in patients with molar pregnancy: a time for re-evaluation. *Obstet Gynecol* 2003; **101**: 732–736.

44 Rotmensch S, Cole LA. False diagnosis and needless therapy of presumed malignant disease in women with false-positive human chorionic gonadotropin concentrations. *Lancet* 2000; **355**: 712–715.

45 Mitchell H, Seckl MJ. Discrepancies between commercially available immunoassays in the detection of tumour-derived hCG. *Mol Cell Endocrinol* 2007; **262**: 310–313.

46 Fisher RA, Soteriou BA, Meredith L, Paradinas FJ, Newlands ES. Previous hydatidiform mole identified as the causative pregnancy of choriocarcinoma following birth of normal twins. *Int J Gynecol Cancer* 1995; **5**: 64–70.

47 Costa H, Doyle P. Influence of oral contraceptives in the development of post-molar trophoblastic neoplasia: a systematic review. *Gynecol Oncol* 2006; **100**: 579–585.

48 World Health Organization. Medical Eligibility Criteria for Contraceptive Use, 3rd edn. [Online]. Geneva, World Health Organization; 2004 [cited 2008 Aug 7]. Available at: URL:http://www.who.int/reproductive_health/publications/mec/mec.pdf

49 Aoki S, Hata T, Hata K et al. Doppler color flow mapping of an invasive mole. *Gynecol Obstet Invest* 1989; **27**: 52–54.

50 Tsukihara S, Harada T, Terakawa N. Ultrasound-guided local injection of methotrexate to treat an invasive hydatidiform mole. *J Obstet Gynaecol Res* 2004; **30**: 202–204.

51 Papadopoulos AJ, Foskett M, Seckl MJ et al. Twenty-five years' clinical experience with placental site trophoblastic tumors. *J Reprod Med* 2002; **47**: 460–464.

52 Kohorn IE. The FIGO 2000 staging and risk factor scoring system for gestational trophoblastic neoplasia. In: Hancock BW, Newlands ES, Berkowitz RS, Cole LA, eds. *Gestational Trophoblastic Neoplasia*, 2nd edn. [Online]. International Society for the Study of Trophoblastic Diseases; 2003 [cited 2008 Aug 7]. Available from: URL:http://www.isstd.org/gtd/07%20word%20for%20print.pdf

53 Newlands ES. Presentation and management of persistent gestational trophoblastic disease (GTD) and gestational trophoblastic tumours (GTT) in the United Kingdom. In: Hancock BW, Newlands ES, Berkowitz RS, Cole LA, eds. *Gestational Trophoblastic Neoplasia*, 2nd edn. [Online]. International Society for the Study of Trophoblastic Diseases; 2003 [cited 2008 Aug 7]. Available from: URL:http://www.isstd.org/gtd/10%20word%20for%20print%20.pdf

54 Wong LC, Ngan HY, Cheng DK, Ng TY. Methotrexate infusion in low-risk gestational trophoblastic disease. *Am J Obstet Gynecol* 2000; **183**: 1579–1582.

55 Kwon JS, Elit L, Mazurka J, Moens F, Schmuck ML. Weekly intravenous methotrexate with folinic acid for nonmetastatic gestational trophoblastic neoplasia. *Gynecol Oncol* 2001; **82**: 367–370.

56 McNeish IA, Strickland S, Holden L et al. Low-risk persistent gestational trophoblastic neoplasia: outcome after initial treatment with low-dose methotrexate and folinic acid from 1992 to 2000. *J Clin Oncol* 2002; **20**: 1838–1844.

57 Foulmann K, Guastalla JP, Caminet N et al. What is the best protocol of single-agent methotrexate chemotherapy in nonmetastatic or low-risk metastatic gestational trophoblastic tumors? A review of the evidence. *Gynecol Oncol* 2006; **102**: 103–110.

58 Kohorn EI. Is lack of response to single-agent chemotherapy in gestational trophoblastic disease associated with dose scheduling or chemotherapy resistance? *Gynecol Oncol* 2002; **85**: 36–39.

59 Bower M, Newlands ES, Holden L et al. EMA/CO for high-risk gestational trophoblastic tumors: results from a cohort of 272 patients. *J Clin Oncol* 1997; **15**: 2636–2643.

60 Turan T, Karacay O, Tulunay G et al. Results with EMA/CO (etoposide, methotrexate, actinomycin D, cyclophosphamide, vincristine) chemotherapy in gestational trophoblastic neoplasia. *Int J Gynecol Cancer* 2006; **16**: 1432–1438.

61 Newlands ES, Mulholland PJ, Holden L, Seckl MJ, Rustin GJ. Etoposide and cisplatin/etoposide, methotrexate, and actinomycin D (EMA) chemotherapy for patients with high-risk gestational trophoblastic tumors refractory to EMA/cyclophosphamide and vincristine chemotherapy and patients presenting with metastatic placental site trophoblastic tumors. *J Clin Oncol* 2000; **18**: 854–859.

20

CHAPTER 20

Abortion for fetal abnormalities or maternal conditions

Jeffrey S. Dungan MD and Lee P. Shulman MD

LEARNING POINTS

- A small but important minority of abortions is performed because of serious fetal abnormalities or serious maternal medical conditions.
- The wide use of prenatal diagnosis with abortion as a backup has been associated with important declines in perinatal and infant mortality in industrialized nations.
- An array of screening and diagnostic tests is used to detect fetal abnormalities, including biochemical tests, ultrasonography, chorionic villus sampling, and amniocentesis.
- Women aborting a wanted pregnancy require not only excellent medical care but also extra emotional support because of the painful ambivalence that can surround their abortion decision.
- In the USA, most women who decide to end a pregnancy affected by fetal abnormalities choose surgical abortion. Women who prefer to deliver an intact fetus for grieving purposes may elect induction abortion or, when available and possible, intact dilation and evacuation.

Introduction

Serious health problems in the pregnant woman or the fetus account for a small but important proportion of induced abortions. Because of the ambivalence that can surround the decision to end a desired pregnancy, women, partners, and families requesting abortion in this setting have unique medical and emotional needs. The emotional response entails grieving for the lost pregnancy, and the recovery can take time.

Most women who learn that they are carrying fetuses with autosomal trisomies or severe structural abnormalities (e.g., anencephaly, Potter's sequence) choose to abort their pregnancies. Abortion is less common for sex chromosome polysomies such as Klinefelter syndrome (49 XXY) that are neither lethal nor severely impairing [1–3]. Wider use of prenatal diagnosis with abortion as a backup has dramatically improved the health of families; reductions in both perinatal and infant mortality rates have been documented in industrialized countries [4,5].

The decision about which screening or testing regimen to use will depend on patient preference, the underlying risk for an abnormality and adverse outcome, availability of resources, stage of gestation, and number of fetuses. In this chapter, we present an overview of prenatal screening and describe abortion options for fetal or maternal indications. Because of the many laws and regulations that govern abortion in the USA, including the Partial-Birth Abortion Ban Act of 2003 [6] and related state laws, providers embarking on second-trimester abortion practice are advised to review Chapters 4, 11, and 12 and consult with legal counsel as appropriate.

Screening for fetal abnormalities

Historically, age greater than 35 years was the most common indication for prenatal diagnosis. The American College of Obstetricians and Gynecologists (ACOG) now recommends that clinicians offer screening for fetal chromosome abnormalities to all pregnant women, not only those aged 35 and older [7]. More recently, abnormal serum screening results or ultrasound abnormalities have led women to consider invasive testing. Alternatively, the diagnostic precision of ultrasonography for some fetal anomalies, such as anencephaly, obviates the need for confirmation.

Management of Unintended and Abnormal Pregnancy, 1st edition. By M Paul, ES Lichtenberg, L Borgatta, DA Grimes, PG Stubblefield, MD Creinin

The distinction between screening and testing

Screening is the testing of the apparently healthy to identify those at increased risk of disease. In contrast, diagnostic testing is performed for specific indications, such as signs, symptoms, or a positive screening test. Thus, screening is not synonymous with diagnosis, and clinicians generally do not intervene based on a screening test.

Screening can provide pragmatic information for patients. Some women choose to undergo prenatal diagnosis despite not desiring an abortion should results indicate serious fetal disease. This information can help them prepare for the birth of a child with special needs. Others will opt for abortion should results return unfavorable. These decisions are inevitably complex and personal, and clinicians should support the woman in whatever choice she makes.

First-trimester screening

The trend toward earlier screening for abnormal fetal genotypes (aneuploidy) emerged with the discovery that reduced levels of pregnancy-associated plasma protein-A (PAPP-A) and elevated levels of human chorionic gonadotropin (β-hCG) were associated with fetal aneuploidy. PAPP-A is secreted from the placenta and is detectable in maternal serum as early as 4 weeks' gestation. The precise function of PAPP-A is unknown, but it is believed to be involved in immune modulation. PAPP-A was originally investigated as a marker for impending spontaneous abortion or ectopic pregnancy, conditions also associated with lower-than-expected values. In initial reports from the early 1990s, serum levels of PAPP-A from a small number of women at 6 to 12 weeks' gestation tended to be significantly lower in most pregnancies affected with trisomy 21 or 18; the median multiple of the mean (MoM) was generally about 0.30 MoM [8]. After other investigators confirmed this association, measurement of PAPP-A in the first trimester was widely incorporated into screening algorithms [9].

β−hCG has also been extensively examined as a serum marker for fetal Down syndrome. In the early 1990s, several reports found that women carrying a trisomy 21 fetus who were screened in the first trimester had levels of free β-hCG, total β-hCG, and intact hCG similar to levels found during the second trimester [9]. Which hCG-related molecule provides the best screening marker remains incompletely resolved; a recent meta-analysis concluded that free β-hCG was preferable [10].

Second-trimester screening

Most centers that offer second-trimester (15 to 20 weeks' gestation) serum screening for trisomy 21 and 18 use either the triple- or quadruple-marker test. The traditional triple-marker test includes maternal serum alphafetoprotein (MSAFP), unconjugated estriol (uE3), and β-hCG. The addition of a fourth marker, dimeric inhibin A, increases sensitivity in the detection rate for fetal trisomy 21 and reduces the false-positive rate [11,12]. Although multiple-marker serum screening is widely used in the USA [13], advances in first-trimester ultrasonography screening may soon change this pattern of practice.

A review of practice patterns among US obstetricians showed that of those who offered genetic screening, about half offered triple screening and half offered the quad test [13]. ACOG's recent Practice Bulletin [7] on screening did not recommend one screening approach over another, but specified that a multi-marker algorithm should be used.

Combining first-trimester and second-trimester screening algorithms

Tests are commonly performed in sequence in medicine, employing a less expensive and often less sensitive screening test first followed by a more costly yet more precise test for positive screens (e.g., syphilis or HIV testing). Combining first- and second-trimester screening leads to better detection than either alone. Sophisticated calculations are necessary to estimate an adjusted risk [14]. Two categories of screening strategies are clinically useful during these two trimesters: integrated screening and sequential screening.

Integrated screening

This form of first- and second-trimester screening involves obtaining information during gestational weeks 10 to 14, but not calculating risk until the second-trimester specimen (typically the four serum markers that comprise the quad screen) has been analyzed, after 15 weeks' gestation [15]. A large trial confirmed the overall high performance of an integrated screening approach [16]. More than 35,000 women were screened during the first and second trimesters, with approximately 20% of the women being older than age 35. The first-trimester screens included sonographic measurement of fetal nuchal translucency, serum PAPP-A, and serum free β-hCG. Results of this screen were not released until calculation of the second-trimester screen risk (quad markers drawn at 15 to 18 weeks' gestation). Data from both screens were then integrated into a single risk calculation, termed *fully integrated screening*. The study also evaluated separate screening performance using biochemistry alone (serum-integrated screening). The addition of second-trimester information enhanced screening performance.

An important disadvantage of the integrated screening approach is the late gestational age at which risk is estimated. This delay precludes chorionic villus sampling (CVS) for women found to have significantly elevated risk based on increased nuchal translucency or an abnormal first-trimester biochemical test. In the large trial described previously [16], women found to have fetal cystic hygroma during the nuchal translucency scan were offered immediate invasive prenatal diagnosis.

Sequential screening

A variation of using both first- and second-trimester screening data is the sequential screening approach, also known as *stepwise sequential screening*. With this algorithm, patients are informed immediately of the first-trimester screening results and offered CVS if the risk calculation is sufficiently elevated (e.g., 1 in 50). Those women with lower risks return for a second-trimester blood draw between weeks 15 and 18, and a second risk calculation is performed similar to that done for integrated screening. In the large trial, a detection rate of about 95% for Down syndrome was achieved at a 5% false-positive rate (2.5% in each trimester)[16]. This compares favorably to the 4% rate with the fully integrated screening approach; indeed, sequential screening is used at our center. If neither nuchal translucency assessment nor facilities with CVS capability are an option for the patient, then a serum-only integrated screen offers the best detection rate.

First-trimester ultrasonography

Nuchal translucency

Ultrasonography assessment of fetal nuchal translucency has become a prominent first-trimester indicator of fetal aneuploidy [17,18]. The measurement is technically challenging, requiring rigorous training to master and ongoing experience to maintain (Fig. 20.1). Quality assurance is critical. The measurement is best performed between 10 and 13 6/7 weeks' gestation. Highest detection rates occur at 12 to 13 weeks [15]. Apparent resolution of abnormally thickened nuchal translucency with serial scanning should not deter further testing, because this abnormal finding can disappear over time in aneuploid fetuses [19].

Nasal-bone assessment

One of the striking phenotypic features of Down syndrome is midface hypoplasia, with underdevelopment of the nasal bridge. In early pregnancy, the fetus with trisomy 21 may have an absent or severely hypoplastic nasal bone on ultrasound when viewed in a sagittal plane. In a series of women at 11 to 14 weeks' gestation undergoing CVS for increased risk of aneuploidy, Cicero and colleagues judged the nasal bone to be absent in 73% of fetuses with trisomy 21 but absent in only 0.5% of normal fetuses [20].

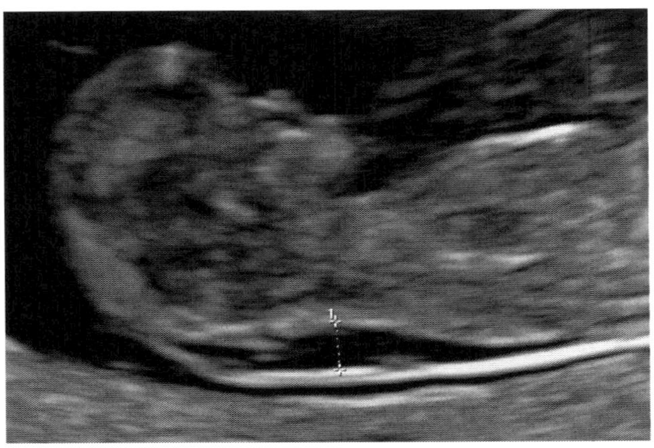

Figure 20.1 Profile view of a first-trimester fetus with increased nuchal translucency (calipers).

Subsequent reports have not been as supportive of this potential marker for trisomy 21[21–23] because nasal features vary by ethnicity. A recent assessment judged this measurement to be useful, but only as a secondary or contingency marker as part of a first-trimester screening program [24].

In summary, during the first trimester the combination of nuchal translucency measurement, when coupled with chemical tests (PAPP-A and free β-hCG), is superior in detecting trisomy 21 when compared to either modality alone. However, where access to first-trimester nuchal translucency measurement or CVS is not available, integrated screening using only chemical markers and maternal age is a reasonable alternative [15].

Second-trimester ultrasonography

In contemporary obstetrical practice in the USA, most prenatal patients undergo ultrasonography screening at about 18 to 20 weeks' gestation [25,26] (Table 20.1). Depending on the experience and skill of the center providing the imaging, many structural anomalies will be detected at this time. Women are then faced with decisions about further prenatal evaluation or abortion. Occasionally the diagnosis in such cases is straightforward, such as with fetal anencephaly (Fig. 20.2). More commonly, structural anomalies detected at the midtrimester ultrasonography examination will result in referral for genetic counseling and consideration of invasive diagnostic testing.

Many women choose to terminate the pregnancy when a structural anomaly is found, even in the presence of a

Table 20.1 Components of fetal anatomy survey (Adapted from American Institute of Ultrasound in Medicine [25] and American College of Radiology [26].)

Fetal cardiac activity, number, and presentation
Amniotic fluid volume
Placental location
Number of vessels in umbilical cord
Biometric measurements to establish gestational age
Head, neck, and face:
Cerebellum
Choroid plexus
Lateral ventricles
Falx
Cavum septum pellucidum
Upper lip
Chest, including four-chamber heart views (and outflow tracts if feasible)
Abdomen, including stomach, kidneys, bladder, cord insertion site
Spine
Extremities
Gender

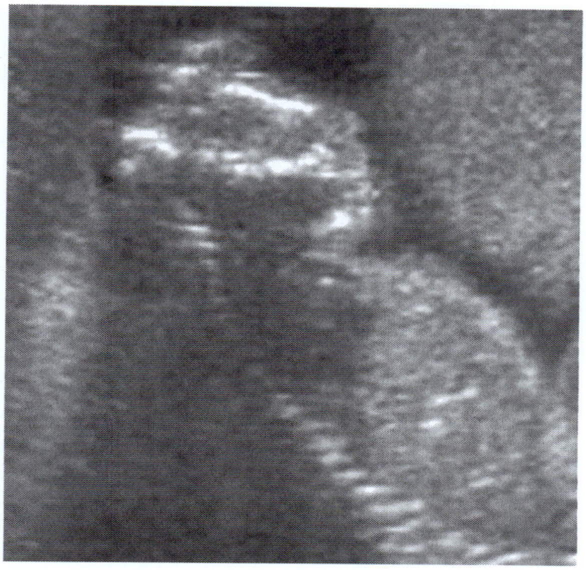

Figure 20.2 Sonogram of a 14-week fetus with anencephaly; cerebral portion of fetal head is absent.

normal chromosome complement [27–29]. The proportions of pregnancies aborted range from about 90% with anencephaly to a low of 30% for disorders requiring surgical repair but generally associated with favorable postrepair prognosis (e.g., gastroschisis)[30]. Women tend to opt for abortion when the abnormality involves the central nervous system (CNS). In a large series reported by Schechtman and colleagues, women found to have fetuses with anencephaly chose abortion in 90% of instances, and nearly 75% of those with fetal encephalocele or other serious CNS malformation chose not to continue their pregnancies [28]. On the other hand, in pregnancies with non-CNS fetal abnormalities, a minority of patients chose abortion unless the diagnosis was severe (e.g., bilateral renal agenesis). If an associated chromosome abnormality is detected via amniocentesis or CVS, women are more likely to abort the pregnancy, especially with the earlier detection afforded by CVS.

Invasive prenatal diagnosis

Invasive prenatal testing, either by CVS or amniocentesis, is performed to obtain a more accurate diagnosis. Counseling should review the patient's risk of having a serious fetal abnormality, the limitations and risks of the procedure (with regard to the health and well-being of the fetus and patient), and the timing of results. Patients need to know that normal results will not guarantee a healthy perinatal outcome; conversely, certain types of abnormal results do not predict a poor outcome.

Chorionic villus sampling

Chorionic villus sampling harvests placental tissue by a transcervical or transabdominal approach. The choice of approach is based on placental location as well as other factors such as fibroids, uterine position, overlying bowel or bladder and, in some cases, vaginal infection. A third approach is transvaginal CVS, a technique reserved for women with a retroverted, retroflexed uterus and a posterior or fundal placenta. In such situations, a transvaginal CVS usually allows sampling of the placenta.

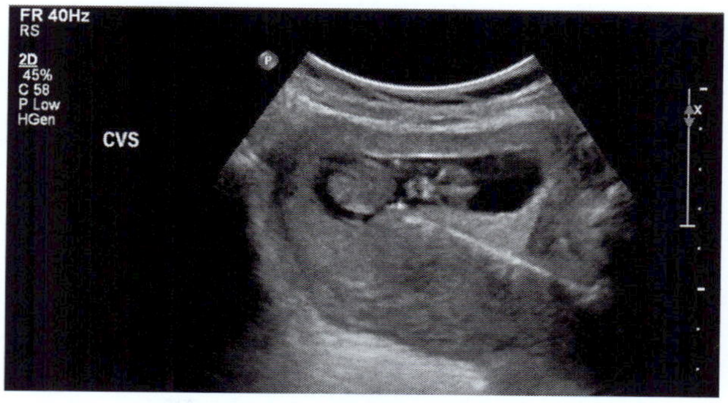

Figure 20.3 Ultrasonography image of transcervical chorionic villus sampling.

Transcervical CVS (Fig. 20.3) is best performed at 10 to 12 weeks' gestation. Contraindications include cervical or vaginal infection (e.g., herpes, chlamydial infection, or gonorrhea) or maternal blood group sensitization. Relative contraindications include a leiomyoma obstructing the cervical canal, bleeding from the vagina within 2 weeks of planned CVS (possibly indicating placental separation or unstable gestation), and a markedly retroverted, retroflexed uterus [31]. Before the CVS is performed, fetal cardiac activity and normal fetal growth must be confirmed by ultrasound. After the procedure, fetal heart activity is verified again by ultrasonography. Patients are monitored for any untoward effects for approximately 10 to 20 minutes. Unsensitized Rh(D)-negative patients are given D-immune globulin 50 μg.

Transabdominal CVS (Fig. 20.4) is used to evaluate pregnancies at the same gestational age as transcervical CVS procedures; however, it also can be performed later in the pregnancy, particularly when ultrasonographic detection of fetal abnormalities warrants rapid diagnosis. This approach may be useful for sampling a placenta in an unusual location or when the transcervical approach is not advisable. Performing CVS through the vagina (Fig. 20.5) is another alternative when uterine anatomy is not conducive to the former approaches [32].

Transcervical CVS and transabdominal CVS appear to be equally safe procedures for first-trimester diagnosis. In a randomized trial comparing transcervical CVS and transabdominal CVS, the loss rates of cytogenetically normal pregnancies through 28 weeks were 2.5 and 2.3%, respectively [33]. In a small randomized trial in Italy, Brambati et al also found no difference in complications between transabdominal and transcervical CVS [34]. By contrast, a randomized comparison of amniocentesis, transabdominal CVS, and transcervical

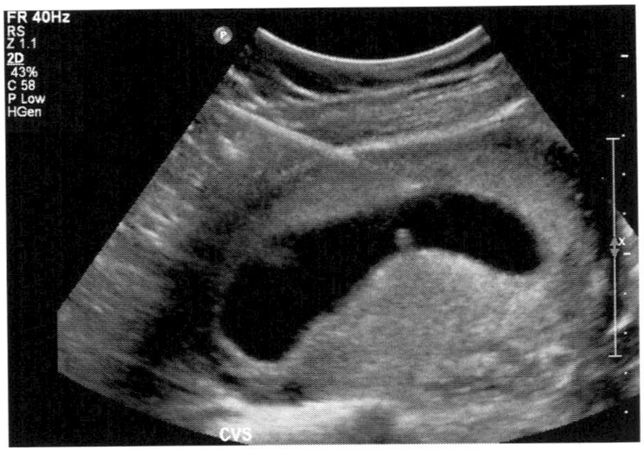

Figure 20.4 Ultrasonography image of transabdominal chorionic villus sampling.

CVS in Denmark found significantly more losses associated with transcervical CVS [35]. More recently, Caughey and colleagues found an association between increasing experience with CVS and reduced risks of fetal loss following CVS, leading to equality in risk for postprocedure loss between CVS and amniocentesis [36].

Several early reports of children with limb reduction defects after maternal CVS led to concerns about fetal safety. However, a comprehensive review of CVS safety sponsored by the World Health Organization evaluated 216,381 CVS cases performed worldwide and found no cause for heightened concern. The authors concluded that "CVS carries no increased risk for fetal loss or congenital malformation, including limb reduction defect" compared to conventional midtrimester amniocentesis [37].

Amniocentesis

An ultrasound examination should be performed immediately before amniocentesis for prenatal diagnosis. This examination serves several purposes: to evaluate fetal number and viability, confirm gestational age, establish placental location, identify uterine structural abnormalities, and estimate amniotic fluid volume.

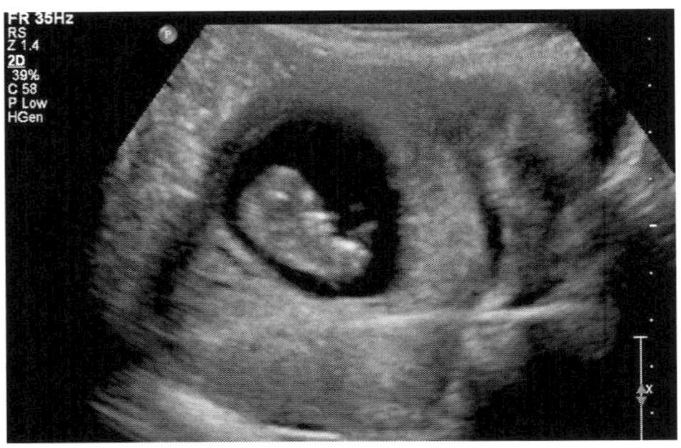

Figure 20.5 Ultrasonography image of transvaginal chorionic villus sampling.

Following the preoperative ultrasound examination, a needle insertion site is chosen. Although a site distant from the placenta is preferable, amniocentesis through the placenta does not compromise the safety of amniocentesis [38]. If reaching the optimal pocket of fluid requires traversing the placenta, selection of the thinnest portion of the placenta may be advisable. The medical team should perform ultrasonography monitoring with continuous visualization of the needle throughout the procedure. Because the first several milliliters of amniotic fluid may contain maternal cells, the initial sample is usually discarded or set aside for serum alpha-fetoprotein (AFP) assay. For a second-trimester amniocentesis performed from 14 to 20 weeks' inclusively, 20 to 25 ml of amniotic fluid suffices. Aspiration of bloody amniotic fluid occurs infrequently (1 to 2% of procedures). The blood, usually maternal, does not impair amniotic cell growth.

Several large collaborative studies have recently addressed the safety of amniocentesis. Eddleman and colleagues evaluated more than 35,000 unselected patients and found a procedure-related loss rate after midtrimester amniocentesis similar to the background frequency [39]. The loss rate in this study was 1 in 1,600 procedures, considerably lower than the risk (1 in 200 to 1 in 300) commonly quoted in texts and counseling materials.

Earlier amniocentesis may be associated with a greater risk of loss. A multicenter randomized trial of amniocentesis allocated 4,374 women to an early amniocentesis cohort ($n = 2{,}183$) or conventional midtrimester amniocentesis cohort ($n = 2{,}185$) [40,41]. In the early amniocentesis group, 1,916 women (87.8%) underwent amniocentesis before 13 weeks' gestation. Loss rates were 7.6% for the early amniocentesis cohort and 5.9% for the midtrimester cohort. Talipes equinovarus (clubfoot deformity) occurred in 1.3% of infants delivered of women in the early amniocentesis group compared to 0.1% in the midtrimester cohort. In addition, amniotic fluid leakage occurred more frequently in the early amniocentesis group (3.5%) than in the midtrimester group (1.7%).

Teratogen exposure

Some women seek or are referred for abortion after exposure to medications, environmental agents, infections, or other exposures during pregnancy. Often such referrals follow innocuous exposures, and after reassurance women may decide to continue their pregnancies. Examples of exposures leading to unnecessary abortion referrals include abdominal x-rays, over-the-counter allergy medicines, and common antibiotics. Many people, including clinicians,

Box A Some Factors to Consider When Counseling Women About Potential Teratogenic Exposures

- *Amount.* Most agents carry a dose-response relationship to production of birth defects, that is, greater doses are more likely to produce manifestations or more severe phenotypic consequences than low doses.
- *Duration.* Prolonged exposure is more likely to result in damage when compared to brief or single exposures.
- *Gestational age.* For agents that cause structural anomalies, the greatest potential for harm occurs during embryogenesis (gestational weeks 5 to 9). Different organ systems develop at different times during this critical period. After this period, exposures may cause other effects such as growth deficits or CNS deficits.

Box B Online Teratogens Databases

TOXNET (Toxicology Data Network)
http://www.toxnet.nlm.nih.gov
Maintained by the National Library of Medicine; accesses multiple databases and provides search engine to investigate specific agents.

Organization of Teratology Information Specialists
http://www.otispregnancy.org
A network of teratology information services and databases organized state-by-state; also enrolls women with potential exposures into surveillance studies.

REPROTOX
http://www.reprotox.org
A subscription service that allows the user to search for specific agents; maintained by the Reproductive Toxicology Center.

TERIS (Teratogen Information System)
http://depts.washington.edu/terisweb/teris
Subscription service maintained by the University of Washington (Seattle) that incorporates one of the standard teratology textbooks, *Shepard's Catalog of Teratogenic Agents*, into its search engine.

overestimate the risk for birth defects caused by medication or other exposures. In fact, only a limited number of medications are known teratogens (Table 20.2). In addition, only about 3 to 6% of all birth defects are attributed to teratogens. Many exposures are completely preventable, particularly if they are recognized and discontinued prior to conception. However, once a concerning exposure occurs during pregnancy, women deciding whether or not to continue a pregnancy need information about possible adverse outcomes and factors that may influence their likelihood.

The counseling of women and their partners in these circumstances is often best done by a genetic counselor or maternal-fetal medicine specialist. Several factors require consideration when addressing the teratogenic potential of any exposure, including dosage, duration, gestational age of the pregnancy, underlying predisposition (genetic background), and use of other agents [42] (Box A). Exposures can sometimes occur via the partner, as when work clothes laden with lead or other agents are laundered at home. Male-mediated developmental toxicity is an area of active investigation [43]. Counseling is not straightforward, and often the counselor is left to quote only a percent range of risk that an abnormality may be present.

The traditional US Food and Drug Administration (FDA) classification system for drug use in pregnancy assigns a letter A, B, C, D, or X to prescription drugs. The FDA is now replacing this system because it has not met the need of either clinicians or women [42]. Numerous textbooks and medical journals are devoted to teratogens and reproductive toxicology, and information is available from the Internet as well (Box B).

The abortion provider must be aware of the potential teratogenic effects of methotrexate and misoprostol. Evidence is limited concerning the potential risk with methotrexate in the first trimester (Chapter 9). Concern exists for misoprostol as well [44], but early reports of potential misoprostol teratogenicity were related to black-market use in large doses and without medical supervision [45]. Ultrasonography may provide some information if detectable anomalies are seen, but a normal sonogram does not exclude anomalies. All

Table 20.2 Examples of agents with evidence of potential teratogenicity.

Angiotensin-converting enzyme (ACE) inhibitors: cardiovascular and central nervous system malformations
Ethanol: growth restriction, microcephaly, facial anomalies, including epicanthal folds, long philtrum, and thin upper lip, cognitive dysfunction
Isotretinoin: craniofacial anomalies, hydrocephalus, microtia, mental retardation
Lithium: heart defects
Methotrexate: craniofacial anomalies, digital anomalies, growth restriction
Misoprostol: Möbius sequence (congenital facial nerve paralysis)
Phenytoin: cleft lip/palate, heart defects, microcephaly, facial dysmorphism
Radiation: requires greater than 5 rad (50 mGy) exposure, microcephaly, growth restriction
Tobacco: growth restriction
Valproic acid: neural tube defects
Warfarin: nasal hypoplasia, eye anomalies, mental retardation

patients electing early medical abortion must receive information about teratogenic potential and the need to follow through until the abortion is completed, by either medical or surgical means.

Maternal conditions

Serious maternal disease or obstetrical conditions can present critical issues for women and couples who may otherwise have a desired pregnancy but are faced with dire prognoses that may lead them to consider abortion. A thorough review is beyond the scope of this book, but we present a few of the many examples here. Chapter 7 addresses evaluation and management of medical conditions as well.

Making decisions about whether or not to continue a pregnancy in these circumstances is often complex and difficult. Conditions that would have absolutely precluded pregnancy a decade ago may now permit pregnancy in certain situations and with appropriate care and monitoring [46]. However, patients with such conditions warrant evaluation by appropriate specialists who can best determine whether the condition, the patient's baseline health, and the physiologic impact of pregnancy can allow for a salutary outcome. Counseling about risks and benefits should include the potential for clinical deterioration or death if the pregnancy continues, as well as the risks of the abortion procedure. If a woman chooses to end the pregnancy, then consultation with maternal-fetal specialists, anesthesiologists, and critical-care specialists may help determine the optimal abortion method.

Cardiovascular disease, whether congenital or acquired, remains one of the most common indications for pregnancy termination for maternal indication [46]. Congenital structural abnormalities, such as Ebstein's anomaly and the cardiac manifestation of Marfan syndrome (widened aortic root), are likely to lead to maternal and fetal problems, regardless of prior surgical repair. Acquired cardiovascular problems, including cardiomyopathy, infectious-related valvular disease, or atherosclerotic disease leading to severe hypertension, can also complicate pregnancy and adversely affect maternal and fetal health. Cystic fibrosis (CF) is another condition that may warrant consideration of pregnancy termination in some circumstances. An inherited and multiorgan condition, CF is characterized by pulmonary, gastrointestinal, and developmental problems. Pregnancy for women with CF may adversely affect pulmonary function, and reduced gastrointestinal absorption can adversely affect fetal growth and development.

Premature preterm rupture of membranes (PPROM) at a pre-viable gestational age is an example of an obstetrical condition that requires prompt emptying of the uterus to minimize the risk of infection, which can be life-threatening. The optimal means of uterine evacuation is unclear, but many centers offer patients the option of either D&E or labor induction with a uterotonic agent, such as misoprostol or oxytocin. A series of 34 patients (14 to 23 weeks' gestation) with rupture of membranes found preoperative laminaria insertion to be safe, although long-term follow-up was not reported [47]. Prophylactic antibiotics are advisable for such patients. If the patient is already infected, aggressive antibiotic therapy with other supportive measures and consultation with intensive care and infectious disease specialists are needed. Prompt uterine evacuation is critical for recovery; indeed, delay is the common theme in deaths from intrauterine infection [48,49].

The abortion procedure

Women having abortions of desired pregnancies for fetal or maternal indications deserve not only excellent medical care but also extra emotional support. Because of the ambivalence that can surround this decision, aborting a wanted fetus can be emotionally wrenching for the woman and her family [50]. Many report that it is the most difficult decision that they have ever faced. During the preoperative discussion, open-ended questions such as, "How difficult did you find the decision to come here today?" or "How are you holding up emotionally with all this?" often elicit tears. Advising the woman that tears are normal and healthy, then just sitting quietly with her and her family as they cry, can be comforting. Some physicians describe for patients the stages of grieving and the emotional fragility that may occur during their recovery. Compassionate, competent care can help these women and their families through this terrible crisis and on toward brighter futures and healthier pregnancies.

The usual range of available abortion methods should be offered as appropriate for the gestational age. In the second trimester, most US women given a choice of D&E or labor induction will choose the former [51]. Certain fetal anomalies may pose technical challenges beyond what is typically encountered with midtrimester pregnancy terminations. For example, large fetal masses (e.g., sacrococcygeal teratomas) or enlargement of the fetal head (hydrocephalus) may necessitate variations in technique. In some instances of fetal hydrocephalus, we have performed transabdominal decompression of cerebral spinal fluid (after injection to cause fetal demise) using a large bore spinal needle to facilitate delivery of the fetus. During D&E procedures, sonographic guidance by a skilled assistant can help immensely when extracting specific structures, ensuring that the jaws of the forceps are properly oriented for efficient use and verifying that perforation has not occurred.

Some women prefer to deliver an intact fetus so they can hold it, take photographs, or make footprints as keepsakes. Intact delivery may also facilitate comprehensive pathologic analysis of an abnormal fetus. Where available and feasible, intact D&E (Chapter 11) may be an alternative to labor-induction abortion in these circumstances. In our experience, having ample cervical dilation prior to D&E is critical for extracting the fetus as intact as possible (after injection to cause fetal demise) in cases where careful pathologic evaluation is necessary to establish a diagnosis. Patients in our center often undergo serial laminaria insertions two or even three times before the D&E procedure. We also have the benefit of a skilled and motivated pathology department experienced in evaluation of post-D&E fetal remains [52].

The same approach to perinatal loss can be used with aborted fetuses as with stillborn infants. For example, even anencephalic fetuses can have a knit cap placed over the posterior aspect of the head, allowing the woman to note how normal was everything else about the fetus. Allowing quiet time for the patient to grieve with her family can be healing. Some abortion services work closely with not only genetic counselors but also perinatal grief counselors. Counselors or hospital chaplains can provide important support to families in this crisis. For example, upon request some chaplains will perform a blessing of the fetus for the patient and her family in the recovery room after D&E or in the patient's room after labor-induction abortion. The service can provide keepsakes for the patient and her family, such as footprints.

Women in emotional crisis merit a seamless transition back to their regular providers. In such cases, telephone calls to the referring clinician can facilitate close follow-up, occasionally as soon as the next day. A short course of sleeping pills may help the patient and her partner if they have been having trouble sleeping.

Two unique patient concerns that may arise in this setting are the potential for fetal suffering and disposition of fetal remains. Preemptive counseling about both topics can be helpful. Women having midtrimester abortions often exhibit a visible sigh of relief when they learn that fetal perception of pain is biologically impossible until later in pregnancy [53]. Regarding fetal disposition, some patients are reassured to learn that a dignified cremation is the default option. Some women want to have the ashes returned after cremation so that they may keep or scatter them personally. Accommodating these wishes helps with the healing process. As noted long ago, "the secret of the care of the patient is in caring for the patient [54]."

Conclusion

A small but important minority of abortions is performed because of serious fetal or maternal conditions. The decision to terminate a pregnancy may follow detection of fetal abnormalities through prenatal screening and diagnostic tests, exposure to teratogenic agents, or the development or worsening of maternal conditions during pregnancy. Often women in these circumstances have desired pregnancies, and many find the decision to end the pregnancy both painful and fraught with ambivalence. The care of pregnant women with fetal abnormalities or serious medical conditions is often complex and may require consultation and intervention from specialists. In addition, involvement of experienced counselors may help address the emotional needs of women and their families as they weather this crisis and prepare to move forward to better days and healthier pregnancies.

References

1 Verp MS, Bombard AT, Simpson JL, Elias S. Parental decision following prenatal diagnosis of fetal chromosome abnormality. *Am J Med Genet* 1988; **29**: 613–622.

2 Grevengood C, Shulman LP, Dungan JS et al. Severity of abnormality influences decision to terminate pregnancies affected with neural tube defects. *Fetal Diagn Ther* 1994; **9**: 273–277.

3 Zlotogora J. Parental decisions to abort or continue a pregnancy with an abnormal finding after an invasive prenatal test. *Prenat Diagn* 2002; **22**: 966–972.

4 van der Pal-de Bruin KM, Graafmans W, Biermans MC et al. The influence of prenatal screening and termination of pregnancy on perinatal mortality rates. *Prenat Diagn* 2002; **22**: 966–972.

5 Liu S, Joseph KS, Kramer MS et al. Fetal and Infant Health Study Group of the Canadian Perinatal Surveillance System. Relationship of prenatal diagnosis and pregnancy termination to overall infant mortality in Canada. *JAMA* 2002; **287**: 1561–1567.

6 Partial-Birth Abortion Ban Act of 2003. 18 U.S.C. §1531, 2003.

7 American College of Obstetricians and Gynecologists Committee on Practice Bulletins. ACOG practice bulletin no. 77: screening for fetal chromosome abnormalities. *Obstet Gynecol* 2007; **109**: 217–227.

8 Wald N, Stone R, Cuckle HS et al. First trimester concentrations of pregnancy associated plasma protein A and placental protein 14 in Down's syndrome. *BMJ* 1992; **305**: 28.

9 MacIntosh MC, Iles R, Teisner B et al. Maternal serum human chorionic gonadotrophin and pregnancy-associated plasma protein A, markers for fetal Down syndrome at 8–14 weeks. *Prenat Diagn* 1994; **14**: 203–208.

10 Evans MI, Krantz DA, Hallahan TW, Galen RS. Meta-analysis of first-trimester Down syndrome screening studies: free β-human chorionic gonadotropin significantly outperforms intact human chorionic gonadotropin in a multimarker protocol. *Am J Obstet Gynecol* 2007; **196**: 198–205.

11 Benn PA, Fang M, Egan JF, Horne D, Collins R. Incorporation of inhibin-A in second-trimester screening for Down syndrome. *Obstet Gynecol* 2003; **101**: 451–454.

12 Ball RH, Caughey AB, Malone FD et al. First- and Second-Trimester Evaluation of Risk (FASTER) Research Consortium. First- and second-trimester evaluation of risk for Down syndrome. *Obstet Gynecol* 2007; **110**: 10–17.

13 Cleary-Goldman J, Morgan MA, Malone FD, Robinson JN, D'Alton ME, Schulkin J. Screening for Down syndrome: practice patterns and knowledge of obstetricians and gynecologists. *Obstet Gynecol* 2006; **107**: 11–17.

14 Hackshaw AK, Wald NJ. Inaccurate estimation of risk in second trimester serum screening for Down syndrome among women who have already had first trimester screening. *Prenat Diagn* 2001; **21**: 741–746.

15 Wald NJ, Rodeck C, Hackshaw AK et al. SURUSS Research Group. First and second trimester antenatal screening for Down's syndrome: the results of the Serum, Urine, and Ultrasound Screening Study (SURUSS). *Health Technol Assess* 2003; **7**: 1–77.

16 Malone FD, Canick JA, Ball RH et al. First- and Second-Trimester Evaluation of Risk (FASTER) Research Consortium. First-trimester or second-trimester screening, or both, for Down's syndrome. *N Engl J Med* 2005; **353**: 2001–2011.

17 Nicolaides KH, Azar G, Byrne D, Mansur C, Marks K. Fetal nuchal translucency: ultrasound screening for chromosomal defects in first trimester of pregnancy. *BMJ* 1992; **304**: 867–869.

18 Snijders RJ, Noble P, Sebire N, Souka A, Nicolaides KH. UK multicentre project on assessment of risk of trisomy 21 by maternal age and fetal nuchal-translucency thickness at 10-14 weeks of gestation. Fetal Medicine Foundation First Trimester Screening Group. *Lancet* 1998; **352**: 343–346.

19 Pandya PP, Snijders RJ, Johnson S, Nicolaides KH. Natural history of trisomy 21 fetuses with increased nuchal translucency thickness. *Ultrasound Obstet Gynecol* 1995; **5**: 381–383.

20 Cicero S, Curcio P, Papageorghiou A, Sonek J, Nicolaides K. Absence of nasal bone in fetuses with trisomy 21 at 11–14 weeks of gestation: an observational study. *Lancet* 2001; **358**: 1665–1667.

21 Prefumo F, Sairam S, Bhide A, Thilaganthan B. First-trimester nuchal translucency, nasal bones, and trisomy 21 in selected and unselected populations. *Am J Obstet Gynecol* 2006; **194**: 828–833.

22 Cicero S, Rembouskos G, Vandecruys H, Hogg M, Nicolaides KH. Likelihood ratio for trisomy 21 in fetuses with absent nasal bone at the 11–14 week scan. *Ultrasound Obstet Gynecol* 2004; **23**: 218–223.

23 Malone FD, Ball RH, Nyberg DA et al. FASTER Research Consortium. First-trimester nasal bone evaluation for aneuploidy in the general population. *Obstet Gynecol* 2004; **104**: 1222–1228.

24 Rosen T, D'Alton ME, Platt LD, Wapner R. Nuchal Translucency Oversight Committee, Maternal Fetal Medicine Foundation. First-trimester ultrasound assessment of the nasal bone to screen for aneuploidy. *Obstet Gynecol* 2007; **110**: 399–404.

25 American Institute of Ultrasound in Medicine. AIUM practice guideline for the performance of obstetric ultrasound examinations [Online]. Laurel, MD: American Institute of Ultrasound in Medicine, 2007 Oct 1 [cited 2008 Aug 18]. Available from: URL:http://www.aium.org/publications/clinical/obstetric.pdf

26 American College of Radiology. ACR practice guideline for the performance of obstetrical ultrasound [Online]. Reston, VA: American College of Radiology, 1990 [modified 2007 Dec 1; cited 2008 Aug 18]. Available from: URL:http://www.acr.org/SecondaryMainMenuCategories/quality_safety/guidelines/us/us_obstetrical.aspx

27 Pryde PG, Isada NB, Hallak M, Johnson MP, Odgers AE, Evans MI. Determinants of parental decision to abort or continue after non-aneuploid ultrasound-detected fetal abnormalities. *Obstet Gynecol* 1992; **80**: 52–56.

28 Schechtman KB, Gray DL, Baty JD, Rothamn SM. Decision-making for termination of pregnancies with fetal anomalies: analysis of 53,000 pregnancies. *Obstet Gynecol* 2002; **99**: 216–222.

29 Rauch ER, Smulian JC, DePrince K, Anath CV, Marcella SW. New Jersey Fetal Abnormalities Registry. Pregnancy interruption after second trimester diagnosis of fetal structural anomalies: the New Jersey Fetal Abnormalities Registry. *Am J Obstet Gynecol* 2005; **193**: 1492–1497.

30 Garne E, Loane M, Dolk H, et al. Prenatal diagnosis of severe structural congenital malformations in Europe. *Ultrasound Obstet Gynecol* 2005; **25**: 6–11.

31 Elias S, Simpson JL, Martin AO, Sabbagha RE, Gerbie AB, Keith LG. Chorionic villus sampling for first trimester prenatal diagnosis: Northwestern University Program. *Am J Obstet Gynecol* 1985; **152**: 204–213.

32 Shulman LP, Simpson JL, Elias S, Felker RE, Emerson DS, Phillips OP. Transvaginal chorionic villus sampling using transabdominal ultrasound guidance: a new technique for first-trimester prenatal diagnosis. *Fetal Diagn Ther* 1993; **8**: 144–148.

33 Jackson LG, Zachary JM, Fowler SE et al. A randomized comparison of transcervical and transabdominal chorionic-villus sampling. The U.S. National Institute of Child Health and Human Development Chorionic-Villus Sampling and Amniocentesis Study Group. *N Engl J Med* 1992; **327**: 594–598.

34 Brambati B, Lanzani A, Tului L. Transabdominal and transcervical chorionic villus sampling: efficiency and risk evaluation of 2,411 cases. *Am J Med Genet* 1990; **35**: 160–164.

35 Smidt-Jensen S, Permin M, Philip J et al. Randomised comparison of amniocentesis and transabdominal and transcervical chorionic villus sampling. *Lancet* 1992; **340**: 1237–1244.

36 Caughey AB, Hopkins LH, Norton ME. Chorionic villus sampling compared with amniocentesis and the difference in the rate of pregnancy loss. *Obstet Gynecol* 2006; **108**: 612–616.

37 Anonymous. Evaluation of chorionic villus sampling safety: WHO/PAHA consultation on CVS. *Prenat Diagn* 1999; **19**: 97–99.

38 Bravo RR, Shulman LP, Phillips OP, Grevengood C, Martens PR. Transplacental needle passage in early amniocentesis and pregnancy loss. *Obstet Gynecol* 1995; **86**: 437–440.

39 Eddleman KA, Malone FD, Sullivan L et al. Pregnancy loss rates after midtrimester amniocentesis. *Obstet Gynecol* 2006; **108**: 1067–1072.

40 Anonymous. Randomised trial to assess safety and fetal outcome of early and midtrimester amniocentesis. The Canadian and Mid-trimester Amniocentesis Trial (CEMAT) Group. *Lancet* 1998; **351**: 242–247.

41 Johnson JM, Wilson RD, Singer J et al. Technical factors in early amniocentesis predict adverse outcome. Results of the Canadian Early (EA) versus Mid-trimester (MA) Amniocentesis Trial. *Prenat Diagn* 1999; **19**: 732–738.

42 Buhimschi CS, Weiner CP. Medications in pregnancy and lactation: Part 1. Teratology. *Obstet Gynecol* **2009**; 113: 166–188.

43 Cordier S. Evidence for a role of paternal exposures in developmental toxicity. *Basic Clin Pharmacol Toxiocol* 2008; **102**: 176–181.

44 Anonymous. Misoprostol and pregnancy: risk of malformations. *Prescrire Int* 2008; **17**: 65–66.

45 Orioli IM, Castilla EE. Epidemiological assessment of misoprostol teratogenicity. *BJOG* 2000; **107**: 519–523.

46 Khairy P, Ouyang DW, Fernandes SM, Lee-Parritz A, Economy KE, Landzberg MJ. Pregnancy outcomes in women with congenital heart disease. *Circulation* 2006; **113**: 517–524.

47 Halperin R, Zimmerman A, Langer R, Bukovsky I, Schneider D. Laminaria dilatation and evacuation for pregnancies with midtrimester premature rupture of membranes: a retrospective cohort study. *Eur J Obstet Gynecol Reprod Biol* 2002; **100**: 181–184.

48 Grimes DA, Cates W Jr, Selik RM. Fatal septic abortion in the United States, 1975–1977. *Obstet Gynecol* 1981; **57**: 739–744.

49 Stubblefield PG, Grimes DA. Septic abortion. *N Engl J Med* 1994; **331**: 310–314.

50 Adler NE, David HP, Major BN, Roth SH, Russo NF, Wyatt GE. Psychological responses after abortion. *Science* 1990; **248**: 41–44.

51 Grimes DA, Smith MS, Witham AD. Mifepristone and misoprostol versus dilation and evacuation for midtrimester abortion: a pilot randomised controlled trial. *BJOG* 2004; **111**: 148–153.

52 Shulman LP, Ling FW, Meyers CM, Shanklin DR, Simpson JL, Elias S. Dilation and evacuation for second-trimester genetic pregnancy termination. *Obstet Gynecol* 1990; **75**: 1037–1040.

53 Lee SJ, Ralston HJ, Drey EA, Partridge JC, Rosen MA. Fetal pain: a systematic multidisciplinary review of the evidence. *JAMA* 2005; **294**: 947–954.

54 Peabody FW. The care of the patient. *JAMA* 1927; **88**: 877–882.

21

CHAPTER 21 Multifetal pregnancy reduction and selective termination

Mark I. Evans MD and David W. Britt PhD

LEARNING POINTS

- Multiple gestations, common with assisted reproductive technologies, carry substantially greater risks of maternal complications and perinatal morbidity and mortality.
- Multifetal pregnancy reduction is an intervention, usually performed in the first trimester, to reduce the overall number of fetuses in a multiple gestation.
- Selective termination is a technique, usually performed in the second trimester, to selectively terminate a fetus with a diagnosed abnormality.
- Techniques for fetal reduction and selective termination include but are not limited to injection of potassium chloride into the fetus or umbilical cord under ultrasound guidance.
- Women or couples considering these procedures may approach their decision with a medical, conceptional, or lifestyle frame.

Introduction

Three decades have passed since the birth of Louise Brown, the first *in vitro* fertilization (IVF) baby. Since then, more than 2 million babies have resulted from assisted reproductive technologies (ARTs). However, these success stories have come at a price. The twin pregnancy proportion, commonly quoted for decades to be 1 in 90, has more than doubled in the USA to 1 in 30 [1]. About 65% of all twins in the USA result from infertility treatments. Some IVF programs create as many multiples as singletons. Depending on the woman's age, from about 9 to 33% of live births following ARTs involve multiple fetuses [2] (Table 21.1). Furthermore, the data suggest that the frequency of monozygotic twinning per se, and as part of higher-order multiples, has continued to rise. This trend translates into dramatically increased risks of fetal anomalies, loss, and prematurity [3,4].

Although ARTs have permitted thousands of women or couples with subfertility to have children, their drawback of multifetal gestation remains a serious concern. Primary prevention of this problem through skillful infertility treatment is the preferable approach. However, when multifetal pregnancies do occur the techniques of multifetal pregnancy reduction (MFPR) and selective termination described in this chapter represent important means of secondary prevention (Box A). The overarching goal is to improve outcomes for the remaining fetuses, as well as the women who carry them.

Box A Terminology

Fetal reduction	A procedure performed in the first trimester to lower the total number of fetuses per se
Selective termination	A procedure, commonly performed in the second trimester, to selectively terminate a fetus with a diagnosed abnormality

Consequences of multifetal pregnancy

The number of pregnancies complicated by multiple fetuses has continued to rise both in the USA and other developed countries [5]. Major factors include delayed childbearing and expanded use of ARTs (Table 21.2).

Although multifetal births constitute a small proportion of all live births, they account for a disproportionate share of perinatal morbidity and mortality, primarily because of prematurity [6]. In the USA, multiple-infant births account

Management of Unintended and Abnormal Pregnancy, 1st edition. By M Paul, ES Lichtenberg, L Borgatta, DA Grimes, PG Stubblefield, MD Creinin
 ISBN: 9781405176965.

Age (yrs)	<35	35–37	38–40	41–42	43–44
Number of cycles	37,178	21,339	18,177	8,632	4,907
Average number of embryos transferred	2.3	2.5	2.9	3.2	3.3
Percentage of live births with twins	32.3	27.7	21.4	15.5	8.5
Percentage of live births with triplets or more	2.0	1.9	1.4	0.6	0.5

Table 21.1 Proportions of twins and triplets from assisted reproductive technologies, USA 2006 (Adapted from Society of Assisted Reproductive Technologies [2].

for approximately 17% of all preterm births, 23% of early preterm births (less than 32 weeks' gestation), and 26% of very-low-birth-weight infants (less than 1,500 grams)[7]. The probability of prematurity and related sequelae correlates with fetal number [1]. In 2005, the proportion of US live-born infants with low birth weight ranged from 9% among singletons to at least 95% among triplets or higher-order multiples [6].

In addition to greater rates of perinatal morbidity and mortality, infants resulting from multifetal pregnancies are more likely to have congenital anomalies and major long-term disabilities [7]. About 20% of babies with birth weights less than 750 g develop cerebral palsy. In Western Australia, Petterson et al showed that the rate of cerebral palsy was 4.6 times greater for twins than for singletons per live births, but 8.3 times greater when calculated per pregnancy [8]. Others calculated cerebral palsy frequency per 1,000 first-year survivors as 2.3 for singletons, 12.6 for twins, and 44.8 for triplets [9]. In a small series in a report of a questionnaire, Dimitiriou et al showed no differences between triplets and twins, but the sample size was too small to draw conclusions [10].

The risk of spontaneous pregnancy loss in multiple gestations increases with the number of fetuses. Data suggest that loss rates through 24 weeks' gestation are approximately 15% for triplet pregnancies, at least 25% for quadruplets, and 50% for quintuplets [11]. Some reports by perinatologists undercount losses because these physicians commonly begin to see patients in the second trimester, by which time many losses have already occurred [12].

Multifetal pregnancies also pose greater risks of maternal morbidity. Women carrying multiple fetuses have a sixfold increased risk of hospitalization because of pregnancy complications such as preterm labor, preterm premature rupture of membranes, preeclampsia, and placental abruption [7]. Multifetal pregnancies are more likely to require delivery by cesarean delivery and to be complicated by postpartum hemorrhage [7,13].

With increasing public, professional, and legal attention to multiple gestations, fewer embryos are being transferred in IVF [14]. The incidence of quadruplets and higher may be slowly diminishing, but the incidence is still too great [3]. Continuing efforts to reduce the proportion of multiple pregnancies resulting from ARTs are critical.

Year	Twins	Triplets	Quadruplets	Quintuplets & Higher Multiples
2005	133,122	6,208	418	68
2004	132,219	6,750	439	86
2003	128,615	7,110	468	85
2002	125,134	6,898	434	69
2001	121,246	6,885	501	85
2000	118,916	6,742	506	77
1999	114,307	6,742	512	67
1998	110,670	6,919	627	79
1997	104,137	6,148	510	79
1996	100,750	5,298	560	81
1995	96,736	4,551	365	57
1993	96,445	3,834	277	57
1991	94,779	3,121	203	22
1989	90,118	2,529	229	40
% change from 1989–2005	47.7%	145.5%	82.6%	70.0%

Table 21.2 Multiple births in the USA selected years, 1989–2005 (Adapted from Martin et al [1].

Multifetal pregnancy reduction

Demographics

Over the past decade, the pattern of patients seeking MFPR has evolved considerably [15]. With the rapid expansion of availability of donor eggs, the number of older women has increased dramatically. At our center, more than 10% of all patients seeking MFPR are more than age 40 years, and nearly half of them are using donor eggs [11].

First-trimester genetic diagnosis by chorionic villus sampling

Genetic counseling and diagnosis are an integral part of the process. By 2001, more than 50% of patients in the USA having ART cycles were older than age 35 years, and the proportion continues to rise. In the 1980s and early 1990s, the most common approach was to offer amniocentesis at 16 to 17 weeks' gestation. A collaborative series showed that fetal losses after amniocentesis were no more frequent than those for comparable MFPR patients who did not have amniocentesis (about 5%)[16].

Subsequently, strategies that combine MFPR and first-trimester prenatal testing emerged. Two approaches have been used: before and after fetal reduction. For the first 10 to 15 years, the approach we used was to perform the reduction first at approximately 10.5 weeks' gestation, reducing down to twins or triplets, followed by chorionic villus sampling (CVS) approximately 1 week later [15,17]. However, for patients reducing to a singleton pregnancy (essentially putting "all of their eggs in one basket"), we preferred the approach of knowing what was "in the basket" before reducing the other fetuses [15]. In these cases, we performed a CVS before reduction, usually on one fetus more than the intended desired number, as well as a fluorescent *in situ* hybridization (FISH) analysis with probes for chromosomes 13, 18, 21, X, and Y. Whereas about 30% of overall anomalies seen on karyotype are not detectable by FISH using these probes [18,19], the absolute risk of an undetected, clinically relevant anomaly is remote. Given both a normal FISH and a normal ultrasound including nuchal translucency (Chapter 20), the residual risk is only about 1 in 400 to 1 in 500. When a discrepancy exists between the FISH and the karyotype, the FISH is more likely to be correct [20]. Most women find this low risk acceptable when weighed against the 2-week wait necessary to obtain the full karyotype.

Our center currently extends this approach to all patients who are appropriate candidates for prenatal diagnosis, regardless of the fetal number. Over the past few years, more than 75% of our patients have combined CVS and fetal reduction procedures. A recent retrospective cohort study involving 758 MFPR patients showed no increased risk of fetal loss among women who had pre-procedure CVS compared to those who did not [21].

Procedures

Patients with desired pregnancies who are considering MFPR must weigh the risks and benefits of carrying all of the fetuses against those associated with reduction techniques. Because each option carries potential consequences, thorough nondirective counseling and informed consent are critical [13]. The ethical dilemma faced by couples and physicians under such difficult circumstances was appreciated even in the earliest reports of fetal reduction [22].

Techniques to achieve fetal reduction have evolved over time. In the mid-1980s, needles were inserted through the abdomen and maneuvered into the fetal thorax for the injection of potassium chloride (KCl). Alternative approaches included mechanical disruption of the fetus or fetal air embolization. Transcervical aspirations were also tried, but they generally were abandoned because of poor results. Some centers used transvaginal mechanical disruption, but data suggested a significantly greater loss rate than with the transabdominal route [23].

Today, virtually all experienced operators perform the procedure by inserting needles through the maternal abdomen under ultrasound guidance. For first-trimester fetal reduction, placement of the needle within the chest cavity suffices for success. Once the needle is appropriately situated, injection of KCl typically results in prompt cardiac asystole.

Outcomes

Several large centers in North America and Europe have aggregated their data. In 1993, the first collaborative report of MFPR indicated a 16% pregnancy loss rate before 24 completed weeks of gestation [24]. This figure represented a major improvement for higher-order multiple pregnancies. Subsequent collaborative papers have shown continued improvements. In the largest collaborative series of 3,513 MFPRs from 11 centers in five countries published in 2001, the loss rate at or before 24 weeks was 9.6% [15]. A recent analysis of 1000 patients undergoing MFPR from 1999 to 2006 at a single center in the USA revealed a loss rate of 4.7% before 24 weeks' gestation [25]. The outcome for triplets reduced to twins and quadruplets reduced to twins is now similar to that of spontaneous twins [15]. The take-home baby proportions for those who start with triplets (95%) and quadruplets (92%) represent dramatic improvements over the outcomes without fetal reduction.

In addition to reductions in the frequency of pregnancy loss, the risk of severe prematurity has declined as well. Both fetal loss and prematurity correlate with the initial number of fetuses [25]. Not surprisingly, the improvements in outcomes are greatest for those with the greater starting numbers.

Early data analyzed by stopping number revealed that the lowest frequency of pregnancy loss was for those pregnancies reduced to twins, with increasing losses for singletons, followed by triplets [15]. However, a recent study found similar loss rates for reduction to twins versus singletons at the same starting number [25]. The frequency of early premature delivery is greatest with triplets followed by twins, then singletons. Gestational age at delivery is also lower for higher-order multiples [25]. Birth weights following fetal reduction decrease with starting and finishing numbers, reflecting increasing prematurity [26].

Monozygotic twins in a higher-order multiple pregnancy pose unique challenges [27]. Provided the "singleton" seems healthy, the best outcomes are achieved by terminating the monozygotic twins. If the singleton is not healthy, then maintaining the twin pregnancy is the next choice.

New data suggest that reducing twins to a singleton may result in better pregnancy outcomes than continuing a twin pregnancy [25,28]. Most women requesting this service are in their 40s or older, are using donor eggs, and want only a singleton pregnancy. The number of experienced centers willing to perform two-to-one reductions is still limited, although some centers have as many as one-third of all reduction patients going to a singleton.

Selective termination

Both chromosomal aberrations and certain structural abnormalities, such as neural tube defects and cardiac anomalies, occur more commonly in twin gestations than in singletons [29]. Monozygotic twins are especially prone to defects of laterality such as situs inversus. Monoamniotic twins have an even greater incidence of abnormalities than do monochorionic/diamniotic fetuses.

Procedures

Selective termination of an anomalous fetus poses challenges different from those associated with reducing the overall number of fetuses. The overriding issue is terminating the affected fetus. Documentation of which fetus is affected can be easy in cases with obvious structural anomalies or a chromosome abnormality in discordant-sex twins. Identification becomes difficult when the defect is a subtle anatomic anomaly, Mendelian disorder, or chromosomal aneuploidy in same-sex twins. Such issues point to the importance of documenting placentation and fetal position when prenatal diagnostic procedures are first undertaken.

Great caution is required in the setting of a single shared placenta and possibly monozygotic twins. The risks of the healthy twin dying are increased under these circumstances [30]. Anderson et al reported four cases of neurologic damage in the surviving monochorionic twin after either spontaneous fetal death or selective termination [31]. Hence, newer methods of umbilical cord ligation and cautery were developed.

The techniques for selective termination have been consistent for nearly two decades, with most experienced operators using transabdominally injected KCl [11,15,22,24,28]. All of the percutaneous techniques require placement of a needle into the fetal cardiac chambers or the umbilical cord. Low-resistance blood return in the operating needle is critical to guarantee vascular access and the subsequent success of the procedure. We generally use a 20-gauge needle, which is positioned carefully above the fetal thorax [32], and use KCl directly out of the vial. Typically, 3 to 10 ml are used in the late first trimester; second-trimester cases can require more than 10 ml. Needle placement is critical, although some leakage of KCl into the amniotic fluid seems to be innocuous. Transvaginal injections of KCl and mechanical disruption have been used, but they generally have been abandoned because of considerably greater loss rates [23].

Outcomes

Data on second-trimester selective terminations are less extensive than those pertaining to first-trimester fetal reduction. However, the procedure can be successfully accomplished in most cases. Concerns include the risk of loss of the remaining fetus prior to viability, death or long-term morbidity of the nonaffected twin secondary to prematurity, and damage from disseminated intravascular coagulopathies or embolization from the decomposing dead twin.

Selective termination in monochorionic twin gestations

Monochorionic placentas invariably have vascular communications that link the circulations of both twins. If one twin dies, the other has a 25 to 30% risk of death and a 25 to 50% risk of severe neurologic morbidity if it survives [33]. Infant morbidity and neurologic handicap may result from hypoperfusion or thromboembolic complications in various organs, particularly the brain. Acute exsanguination of the surviving twin into the circulation of the dead twin through placental vascular anastomoses has been proposed to cause acute hypotension and irreversible hypoxic brain damage [34]. Thromboplastic proteins transfused from the dead twin to the remaining twin's circulation through these placental vascular anastomoses also could result in thrombotic damage to the liver, spleen, kidneys, and brain of the remaining twin [35,36].

Intracardiac injection of KCl is not an option in monochorionic twin gestations, because the agent could transfer to the nonaffected twin through the vascular communications. Alternative techniques have aimed at interrupting umbilical cord flow in the anomalous twin completely and permanently. If the occlusion is not complete or reopens over time, then persistent fetal-to-fetal transfusion or acute hemorrhage between fetuses may occur. Both conditions can cause fetal death in monochorionic twins. Vascular embolization, intrahepatic alcohol injection, laser and monopolar thermocoagulation, radiofrequency ablation, and fetoscopic umbilical cord ligation have been used to attempt permanent occlusion, but none has met with consistent success [32].

Societal issues

Although MFPR reduction has been integrated into infertility therapies, it will remain controversial because of widely divergent religious and ethical positions. Opinions about fetal reduction do not follow the classic "pro-choice/pro-life" dichotomy [11,15,17,24]. Most proponents see it in terms of the principle of proportionality (i.e., therapy to achieve the most good for the least harm)[37,38].

The debate over reducing triplets to improve outcomes is largely resolved. However, debate continues over offering fetal reduction routinely for twins, even spontaneous twins, for which the outcome has commonly been considered "good enough [28]." Data suggest that reduction of twins to a singleton improves the outcome of the remaining fetus [25,28], and we expect that requests for reduction from twins to singleton will increase in the years ahead.

Where controversial, high-anxiety decisions are concerned, patients treat these decisions as an ongoing part of the social reality that they are creating to live in and raise a family [39]. This reality-construction process is proactive, with couples aware of the potential consequences of sharing with others what they are going through. In a recent study of sharing strategies among MFPR patients, four patterns of information sharing emerged [40]. Selective strategies included:

- A *defended-relationship approach*, in which only the partner and patient know about the problems and treatments.
- A *qualified family and friends strategy*, in which information is shared only with those who appear to be trustworthy in terms of their reactions.

Two less selective strategies also were evident:

- *Both sets of parents* are privy to what the couple is going through.
- An *extended, open network strategy* that involves informing family, friends, and colleagues.

Women or couples considering MFPR may encounter various reactions from those they have told, ranging from support and compassion to opposition or even hostility. No sharing strategy completely avoids the risk of encountering negative reactions. However, informing patients who anticipate or fear negative reactions about the option of selectively sharing what they are going through may help to decrease their anxieties.

However, the social realities in which people live involve more than people; they also involve values, norms, and attitudes. These elements play a role in how patients frame the decisions that they make regarding medical technologies and procedures, including MFPR. Three general frames are evident [40]. The first, a *rational medical frame*, focuses on evidence regarding statistical outcomes. The commitment to factual analysis typically comes from patients' involvement in disciplines in which an appreciation of and trust in facts form a fundamental part of their disciplinary identity (e.g., engineering or medicine). Such women are more likely to want quantitative estimates of risk associated with different reduction choices. They will want to engage in a rigorous discussion of the data and their implications, even if it is relatively painful to do so. Women prone to a rational medical frame will be likely to choose a final number for reduction that maximizes the chances of a "take-home" baby.

The *conceptional frame* assumes that life begins at conception. For those opposed to abortion or reduction, a detached examination of the evidence is simply not possible. These facts hold no special moral authority and are not trusted in and of themselves. The patients' beliefs and those of the individuals and social institutions to which they relate have a moral authority as well. Such women will likely seek a balance that reduces their relative risk to acceptable limits. Unless the consequences are dire, they likely will not reduce at all or choose to reduce only to three.

The third is termed the *lifestyle frame*. For some women, the demands of career and existing children constitute powerful elements in their constructed realities. They seek to balance having a family with working, although the commitment to working is less than that seen among medical frame patients. Such women may choose reduction to two or even one fetus, depending on the number of existing children they have and the level of resources that the family has.

For women using a medical frame, reduction choices can be straightforward. However, this is not usually the case for women who must forge a resolution among potentially incompatible elements, as for women who are struggling to reconcile the potentially oppositional elements of certain religious beliefs with the risks associated with higher-level pregnancies (conceptional frame), or those who are struggling to reconcile the potentially conflicting identities of home and work (lifestyle frame).

Conclusion

Although fertility therapies hold important benefits for women and couples, they also increase the risk of multifetal pregnancy with its attendant maternal complications and perinatal morbidity and mortality. Ongoing efforts to reduce the frequency of ART-related multiple gestations represent the best approach to addressing this important public health problem. However, when multifetal pregnancies do occur, MFPR and selective termination are important means of improving pregnancy outcomes. Increasing experience with these techniques over the past two decades has substantially lowered the risk of pregnancy loss. Patients' decisions regarding these options involve multiple considerations and may be influenced by the lens through which they view the data. Practitioners can support women in these difficult circumstances by providing thorough and accurate information, nondirective counseling, and support, as well as excellent and compassionate medical care.

References

1 Martin JA, Hamilton BE, Sutton PD et al. Births: final data for 2005. National Vital Statistics Reports 56(6) [Online]. Hyattsville (MD): National Center for Health Statistics, 2006 [cited 2008 Aug 18]. Available from: URL:http://www.cdc.gov/nchs/data/nvsr/nvsr56/nvsr56_06.pdf

2 Society of Assisted Reproductive Technologies. Clinic Summary Report, 2006 [Online]. Birmingham (AL): Society of Assisted Reproductive Technologies, 2006 [cited 2008 Aug 11]. Available from: URL:https://www.sartcorsonline.com/rptCSR_PublicMultYear.aspx?ClinicPKID=0

3 Blickstein I, Keith LG. The decreased rates of triplet births: temporal trends and biologic speculations. *Am J Obstet Gynecol* 2005; **193**: 327–331.

4 Toledo MG. Is there increased monozygotic twinning after assisted reproductive technology? *Aust N Z J Obstet Gynaecol* 2005; **45**: 360–364.

5 Blondel B, Kogan MD, Alexander GR et al. The impact of the increasing number of multiple births on rates of preterm birth and low birthweight: an international study. *Am J Public Health* 2002; **92**: 1323–1330.

6 Wright VC, Chang J, Jeng G, Macaluso M. Assisted reproductive technology surveillance—United States, 2005. *MMWR Surveill Summ* 2008; **57**: 1–23.

7 American College of Obstetricians and Gynecologists, Committee on Practice Bulletins-Obstetrics; Society for Maternal-Fetal Medicine; ACOG Joint Editorial Committee. ACOG practice bulletin #56: multiple gestation: complicated twin, triplet, and high-order multifetal pregnancy. *Obstet Gynecol* 2004; **104**: 869–883.

8 Petterson B, Nelson K, Watson L, Stanley F. Twins, triplets, and cerebral palsy in births in Western Australia in the 1980s. *BMJ* 1993; **307**: 1239–1243.

9 Pharoah PO, Cooke T. Cerebral palsy and multiple births. *Arch Dis Child Fetal Neonatal Ed* 1996; **75**: F174–F177.

10 Dimitriou G, Pharoah PO, Nicolaides KH, Greenough A. Cerebral palsy in triplet pregnancies with and without iatrogenic reduction. *Eur J Pediatr* 2004; **163**: 449–451.

11 Evans MI, Rodeck CH, Stewart KS, Yaron Y, Johnson MP. Multiple gestation: genetic issues, selective termination, and fetal reduction. In: Gleicher SP, Buttino L Jr, Elkayam U et al., eds. *Principles and Practices of Medical Therapy in Pregnancy*, 3rd edn. Norwalk, CT: Appleton & Lange Publishing, 1998, 235–242.

12 Evans MI, Wapner RJ, Ayoub MA, Shalhoub AG, Feldman B, Yaron Y. Spontaneous abortions in couples declining multifetal pregnancy reduction. *Fetal Diagn Ther* 2002; **17**: 343–346.

13 American College of Obstetrics and Gynecologists, Committee on Ethics. ACOG committee opinion. Number 369. June 2007. Multifetal pregnancy reduction. *Obstet Gynecol* 2007; **109**: 1511–1515.

14 Corbellini G. Scientists, bioethics, and democracy: the Italian case and its meanings. *J Med Ethics* 2007; **33**: 349–352.

15 Evans MI, Berkowitz R, Wapner R et al. Improvement in outcomes of multifetal pregnancy reduction with increased experience. *Am J Obstet Gynecol* 2001; **184**: 97–103.

16 McLean LK, Evans MI, Carpenter RJ Jr, Johnson MP, Goldberg JD. Genetic amniocentesis (AMN) following multifetal pregnancy reduction does not increase the risk of pregnancy loss. *Prenat Diagn* 1998; **18**: 186–188.

17 Evans MI, Littman L, St. Louis L et al. Evolving patterns of iatrogenic multifetal pregnancy generation: implications for aggressiveness of infertility treatments. *Am J Obstet Gynecol* 1995; **172**: 1750–1753.

18 Evans MI, Henry GP, Miller WA et al. International, collaborative assessment of 146,000 prenatal karyotypes: expected limitations if only chromosome-specific probes and fluorescent in-situ hybridization were used. *Hum Reprod* 1999; **14**: 1213–1216.

19 Homer J, Bhatt S, Huang B, Thangavelu M. Residual risk for cytogenetic abnormalities after prenatal diagnosis by interphase fluorescence in situ hybridization (FISH). *Prenat Diagn* 2003; **23**: 566–571.

20 Evans M, Andriole S, Pergament E. Changing the paradigm: both FISH and karyotype should be routine for prenatal diagnosis. *Am J Obstet Gynecol* 2007; **197**: S167.

21 Ferrara L, Gandhi M, Litton C et al. Chorionic villus sampling and the risk of adverse outcome in patients undergoing multifetal pregnancy reduction. *Am J Obstet Gynecol* 2008; **199**: 408.e1–408.e4.

22 Evans MI, Fletcher JC, Zador IE, Newton BW, Quigg MH, Struyk CD. Selective first-trimester termination in octuplet and quadruplet pregnancies: clinical and ethical issues. *Obstet Gynecol* 1988; **71**: 289–296.

23 Timor-Tritsch IE, Peisner DB, Monteagudo A, Lerner JP, Sharma S. Multifetal pregnancy reduction by transvaginal puncture: evaluation of the technique used in 134 cases. *Am J Obstet Gynecol* 1993; **168**: 799–804.

24 Evans MI, Dommergues M, Wapner RJ et al. Efficacy of transabdominal multifetal pregnancy reduction: collaborative experience among the world's largest centers. *Obstet Gynecol* 1993; **82**: 61–67.

25 Stone J, Ferrara L, Kamrath J et al. Contemporary outcomes with the latest 1000 cases of multifetal pregnancy reduction (MPR). *Am J Obstet Gynecol* 2008; **199**: 406e1–406e4.

26 Torok O, Lapinski R, Salafia CM, Bernasko J, Berkowitz RL. Multifetal pregnancy reduction is not associated with an increased risk of intrauterine growth restriction, except for very-high-order multiples. *Am J Obstet Gynaecol* 1998; **179**: 221–225.

27 Yakín K, Kahraman S, Cömert S. Three blastocyst stage embryo transfer resulting in a quintuplet pregnancy. *Hum Reprod* 2001; **16**: 782–784.

28 Evans MI, Kaufman MI, Urban AJ, Britt DW, Fletcher JC. Fetal reduction from twins to a singleton: a reasonable consideration? *Obstet Gynecol* 2004; **104**: 102–109.

29 Bronsteen RA, Evans MI. Multiple gestation. In: Evans MI, Fletcher JC, Dixler AO, Schulman JD, eds. *Fetal Diagnosis and Therapy: Science, Ethics, and the Law.* Philadelphia: Lippincott Harper Publishing, 1989, 242–266.

30 Golbus MS, Cunningham N, Goldberg JD, Anderson R, Filly R, Callen P. Selective termination of multiple gestations. *Am J Med Genet* 1988; **31**: 339–348.

31 Anderson RL, Golbus MS, Curry CJ, Callen PW, Hastrup WH. Central nervous system damage and other anomalies in surviving fetus following second-trimester antenatal death of co-twin. Report of four cases and literature review. *Prenat Diagn* 1990; **10**: 513–518.

32 Evans MI, Rodeck CH, Johnson MP, Berkowitz RL. Selective termination. In: Evans MI, Johnson MP, Yaron Y, Drugan A, eds. *Prenatal Diagnosis: Genetics, Reproductive Risks, Testing, and Management.* New York: McGraw-Hill Publishing, 2006, 571–578.

33 Bajoria R, Wigglesworth J, Fisk NM. Angioarchitecture of monochorionic placentas in relation to the twin-twin transfusion syndrome. *Am J Obstet Gynecol* 1995; **172**: 856–863.

34 Van Heteren CF, Nijhuis JG, Semmekrot BA, Mulders LGM, van den Berg PP. Risk for surviving twin after fetal death of co-twin in twin-twin transfusion syndrome. *Obstet Gynecol* 1998; **92**: 215–219.

35 Fusi L, McFarland P, Fisk N, Nicolini U, Wigglesworth J. Acute twin-twin transfusion: a possible mechanism for brain-damaged survivors after intrauterine death of a monochorionic twin. *Obstet Gynecol* 1991; **78**: 517–520.

36 Pharoah PO. Cerebral palsy and multiple births. In: Blickstein I, Keith LG, eds. *Multiple Pregnancies: Epidemiology, Gestation, and Perinatal Outcome*, 2nd edn. London: Taylor & Francis, 2005, 807–816.

37 Britt DW, Risinger ST, Mans M, Evans MI. Devastation and relief: conflicting meanings in discovering fetal anomalies. *Ultrasound Obstet Gynecol* 2002; **20**: 1–5.

38 Britt DW, Evans WJ, Mehta SS, Evans MI. Framing the decision: determinants of how women considering multifetal pregnancy reduction as a pregnancy-management strategy frame their moral dilemma. *Fetal Diagn Ther* 2004; **19**: 232–240.

39 Britt DW, Campbell EQ. Assessing the linkage of norms, environments and deviance. *Social Forces* 1977; **56**: 532–550.

40 Britt DW, Evans MI. Sometimes doing the right thing sucks: frame combinations and multi-fetal pregnancy reduction decision difficulty. *Soc Sci Med* 2007; **65**: 2342–2356.

22

CHAPTER 22

Providing abortion in low-resource settings

Laura Castleman MD, MPH, MBA, Beverly Winikoff MD, MPH, and Paul Blumenthal MD, MPH

LEARNING POINTS

- Current abortion technologies, including manual vacuum aspiration (MVA) and medical abortion, permit provision of safe abortion in decentralized settings, even in remote areas.
- Flexibility in protocols for medical abortion increases its availability in restrictive or low-resource settings.
- Inability to offer tests or services that are nice to have but not essential, such as laboratory tests or ultrasound for pregnancy dating, should not impede delivery of abortion care in low-resource settings. Similarly, eliminating routine follow-up examinations can reduce the number of required clinic visits and thus increase women's access to safe abortion.
- Perhaps the most important step health care facilities can take to improve the quality of abortion care is to replace dilation and sharp curettage (D&C) with aspiration or medical abortion, as recommended by the World Health Organization.

Introduction

Low-resource settings are defined as those with inadequate infrastructure, commodities, personnel, finances, or other elements commonly integral to high-quality services. Facilities in such settings may be characterized by the lack of:

- Physical infrastructure, such as electricity, running water, and roads
- Medications, equipment, and other essential supplies, as well as the systems that support their availability (Fig. 22.1)
- Health care staff with the training, credentials, and experience appropriate for providing abortion services.

In addition, low-resource settings are commonly characterized by other factors that limit access to safe abortion care. These factors may include poverty, low literacy rates, legal restrictions, gender inequity, and social norms that stigmatize abortion.

Although the World Health Organization (WHO) does not recognize a "correct" level of health financing, some groups living within countries whose national governments spend less than about $60 per person per year on health "are unable to access health services from an adequately performing health system [1]." Few countries in Africa, Asia, and Latin America are able to spend more than $60 per person per year; in such settings, adhering to standards of practice recommended for wealthier communities may not be feasible.

This chapter is intended for health care personnel seeking to improve the quality and accessibility of abortion care while working within considerable resource constraints. We describe factors that influence abortion access and safety in low-resource settings, discuss specific clinical and health system issues relevant to abortion provision in such settings, and offer recommendations for clinicians and program managers.

Factors affecting access and safety in low-resource settings

Impact on access

Much variability exists in access to health care services among populations within regions, even in wealthy countries. For example, good diagnostic and treatment options may be available to individuals living in urban centers but not rural ones. Low-income and disadvantaged women have more trouble accessing abortion services and tend to present for care at later gestational ages [2,3]. Although medical and aspiration abortion are very safe, the risk of complications rises as pregnancy advances [3]. Thus, those who are most lacking in resources are subject to increased risk and cost [4,5].

Management of Unintended and Abnormal Pregnancy, 1st edition. By M Paul, ES Lichtenberg, L Borgatta, DA Grimes, PG Stubblefield, MD Creinin
 ISBN: 9781405176965.

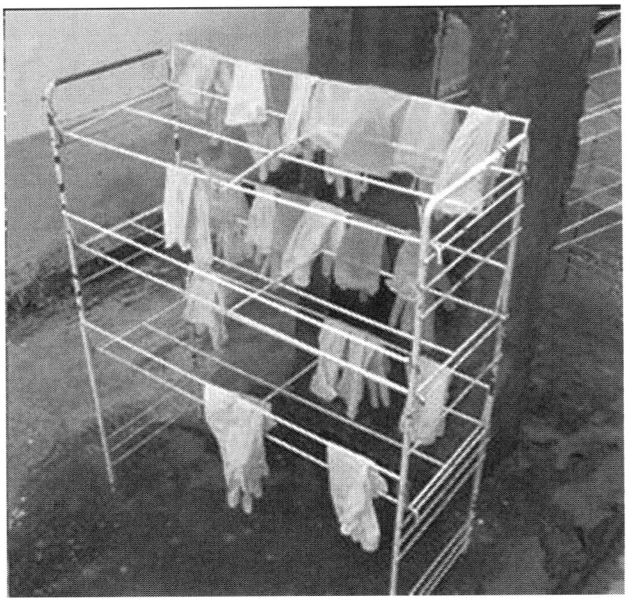

Figure 22.1 Gloves processed for reuse, Vietnam (see Plate 22.1).

Intangible factors such as the legal, political, and social environment also affect abortion access and quality of care. Restrictive regulations may compromise clinicians' ability to follow internationally accepted or evidence-based guidelines. National standards with ambiguous language about abortion can create obstacles when women do not know to what services they are entitled and clinicians do not know what they may legally do [6]. Health workers involved in abortion provision in remote settings often have limited opportunities for professional exchange. Medical meetings may be difficult to attend, and lack of support within the immediate surrounding community may inhibit networking with other abortion providers. Such professional isolation negatively affects morale and clinical performance [7]. Lack of social support for abortion or for women's rights can create additional barriers for women and clinicians. For instance, in settings where patriarchal values inhibit women's autonomy, a pregnant woman may not be allowed to decide for herself whether to have an abortion. Access to safe abortion services is even more problematic when the level of reproductive health knowledge in the community is low; women may not know what is available or how to ask for it [8].

Impact on safety

Whether caused by resource constraints, legal restrictions, or other factors, lack of access to high-quality abortion care harms women. The full extent of this impact is difficult to quantify because reliable information on abortion-related complications is often limited in settings with low resources or restrictive laws [9,10]. Researchers estimate that 98% of the approximately 20 million unsafe abortions performed globally each year occur in developing countries [11].

Complications from unsafe abortion contribute disproportionately to maternal mortality and account in part for the enormous disparity in maternal mortality ratios between high- and low-resource settings [11] (Chapter 2). The difference in maternal mortality ratios between wealthy and poor countries is larger than that of any other health indicator [12]. Complications from unsafe abortion in low-resource settings cause more admissions to gynecologic wards than any other factor [10].

These discouraging circumstances mask the fact that safe abortion can be provided effectively even in challenging situations. The following sections describe strategies used in a variety of settings worldwide to facilitate women's access to safe abortion care. Rather than being immobilized by a model of abortion care that is perfect but impossible to reach, clinicians can take small, achievable steps toward the goal of improving the quality of care. The WHO reinforces the concept that even seemingly small improvements in abortion care can yield significant results: "In most cases, minor adaptations of existing facilities, acquisition of minimal additional equipment, or provision of basic training can allow for services to be provided where none previously existed or can improve the quality, safety, efficiency, and capacity of existing services [6]."

Clinical considerations

First-trimester abortion

Abortion is safest when performed early in pregnancy [3]. Making abortion widely accessible, including in rural decentralized areas, enables women to secure services more easily and earlier. Current abortion technologies facilitate this goal, even in low-resource settings. The WHO-recommended methods in the first trimester are vacuum aspiration and medical abortion [6]. Ideally, a woman wanting to end her pregnancy should be given a choice between these methods.

Generally speaking, the simpler the method, the more accessible it is for women and clinicians. The medical system and patients themselves may be unable to afford tests and visits that are not essential. Most women seeking early medical or aspiration abortion can be safely treated using only clinical assessment, saving ultrasound and laboratory tests for the occasional patient who cannot be evaluated otherwise [6,13].

Medical abortion

Medical abortion can expand access to safe abortion care, especially in restrictive or low-resource settings that lack other safe options. This method enables women to avoid operating rooms, anesthesia, and uterine instrumentation. Using medications to induce abortion can lower costs and transfer control from the clinician to the woman [14,15]. Empowering women may be particularly important where large social gaps exist between patients and clinicians, as is often the

Box A First-trimester medical abortion success rates [17,18]

Mifepristone + misoprostol: 91–99%

Misoprostol alone: 77–93%

case in low-resource settings and where abortion is legally restricted and socially stigmatized [15].

When medical abortion is first introduced into a system, clinicians tend to intervene to complete the abortion more frequently than is necessary [16]. With experience, medical personnel become more comfortable supporting women during the course of medical abortion, thus enabling them to complete the process on their own. This "learning curve" is evident in medical abortion studies, with more recent studies tending to have greater rates of success [17,18] (Box A). The success rate drops as pregnancy advances, but even in the late first trimester, the rate of complete abortion is still high. For instance, success rates at 9 to 13 weeks' gestation approximate 95% with mifepristone and misoprostol and 85% with misoprostol alone [19–23].

Protocol options

Significant flexibility exists in the way that medical abortion can be provided, thereby increasing the likelihood that women and practitioners will find approaches that meet their needs. Mifepristone regimens are in widespread use worldwide, with numerous country-specific adaptations [17,24–26] (Table 22.1). Although many different protocols can be utilized to achieve high success rates, some confer specific advantages in certain settings. For example, nonvaginal routes of misoprostol administration may be preferable where a woman must maintain utmost secrecy about having sought an induced abortion, even in the event that she needs to seek emergency care from another provider. For women at 9 weeks' gestation or less, the following commonly used regimens achieve success rates ranging from 93 to 99%: mifepristone 200 mg orally on day 1, followed on day 2 or 3 by misoprostol 800 μg buccally or vaginally, at home or in the clinic [24,27].

Assessment and confirmation of completion

Although readily available ancillary tests may aid decision-making during medical abortion, mandating tests for all women creates obstacles if such tests are difficult to obtain. Recommendations for which tests to do should consider local resources and treatment alternatives.

In most cases, the patient's history and pelvic examination suffice to date a pregnancy [13,28–30]. For example, a prospective study of mifepristone and misoprostol in Albania used inclusion criteria of reported amenorrhea up to 8 weeks and clinical examination, with optional use of ultrasound [31]. This regimen was successful in almost 97% of cases. Exact dating is not necessary, as the medications are effective throughout a range of gestational ages.

For many women, the history and pelvic examination can also confirm completion of the abortion, particularly when the evaluation occurs no sooner than 1 to 2 weeks after treatment [13,29,32]. If this clinical evaluation is inconclusive, then clinicians can use ultrasound or pregnancy tests to avoid missing a continuing pregnancy. In the absence of ongoing pregnancy, intervention should be based on clinically concerning symptoms rather than ultrasound findings (Chapter 9). Endometrial thickness and echogenicity on ultrasound after medical abortion do not correlate well with patient symptoms, do not indicate incomplete abortion, and do not warrant intervention [33].

Table 22.1 Commonly used mifepristone-misoprostol regimens for first-trimester abortion (Data from Abuabara et al [17], Fiala and Gemzell-Danielsson [24], Cheng [25], Tang and Ho [26].)

Mifepristone (mg, orally)	Misoprostol (μg)	Where Used
600	400 orally	Labeled[a] in India, the USA, Tunisia, South Africa, France, and most other European countries
200	400 orally	Used in Tunisia and occasionally the USA
200	800 vaginally	Most commonly used regimen in the UK and Sweden, and used in the USA
200	800 buccally	Most commonly used regimen in the USA
200	800 orally	Marie Stopes International[b]
150 (repeated 25-mg doses)	600 orally	Most commonly used regimen in China

[a] The term *labeled* refers to what regulatory bodies have authorized; what is actually used in common practice may differ substantially.

[b] Marie Stopes International (MSI) is a global organization with clinics in many countries; the regimen here refers to that used by MSI in the UK.

Medical abortion protocols also can be simplified by minimizing the number of clinic visits. Researchers are investigating alternatives to the traditional clinic-based follow-up examination [13,29], including using urine pregnancy tests to confirm completion [34,35]. Although still considered investigational, semiquantitative urine pregnancy tests are receiving attention as a way to reduce mandatory follow-up visits after medical abortion; only women with positive results on a home screening test would require follow-up [35]. This approach already exists at Marie Stopes International UK clinics, where women having medical abortions receive a high-sensitivity pregnancy test to perform at home 3 weeks after the abortion. If the test is positive, a follow-up visit is scheduled; if it is negative, the woman's abortion care is complete. (Worsley K, personal communication, 2008).

Rather than requiring additional tests and follow-up visits for all, specialized testing can be targeted toward those who fall into a concerning clinical course. Usually, a woman undergoing medical abortion knows if she is experiencing a problem before the follow-up visit diagnoses a complication [36]. For example, women who do not have vaginal bleeding after taking misoprostol warrant evaluation for ongoing pregnancy.

Concerns have arisen about potential teratogenicity should the pregnancy continue after medical abortion (Chapter 9). No evidence indicates that mifepristone causes birth defects [17]. Misoprostol may be associated with a low rate of malformations; the absolute risk is estimated to be less than 10 malformations per 1,000 live births [37]. Concerns about teratogenicity should take into account medical abortion's high rate of effectiveness; the low but possible risk of birth defects should the pregnancy continue after taking misoprostol; and the fact that, because the pregnancy is clearly unwanted, vacuum aspiration is usually performed if medical abortion fails.

Regimen alternatives

Vaginal, oral, sublingual, and buccal routes of misoprostol administration have all been used successfully after mifepristone [26,38,39] (Chapter 9). Flexibility also exists regarding the timing of misoprostol administration after mifepristone, giving women options as to when they will experience the bleeding and cramping associated with misoprostol. For example, one randomized trial found comparable efficacy when vaginal misoprostol was used 1, 2, or 3 days after mifepristone up to 8 weeks' gestation [40], and recent studies suggest that even shorter intervals are effective (Chapter 9). Buccal misoprostol provided 1 or 2 days after mifepristone has been found to be equally effective and satisfactory as vaginal misoprostol through 9 weeks' gestation [27,38].

In settings where mifepristone is not available, misoprostol-alone protocols may be used to induce an abortion with success rates of approximately 85 to 90% [18] (Chapter 9). Although protocols vary, options through 9 weeks' gestation include:

- Misoprostol 800 μg vaginally every 6, 12, or 24 hours up to three doses [41,42]
- Misoprostol 800 μg sublingually every 3 hours up to three doses [41,42]
- Misoprostol 800 μg buccally with one repeat dose given 4 to 12 hours later. Although no studies have been published to date on this regimen, it is commonly used in Mexico.

Sublingual administration is associated with a slightly greater rate of side effects. For pregnancies at 10 to 13 weeks, not enough evidence currently exists to recommend a specific regimen.

Medical abortion also offers flexibility in where the drugs are taken and where the woman experiences the abortion. That misoprostol can be administered either in the clinic or in a different location of the woman's choosing enhances her ability to ensure privacy. The method also gives the woman the option of carrying out much of the process in her own home, which is especially relevant if she lives far from a clinic or has childcare or work issues that make being away from home difficult [17,43,44].

Medical abortion provides options in terms of staffing, as it can be administered and managed by nurses, midwives, and other trained personnel [15,17,45–50] (Box B). Trained midlevel providers can safely and effectively perform vacuum aspiration, the standard treatment for failed medical abortion [51–53], thus enabling delivery of medical abortion in decentralized areas that have few or no doctors. Manual vacuum aspiration (MVA) and medical abortion are complementary technologies, because the ability to perform MVA enables the practitioner to administer medical abortion more independently. Practitioners with MVA skills can treat most medical abortion complications privately in their own clinics, which is highly desirable in restrictive and remote practice settings.

Aspiration abortion

Historically, uterine evacuation was accomplished with sharp curettage, a practice that still persists in many low-resource settings. Repeated studies have shown that vacuum aspiration is safer, less expensive, and more acceptable to women than sharp curettage [54,55]. The latter also is associated with greater risk of bleeding, more pain, longer duration of procedures, and increased consumption of health system resources [6,56–58]. The greater risk of clinical complications associated with sharp curettage is a particularly important argument against its use at lower levels of the health care system, because some complications may require treatment that small rural facilities are not equipped to offer. The WHO recommends vacuum aspiration rather than sharp curettage for uterine evacuation [6].

Box B Integrating medical abortion services into the Tunisian National Family Planning Program [48–50]

Tunisia is the only country in North Africa with legal access to abortion. First-trimester abortion is available upon request in a range of settings, including public family planning clinics. Medical abortion was introduced in 2001 after a series of clinical studies demonstrated high efficacy, safety, and acceptability of mifepristone 200 mg and misoprostol 400 μg orally through 56 days' gestation.

The drugs were registered in the usual way as mifepristone 600 mg and misoprostol 400 μg orally to 49 days' gestation. Yet from the outset, 200 mg of mifepristone has been used based on evidence of its equal efficacy. Other innovations studied to improve access included sublingual misoprostol administration, extending medical abortion to 63 days' gestation, optional home use for misoprostol, and offering care via mobile clinics and in the private sector. In some sites, midwives are responsible for almost all components of medical abortion services, including pregnancy dating based on menstrual history and ultrasound, physical examination to determine eligibility, patient education, and follow-up.

Efficacy increased from 91% in introduction trials to approximately 96% in more recent evaluations, demonstrating the importance of provider experience and confidence. Repeatedly, women have reported high rates of satisfaction (about 95% in clinical studies), and most said they would choose the method again or recommend the method to a friend—including both married and unmarried women who, research suggests, have different motivations for selecting medical abortion. Women appreciate the method's discreet and noninvasive nature.

Despite limited availability of medical abortion in 2007, it comprised 30% of the almost 18,000 public sector abortions provided nationally. Where offered, medical abortion is selected by at least 60% of women seeking abortion in family planning clinics. To meet the growing demand for a choice of abortion methods and to reduce the burden on surgical wards, expansion of medical abortion is planned throughout Tunisia.

Contributed by Rasha Dabash, MPH

Studies indicate that manual vacuum aspiration is equivalent to electric vacuum aspiration in terms of effectiveness, safety, and acceptability for first-trimester abortions [59–62]. A systematic review of 10 randomized controlled trials involving 1,660 women who had first-trimester abortions with manual or electric suction found no statistically significant differences in complete abortion rates or participants' satisfaction [62]. MVA is particularly appropriate for rural and decentralized settings because the instruments used are portable, inexpensive, reusable, and do not require electricity [58,63–65] (Box C).

Clinicians performing aspiration abortion should identify products of conception (POC) after evacuation to ensure complete abortion and to rule out ectopic pregnancy (Chapter 10). Resource constraints such as no electricity for backlighting make this practice more difficult, but with creative problem-solving, products of conception can usually be identified. For example, tissue can be floated in a glass-bottom dish that is then held up to the window to provide backlighting. Placing the tissue on a sieve or cloth and pouring water over it often enables the sac or villi to stand out. Some clinicians mix the POC with sterile water, which lyses the blood and often accentuates that portion of the tissue most promising for villi. By placing such tissue on the back of a gloved hand for closer inspection, clinicians can often identify the sac or villi. Although the topic has not been formally studied, experience with MVA suggests that it may help the clinician to identify the POC after very early aspiration abortions due to less tissue shredding (Goldberg A, personal communication, 2008). When in doubt about visualizing POC after aspiration abortion conducted in a setting without ancillary testing, the provider should counsel the woman about the warning signs of ectopic pregnancy and the need for close follow-up.

Clinicians often worry about complications occurring if the patient does not have a follow-up visit after aspiration abortion. However, this visit usually occurs about 2 weeks after the abortion, which is past the time when most serious complications occur (Chapter 14). A review of the literature found no evidence to support a routine follow-up visit after aspiration abortion [36]. Marie Stopes International suggests that a woman undergo a follow-up visit after aspiration

Box C Bringing safe abortion to the primary-care level with MVA [65] (Iyengar K, personal communication, 2008)

In rural areas of Rajasthan, India's largest state, people are generally poor, with only a 17% literacy rate. Most cannot afford to travel to the city for care. Electricity supply is intermittent; there is no piped water; and, at the time of the intervention described here, most government health centers lacked equipment and trained providers needed to offer safe abortion.

A demonstration project at a private clinic run by Action Research Training in Health (ARTH) introduced MVA for abortion into this setting. The protocol consisted of MVA with ibuprofen and diazepam for patient comfort, along with strong verbal reassurance during the procedure. To decrease barriers to care, services were organized such that women received abortions on the same day that they presented to the clinic. Over the course of 4 years, clinic staff delivered safe first-trimester abortions to 534 women in this very low-resource setting while successfully implementing key elements of high-quality care such as privacy, confidentiality, infection prevention, and counseling. During in-depth interviews, women said they particularly valued the convenience and confidentiality of the service, including their ability to return home or to work on the same day that they had an abortion.

The clinics began offering medical abortion in addition to MVA once the appropriate drugs were approved for use in India. Between 1999 and 2007, ARTH clinics provided safe abortion services to more than 2,000 women.

only if she experiences a problem or otherwise wants to be seen [66].

Second-trimester abortion

Although many factors contribute to women needing second-trimester abortions, difficulty finding an abortion provider is a primary reason in both high- and low-resource settings [67–69]. Women participating in studies have described going from clinic to clinic trying to find care, as well as delaying abortion because of failure to recognize pregnancy earlier, difficulty deciding what to do, or logistical problems getting to the clinic (e.g., cost, child care, difficulty getting time off work).

Second-trimester abortion accounts for a disproportionate share of abortion-related morbidity and mortality [3,70]. The 10 to 15% of all abortions that take place after the first trimester cause approximately two-thirds of all major complications and half of all abortion-related maternal deaths [70–73]. Accurate, updated information on morbidity and mortality associated with second-trimester abortion specifically in low-resource settings is difficult to obtain, in part because many poor countries do not tabulate these data. Complications are more likely to occur when abortions are performed outside of the medical system or when recommended protocols are not followed. In one review from Russia, second-trimester abortion accounted for 6.6% of all abortions but 76% of all abortion-related mortality, primarily from so-called criminal abortions performed by untrained clinicians or in unauthorized settings [74]. Methods used included saline induction, sharp curettage, and insertion of various objects, including even a toothbrush.

This heavy burden of complications in the second trimester is preventable. When experienced clinicians follow recommended protocols, second-trimester abortion has a low rate of complications [6,75–78].

Induction

Very effective regimens have been described for induction abortion in the second trimester (Chapter 12), although variability exists in the literature regarding protocols, inclusion criteria, and definitions of success. Regimens are the same regardless of the resource level in the community.

In addition to misoprostol-based protocols, many other regimens for second-trimester abortion exist. For example, extra-amniotic ethacridine lactate instillation is being used in Germany, India, Turkey, and Vietnam [79–82]. Few studies have directly compared ethacridine lactate to misoprostol. The limited evidence available suggests that ethacridine lactate is relatively successful (93%) at inducing uterine evacuation but that it is a slow process, usually taking at least several days [81]. A study in Uzbekistan compared misoprostol to intrauterine hypertonic saline plus intravenous prostaglandin $F_{2\alpha}$ for second-trimester termination [83]. Both methods were effective (99 and 100%, respectively), but the saline approach took approximately 16 hours longer and was associated with significantly greater rates of retained placenta and hemorrhage. Patient and provider satisfaction was greater in the misoprostol group. In very low-resource settings that lack adequate means of infection prevention, misoprostol-based induction regimens are preferable to regimens that require intrauterine instrumentation.

Dilation and evacuation (D&E)

The technique of dilation and evacuation (Chapter 11) may be adapted for settings that lack laminaria and electricity. Cervical preparation with buccal misoprostol followed by evacuation with MVA and forceps was shown to be safe and effective for women seeking pregnancy termination at 13 to 18 weeks' gestation [84–86] (Table 22.2). If no means of cervical preparation is available, then induction may represent a safer option.

After a WHO assessment in Vietnam revealed that women had difficulty obtaining second-trimester abortions, the Vietnamese Ministry of Health supported introduction of this adapted D&E technique [86,87]. Subsequently, Vietnam also adopted misoprostol for induction abortion. These interventions have led to improved accessibility, safety, reduced procedure time, and resource savings. The D&E approach is also being introduced in Nepal, Cambodia, and South Africa. The ability to perform D&E safely depends on experience, training, and adequate caseload to ensure that providers have the opportunity to maintain their skills. If any of these factors is lacking, induction with medications should be used instead [6].

Systems considerations

In addition to establishing clinical protocols and options that facilitate access to care, the sustainable provision of abortion in low-resource settings requires attention to a number of service delivery issues. Following are selected examples of pertinent system considerations; numerous resources provide more detailed information [6,88] (http://www.ipas.org, http://www.pathfind.org, http://www.gynuity.org).

Preparing the site: Staffing and physical space

Facilities in low-resource settings may have limited physical space (Fig. 22.2). Nonetheless, health care staff should respect the woman's privacy throughout the abortion process. Speaking to the woman one-on-one before the abortion helps to ensure autonomous decision-making. If a room is not available for the entire process, installing curtains or other dividers to create a separate space can enhance privacy and confidentiality.

Space and staffing considerations are especially important for a woman undergoing second-trimester induction abortion; she requires a place to labor, rest, and expel the pregnancy. The woman will need to remain at the facility

Table 22.2 Sample protocol for D&E in low-resource setting, 13 to 18 weeks' gestation.

Before the procedure

1. Obtain medical history and perform examination (including pelvic examination).
2. Conduct ultrasound to confirm gestational age.
3. Provide woman with information on what to expect and obtain informed consent.
4. Administer misoprostol 400 μg vaginally or buccally 3 to 4 hours before the procedure.
5. When feasible, a nurse or other trained staff person should monitor the patient while waiting for the misoprostol to take effect.
6. Prior to evacuation, provide pain-relief medication.

In the procedure room

Doctor and assistant should maintain communication with patient throughout the procedure.

1. Wash hands, put on gloves, gown, and goggles.
2. Confirm that all instruments are ready including speculum, tenaculum, local anesthetic, cannulae, Sopher and Bierer forceps, suction apparatus (MVA with adaptor if necessary for 14-mm cannula, or electric pump).
3. Insert speculum, clean cervix, and apply local anesthetic and tenaculum.
4. Use dilators to check adequacy of dilation; if not adequately dilated, repeat misoprostol administration and wait for ripening.
5. Dilate cervix sufficiently to insert a 12-mm cannula for gestations of 14 weeks or less; use at least a 14-mm cannula for gestations past 14 weeks.
6. Insert cannula through cervix, attach aspirator, and remove as much amniotic fluid as possible.
7. Remove cannula and use forceps to evacuate tissue.
   - Always withdraw forceps with a rotary motion.
   - Avoid excessive traction against the internal os by re-grasping the tissue as necessary to reduce its bulk.
   - Complete most extractions from the low portion of the uterine cavity; avoid reaching high into the uterus to minimize the risk of perforation.
   - Open forceps in antero/posterior orientation just inside the internal os
   - Drop the handle of the forceps posteriorly, so that the blades are more anterior, consistent with the orientation of the uterus.
   - Use ultrasound if unable to rapidly (less than 10 minutes) locate and remove fetus.
   - If fetal parts such as calvarium cannot be readily removed, administer 400 μg buccal misoprostol and wait 2 to 3 hours. Attempt procedure again.
8. Evacuate any remaining tissue or placenta with forceps or suction.
9. Examine fetal tissue to ensure complete evacuation. Identify fetal parts and placenta. If any doubt exists about the presence of all fetal parts, confirm complete evacuation with ultrasound.
10. Treat fetal tissue discreetly, remaining mindful of patient and staff sensibilities.
11. Assist patient to the recovery area, where she should be monitored for at least 1 hour before discharge.

throughout the induction, which can last from 6 hours to a few days. Clinicians should provide care in a nonjudgmental way. In many sites, second-trimester induction abortion commonly occurs in labor and delivery wards, where nurses are used to caring for women with desired pregnancies at term. Values clarification work may help staff respond appropriately to women seeking abortions and minimize the possibility of their treating such patients judgmentally or punitively.

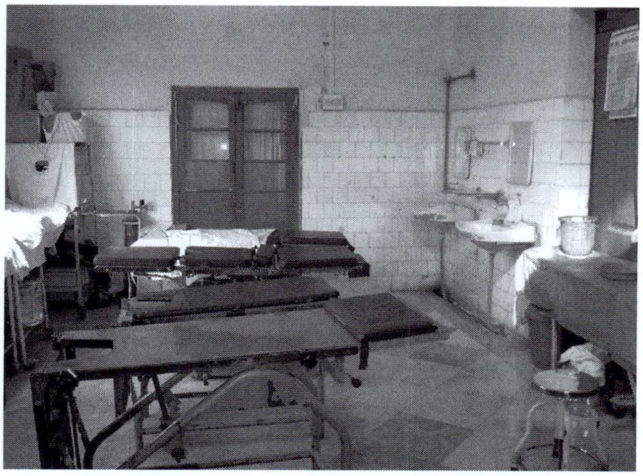

Figure 22.2 Procedure room in India. Note the presence of multiple tables because of lack of space.

Pain management

According to the WHO, "Providing adequate pain management does not require a large investment in drugs, equipment, or training. Neglecting this important element needlessly increases women's anxiety and discomfort and seriously compromises quality of care [6]." All health care facilities offering abortion should offer options for pain management along with verbal reassurance and support. During both medical and aspiration abortion, the following simple approaches improve the woman's comfort [89].

- A clear explanation of what to expect before, during, and after the procedure.
- Health care staff who are:
  - Calm, empathetic, gentle, and unhurried
  - Attentive to the woman, listen to her, and make her needs their first priority
  - Respectful of the woman's privacy and confidentiality

- ◦ Capable of conversing with the woman throughout the entire procedure (for vacuum aspiration), providing both a distracting dialogue and verbal reassurance.

Women having aspiration abortions benefit from a procedure room that is quiet [60,90] and not intimidating in appearance, preferably not in the operating theater. Cervical anesthesia helps to alleviate discomfort (Chapter 8). For both aspiration and medical abortion, nonsteroidal antiinflammatory agents help to decrease pain; some women prefer stronger analgesics.

Infection prevention

The temptation to cut corners when resources are scarce is especially detrimental when it relates to infection prevention. Effective infection prevention need not be costly or difficult. To minimize the risk of infection for both patients and health care staff, the following essential principles should be observed in any abortion-care setting:

- Proper processing of any items intended for reuse, which means cleaning followed by either high-level disinfection, in which boiling or chemical agents are used to inactivate all microorganisms except for some bacterial endospores, or sterilization through pressurized steam, chemical methods, or gas to eliminate all microorganisms including endospores (Fig. 22.3) [6]. New models of MVA equipment can be autoclaved [58].
- Handwashing or, where running water is not available, use of antiseptic scrubs.
- Use of "no touch" technique (Chapter 10), in which instruments entering the uterus are sterile and the tip of anything inserted through the cervix is kept from touching vaginal walls or other nonsterile surfaces. Clinicians can accomplish this objective by touching the handle end of instruments only, avoiding the vaginal walls, minimizing the number of instruments passing through the cervix, and by being mindful of where the cannula is placed. Avoid touching the tips of cannulas or forceps with gloves; instead, use a sterile sponge or gauze to remove tissue from the cannula or forceps.
- Proper waste disposal [91].
- Antibiotics are recommended at the time of aspiration abortion to decrease the risk of postabortal infection [6,92] (Chapter 14). However, lack of antibiotics should not be an obstacle to care; where antibiotics are not available, safe abortion care can still be provided.

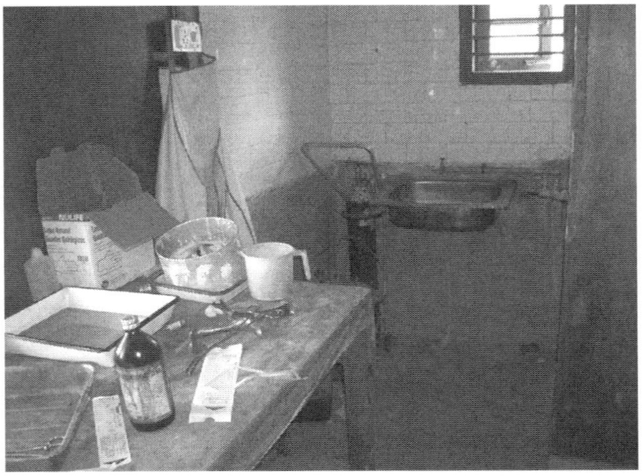

Figure 22.3 Instrument processing, India.

Contraception

Poor, marginalized, and less-educated women are at increased risk for unwanted pregnancy and abortion [2]. Contributing factors include cultural issues, such as myths overemphasizing the dangers of modern contraceptive methods and traditional and patriarchal values that inhibit women's ability to control their own fertility. In many low-resource settings, women have only rare contact with the health care system, making provision of abortion care a valuable opportunity for attending to contraceptive needs. Yet often abortion and contraceptive services are physically and administratively separated [58]. Most contraceptive methods can be started immediately after either aspiration or medical abortion [93] (Chapter 14). Making contraceptive counseling and methods available immediately after an abortion increases contraceptive use and helps prevent future unintended pregnancies and abortions [94]. It allows the woman to obtain contraception even if she does not return for a follow-up visit [36]. Integrated abortion and contraceptive services should be incorporated into health system planning.

Postabortion care (incomplete abortion)

When access to safe abortion is limited, a woman may resort to unsafe methods that result in incomplete abortion, hemorrhage, or infection [64,95]. Complications from unsafe abortion take an especially tremendous toll on already overburdened health care systems and facilities in low-resource settings. Ironically, almost all complications from unsafe abortion are preventable through access to contraception and safe abortion, which also are far less costly to provide. Liberalizing abortion laws and making safe abortion accessible reduce the stigma that drives women to seek clandestine and often dangerous services. Certainly, it is far better for women's health to prevent the problem of unsafe abortion than to treat its complications [10,64].

Postabortion care (PAC) is a programmatic approach to help women who present for treatment of incomplete abortion or other complications resulting from unsafe abortion. PAC consists of several elements [58,96]: uterine evacuation with appropriate pain management and emergency treatment, counseling to address a woman's emotional and physical health needs, contraceptive provision if desired, related

Box D Improving postabortion care in El Salvador [57]

El Salvador has limited resources and no indications for legal abortion, even to save a woman's life. In this setting, where many women present to hospitals with incomplete abortions, women were being kept in the hospital overnight after receiving sharp curettage in the operating room under general anesthesia. No formal connection existed between PAC and family planning services.

In a prospective nonrandomized controlled trial in El Salvador, 154 women presenting with incomplete abortion received either traditional sharp curettage services or MVA with local anesthesia and subsequent contraceptive counseling. MVA treatment with contraceptive counseling was associated with a significant decrease in cost, a shorter hospital stay, and greater contraceptive use after the procedure.

Researchers concluded that improving PAC services by introducing a clinic-based model, such as that facilitated by MVA or misoprostol, offers a good opportunity to simultaneously link services to contraceptive counseling and provision.

reproductive health services, and community partnerships to prevent unwanted pregnancies and unsafe abortion.

Ideally, a woman presenting for PAC should be given a choice between vacuum aspiration and medication for uterine evacuation. Vacuum aspiration and misoprostol, rather than sharp curettage, are preferred methods for uterine evacuation [6,54,56]. MVA and misoprostol are safe and effective for PAC and reduce costs to the medical system compared to provision of sharp curettage (Box D). A study reviewing results from 10 major PAC projects in public-sector hospitals in Latin America found that moving uterine evacuation services from the operating room into an outpatient setting substantially reduced resources used, cost, and length of stay for the woman [97]. Data from hospitals in Bolivia, Mexico, and Peru showed cost reductions ranging from 32 to 72% with the transition to outpatient MVA services for PAC. Eliminating most of the need for PAC by preventing unsafe abortion saves even more resources. For example, according to one model utilizing data from Uganda, offering safe legal abortion would reduce the cost per patient by an estimated 86% compared to providing sharp curettage for PAC in a restrictive legal setting [98].

Misoprostol for PAC is especially appropriate for meeting the needs of women in remote areas or other settings that do not offer vacuum aspiration [54] (Box E). Misoprostol is highly satisfactory to women requiring care for incomplete abortion. It can be safely administered to complete uterine evacuation using only clinical history and examination to assess women, without routine use of ultrasound [99,100]. Published studies support the following protocols for the treatment of incomplete abortion in women with uterine size of 12 weeks or less:

- Misoprostol 600 μg orally (one-time dose) [100–105]
- Misoprostol 400 μg sublingually (one-time dose) is a promising alternative but supporting publications are limited [101,104,106].

Success rates range from 90 to 99%[99,100,102]. Most studies confirm completion during a follow-up visit; in general, the woman should be seen no earlier than 7 to 10 days after misoprostol administration to minimize unnecessary intervention [101].

Sustainable supplies, medications, and equipment

Providing abortion services on an ongoing basis requires a continuous supply of medications and instruments, a task that may be especially challenging in low-resource settings and where abortion is highly controversial [58,107]. In some settings, low-volume markets and narrow distributor profit margins make integration into commercial marketing mechanisms difficult [58].

Menstrual regulation

In legally restrictive settings, options may still be available for women, including menstrual regulation. In this practice, women experiencing a delay in their menses are offered aspiration or medication to evacuate the uterine contents or, effectively, "bring down menses [108]." This service is extensive in contexts such as Bangladesh, a country where abortion is prohibited in most scenarios and an estimated 500,000 women per year undergo menstrual regulation.

Training

Ideally, doctors and midlevel practitioners learn to provide abortions during preservice training. These lessons can be supplemented by courses throughout the clinician's career to update skills and knowledge. For best results, in-service trainings should be provided to health care teams including clinicians, counselors, medical assistants, and managers from the same facility. This team approach facilitates the implementation of a new service, as trainees can provide ongoing support to each other. If one of the trained individuals must leave, other members of the team can work together to fill the void and sustain services. Training a team also increases the chance that the new skills will be passed on to other colleagues. This type of reinforcement may be especially important where abortion care is stigmatized.

Midlevel providers can perform uterine evacuation procedures safely and effectively in clinic settings, and they should be included as an essential part of the trainee team [46,52,109,110]. In a prospective randomized controlled trial in South Africa and Vietnam, 2,894 women received first-trimester MVA procedures performed either by a doctor or a midlevel provider; no difference was found in the rate of complications [53]. Midlevel providers should also be included in medical abortion training and service delivery [15,111].

Box E Introducing misoprostol for postabortion care in Madagascar [106]

A randomized controlled trial at a large maternity center in Madagascar's capital compared two different misoprostol regimens for treatment of incomplete abortion. Two hundred women were diagnosed with incomplete abortion on purely clinical grounds because neither sonography nor pregnancy tests are consistently available in such a low-resource setting. Women then received either 600 μg of misoprostol orally or 400 μg sublingually. Both regimens resulted in high success rates: 93.0% for the oral route and 93.9% for the sublingual route. These findings confirmed earlier results establishing the efficacy and acceptability of oral misoprostol [100,102,105].

Stakeholders were enthusiastic about the prospect of using a single-dose medication such as misoprostol to manage incomplete abortion and immediately realized the advantages of a method that could be provided by practitioners without surgical skills. With just minimal training, nurses managed most of the care from the initial visit to the follow-up assessment.

Study results underscore that misoprostol is a safe, effective, and acceptable treatment for incomplete abortion that can help expand postabortion care services in low-resource settings. In addition, establishing a reduced-dose regimen may have important implications in terms of cost and availability, especially in settings where resources are constrained. Madagascar's Ministry of Health has now incorporated misoprostol for incomplete abortion into official reproductive health norms and standards.

Training combined with follow-up after the initial intervention is an especially important educational approach in low-resource settings [112]. Clinicians who travel from isolated, rural areas to participate in trainings held in central locations may have relatively few support services to back them up when they return to their communities. Ideally, participants should achieve confidence and proficiency before leaving the training. This objective can be difficult to achieve in training courses characterized by inadequate time or in settings with low patient volume. Research and experience in other areas of medicine have shown that practice on simulation models is an effective way for trainees to acquire procedural skills before they perform them on patients [113]. The papaya has proven to be a low-cost, readily available model to simulate the uterus in trainings sessions on vacuum aspiration [114] (Fig. 22.4). Pelvic models also have been used effectively in D&E trainings in Vietnam [86], where trainees were required to show proficiency on such models before performing procedures on women. Trainees learning to provide medical abortion may benefit from interactive exercises, such as role-playing and discussing case histories.

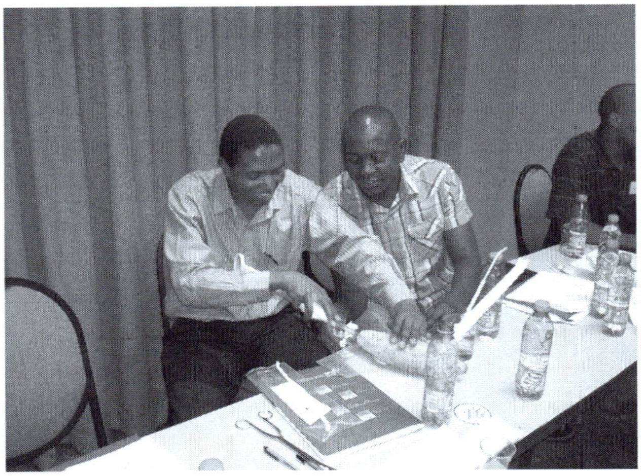

Figure 22.4 Trainees in South Africa learning vacuum aspiration on fruit used as a uterine model (see Plate 22.2) (Courtesy of Dr. Alison Edelman)

To the extent possible, trainings should mirror trainees' working conditions and the resources that will be available to them on an ongoing basis. For example, teaching that an abortion procedure is dependent on ultrasound is not useful if providers will have very limited access to ultrasound after the training. Trainers should also model other important aspects of service delivery during training, including showing respect for women seeking abortions, remaining sensitive to their needs for privacy, ensuring informed consent prior to treatment, and requiring that women receive treatment for pain.

Finally, efforts to implement and sustain abortion care benefit tremendously from involving local leaders from the earliest stages of a training-based intervention. Many low-resource communities are tightly knit, and community leaders wield considerable influence. Gaining their support in strengthening abortion services increases the likelihood of success [8]. Even one committed insider can make all the difference in implementing local strategies to improve women's access to safe abortion services.

Numerous resources are available to assist in the training efforts, including full training curricula designed to maximize women's access to high-quality care in low-resource settings [115–118] (Appendix).

Recommendations

In low-resource settings, existing health care funds should be used judiciously and in ways that favor simple, sustainable, and effective approaches [119]. Following are some general recommendations based on related publications to guide health care providers seeking to improve abortion care in the face of considerable resource constraints:

1 ***Decrease burdensome regulations*** [6]. Standards designed to ensure quality should not have the effect of confining services to high-cost, high-resource settings. Rather, standards and technologies should be adapted with the goal of making

medical and aspiration abortion available at primary health care levels and in communities that otherwise lack safe options [65]. For example, in South Africa a liberal law, the Choice on Termination of Pregnancy Act, initially required facilities to be designated by the central Ministry of Health as able to provide abortion services [8]. This centralized authorization process translated into a lengthy wait, ranging from 6 months to 2 years, before clinics could provide abortions (Trueman K, personal communication, 2008). The policy stood in the way of some sites providing services, thereby decreasing access to safe care in many remote areas where clinics had yet to be authorized [69]. Fortunately, a subsequent amendment to the act decentralized the authorization process. Similar processes occurred in India [65].

2 ***Limit exclusion criteria.*** Even well-intended exclusion criteria can hinder access to safe abortion care; demedicalizing services increases women's access [15]. For example, breastfeeding women are often excluded from receiving medical abortion despite lack of evidence that drugs used in medical abortion harm infants [17]. Small amounts of the medications likely do appear in breast milk, but providers can counsel women to consider discarding the breast milk for a short time after taking the medications rather than excluding them from services. Similarly, anemia is not an absolute contraindication for abortion; women with chronic anemia usually may undergo medical abortion or MVA safely as long as they have appropriate instructions for addressing heavy bleeding [17,120]. Women with fibroids, asthma, previous cesarean section, and hepatitis all may receive medical abortion [16,17].

3 ***Simplify protocols to facilitate usage.*** Simple, confidential protocols for abortion care are essential to discourage women in restrictive and low-resource settings from turning to private yet unsafe abortions [15]. Some clinicians believe that they are less likely to miss problems if they require women to be seen many times. Yet requiring multiple clinic visits makes the whole process more difficult and particularly affects the most marginalized women for whom travel distances, financial constraints, or confidentiality concerns may make multiple visits impossible [65].

4 ***Increase women's and clinicians' knowledge of indications for which abortion is legally permitted.*** In settings where the law governing abortion is liberal yet access is poor, many women and clinicians may not know that abortion is legal [65]. Even restrictive settings usually allow legal abortion for some indications [121]. Health system administrators, clinicians, and women should be made aware of the widest range of circumstances in which safe abortion care can be provided; additionally, women should know where services are available and how to access care. A study from a Latin American restrictive setting examining ways to reach women directly found that women considered physicians the most appropriate source for information about abortion; midwives, pharmacists, and women's groups were regarded as good referral agents but not providers of information [122]. In some restrictive settings in parts of Africa, community members themselves were active in developing initiatives in which trained religious leaders and groups used their weekly sermons to communicate relevant reproductive health messages, and community-based organizations reached youth at sporting events and other venues where young people gather (Daroda R, personal communication, 2008).

5 ***Emphasize decentralization of services.*** The WHO recommends that the following elements of abortion care be available at the primary-care level [6]:

- Health care workers trained to provide counseling on contraception, unwanted pregnancy, and abortion
- A broad range of contraceptive methods
- Medical abortion and vacuum aspiration
- Treatment for incomplete abortion
- Staff with the ability to recognize stages of abortion
- Prompt treatment or referral for abortion complications that are beyond the capacity of the facility to handle.

Providing uterine evacuation in clinic-based settings rather than hospitals is often less costly for the health care system and more convenient, faster, and more private for the woman [57,123,124]. In a clinic, the woman may be more likely to receive care from a clinician with whom she already has a relationship, a reassuring prospect to many patients [55,123]. Midlevel providers have been essential in decentralizing services. In Ghana, where physicians tend to concentrate in urban areas [109], midwives safely and enthusiastically expanded postabortion care and family planning services to rural areas, where the services were most needed. Medical abortion is safe and appropriate for use in even the most remote sites.

Some clinicians withhold medical abortion from poor or illiterate women, asserting that they are neither smart enough nor sophisticated enough to undergo the procedure safely [125]. One doctor in rural India said, "This method is not appropriate for rural women. They are less knowledgeable, lack awareness, and are not cooperative with the doctors. This method might be more suitable for educated urban people." Such attitudes and resulting practices are not evidence-based, and they restrict access for the most vulnerable women who probably could derive the greatest benefit from a safe and straightforward method such as mifepristone-misoprostol abortion. Even if women cannot read, effective communication can occur through picture-based instructions. Presenting patient instructions in a simple and straightforward way at the start of a medical abortion service helps to increase staff comfort with the method as well. Initial instructions that seem complicated only confuse patients and intimidate staff (Fjerstad M, personal communication, 2008).

6 ***Build opportunities for professional exchange.*** Networking enables health care workers to learn from each other about new techniques, problem-solve around shared challenges, and support each other psychologically. Clinicians working in remote areas or restrictive settings may lack networking opportunities, making it difficult for them to feel confident and knowledgeable in their practice. Although data specific to abortion is limited, the medical literature suggests several approaches that, where appropriate, can counter such isolation:

- Promote access to updated clinical information and peer support through online educational opportunities and communities; the Internet may provide a lifeline to virtual communities of practice [126] (Appendix). Disseminate interactive CD-ROMs, including videos from professional conferences, that encourage online interaction among practitioners [127].
- Create regional resource centers where health care workers can access current literature and interact with peers.
- Managers of individual health care facilities should explore ways to provide on-site support for abortion-care workers, including creating time and facilities for clinicians to network in such communities of practice.

7 ***Use data to improve quality of abortion care.*** To track both needs and results of program interventions in low-resource settings, abortion trends must be assessed better. Health facilities and systems should develop data collection and assessment systems to ensure adequate services for the population including safe abortion for all legal indications, treatment of abortion complications, and contraception after abortion [128,129]. One recommended guideline is to have five facilities offering each of these services per 500,000 people. Use of monitoring indicators, such as the proportion of women treated for abortion-related complications, enables health care systems to know if gaps exist in services and where specific strengthening is required.

Conclusion

Safe abortion services, which are legally permitted for at least some indications almost everywhere in the world, are essential to protecting women's lives and health. Providing this critical care is especially important in low-resource settings, where women are at the greatest risk of unintended pregnancy and unsafe abortion. In such settings, using resources in ways that favor simplicity and sustainability can improve access to services and the safety and quality of care.

Acknowledgments

The authors thank Rasha Dabash MPH, Ayisha Diop MPH, Sharad Iyengar MD, Elese Stutts MLS, and Merrill Wolf MA for their contributions to this chapter.

References

1 World Health Organization. Health Systems: Improving Performance. World Health Report 2000. Geneva: World Health Organization. 2000.

2 Finer LB, Henshaw SK. Disparities in rates of unintended pregnancy in the United States, 1994 and 2001. *Perspect Sex Reprod Health* 2006; **38**: 90–96.

3 Bartlett LA, Berg CJ, Shulman HB et al. Risk factors for legal induced abortion-related mortality in the United States. *Obstet Gynecol* 2004; **103**: 729–737.

4 Boonstra HD, Gold RB, Richards CL, Finer LB. Abortion in Women's Lives. New York: Guttmacher Institute, 2006.

5 Finer LB, Frohwirth LF, Dauphinee LA, Singh S, Moore AM. Timing of steps and reasons for delays in obtaining abortions in the United States. *Contraception* 2006; **74**: 334–344.

6 World Health Organization. Safe Abortion: Technical and Policy Guidance for Health Systems. Geneva: World Health Organization, 2003.

7 Held MB, Brann M. Recognizing HIV/AIDS volunteers' stressors and desire for support. *AIDS Care* 2007; **19**: 212–214.

8 Trueman K. Finding community-based solutions for overcoming barriers to safe abortion care in rural South Africa. *Ipas Dialogue* 2003; **7** (1).

9 Sedgh G, Henshaw S, Singh S, Ahman E, Shah IH. Induced abortion: estimated rates and trends worldwide. *Lancet* 2007; **370**: 1338–1345.

10 Singh S. Hospital admissions resulting from unsafe abortion: estimates from 13 developing countries. *Lancet* 2006; **368**: 1887–1892.

11 World Health Organization. Unsafe Abortion: Global and Regional Estimates of the Incidence of Unsafe Abortion and Associated Mortality in 2003. Geneva: World Health Organization, 2007.

12 Hill K, Thomas K, AbouZahr C et al. Maternal Mortality Working Group. Estimates of maternal mortality worldwide between 1990 and 2005: an assessment of available data. *Lancet* 2007; **370**: 1311–1319.

13 Clark W, Panton T, Hann L, Gold M. Medication abortion employing routine sequential measurements of serum hCG and sonography only when indicated. *Contraception* 2007; **75**: 131–135.

14 Fjerstad M. What does it cost to provide medical abortion? [PowerPoint presentation]. Seattle, WA: National Abortion Federation, 2003.

15 Iyengar SD. Introducing medical abortion within the primary health system: comparison with other health interventions and commodities. *Reprod Health Matters* 2005; **13**: 13–19.

16 von Hertzen H, Baird D. Frequently asked questions about medical abortion. *Contraception* 2006; **74**: 3–10.

17 Abuabara K, Blum J. Providing Medical Abortion in Developing Countries: An Introductory Guidebook. Results of a Team Residency at the Bellagio Study and Conference Center. New York: Gynuity, 2004.

18 Clark W, Shannon C, Winikoff B. Misoprostol for uterine evacuation in induced abortion and pregnancy failure. *Expert Rev Obstet Gynecol* 2007; **2**: 67–108.

19 Hamoda H, Ashok PW, Flett GM, Templeton A. Medical abortion at 64 to 91 days of gestation: a review of 483 consecutive cases. *Am J Obstet Gynecol* 2003; **188**: 1315–1319.

20 Hamoda H, Ashok PW, Flett GM, Templeton A. Medical abortion at 9–13 weeks' gestation: a review of 1076 consecutive cases. *Contraception* 2005; **71**: 327–332.

21 Ashok PW, Kidd A, Flett GM, Fitzmaurice A, Graham W, Templeton A. A randomized comparison of medical abortion and surgical vacuum aspiration at 10–13 weeks gestation. *Hum Reprod* 2002; 17: 92–98.

22 Carbonell JL, Varela L, Velazco A, Tanda R, Sánchez C. Vaginal misoprostol for abortion at 10–13 weeks' gestation. *Eur J Contracept Reprod Health Care* 1999; **4**: 35–40.

23 Carbonell JL, Velazco A, Varela L et al. Misoprostol for abortion at 9–12 weeks' gestation in adolescents. *Eur J Contracept Reprod Health Care* 2001; **6**: 39–45.

24 Fiala C, Gemzel-Danielsson K. Review of medical abortion using mifepristone in combination with a prostaglandin analogue. *Contraception* 2006; **74**: 66–86.

25 Cheng L. Medical abortion in early pregnancy: experience in China. *Contraception* 2006; **74**: 61–65.

26 Tang OS, Ho PC. The pharmacokinetics and different regimens of misoprostol in early first-trimester medical abortion. *Contraception* 2006; **74**: 26–30.

27 Winikoff B, Dzuba IG, Creinin MD et al. Two distinct oral routes of misoprostol in mifepristone medical abortion: a randomized controlled trial. *Obstet Gynecol* 2008; **112**: 1303–1310.

28 Mundle S, Elul B, Anand A, Kalyanwala S, Ughade S. Increasing access to safe abortion services in rural India: experiences with medical abortion in a primary health center. *Contraception* 2007; **76**: 66–70.

29 Clark WH, Gold M, Grossman D, Winikoff B. Can mifepristone medical abortion be simplified? A review of the evidence and questions for future research. *Contraception* 2007; **75**: 245–250.

30 Fielding SL, Schaff EA, Nam NY. Clinicians' perceptions of sonogram indication for mifepristone abortion up to 63 days. *Contraception* 2002; **66**: 27–31.

31 Bracken H, Gliozheni O, Kati K et al. Medical Abortion Research Group. Mifepristone medical abortion in Albania: results from a pilot clinical research study. *Eur J Contracept Reprod Health Care* 2006; **11**: 38–46.

32 Rossi B, Creinin MD, Meyn LA. Ability of the clinician and patient to predict the outcome of mifepristone and misoprostol medical abortion. *Contraception* 2004; **70**: 313–317.

33 Markovitch O, Tepper R, Klein Z, Fishman A, Aviram R. Sonographic appearance of the uterine cavity following administration of mifepristone and misoprostol for termination of pregnancy. *J Clin Ultrasound* 2006; **34**: 278–282.

34 Godfrey EM, Anderson A, Fielding SL, Meyn L, Creinin MD. Clinical utility of urine pregnancy assays to determine medical abortion outcome is limited. *Contraception* 2007; **75**: 378–382.

35 Grossman D, Berdichevsky K, Larrea F, Beltran J. Accuracy of a semi-quantitative urine pregnancy test compared to serum beta-hCG measurement: a possible screening tool for ongoing pregnancy after medication abortion. *Contraception* 2007; **76**: 101–104.

36 Grossman D, Ellertson C, Grimes DA, Walker D. Routine follow-up visits after first-trimester induced abortion. *Obstet Gynecol* 2004; **103**: 738–745.

37 Philip N, Shannon C, Winikoff B, eds. Misoprostol and teratology: reviewing the evidence. Report of a meeting [Online]. New York: Population Council, 22 May 2002 [cited 21 Aug 2008]. Available from: URL:http://www.popcouncil.org/pdfs/ebert/Misoterat.pdf

38 Middleton T, Schaff E, Fielding SL et al. Randomized trial of mifepristone and buccal or vaginal misoprostol for abortion through 56 days of last menstrual period. *Contraception* 2005; **72**: 328–332.

39 Shannon C, Wiebe E, Jacot F et al. Regimens of misoprostol with mifepristone for early medical abortion: a randomised trial. *BJOG* 2006; **113**: 621–628.

40 Schaff EA, Fielding SL, Westhoff C et al. Vaginal misoprostol administered 1, 2, or 3 days after mifepristone for early medical abortions: a randomized trial. *JAMA* 2000; **284**: 1948–1953.

41 Instructions for use—abortion induction with misoprostol in pregnancies through 9 weeks LMP [Online]. Washington, DC: Reproductive Health Technologies Project and Gynuity Health Projects, 28 July 2003 [cited 23 July 2008]. Available from: URL:http://www.rhtp.org/news/publications/documents/Miso%20for%20Pregnancy%20Termination.IFU.English.pdf

42 Faúndes A, Fiala C, Tang OS, Velasco A. Misoprostol for the termination of pregnancy up to 12 weeks of pregnancy. *Int J Gynaecol Obstet* 2007; **99**: S172–S177.

43 Berer M. Why medical abortion is important for women. *Reprod Health Matters* 2005; **13**: 6–10.

44 Shannon CS, Winikoff B, Hausknecht R et al. Multicenter trial of a simplified mifepristone medical abortion regimen. *Obstet Gynecol* 2005; **105**: 345–351.

45 Coyaji K. Early medical abortion in India: three studies and their implications for abortion services. *J Am Med Womens Assoc* 2000; **55**: 191–194.

46 Joffe C, Yanow S. Advanced practice clinicians as abortion providers: current developments in the United States. *Reprod Health Matters* 2004; **12**: 198–206.

47 Parrado R. Promoting midlevel medical abortion provider provision rather than ob-gyn provision. Presented 18th FIGO World Congress of Gynecology and Obstetrics, Kuala Lumpur, Malaysia, November, 2006.

48 Elul B, Hajri S, Ngoc NN et al. Can women in less-developed countries use a simplified medical abortion regimen? *Lancet* 2001; **357**: 1402–1405.

49 Blum J, Hajri S, Chélli H, Mansour FB, Gueddana N, Winikoff B. The medical abortion experiences of married and unmarried women in Tunis, Tunisia. *Contraception* 2004; **69**: 63–69.

50 Hajri S, Blum J, Gueddana N et al. Expanding medical abortion in Tunisia: women's experiences from a multi-site expansion study. *Contraception* 2004; **70**: 487–491.

51 Dickson-Tetteh K, Billings DL. Abortion care services provided by registered midwives in South Africa. *Int Family Planning Perspect* 2002; **28**: 144–150.

52 Goldman MB, Occhiuto JS, Peterson LE, Zapka JG, Palmer RH. Physician assistants as providers of surgically induced abortion services. *Am J Public Health* 2004; **94**: 1352–1357.

53 Warriner IK, Meirik O, Hoffman M et al. Rates of complication in first-trimester manual vacuum aspiration abortion done by doctors and mid-level providers in South Africa and Vietnam: a randomised controlled equivalence trial. *Lancet* 2006; **368**: 1965–1972.

54 Gemzell-Danielsson K, Fiala C, Weeks A. Misoprostol: first-line therapy for incomplete miscarriage in the developing world. *BJOG* 2007; **114**: 1337–1339.

55 Johnson BR, Benson J, Bradley J, Ordonez AR. Costs and resource utilization for the treatment of incomplete abortion in Kenya and Mexico. *Soc Sci Med* 1993; **36**: 1443–1453.

56 Forna F, Gulmezoglu A. Surgical procedures to evacuate incomplete abortion. *Cochrane Database Syst Rev* 2001: CD001993.

57 Koontz SL, de Perez OM, Leon K, Foster-Rosales A. Treating incomplete abortion in El Salvador: cost savings with manual vacuum aspiration. *Contraception* 2003; **68**: 345–351.

58 Rogo K. Improving technologies to reduce abortion-related morbidity and mortality. *Int J Gynaecol Obstet* 2004; **85**: S73–S82.

59 Dean G, Cardenas L, Darney P, Goldberg A. Acceptability of manual versus electric aspiration for first trimester abortion: a randomized trial. *Contraception* 2003; **67**: 201–206.

60 Edelman A, Nichols MD, Jensen J. Comparison of pain and time of procedures with two first-trimester abortion techniques performed by residents and faculty. *Am J Obstet Gynecol* 2001; **184**: 1564–1567.

61 Goldberg AB, Dean G, Kang MS, Youssof S, Darney PD. Manual versus electric vacuum aspiration for early first-trimester abortion: a controlled study of complication rates. *Obstet Gynecol* 2004; **103**: 101–107.

62 Wen J, Cai QY, Deng F, Li YP. Manual versus electric vacuum aspiration for first-trimester abortion: a systematic review. *BJOG* 2008; **115**: 5–13.

63 Baird TL, Flinn SK. Manual Vacuum Aspiration: Expanding Women's Access to Safe Abortion Services. Chapel Hill, NC: Ipas, 2002.

64 Grimes DA, Benson J, Singh S et al. Unsafe abortion: the preventable pandemic. *Lancet* 2006; **368**: 1908–1919.

65 Iyengar K, Iyengar SD. Elective abortion as a primary health service in rural India: experience with manual vacuum aspiration. *Reprod Health Matters* 2002; **10**: 54–63.

66 Marie Stopes International. Marie Stopes International Partnership Manual, Clinical Standards—Section 5. August, 2006.

67 Drey EA, Foster DG, Jackson RA, Lee SJ, Cardenas LH, Darney PD. Risk factors associated with presenting for abortion in the second trimester. *Obstet Gynecol* 2006; **107**: 128–135.

68 Gallo MF, Nghia NC. Real life is different: a qualitative study of why women delay abortion until the second trimester in Vietnam. *Soc Sci Med* 2007; **64**: 1812–1822.

69 Harries J, Orner P, Gabriel M, Mitchell E. Delays in seeking abortion until the second trimester: a qualitative study in South Africa. *Reprod Health* 2007; **4**: 7.

70 World Health Organization. Medical Methods for Termination of Pregnancy. Report of a WHO Scientific Group. Geneva: World Health Organization Technical Report Series, 1997: 871.

71 Tietze C. Induced Abortion: A World Review. New York: Population Council, 1981.

72 Democratic Nursing Organisation of South Africa. Memorandum on the implementation of the Choice of Termination of Pregnancy Act, Act 92 of 1996 [Online]. Denosa, South Africa: Democratic Nursing Organisation of South Africa, 7 Jun 2000 [cited 15 Jul 2008]. Available from: URL:http://www.pmg.org.za/docs/2000/appendices/000607DENOSA.htm

73 Ho PC, Blumenthal PD, Gemzell-Danielsson K, Gomez PLR, Mittal S, Tang OS. Misoprostol for the termination of pregnancy with a live fetus at 13–26 weeks. *Int J Gynaecol Obstet* 2007; **99**: S178–S181.

74 Zhirova IA, Frolova OG, Astakhova TM, Ketting E. Abortion-related maternal mortality in the Russian federation. *Stud Fam Plann* 2004; **35**: 178–188.

75 Grimes DA, Schulz KF. Morbidity and mortality from second-trimester abortions. *J Reprod Med* 1985; **30**: 505–514.

76 Autry AM, Hayes EC, Jacobson GF, Kirby RS. A comparison of medical induction and dilation and evacuation for second-trimester abortion. *Am J Obstet Gynecol* 2002; **187**: 393–397.

77 Ashok PW, Templeton A, Wagaarachchi P, Flett G. Midtrimester medical termination of pregnancy: a review of 1002 consecutive cases. *Contraception* 2004; **69**: 51–58.

78 Lohr PA, Hayes JL, Gemzell-Danielsson K. Surgical versus medical methods for second trimester induced abortion (review). *Cochrane Database of Syst Rev* 2008; **1**: CD006714.

79 Järnbert A, Klang B, Vinh NT, Ham NN. Comparative study of cervical laminar tents prior to extra-amniotic injection of ethacridine lactate (Rivanol) and a condom-nelathon catheter method for second-trimester pregnancy interruption in Vietnam. *Gynecol Obstet Invest* 1999; **48**: 113–118.

80 Kelekci S, Erdemoglu E, Inan I. Randomized study on the effect of adding oxytocin to ethacridine lactate or misoprostol for second-trimester termination of pregnancy. *Acta Obstet Gynecol Scand* 2006; **85**: 825–829.

81 Berg C, Ludwig M, Sturm N, Diedrich K, Gembruch U, Geipel A. Intraamniotic ethacridine lactate instillation versus vaginal PGE1 in second trimester termination of pregnancy. *Eur J Obstet Gynecol Reprod Biol* 2006; **126**: 193–196.

82 Malhotra N, Chanana C. Silent rupture of unscarred uterus: an unusual presentation at second trimester abortion. *Arch Gynecol Obstet* 2007; **275**: 283–285.

83 Kapp N, Todd CS, Yadgarova KT et al. A randomized comparison of misoprostol to intrauterine instillation of hypertonic saline plus a prostaglandin F2alpha analogue for

second-trimester induction termination in Uzbekistan. *Contraception* 2007; **76**: 461–466.

84 Todd CS, Soler M, Castleman L, Rogers MK, Blumenthal PD. Buccal misoprostol as cervical preparation for second trimester pregnancy termination. *Contraception* 2002; **65**: 415–418.

85 Todd CS, Soler ME, Castleman L, Rogers MK, Blumenthal PD. Manual vacuum aspiration for second-trimester pregnancy termination. *Int J Gynaecol Obstet* 2003; **83**: 5–9.

86 Castleman LD, Oanh KT, Hyman AG, Thuy le T, Blumenthal PD. Introduction of the dilation and evacuation procedure for second-trimester abortion in Vietnam using manual vacuum aspiration and buccal misoprostol. *Contraception* 2006; **74**: 272–276.

87 World Health Organization. Abortion in Viet Nam: An Assessment of Policy, Programme and Research Issues. Geneva: World Health Organization, 1999.

88 Berwick DM. Lessons from developing nations on improving health care. *BMJ* 2004; **8**: 1124–1129.

89 Castleman L, Mann C. Manual Vacuum Aspiration for Uterine Evacuation: Pain Management. Chapel Hill, NC: Ipas, 2002.

90 Bird ST, Harvey M, Nichols MD, Edelman A. Comparing the acceptability of manual vacuum aspiration and electric vacuum aspiration as methods of early abortion. *JAMA* 2001; **56**: 124–126.

91 Tietjen L, Dossemeyer D, McIntosh N. Infection Prevention: Guidelines for Healthcare Facilities with Limited Resources. Baltimore, MD: JHPIEGO, 2003.

92 Sawaya GF, Grady D, Kerlikowske K, Grimes DA. Antibiotics at the time of induced abortion: the case for universal prophylaxis based on a meta-analysis. *Obstet Gynecol* 1996; **87**: 884–890.

93 World Health Organization. Medical Eligibility Criteria for Contraceptive Use, 3rd edn. Geneva: World Health Organization, 2004.

94 Johnson BR, Ndhlovu S, Farr S, Chipato T. Reducing unplanned pregnancy and abortion in Zimbabwe through postabortion contraception. *Stud Fam Plann* 2002; **33**: 195–202.

95 Berer M. National laws and unsafe abortion: the parameters of change. *Reprod Health Matters* 2004; **12**: 1–8.

96 Corbett MR, Turner KL. Essential elements of postabortion care: origins, evolution and future directions. *Int Fam Plann Perspect* 2003; **29**: 106–111.

97 Billings D, Benson J. Postabortion care in Latin America: policy and service recommendations from a decade of operations research. *Health Policy Plan* 2005; **20**: 158–166.

98 Johnston HB, Gallo MF, Benson J. Reducing the costs to health systems of unsafe abortion: a comparison of four strategies. *J Fam Plann Reprod Health Care* 2007; **33**: 250–257.

99 Bique C, Usta M, Debora B, Chong E, Westheimer E, Winikoff B. Comparison of misoprostol and manual vacuum aspiration for the treatment of incomplete abortion. *Int J Gynaecol Obstet* 2007; **98**: 222–226.

100 Shwekerela B, Kalumuna R, Kipingili R et al. Misoprostol for treatment of incomplete abortion at the regional hospital level: results from Tanzania. *BJOG* 2007; **114**: 1363–1367.

101 Blum J, Winikoff B, Gemzell-Danielsson K, Ho PC, Schiavon R, Weeks A. Treatment of incomplete abortion and miscarriage with misoprostol. *Int J Gynaecol Obstet* 2007; **99**: S186–S189.

102 Dao B, Blum J, Thieba B et al. Is misoprostol a safe, effective and acceptable alternative to manual vacuum aspiration for postabortion care? Results from a randomized trial in Burkina Faso, West Africa. *BJOG* 2007; **114**: 1368–1375.

103 Nguyen NT, Blum J, Durocher J, Quan TTV, Winikoff B. A randomized controlled study comparing 600 versus 1200 μg oral misoprostol for the medical management of incomplete abortion. *Contraception* 2005; **72**: 438–442.

104 Rizzi RG. Capitulo 5. Tratamiento del aborto incompleto. In: Faúndes A, ed. Uso de Misoprostol en Obstetricia y Ginecología, 2nd edn. Santa Cruz de la Sierra, Bolivia: FLASOG, 2007.

105 Weeks A, Alia G, Blum J et al. A randomized trial of oral misoprostol versus manual vacuum aspiration for the treatment of incomplete abortion. *Obstet Gynecol* 2005; **106**: 540–547.

106 Diop A, Raghavan S, Rakotovao J, Comendant R, Blumenthal P, Winikoff B. Two routes of administration for misoprostol in the treatment of incomplete abortion: a randomized clinical trial. *Contraception*, in press.

107 Abernathy M. Planning for a Sustainable Supply of Manual Vacuum Aspiration Instruments: A Guide for Program Managers, 2nd edn. Chapel Hill, NC: Ipas, 2007.

108 Chowdhury SNM, Moni D. Situation analysis of the menstrual regulation programme in Bangladesh. *Reprod Health Matters* 2004; **12**: 95–104.

109 Billings DL, Ankrah V, Baird TL, Taylor JE, Ababio KPP, Ntow S. Midwives and comprehensive postabortion care in Ghana. In: Huntington D, Piet-Pelon NJ, eds. Postabortion Care: Lessons from Operations Research. New York: Population Council, 1999.

110 Wolf M. Deciding women's lives are worth saving: expanding the role of midlevel providers in safe abortion care. Issues in abortion care 7. Chapel Hill, NC: Ipas and IHCAR, 2002.

111 Swedish Board of Health and Welfare. Medicinska aborter, fördelning av arbetsuppgifter—praxis och regelverk [Online], 2008 [cited 15 Jul 2008]. Available from: URL:http://www.socialstyrelsen.se/NR/rdonlyres/E9BD5EC0-D272-40DF-AC76-623068B400AE/9503/20081032.pdf

112 Rowe AK, de Savigny D, Lanata CF, Victora CG. How can we achieve and maintain high-quality performance of health workers in low-resource settings? *Lancet* 2005; **366**: 1026–1035.

113 Ziv A, Wolpe PR, Small SD, Glick S. Simulation-based medical education: an ethical imperative. *Acad Med* 2003; **78**: 783–788.

114 Paul M, Nobel K. Papaya: a simulation model for training in uterine aspiration. *Fam Med* 2005; **37**: 242–244.

115 Hyman AG, Castleman L. Woman-centered abortion care: reference manual [Online]. Chapel Hill, NC: Ipas, 2005 [cited 15 Jul 2008]. Available from: URL:http://www.ipas.org./Publications/Woman-centered_abortion_care_Reference_manual.aspx

116 Hyman AG, McInerney T, Turner K. Woman-centered abortion care: trainer's manual [Online]. Chapel Hill, NC: Ipas, 2005 [cited 15 Jul 2008]. Available from: URL:http://www.ipas.org./

Publications/Woman-centered_abortion_care_Trainers_manual.aspx

117 Turner K, McInerney T, Herrick J. Woman-centered postabortion care: trainer's manual. Chapel Hill, NC: Ipas, 2004 [cited 15 Jul 2008]. Available from: URL:http://www.ipas.org./Publications/Woman-centered_postabortion_care_Trainers_manual.aspx

118 Herrick J, Turner K, McInerney T, Castleman L. Woman-centered postabortion care: reference manual. Chapel Hill, NC: Ipas, 2004 [cited 15 Jul 2008]. Available from: URL:http://www.ipas.org./Publications/Woman-centered_postabortion_care_Reference_manual.aspx

119 Anderson BO. Guidelines for limited resource settings. In: Bridging the gap: transforming knowledge into action. Washington, DC, 2006 [cited 15 Jul 2008]. Available from: URL: http://2006.confex.com/uicc/uicc/techprogram/P278.HTM.

120 Harper C, Winikoff B, Ellertson C, Coyaji K. Blood loss with mifepristone–misoprostol abortion: measures from a trial in China, Cuba and India. *Int J Gynaecol Obstet* 1998; **63**: 39–49.

121 Cook R, Dickens B, Fathalla M. Reproductive Health and Human Rights. New York: Oxford University Press, 2003.

122 Cohen J, Ortiz O, Llaguno SE, Goodyear L, Billings D, Martinez I. Reaching women with instructions on misoprostol use in a Latin American country. *Reprod Health Matters* 2005; **13**: 84–92.

123 Dalton VK, Castleman L. Manual vacuum aspiration for treatment for early pregnancy loss. *Postgraduate Obstetrics and Gynecology* 2002; **22**: 19.

124 Dalton VK, Harris L, Weisman CS, Guire K, Castleman L, Lebovic D. Patient preferences, satisfaction, and resource use in office evacuation of early pregnancy failure. *Obstet Gynecol* 2006; **108**: 103–110.

125 Ramachandar L, Pelto PJ. Medical abortion in rural Tamil Nadu, South India: a quiet transformation. *Reprod Health Matters* 2005; **13**: 54–64.

126 Nagy P, Kahn CE Jr, Boonn W et al. Building virtual communities of practice. *J Am Coll Radiol* 2006; **3**: 716–720.

127 Kurzydlo AM, Casson C, Shumack S. Reducing professional isolation: Support Scheme for Rural Specialists. *Australas J Dermatol* 2005; **46**: 242–245.

128 Healy J, Otsea K, Benson J. Counting abortions so that abortion counts: indicators for monitoring the availability and use of abortion care services. *Int J Gynaecol Obstet* 2006; **95**: 209–220.

129 Setel PW, Macfarlane SB, Szreter S et al. Monitoring of vital events. A scandal of invisibility: making everyone count by counting everyone. *Lancet* 2007; **370**: 1569–1577.

23

CHAPTER 23

Ensuring quality care in abortion services

Beth Kruse MS, CNM, ARNP and Carla Eckhardt CPHQ

LEARNING POINTS

- The broader health care quality movement informs the pursuit of excellence in abortion care.
- The Institute of Medicine's "Six Aims for Quality in Health Care" can be applied to the process of developing a quality management program for abortion services; namely, care should be safe, effective, timely, patient-centered, efficient, and equitable.
- A quality management program includes the following broad areas of oversight: structure and environment, equipment and technologies, processes, and people.
- Quality management methodology is designed to identify opportunities and implement measures to reduce patient complications and improve satisfaction with care. A number of methods are available to analyze quality indicators, including sentinel-event indicators, rate-based indicators, process measures, and outcome indicators.
- The integration of quality management resources into the clinical setting will help facilities meet and maintain standards that are subject to professional and government regulation.

Introduction

Abortion care encompasses a broad range of services, beginning with the first contact a woman makes with a health care provider after she suspects or determines that she is pregnant. The provision of abortion is located within the larger framework of health care, and accordingly it is subject to the same matrix of sociocultural, professional, economic, political, and regulatory forces. Abortion providers must be cognizant of trends and compliant with standards of care that stem from a number of relevant health-related professions, including those pertinent to the emerging discipline of health care quality management.

Providing services that are safe, effective, and appropriate improves patient outcomes and enhances patient and staff satisfaction. This chapter provides a broad framework for quality care that emphasizes establishing quality as a strategic priority; building an organizational culture that supports quality at all levels; and fostering teamwork, communication, transparency, and systems thinking. Topics include human resources and environmental issues such as equipment and supplies, patient flow, safety and privacy, staff training and competency, documentation, and how to design systems for continuous quality improvement. Abortion provision in low-resource settings is addressed in Chapter 22.

Management of Unintended and Abnormal Pregnancy, 1st edition. By M Paul, ES Lichtenberg, L Borgatta, DA Grimes, PG Stubblefield, MD Creinin

Historical overview

Philosophy, standards, and management approaches

The Institute of Medicine (IOM) has defined health care quality as the extent to which health services increase the likelihood of desired health outcomes [1]. The field of quality management (sometimes referred to as *total quality management*) in health care encompasses all of the following: fundamental management techniques, assessment and assurance methods, and technical tools in a dynamic multidisciplinary environment focusing on continuous process improvement [2]. The three main areas of quality management include quality improvement, quality assessment, and quality assurance (Box A).

In the USA, the field of modern health care quality management gained momentum in the latter half of the 20th century. Although manufacturing industries previously had embraced concepts and tools for quality management in production and customer satisfaction, not until 1966 with

Box A Components of Quality Management

Quality Improvement	Quality Assessment	Quality Assurance
The processes used in developing and relating a body of knowledge to the continuous improvement of systems, policies, and procedures that will direct these services toward the goal of improved patient outcomes.	The collection of data that measures the effectiveness of current systems and links structure and process to the improvement of clinical outcomes.	The utilization of assessment and improvement strategies to identify, monitor, and provide feedback on performance in a continuous cycle.

publication of Donabedian's groundbreaking article, "Evaluating the Quality of Medical Care [3]," did interest emerge in transferring models of structure, process, and outcome measurements to the health care industries.

The 1970s and 1980s brought rapid and increasingly widespread awareness of the need for more sophisticated assessments of health care practices. During this time, the IOM was established to analyze clinical evidence and develop recommendations for US health care policies. Concurrently, the American College of Obstetricians and Gynecologists (ACOG), the American Medical Association (AMA), and the American Nursing Association issued their first peer-review guidelines and established professional standards committees. State medical societies and associations developed and supported peer-review protection laws to safeguard credentials committees and peer-review documents from litigation. Professional associations such as ACOG and the American College of Nurse Midwives published their first quality assurance guidelines, and they expected their members to participate in quality assurance, continuing competency, and peer-review programs. The Agency for Health Care Policy and Research (AHCPR), forerunner of the current Agency for Healthcare Research and Quality (AHRQ), was founded specifically to engage in quality-related research that would inform health care policies through the best scientific evidence.

In 1996, the IOM convened a National Roundtable on Health Care Quality, and by 1999 it had gathered enough supportive evidence to publish the revolutionary treatise, "To Err is Human: Building a Safer Health System [1]." This document exposed the alarming extent of medical error and its toll on public health in the USA. By doing so, the IOM shifted quality management for the new millennium, focusing more closely on safety, patient satisfaction, and clinical outcomes. In 2001, a second report from the IOM's Committee on Quality of Health Care in America, "Crossing the Quality Chasm [4]," investigated health systems' deficits in greater depth and made recommendations for change, delineating "Six Aims for Quality in Health Care" (Box B).

The Six Aims became a rallying cry for quality program design that has since been adopted by major governmental and nongovernmental organizations and small facilities alike. The publication in 2006 of a third IOM report, "Performance Measurement: Accelerating Improvement [5]," has generated similar excitement and controversy as it calls for innovative techniques to examine measurable change according to the Six Aims.

The US Health Information Portability and Accountability Act (HIPAA) of 1996 (amended in 2002) regulates access to care as well as its continuity and privacy, and it affects providers in both the public and private sectors. Canada expanded its corollary legislation, the Personal Information Protection and Electronic Documents Act (PIPEDA), to include the health care sector in 2002. These federal-level regulations exemplify how the economic shift necessitating relationships with third-party payers has drawn independent practitioners into a new and complex arena of oversight. Third-party payers, as well as numerous accrediting bodies, are increasingly interested in the quality management systems of their affiliated institutions.

The focus on safety and its informatics corollary, privacy, has wrought vast changes in the provision of health care services. Ensuring that patients and personnel remain safe from injury essentially extends the maxim, "First, do no harm"; however, the myriad systems that this formula encompasses go far beyond taking care to give the correct medicine in the correct amount to the correct patient. These systems include physical plant structures and equipment maintenance, emergency evacuation procedures, food safety and hygiene, and competent and properly licensed caregivers. Protection from infection, discrimination, and violence constitute other crucial concerns. Information technology systems, whether simple (telecommunications) or more complex (e.g.,

Box B Six Aims for Quality in Health Care (From Institute of Medicine [4]).

All health care should be:

- Safe
- Effective
- Timely
- Patient-centered
- Efficient
- Equitable

electronic health records, computerized billing), are essential to the infrastructure of any modern service. Maintaining compliance with guidelines for health information protection may be a highly complex undertaking, dependent on technology systems as well as state, provincial, and federal regulations.

Over the past 15 years, the recognition that quality management must lie at the foundation of modern health care provision has increased remarkably. Historical quality assurance processes that affect only one component of total quality management, such as peer review and continuing education, no longer suffice to meet professional standards or the expectations of health care consumers and their representatives in community, state, and federal regulatory agencies for safe and effective health care services. Indeed, assuring safe and effective services in the modern health care environment requires that the administration of each health care facility and its workforce pursue the goals of quality assurance and continuous improvement.

Essential goals for health care policy as applied to point-of-care (POC) delivery

Escalating costs, regulatory pressures, and the demands of quality improvement require an orchestrated approach. Public and private organizations are undertaking national projects that focus on the Six Aims identified by the IOM, thereby catalyzing the development and evaluation of new management techniques. New models of organizational commitment to quality care are patient-centered, evidence-based, consensus-based, performance-based, and transparent.

Patient-centered care: Listening and learning from patients

Under the combined influence of the consumers' rights and women's self-health movements of the 1960s and 1970s, providers in the fields of reproductive rights and abortion readily embraced the tenets of a new philosophy in health care. This philosophy recognized that patients have both responsibilities and rights in relation to the care that they receive, entailing a commitment on the part of both patients and staff to communicate expectations. A US Advisory Commission on Consumer Protection and Quality in the Health Care Industry convened in 1997 to develop guidance for health systems striving to "promote and assure health care quality and value, and protect consumers and workers [6]." Its mission included creating a Consumer Bill of Rights and Responsibilities, which served as the template for the individualized Patient's Bill of Rights developed by national health organizations, insurance companies, health maintenance organizations, and many states and individual facilities. These same protections apply in office or clinic settings that provide abortion care.

Evidence-based care: Using research to guide practice

In 1989, the newly formed Agency for Health Care Policy and Research was charged with overseeing the nationwide adoption of scientifically based practice guidelines. Subsequently, organizations including the AMA, the IOM, the American Academy of Family Physicians, ACOG, and the National Abortion Federation (NAF) promoted clinical practice guidelines as a means of furthering quality care, decreasing health care costs through appropriate treatment, and reducing professional liability [7]. In response to the growing evidence base supporting health care quality, organizational structures have evolved rapidly over the last decade. The old rules of physician autonomy and opacity no longer apply. Governments as well as the private sector have active roles in setting the agenda for health care quality and cost containment.

Consensus-based care: A teamwork approach to quality

Effective teams for achieving consensus are composed of system leaders (administrators), technical leaders (physicians, clinicians), and staff leaders (clinical coordinators), as well as other key staff. Standards of care are established through the collaborative efforts of experts in the evidence-based fields of both quality and clinical practice. In abortion care, organizations such as NAF maintain current clinical practice guidelines, and quality professionals experienced in reproductive health care systems assist internal teams with total quality management programs. These systems function together to ensure that facilities focus on the quality of services everyday. This approach is called the *continuous readiness model*: facilities do not perform differently during bi- or tri-annual quality audits than they do on any day when patients are receiving care.

Performance-based care and transparency: How well are we doing?

The contemporary concept of "transparency," whereby patients (consumers) as well as third-party payers will have the right to access the performance data of hospitals and individual practitioners, is rapidly gaining ground. Over the last few years, many health care professionals have experienced the inroads made by the controversial "pay-for-performance" model of reimbursement. All health care providers, whether or not their budgets are directly subject to this model, will be affected by increasing public awareness of consumers' rights to access this information. Beginning in 2008, hospital performance reporting in the USA will be public information, and the Centers for Medicare and Medicaid Services will no longer reimburse for costs of "reasonably preventable" injuries [8].

Patient safety: A health care quality framework applied to abortion care [9]

Structure and environment

Providers can offer high-quality abortion care in a variety of settings. In the USA, most abortions occur in freestanding clinics [10]. In Canada and many Western European countries, abortions take place primarily in hospital settings. Regardless of the institution, facilities that provide abortions must have appropriate space, equipment, and supplies to meet all routine and emergency needs. They may be further designed to enhance efficiency, as well as the comfort and security of patients and staff, as part of promoting the Six Aims [4].

Workplace violence policies are becoming widespread in many industries. In abortion facilities, the threat of antiabortion violence amplifies security risks [11]. Security planning must consider safeguarding both patients and staff when the facility is open, and securing the facility when it is unoccupied. The facility planner may wish to retain a security consultant or work with local law enforcement agencies to assess risk and devise security measures. Policies and procedures related to a range of safety issues (e.g., security, occupational health, privacy) must accord with government and labor regulations and be available to all staff.

Form meets function: Patient flow

A patient flow chart (Fig. 23.1) helps to optimize the number, type, and duration of patient/staff interactions and plan where each step will occur. For staff, smooth patient flow results in efficient use of time and energy, leaving more of both for patient care. For patients, improved care delivery translates into better outcomes and heightened satisfaction.

Although patient flow models vary, a design that minimizes patient waiting time is optimal. This objective can be accomplished by eliminating redundancy in the steps of the process and consolidating patient "stops." A desirable physical layout promotes a one-way, sequential pattern of patient flow. To protect confidentiality and minimize anxiety, facilities should arrange internal seating areas so that waiting areas for patient education, counseling, and laboratory work are not near procedure or recovery rooms. The principle areas of staff activity or patient "stops" in the patient flow process (Fig. 23.1) are addressed next.

Telephone screening and appointments. "Patients often measure the clinic's diligence in pursuing their best interest based simply on their perception of the clinic's efforts in explaining and scheduling their appointments" (VanDerhei and Randall [12]). Facilities should aim to minimize the time between the patient's request for an appointment and their procedure, as well as the number of visits required. Although abortion providers must observe waiting requirements where they exist (Chapter 4), additional visits may add stress and delay care [13].

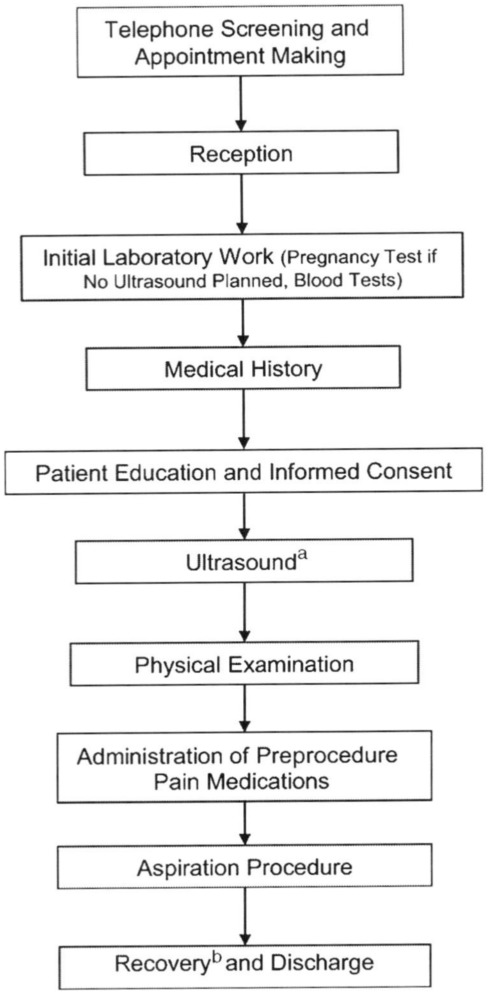

Figure 23.1 Patient flow chart for aspiration abortion.
[a] Routine ultrasound is not required for first-trimester aspiration abortion as long as the patient's reported onset of her last menstrual period (LMP) accords with uterine size by pelvic examination.
[b] A dedicated recovery area may not be needed for patients receiving only local cervical anesthesia or mild sedation; recovery in the procedure room is acceptable as long as trained staff is available to observe and discharge the patient.

Providing a private space for appointment/screening services may require separating it from the reception window. Occasionally, a facility will not be able to offer the services most appropriate for a given patient. In this situation, staff should be able to provide referrals for the following:

- Other abortion providers (including gestational age limits, pain management options, general fee structures)
- Pregnancy options information services (phone-based and local)
- Adoption and foster parenting services
- Translator services
- Domestic violence hotlines and shelters

- Rape and sexual abuse/assault hotlines
- Individual/group therapists
- Postabortion counseling (phone-based and local)
- Child Protective Services
- Crisis hotlines (e.g., domestic violence).

Patient intake/front-desk registration. This area should facilitate confidential staff-patient interactions and payment of fees. Receptionists should have access to pertinent medical records while observing guidelines for information protection.

Reception area. The size of the reception area will depend upon patient volume and the facility's policies for accompanying support persons. Issues of security, privacy, and patient satisfaction must be considered.

Patient education/counseling rooms. Privacy and confidentiality are paramount considerations. Although common educational topics may be covered in a group setting, the NAF Clinical Policy Guidelines [14] require that each patient have the opportunity for an individual conversation with a staff member.

Laboratory areas. Each practice must determine which tests will be done on-site and which will be sent to outside laboratories. Some facilities have a convenient pass-through window that allows patients to pass urine samples from the restroom directly into the laboratory. In small abortion practices, blood sampling may occur in an interview or examination room; however, as patient volume increases, creating laboratory space for phlebotomy enhances efficiency. Some laboratories accommodate multiple functions, and they may be subject to additional regulation. Under all circumstances, infection control measures must be strictly observed to prevent nosocomial infections. Infection control can be challenging when contamination-prone processes take place in otherwise "clean" areas, such as interview rooms, or when the laboratory has minimal space for "clean" tasks, such as charting or instrument processing. These settings require that staff maintain heightened awareness and that administrators take all possible precautions to minimize risk.

Physical examination, ultrasound, and procedure rooms. The number and size of rooms reflect patient volume, the methods of abortion and pain management provided, and in some cases external regulations. In some practices, a patient has her physical examination, ultrasound, and abortion procedure in one room; in other settings, these steps occur in different rooms or perhaps on different days. Minimizing the number of times a patient must dress and undress during any given visit enhances efficiency, as well as patient privacy and convenience.

External regulations may specify the dimensions of the procedure room, door size, ventilation, and equipment. In other circumstances, regulations may apply only when certain methods of abortion, sedation, or anesthesia are utilized. Unless otherwise regulated, the optimal size of the procedure room will depend upon the equipment and number of staff required for the abortion methods used. Anticipating space for an ultrasound machine is prudent.

Examination of evacuated uterine contents. Many facilities have a dedicated space in close proximity to the patient care area for inspection of the fresh tissue aspirate. Pass-through windows or doors from the procedure room to the tissue work area are an added convenience. The NAF Clinical Policy Guidelines [14] require examination of evacuated tissue for products of conception prior to patient discharge.

Recovery area. Recovery time and space are essential in facilities that provide surgical abortion care. A patient's stay in the recovery area varies according to the type of abortion procedure and the drugs used. In facilities providing only local anesthesia and mild sedation, patients may recover in the procedure room as long as appropriately trained staff are available to observe and discharge them.

In busy abortion facilities or those providing second-trimester procedures with moderate sedation or general anesthesia, a dedicated recovery area typically consists of a room with several reclining chairs or beds. Curtains that pull around the beds or chairs assure privacy when needed, but they must not obscure the view of the recovery room staff. Ideally, the recovery area will have at least one patient restroom that is large enough to be used as a changing room if needed.

Equipment and technologies

Equipment, technologies, and supplies depend on the services offered. They may include instruments used for evaluating patients (e.g., blood pressure cuffs, scales, ultrasound machines, laboratory equipment) or treating patients (e.g., suction and anesthesia apparatus); storage for medical and patient care supplies (e.g., medication and laboratory diagnostics refrigerators, patient snack refrigerators); instrument processing devices (e.g., autoclaves); as well as emergency equipment and supplies (e.g., fire extinguishers, oxygen delivery systems, backup generators). Suggested equipment and supply lists are available from several professional organizations (Appendix).

Equipment and supplies should be well maintained; some devices may require service by qualified bioengineering firms. The volume of supplies should suffice for daily operations; excessive supplies may take up critical storage space and make monitoring for expiration dates cumbersome.

Health care facilities must have readily accessible emergency equipment and supplies, as well as staff trained in policies and procedures for handling medical, security, and environmental emergencies. The NAF Clinical Policy Guidelines [14] mandate that a cardiopulmonary resuscitation (CPR)-certified staff member be available on-site for emergency care whenever surgical abortions are performed. These Guidelines also list the supplies necessary for ensuring patients' safety during medical care. Additional useful emergency considerations include the following:

- External regulations may specify the location and content of emergency carts and oxygen-delivery systems.
- Adequate backup power and lighting sources permit clinicians to complete any surgical procedure in progress at the time of a power outage.
- An intercom or paging system facilitates communications during emergencies.
- Posting emergency exits prominently and training staff in procedures for evacuating the facility improve emergency response.
- An emergency exit located near the procedure and recovery areas will allow an ambulance team direct patient access, if needed.
- Periodic staff drills in emergency procedures are highly recommended.

Health and safety agencies will assist in protecting the public's safety during environmental disasters; abortion facilities may also choose to consult with experts in security related to antiabortion threats and terrorist activities.

Cleaning and sterilization

Facilities need space for washing and sterilizing instruments and processing other reusable supplies. Ideally, these spaces are located conveniently close to patient care areas yet out of patients' view. When storage and processing share a common room, the space must be divided into *clean* and *dirty* areas to comply with infection control regulations. *Dirty* procedures include handling potentially infectious materials (e.g., blood, tissue samples) and washing contaminated instruments. *Clean* procedures include the preparation of clean instruments for sterilization and preparation of sterile and disposable supplies. Facilities with space restrictions may perform blood and urine sample testing, tissue examination, and instrument cleaning and sterilization procedures in the same room, as long as clean processes are protected by a virtual boundary and staff remains vigilant. This boundary may be further delineated by a visual aid, such as a line on the countertop or the use of clean and dirty signs.

Proper decontamination, cleaning, disinfection, and sterilization are essential to reducing the risk of nosocomial infections. The required level of processing differs for surfaces and various types of equipment and supplies (Table 23.1). Providers must observe regulations; complete technical resources are available from manufacturers, government agencies such as the Centers for Disease Control and Prevention (CDC), and other sources [15,16]. Biological indicators should be utilized regularly to test the adequacy of autoclave sterilization. The US Food and Drug Administration (FDA) offers a list of chemical germicides approved for high-level disinfection [17]. Facility administrators should consider environmental and occupational health and safety features when choosing products for these purposes. Material Safety Data Sheets (MSDS) for all chemicals must be readily available to employees.

Table 23.1 Processing of equipment and supplies.

Equipment and Instruments	Level of Cleaning, Disinfection, or Sterilization[a]	Comments
Speculum	High-level disinfection[b]	
Ultrasound vaginal probe	High-level disinfection	Must also be covered with a single-use sheath or unlubricated condom
Ultrasound abdominal probe	Cleaning or general disinfection	
Manual vacuum aspirator	High-level disinfection; some models autoclavable	All cannulae must be sterile and single-use only
Cervical dilators	Sterilization[c]	Processing staff must be trained to competency in cleaning, wrapping, and sterilizing techniques, as well as the hallmarks of contamination (e.g., wet or ripped packaging)
Electric vacuum aspiration glass collection bottles	Cleaning or general disinfection	
Abortion suction tubing	High level disinfection (reusable tubing only)	Tubing labeled as single-use should not be reprocessed
Procedure room surfaces (e.g., exam table, countertops)	Cleaning or general disinfection	Germicidal wipes are environmentally safer than aerosol sprays

[a] All listed instruments and supplies require thorough cleaning prior to any higher level of disinfection or sterilization.

[b] High-level disinfection eliminates all recognized pathogenic microorganisms, except for high levels of bacterial endospores, and is accomplished with chemical germicides cleared for marketing by the US Food and Drug Administration [15].

[c] Sterilization uses physical or chemical procedures to destroy all microorganisms, including highly resistant bacterial endospores. In general, reusable medical devices or patient-care equipment that enters normally sterile tissue or the vascular system require sterilization [15].

Processes

Quality medical services require administrative procedures to ensure safety, confidentiality, and accountability. As part of the overall quality program, reviewing these processes at least annually helps to ensure that all components are functioning and that they meet the needs of patients.

Important policies and procedures requiring oversight within the quality management infrastructure include the following:

- Medical records (e.g., documentation, confidentiality, records release, storage)
- Office procedures (e.g., equipment, supplies, telephone services)
- Safety and security (e.g., building codes, disaster preparedness, handicap access, biohazardous waste, bioengineering logs)
- Infection control (e.g., precautions; environmental; laundry; instrument cleaning, disinfection and sterilization; waste management; staff health files and incident reports; policies from regulatory agencies, such as the US Occupational Safety and Health Administration or the Canadian Centre for Occupational Health and Safety)
- Medications (e.g., protocols, inventory, controlled substance logs)
- Laboratory (e.g., equipment and test result logs, inventory, policies of regulatory agencies such as the Clinical Laboratory Improvement Amendments)
- Equipment and instruments (e.g., quality, maintenance, inventory)
- Personnel (e.g., licensing, training, health records, other human resources documents)
- Patient care (e.g., policies and procedures, clinical policy guidelines, statistics, complications logs, triage logs, communications, scheduling, education, satisfaction and complaints, flow).

Developing a "daily procedures" manual for abortion care may be helpful. Daily procedures include tasks that staff must accomplish each time a patient receives abortion care. The manual will facilitate training of new staff or temporary personnel, and it also will serve as a useful reference for regular staff.

Clinical Practice Guidelines

"Well-developed, scientifically based practice guidelines have an important role to play in assessing, assuring, and improving the quality of health care services provided in this country. Clear, specific guidelines and associated review criteria should help prevent, or alternatively, identify and remedy problems of overuse of care, underuse of care, and poor technical and interpersonal provision of care" (Institute of Medicine [18]).

Practice guidelines distill medical knowledge into a convenient and readily usable format [19]. They are an important component of quality assurance programs mandated by many insurers and accreditation or licensing agencies. NAF pioneered efforts to establish clinical guidelines for abortion practice in 1978, and since 1991 the NAF Clinical Policy Guidelines Committee has convened several times a year to review the scientific evidence, develop and revise relevant standards, and ensure accountability. NAF revises its Clinical Policy Guidelines annually and submits them to the AHRQ National Guidelines Clearinghouse; they are also available to the medical community and the public at large [14]. Quality management processes may incorporate measurement tools derived from clinical policy guidelines as a means of ensuring compliance, documenting actual practices, and implementing educational remedies as necessary.

A system for maintaining key reference documents

Documents that should be easily accessible include all applicable protocols and procedure manuals, standards and clinical guidelines, regulations, reporting requirements and forms, patient education handouts, and a complete set of blank chart forms. Placing the reference set in an electronic format on a shared drive, or in clearly labeled binders or files in a designated area, facilitates access. Appropriate personnel should review these reference documents at least annually and update them on a periodic basis as needed. An archival system to maintain obsolete documents is helpful; for example, during a review or legal proceeding, archived documents assist in establishing the usual practice of the facility at a previous period. Requirements for documentation and reporting vary greatly by locale and by the number of external regulatory bodies a medical provider must satisfy.

Patient records and written materials

Requirements vary as to what forms and consents must appear in the patient record. With the widespread implementation of electronic health records, forms management entails new challenges. Although many health care facilities aim to be "paperless," informed consent documents still require a patient's signature and paperless systems still need auditing to ensure completeness and accuracy. Documentation, whether electronic or in paper form, should include the following:

- History and physical examination
- Documentation of patient education/counseling
- Ultrasound report with images (if done)
- Procedure/operative record
- Anesthesia/medication record
- Recovery and discharge record
- Medication order forms
- Problem lists
- Consent forms
- Follow-up care

Facilities without electronic health records need a designated, secure area for current patient charts and a system for easy retrieval of records when needed. For facilities using electronic health records, a staff member well versed in information technology is an invaluable asset. Well-designed software meets clinical needs, legal standards, and privacy regulations while incorporating security protections against tampering and intrusion.

Having written material available to patients allows them to reference instructions at a later time. Fact sheets, including the following topics, will support efficient patient education and reinforce in-person instructions:

- Abortion aftercare instructions
- Warning signs for abortion complications
- Explanation of various procedures (laminaria placement, abortion)
- Comparison of medical versus aspiration abortion
- Home use of medications dispensed for medical abortion and what to expect
- "Insufficient tissue" and ectopic precautions
- Rh factor
- Contraceptive information, including directions for use and warning signs for rare but serious risks
- Emergency contraception instructions.

A system for abortion-related calls during and after office hours

Although serious postabortion problems occur rarely, providers must establish a system for responding to patient calls at any time. The NAF Clinical Policy Guidelines [14] mandate that patients receive written instructions for contacting the medical facility at any time. When setting up a system, clearly delineate staff responsibilities for triaging and handling calls. If a patient calls during office hours, telephone staff must know how to route complications calls to appropriately trained and licensed staff. After-hours calls require a system for prompt response. An answering service can relay calls to staff, or on-call staff can carry a pager or cellular telephone that patients can access directly. Some facilities use a combination of communication methods. A licensed clinician must always be available for consultation [14].

Nonlicensed personnel who handle postabortion calls need clear written protocols for triaging patients. When licensed providers are not taking "first call," the medical director may choose to develop standing orders for triage management because nonlicensed staff should not make medical decisions. Important documentation includes the time of the patient's call; when the staff member reached the patient; her questions, symptoms, and responses to focused history taking; any new instructions; medical consultation (if applicable); and follow-up. This information must be transferred to the patient's record, and a clinician should review the record in a timely fashion.

Infection control

Each facility must establish policies and procedures for infection control that address such issues as environmental and equipment cleaning, instrument cleaning and processing, correct handwashing and use of personal protective equipment (PPE), blood and body fluid exposure management, and incident reporting. A complete listing is beyond the scope of this chapter. Administrators must be familiar with relevant health regulations. Personnel are responsible for protecting themselves, their patients, and their coworkers by observing infection prevention measures. Communicating the rationale for occupational health and safety precautions to staff, including infection prevention measures and the use of appropriate PPE, helps to enhance compliance.

In the USA, each employer is responsible for complying with the federal Occupational Safety and Health Administration (OSHA) Bloodborne Pathogens Standard [20]. The Standard requires training of all employees at hire and annually thereafter. Furthermore, each facility must have an exposure plan that identifies and provides appropriate PPE for all tasks and ensures that precautions are followed. Among other precautions, OSHA mandates the proper use of gloves, fluid-barrier gowns, masks or face shields, eye protection, and shoe covers in situations that pose a potential risk of splashing or exposure to bodily fluids. In abortion care, such exposures may occur during surgical procedures, when examining the tissue aspirate, and when washing instruments. Other activities may require some but not all of the listed PPE. The CDC also has developed rigorous hand hygiene guidelines [21] that are a key part of the overall strategy to reduce infections in health care settings and promote patient safety. A simple and useful hand-washing video is available online at http://www.youtube.com/watch?v=1Rx5UNLDlw4. Posting appropriate handwashing reminders in staff restrooms, laboratory areas, and patient rooms helps to reinforce proper hygiene practices among practitioners, staff, and visitors.

People

Quality abortion services require appropriately skilled and experienced personnel. On a subtler level, models of care that promote positive relationships between patients and staff enhance health outcomes and patient satisfaction.

Provider availability and training

In the USA, the number of facilities that provide abortion services has been declining for decades [10,22,23]. According to the Guttmacher Institute, 87% of US counties and 69% of metropolitan areas have no abortion provider [10]. In 1990, NAF and ACOG convened a national symposium to explore the shortage of abortion providers and devise strategies to address the problem [24]. Many reasons were identified for the shortage, including the "graying" of committed physicians who had witnessed the morbidity and mortality associated with illegal abortion, the stigmatization and isolation of abortion providers, low pay and repetitive work for physicians in specialized clinics, the underrepresentation of physician specialists in rural areas, and lack of training in residency programs. To address the training deficit, the Accreditation Council for Graduate Medical Education (ACGME) issued guidelines in 1996 that included a requirement for OB-GYN residency programs to offer residents experience with induced abortion, with an opt-out provision for those with religious or moral objections [25].

Due to these efforts and others, the proportion of obstetrics and gynecology and family medicine programs that offer abortion training has increased, and family planning fellowships have also been established. According to a survey of OB-GYN residency directors in the USA, 51% of OB-GYN residency programs provided routine abortion training in 2004 [26] compared to only 12% in 1992 [22]. "This shift in training is significant, because routine status clearly leads to training in a greater variety of abortion techniques for the management of both first and second trimester pregnancies" (Eastwood et al [26]). Furthermore, abortion training during residency correlates positively with future abortion provision [27]. Notwithstanding these advances, the ACOG committee on Health Care for Underserved Women recently published a Committee Opinion that recognized the continuing inadequacy of training opportunities in family planning and abortion and supported the integration of these topics into medical school and OB-GYN residency program curricula [28].

Additional ongoing initiatives seek to enhance access to services by increasing the role of primary care practitioners in abortion provision. Several states currently acknowledge medical abortion or aspiration abortion as within the scope of practice of nurse practitioners, nurse midwives, and physician assistants; however, in many other states legal and regulatory barriers to abortion provision by nonphysicians remain in effect (Chapter 4).

Selecting and evaluating providers

Before hiring an abortion provider, a facility must determine that the clinician has the expertise to perform procedures competently. Disciplinary boards for medical professionals may provide information about complaints or deficiencies, but they do not establish competence.

Initial methods of evaluation include reviewing credentials, training, and work experience as well as direct observation by an experienced provider. The ACGME has established six domains of competency for medical residency evaluation purposes [29] that can be adapted to the abortion setting [30] (Table 23.2). The medical director is responsible for ensuring the continuing competency of all providers and their compliance with clinical policies and procedures. Medical record reviews and analysis of complications logs may help with this process.

Staff selection

Selecting staff to provide quality abortion care is more complex than matching professional licenses and work skills to tasks. Qualified applicants should also exhibit positive attitudes toward sexuality and abortion, which contribute to patient care and staff morale.

Like many medical practices, abortion facilities often rely on a mixture of licensed and nonlicensed staff to perform various duties. Regulations governing the level of licensure and supervision required for specific tasks vary. Planning an abortion service includes delineating each function in the abortion process and determining if government or licensing agencies mandate a specific medical or laboratory professional to provide that care.

Staff training, evaluation, and retention

"Keeping staff educated, involved, and satisfied is the key to keeping patients safe" (Perry-Ewald, 2007, personal communication). Training staff who are new to abortion services involves addressing both medical and psychosocial issues. Many organizations offer educational materials to assist in training (Appendix).

During orientation and training, a buddy system using structured activities helps to build skills and integrate the new employee into the culture of the organization. One effective model uses a 30-60-90-day plan for training and evaluation, customizing the training program to each employee's prior knowledge and experience (Perry-Ewald, 2007, personal communication). A checklist for skills acquisition and key performance indicators can be helpful. Following the initial 90-day period, facilities may choose to follow an annual schedule for formal performance review, which sometimes involves a self-assessment as well as a manager's review of strengths, areas for growth, accomplishments, goals, and other issues. The evaluation may include the results of chart reviews, relevant patient satisfaction/complaint responses, incident reports, or feedback regarding communications problems with other staff or providers.

Regular staff meetings and in-services offer opportunities to provide positive feedback and engage in shared problem-solving and planning activities, as well as to share new information and advance skills. Providing opportunities for decision-making by consensus, leadership through facilitation, and task-sharing among the team encourages participation, which in turn enhances success [31].

Leadership/culture

A quality management program can only thrive with active support and guidance from the leaders of the organization. The role of leadership in the quality program is to balance the setting and achieving of collective goals. Leaders will

Table 23.2 Sample performance evaluation measures for abortion providers. (Adapted with permission from Goodman et al [30].)

Medical Knowledge

- Identifies factors pertinent to abortion care during patient history review
- Knows appropriate use of medications
- Knows appropriate use and interpretation of laboratory tests
- Identifies features of ectopic pregnancy
- Knows contraceptive options and contraindications to specific methods
- Knows indications for sonography

Patient Care

- Reviews history thoroughly, asks additional questions as indicated
- Confirms patient consent
- Accurately estimates uterine size and position from pelvic examination
- Interprets sonogram findings for dating and completion of abortion
- Asks and answers questions in a patient-centered manner (i.e., one that is free of judgments and is focused on meeting the patient's expressed needs)
- Administers analgesics/sedatives in appropriate doses
- Provides effective paracervical anesthesia
- Safely dilates cervix to correct size for gestational age
- Consistently uses "no-touch" technique for instruments inserted into the uterus
- Accurately assesses when uterus is empty
- Completes procedure in a timely manner
- Examines tissue aspirate and identifies pregnancy elements accurately
- Prescribes appropriate postprocedure medications as needed
- Effectively manages difficulties encountered during the procedure (e.g., dilation, cervical laceration, anatomical variations)

Communication and Interpersonal Skills

- Consistently introduces herself or himself to patients
- Consistently uses open-ended questions when counseling patients
- Establishes rapport with the patient

Professionalism

- Demonstrates respect for patients and staff
- Maintains strict patient confidentiality
- Documents all relevant patient data legibly
- Is aware of his or her limitations

Systems-Based Practice

- Demonstrates knowledge of range of access issues related to abortion services, including billing and insurance

Practice-Based Learning and Improvement

- Demonstrates ability to appraise and assimilate evidence from scientific studies to support patient care decisions

hold high-level and mid-level staff accountable for quality outcomes, and they should provide appropriate resources for improvement initiatives in clinical programs. An ideal leader "maintains constancy of purpose, establishes clear goals and expectations, and fosters a respectful positive culture. Leaders take time to build knowledge, review and reflect, and take action on the microsystem level or in the larger organization" (Mohr [32]).

Identifying all of the formal and informal leadership influences on a clinical process may be challenging. For example, even when key staff members are not officially part of the leadership team, their motivation, attitudes, and informal influences will affect the success of an improvement initiative. "Achieving results at the system or organizational level requires will at all levels, but especially the will of top management to make a new way of working attractive and the status quo uncomfortable. . . The responsibility of managers and supervisors includes continual improvement of the work processes under their control" (Nolan [33]).

Lastly, the culture of change and improvement must be positive and respectful. A tendency exists in any system to overlook problems or mistakes. A successful quality program rewards staff for uncovering errors, reporting incidents, and helping to correct systems. In a culture of transparency with collective goals for improvement, staff will identify and solve many day-to-day problems that might otherwise go unnoticed and have a negative impact on patient outcomes.

Designing and implementing an evidence-based quality management program

Many regulatory agencies and national organizations outline standards for how to deliver health care. These standards often serve as references for the development of audit tools that measure a facility's clinical performance and compliance. The Joint Commission recommends prioritizing quality management activities that affect a large population of patients, place patients at risk, or are problem prone [34]. The following six simple questions lead to a framework for a Quality Management Program:

- Did the patient get the treatment she was seeking?
- Was the facility clean?
- Was the patient safe?
- Was her pain managed to her satisfaction?
- Was her care delivered in a respectful manner?
- Were her questions answered sufficiently?

Although not difficult to build, quality management programs will work only if they incorporate systems for auditing and reflection into routine operations. By maintenance and oversight, quality managers can identify opportunities and implement measures to reduce patient complications and improve satisfaction with care. For example, by continually monitoring infection rates, facilities can identify any increase quickly, examine potential causes, and institute remedies. As the quality evidence attests, this time is well spent when services become more efficient, satisfied patients refer other patients, and clinical outcomes are improved.

Methodology

"All improvement requires change, but not all change is improvement" (Institute for Healthcare Improvement [35]). Any general quality initiative could use the following basic methodology:

- Define the indicator (the problem you want to solve)
- Identify the goal or benchmark you would like to achieve
- Conduct a surveillance process (auditing, scoring, data report) at regular intervals
- Identify one to three interventions that will change the process or improve the outcome
- Establish a baseline
- Implement interventions
- Perform continuous monitoring
- Measure improvement
- Provide feedback to staff.

This methodology allows the clinical team to identify a problem, measure it, fix it, and determine whether the solution requires implementation of new processes. As a rigorous methodology, it may carry more credibility with providers and the accrediting community, and it can quantify success. However, other simplified and equally successful methodologies can be used (Fig. 23.2). The important issue is to start somewhere, and not to worry too much about which method you use.

When launching any quality improvement program, another important consideration entails who will be involved in the design. The literature provides strong support for including a broad group. Quality initiatives that come solely from managers often fail to address practical issues that affect frontline personnel. Having administration and staff work together on improvement processes helps to ensure success and sustainability. Staff can provide valuable information, identify details that are not readily apparent, and may even uncover traditions passed on to them during training (for example, "I was told we always did it this way because that was how the doctor liked it").

The quality management literature refers to quality teams as local microsystems [36]. In a local microsystem, the team:

- Understands the purpose of its work as it relates to patients ("internal customers")
- Measures the performance of its work against this purpose
- Recognizes that the performance of its unit depends on processes and how they are linked to each other.

Examples of microsystems might include the back-office staff in a freestanding clinic, one clinic site in a multisite organization, or the team that provides abortion services in a hospital setting. "Good microsystems leaders have the capability to make improvement work an attractive way for all to accomplish the purpose of the work unit" (Nolan [36]).

Once the team has assembled, the next step is to begin framing the structure of the quality management program. Like most programs, quality management programs have multiple components. Identifying performance goals, monitoring performance indicators, responding to clinical incidents, managing patient complaints, and conducting improvement projects all must be part of the program. The following sections discuss these components in more detail.

Performance measures and indicators

Quality indicators are those aspects of care that warrant monitoring and evaluation [37]. These indicators typically apply to three areas of care: the structure of the care delivery system, the process, and the outcomes (Table 23.3). Quality indicators may be objective, such as rates of complications or hospitalization, or subjective, such as patient satisfaction. Quality managers must choose specific indicators to serve as a basis for monitoring (Box C). The indicator data will provide the evidence base by which quality managers and staff may:

- Make decisions
- Help prioritize areas for improvement
- Recognize success
- Evaluate performance.

The microsystem team may encounter a common pitfall of any quality management program if it attempts to address too many indicators simultaneously. The literature in quality management suggests modifying no more than three to five specific indicators within a year's time. If indicators are prioritized as high volume, high risk, high cost, or problem prone, the team can feel more confident that improvement

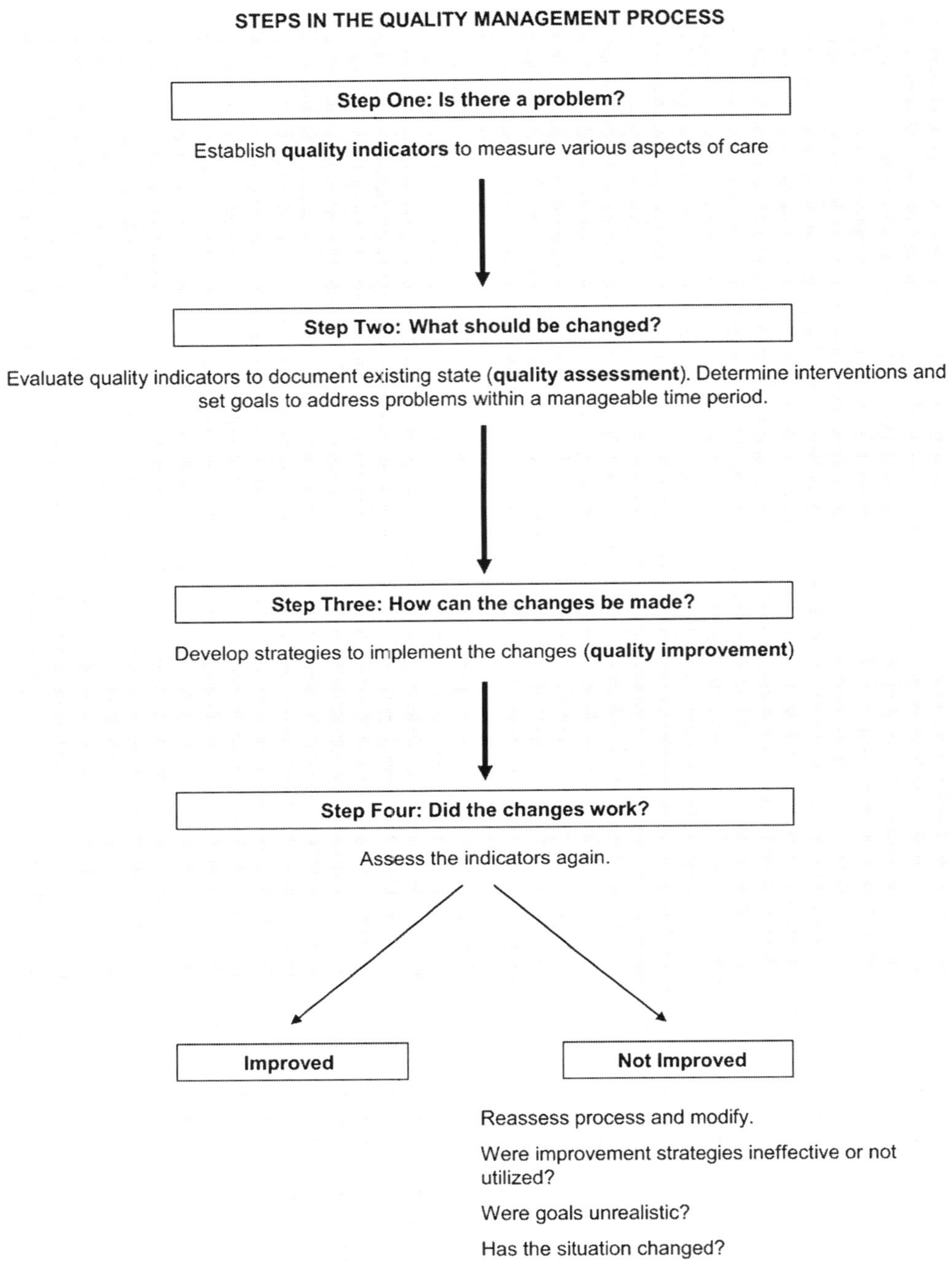

Figure 23.2 Steps in the quality management process.

efforts will have an impact. Additional indicators can be measured, depending on the resources available, but change efforts should be limited.

Using and sharing reliable indicator data on a regular basis are important cornerstones to the quality program. When staff members are unable to identify differences in outcomes of care, they may not feel motivated to maintain the change. Most people can be motivated to improve their performance if they are provided with relevant feedback. Presenting feedback in a collaborative and nonpunitive manner helps to build the trust that is essential for change (Box D).

Process and outcomes measurement and data interpretation

A number of methods are available to analyze quality indicators, including sentinel event indicators, rate-based indicators, process measures, and outcome indicators.

Table 23.3 Examples of quality indicators.

Care Delivery System Indicators

Physical Plant

- The physical environment is clean, inviting, and comfortable. The facility's approach to patients (e.g., woman-centered, compassionate, efficient) is evident to the patient in all steps of the process.
- Equipment is maintained on a routine basis.
- Adequate security is ensured for staff and patients.

Personnel Policies and Practices

- Hiring, selection, and supervision practices are consistent. Staff turnover is low and demonstrates a good working environment.
- Clear and appropriate job descriptions are tied to performance evaluations.
- Staff understands the supervision chain and the grievance process.
- Continuous training and education are offered to staff.
- Assessment of technical competence of staff is documented.

Cost Effectiveness

- Resources are utilized effectively.

Process Indicators

- Clinical practice guidelines compliance
- Emergency equipment preparedness
- Documentation of interpreter services
- Length of visit
- Number of needlestick injuries
- After-hours emergency care, triage availability, and utilization

Outcome Indicators

- Patient satisfaction (measured by surveys or telephone calls)
- Patient complaints
- Complication rates (utilizing NAF data or other criteria)
- Adverse events related to anesthesia or analgesia

Box C Utilizing an Outcome Indicator Relevant to Abortion Care: Measuring the Total Time of a Visit

1. *Identify criteria*: Time from check-in to discharge. It will be helpful to subcategorize those distinct service areas where patients spend a substantial amount of time during their visit (e.g., waiting room/paperwork, ultrasound, education or counseling, laboratory, procedure room, recovery).
2. *Set performance goals*: No more than 1.5 to 2.5 hours for each visit.
3. *Collect data*: Create a small form to document patient name, date, and time spent in each service area. Set the duration interval for data collection (e.g., 2 weeks).
4. *Analyze data*: Input all of the data on a spreadsheet to visualize the time patients spend in each step of the process. Find out where the bottlenecks occur within each visit. Identify patterns and discuss possible causes with the team.
5. *Identify areas for improvement*: Are there ways to streamline patient education, consents, or procedures? Could you create a handout to help with your patients' most frequently asked questions? Does each room contain the necessary supplies in ample quantities?
6. *Implement improvement activities*: Initiate possible solutions for the identified problems.
7. *Evaluate*: Collect data (for a similar time frame) once changes have been made. Has there been a net positive effect? Did different bottlenecks appear?

Box D

A goal of the quality management team is to reduce the rate of retained products of conception. In this clinic, the laboratory staff is responsible for setting up the tissue examination station and preparing the tissue for inspection by the physician. The review process reveals that the staff is not adequately preparing the tissue for examination, making it difficult for the examiner to distinguish the presence or absence of early pregnancy tissue. Background information gathered from the staff in the tissue laboratory reveals that they have not been setting up the counters every morning with backlighting and a float dish, because setting up the tissue examination area properly is time-consuming. The identified intervention is that the room will be set up at the end of each clinic day, when the staff is perceived to have more time. However, unless the laboratory staff is aware of the reason for the change, they may not consistently follow through, thus corrupting the intervention and making it impossible to achieve the desired result of reducing the complication rate. Imagine the difference if the staff knew about the clinical data that triggered the improvement project, and how the change in their performance might improve patient care!

Box E Example of a Root Cause Analysis Using the Five "Why's"

Level of the Problem		Corresponding Level of Improvement Activity
Patient visits have decreased markedly in the last 2 months.	Why? #1	Appointment schedules are not filling.
Appointments are not filling because patients cannot get through on the phone lines.	Why? #2	Patients are complaining that they get a busy signal.
Manager decides to conduct mystery calls over the next 2 weeks.	Why? #3	To experience what the patients experience.
Phones often go to a busy signal during the business day.	Why? #4	Because the staff put the phones on hold.
Staff is putting the phones on hold because the front desk is short-staffed; the staff cannot answer phones and check in patients at the same time.	Why? #5	Hire more staff for the front desk and discuss telling management about problems more openly.

Sentinel event indicators are rare occurrences with grave consequences. They require immediate response and resolution. Sentinel event indicators lend themselves to performing a root cause analysis. The most basic way to conduct a root cause analysis is to ask "Why?" five consecutive times (often referred to as "The Five Why?s") (Box E).

Frequency-based indicators are used to monitor many events or a process over a specified period of time. They measure the frequency of events in relation to the population at risk. Complication rates are an example of this type of indicator. The rate (commonly reported in percentages) is determined by dividing the number of complications that occurred during a specified period of time (numerator) by the total number of abortions performed during that time interval (denominator).

Process and outcome indicators. Process measures answer the question, "Are we doing the right thing?" (e.g., we saw 20 patients today, and no visit time exceeded 2.5 hours). Outcome measures answer the question, "Are we doing the right thing well?" (e.g., we saw 20 patients today; no visit time exceeded 2.5 hours; we did not receive any patient complaints; and no complications occurred). In both cases, the indicator must be measured against a specified goal or practice benchmark.

Continuous measurement data collection represents another reliable way to determine if an improvement intervention has had an impact. The data will reveal if improvement has occurred over time. This methodology can be used instead of, or in concert with, benchmarking. Benchmarking is defined as the process of improving performance by continuously identifying and adapting outstanding practices and processes found both inside and outside the organization. By using benchmarking, a quality program can compare internal improvements to past performance and to the performance of other like organizations.

Many of the previous indicators can benefit from a thorough investigation or root cause analysis. This interdisciplinary process is a requirement of the Joint Commission in response to sentinel events, but it also has utility in other situations. Root cause analysis involves determining all of the possible causes for an undesirable variation to identify where change will have the greatest possible effect. Taking the time to develop a detailed understanding of any health care process will help to identify the type of data analysis most useful to the improvement process. The greater the understanding of the data and the problem, the greater the likelihood of finding the correct solution.

Tools

Once the team has determined indicators and outlined a program, it can use a number of tools to assist in the achievement of performance goals. Examples include:

- Patient charts and written materials
- Self-assessment tools
- Medical record review/audit indicators
- Peer review (Health Care Quality Improvement Act and National Practitioner Data Bank materials)
- Outside auditors (National Abortion Federation, Planned Parenthood Federation of America, Accreditation Association for Ambulatory Health Care)
- Decision support systems, patient-specific risk adjustment, and benchmarking.

Change models and management

Two recognized and effective change and monitoring frameworks include the Plan-Do-Study-Act (PDSA) Cycle and the Six Sigma Framework.

Plan-Do-Study-Act Cycle

The PDSA model (Fig. 23.3) is used to test change initiatives against performance improvement [35]. Completing an improvement cycle usually entails multiple repetitions of PDSA; in other words, achieving sustainable change takes time (Box F).

For example, if a team decides that redesigning a clinical form will improve documentation, the new form rarely will be perfect after its first revision. Typically, several trials of different versions of the form will occur before achieving the improved documentation. The PDSA model provides a simple but effective way of measuring if change has taken

Box F Using the Plan-Do-Study-Act (PDSA) Cycle to Improve Compliance in Obtaining Signatures for Informed Consent

- Define the indicator: Signed and witnessed consents.
- Identify the goal: 100% of all abortion consent forms must be signed prior to the procedure.
- Conduct surveillance: Daily chart audit.
- Identify the interventions: Staff training, provider refresher, change the location of the consent forms in the chart.
- Establish a baseline: Based on 1 week of chart audits.
- Implement the quality management interventions.
- Conduct a staff in-service.
- Meet with the providers to discuss expectations (e.g., that each provider will check the chart in advance and will complete the informed consent process with the patient prior to proceeding with any further services).
- Supervise front desk staff until the new chart form sequence is routine.
- Perform continuous monitoring: Audit charts for 2 weeks post-implementation. If the goal has not been met, reevaluate the content of the interventions, conduct further training, and monitor again until compliance reaches 100%. After a 6-month interval, audit charts again to ensure sustained improvement. Continue to monitor this indicator on a regular basis.
- Utilize regular staff meetings to engage staff and providers in updates on challenges and successes and to celebrate sustaining the goal.

place, if it has resulted in improvement, and if that improvement is sustainable. It requires a commitment to measuring the process over time. Most improvement projects have a delay between implementing an intervention and seeing an improvement in performance. To use another example, a facility may introduce online versions of medical history and financial forms to lessen patient waiting time, but attaining a measurable reduction in waiting-room time still may take weeks or months.

Six Sigma framework

The Six Sigma framework is a means of structuring a data-driven approach and methodology for process improvement. Of the many Six Sigma models, the one used most commonly in health care elaborates on the PDSA cycle and is known as the DMAIC Cycle: Define, Measure, Analyze, Improve, and Control. In simplified terms, the basic theory underlying Six Sigma is that controlling for variation in a work process results in increased efficiency [38]. This tool can be useful in abortion care because although each patient's experience varies, the clinical process for abortion service delivery is often consistent. Reducing variation may include such standardization measures as mailing or connecting patients to a telephone recording for preprocedure instructions, video versions of patient education materials, redesigned forms with checkboxes replacing narrative space, or preprinted discharge instructions. This model suggests that the reduction of repetitive actions by staff will increase clinical efficiency, reduce error, and reduce waste.

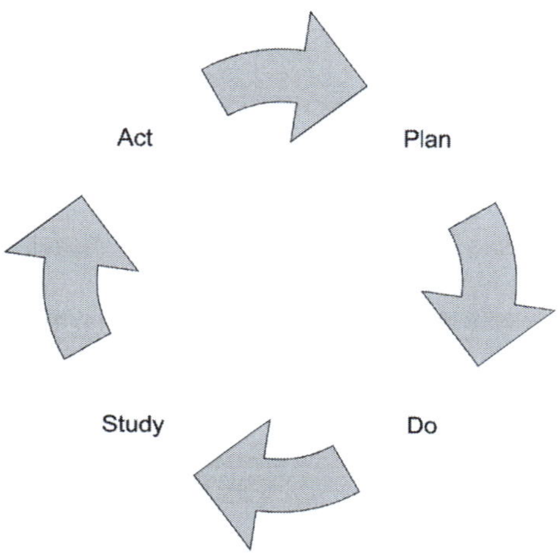

Figure 23.3 Plan-Do-Study-Act (PDSA) Cycle.

Managing patient complaints

In a patient-centered environment, concerns and complaints are not a measure of failure but an opportunity for improvement. Discussing any problems in a nonpunitive and supportive atmosphere promotes transparency and problem-solving.

A patient with a complaint, whether dissatisfied with her experience or unhappy with an outcome, wants to know that someone has listened to her issue and will help her. Useful suggestions for addressing complaints are as follows [30]:

- Acknowledge the problem being described and reflect back your understanding of the issues, letting the patient know that you take her comments seriously.
- Take responsibility for the problem instead of shifting blame. Find out what you can do to resolve the situation for this patient. Ask her what she would like to see changed. Do not assume or make suggestions for her.
- Thank her for bringing the issue to your attention. Let her know that her willingness to voice her concerns helps improve services for everyone.

- Be committed to respond in a timely manner (within 48 hours, if possible).
- Document complaints, including the date, time, and type of complaint.
- Review a complaints log intermittently to identify improvement opportunities.

Conducting performance improvement projects

To most accrediting or auditing bodies, having a well-defined improvement project is representative of a robust quality program. The goal of improvement projects is to create sustainable change in clinical practice or staff behavior that positively affects the patient and her experience. Performance improvement projects should be tailored to the individual setting. The indicators most suitable for a performance improvement project include those that affect a large population, are affiliated with patient risk, or are chronically problematic. The steps for any given project may be simple or complex. Identifying one or two projects each year keeps quality "top of mind" for employees while they work toward a common goal. It also demonstrates the impact that each individual can have on patient care and allows staff to focus on a new project, and hopefully a new success, each year.

Conclusion

Quality improvement in abortion care is composed of intricate networks of multiple processes, ranging from the most basic problem-solving techniques to fine adjustments of high-functioning systems. It provides women with safe, effective, and appropriate care and ensures that those who deliver this care do so within a safe, efficient, and supportive organizational environment. Total quality benefits patients, staff and providers, the organization, and the larger community.

References

1 Kohn LT, Corrigan JM, Donaldson MS, eds. *To Err Is Human: Building a Safer Health System.* Washington (DC): National Academy Press, 1999.

2 Pelletier LR, Beaudin CL, eds. *Q Solutions: Essential Resources for the Healthcare Quality Professional.* Glenview (IL): National Association for Healthcare Quality, 2005.

3 Donabedian A. Evaluating the quality of medical care. *Milbank Mem Fund Q* 1966; **44**: 166–206.

4 Institute of Medicine, Committee on Quality of Health Care in America. *Crossing the Quality Chasm: A New Health System for the 21st Century.* Washington (DC): National Academy Press, 2001.

5 Institute of Medicine, Committee on Redesigning Health Insurance Performance Measures, Payment, and Performance Improvement Programs. *Performance Measurement: Accelerating Improvement.* Washington (DC): National Academy Press, 2006.

6 President's Advisory Commission on Consumer Protection and Quality in the Health Care Industry. Consumer bill of rights and responsibilities [Online]. Washington (DC): President's Advisory Commission on Consumer Protection and Quality in the Health Care Industry, 17 Jul 1998 [cited 20 Aug 2008]. Available from: URL:http://www.hcqualitycommission.gov/final/append_a.html

7 American College of Obstetricians and Gynecologists. *Reading the Medical Literature: Applying Evidence to Practice.* Washington (DC): American College of Obstetricians and Gynecologists, 1998.

8 US Department of Health and Human Services, Centers for Medicare and Medicaid Services. Hospital-acquired conditions and present on admission indicator reporting listening session [Online]. Baltimore (MD): Department of Health and Human Services, 2007 Dec 17 [cited 20 Aug 2008]. Available from: URL:http://www.cms.hhs.gov/HospitalAcqCond/Downloads/HAC-POA-Listening12-17-2007.pdf

9 Byers JF, White SV. *Patient Safety: Principles and Practice.* New York: Springer Publishing, 2004.

10 Jones RK, Zolna MRS, Henshaw SK, Finer LB. Abortion in the United States: incidence and access to services, 2005. *Perspect Sex Reprod Health* 2008; **40**: 6–16.

11 National Abortion Federation. Violence and disruption statistics: Incidents of violence and disruption against abortion providers in the U.S. and Canada [Online]. Washington (DC): National Abortion Federation, 31 Oct 2008 [cited 17 Jan 2009]. Available from: URL:http://www.prochoice.org/pubs_research/publications/downloads/about_abortion/violence_statistics.pdf

12 VanDerhei D, Randall L. *Striving for Excellence in Abortion Care: A Self-Assessment Tool.* St. Petersburg, FL: CAPS Project, 2001.

13 Henshaw SK. Factors hindering access to abortion services. *Fam Plann Perspect* 1995; **27**: 54–59.

14 National Abortion Federation. Clinical policy guidelines [Online]. Washington (DC): National Abortion Federation, 2008 [cited 5 Jun 2008]. Available from: URL:http://www.prochoice.org/pubs_research/publications/downloads/professional_education/CPG2008.pdf

15 Centers for Disease Control and Prevention. Sterilization or disinfection of medical devices [Online]. Atlanta (GA): Centers for Disease Control and Prevention, 20 Aug 2002 [cited 17 Jan 2009]. Available from: URL:http://www.cdc.gov/ncidod/dhqp/bp_sterilization_medDevices.html

16 Centers for Disease Control and Prevention. Guideline for environmental infection control in health-care facilities [Online]. Atlanta (GA): Centers for Disease Control and Prevention, 15 Dec 2005 [cited 17 Jan 2009]. Available from: URL:http://www.cdc.gov/ncidod/dhqp/gl_environinfection.html

17 US Food and Drug Administration. FDA-cleared sterilants and high-level disinfectants with general claims for processing reusable medical and dental devices [Online]. Rockville (MD): US Food and Drug Administration, 28 Sep 2006 [cited 20 Aug 2008]. Available from: URL:http://www.fda.gov/cdrh/ode/germlab.html

18 Institute of Medicine. *Guidelines for Clinical Practice: From Development to Use*. Washington (DC): National Academy Press, 1992.

19 Hayward RS, Wilson MC, Tunis SR, Bass EB, Guyatt G. Users' guides to the medical literature. VIII. How to use clinical practice guidelines. A. Are the recommendations valid? *JAMA* 1995; **274**: 570–574.

20 US Department of Labor, Occupational Safety and Health Administration. Bloodborne pathogens standards 29 CFR 1910.1030 [Online]. Washington (DC): US Department of Labor, Occupational Safety and Health Administration, 17 Sep 2007 [modified 2 Jun 2008; cited 20 Aug 2008]. Available from: URL:http://osha.gov/SLTC/bloodbornepathogens/standards.html

21 Boyce JM, Pittet D, Healthcare Infection Control Practices Advisory Committee, HICPAC/SHEA/APIC/IDSA Hand Hygiene Task Force. Guidelines for hand hygiene in health-care settings: recommendations of the Healthcare Infection Control Practices Advisory Committee and the HICPAC/SHEA/APIC/IDSA Hand Hygiene Task Force. Guideline for Hand Hygiene in Health-Care Settings. *MMWR Recomm Rep* 2002; **51**: 1–45.

22 MacKay HT, MacKay AP. Abortion training in obstetrics and gynecology residency programs in the United States, 1991–1992. *Fam Plann Perspect* 1995; **27**: 112–115.

23 Grimes DA. Clinicians who provide abortions: the thinning ranks. *Obstet Gynecol* 1992; **80**: 719–723.

24 National Abortion Federation, American College of Obstetricians and Gynecologists. *Who Will Provide Abortions: Ensuring the Availability of Qualified Practitioners*. Washington (DC): National Abortion Federation, 1991.

25 Accreditation Council for Graduate Medical Education. Obstetrics/gynecology program requirements [Online]. Chicago (IL): Accreditation Council for Graduate Medical Education, 1 Jan 2008 [cited 20 Aug 2008]. Available from: URL:http://www.acgme.org/acWebsite/RRC_220/220_prIndex.asp

26 Eastwood KL, Kacmar JE, Steinauer J, Weitzen S, Boardman LA. Abortion training in United States obstetrics and gynecology residency programs. *Obstet Gynecol* 2006; **108**: 303–308.

27 Steinauer J, Landy U, Filippone H, Laube D, Darney PD, Jackson RA. Predictors of abortion provision among practicing obstetrician-gynecologists: a national survey. *Am J Obstet Gynecol* 2008; **198**: 39.e1–39.e6.

28 American College of Obstetricians and Gynecologists, Committee on Health Care for Underserved Women. Abortion access and training. ACOG Committee Opinion No. 424, January 2009. *Obstet Gynecol* 2009; **113**: 247–250.

29 Accreditation Council for Graduate Medical Education. Common program requirements: general competencies [Online]. Chicago (IL): Accreditation Council for Graduate Medical Education, 13 Feb 2007 [cited 20 Aug 2008]. Available from: URL:http://www.acgme.org/outcome/comp/GeneralCompetenciesStandards21307.pdf

30 Goodman S, Wolfe M, TEACH Trainers Collaborative Working Group. *Early Abortion Trainer's Workbook*, 2nd edn. San Francisco: University of California, San Francisco Center for Reproductive Health Research and Policy, 2007, 164–165.

31 Lanza ML. Feminist leadership through total quality management. *Health Care Women Int* 1997; **18**: 95–106.

32 Mohr JJ. *Clinical Microsystem Assessment Tool*. Hanover (NH): Dartmouth University, 2003.

33 Nolan TW. *Execution of Strategic Improvement Initiatives to Produce System-Level Results*. Cambridge (MA): Institute for Healthcare Improvement, 2007.

34 Claflin N, ed. *National Association for Healthcare Quality Guide to Quality Management*, 8th ed. Glenview (IL): National Association for Healthcare Quality, 1998, 145.

35 Institute for Healthcare Improvement. How to improve: improvement methods [Online]. Cambridge (MA): Institute for Healthcare Improvement [cited 6 Jun 2008]. Available from: URL:http://www.ihi.org/IHI/Topics/Improvement/ImprovementMethods/HowToImprove

36 Nolan TW. Execution of strategic improvement initiatives to produce system-level results. IHI Innovation Series white paper. Cambridge (MA): Institute for Healthcare Improvement, 2007, 18.

37 Institute for Healthcare Improvement. Measures [Online]. Cambridge (MA): Institute for Healthcare Improvement [cited 17 Jan 2009]. Available from: URL:http://www.ihi.org/IHI/Topics/Improvement/ImprovementMethods/Measures

38 Lloyd DH II, Holsenback JE. The use of sigma in health care operations: application and opportunity. Academy of Health Care Management Journal, 2006.

Appendix: Resources for abortion providers

Melissa Werner MPH, MAT

This chapter includes several resources that can support clinicians in providing abortion care. The first section lists basic provisions for any facility offering first-trimester aspiration abortions, as well as additional equipment useful for second-trimester abortions. The types and numbers of instruments, equipment, and medications that a facility needs depend in part on the practice setting, volume of patients seen, the types of abortion procedures offered, and the facility's gestational age limits for abortion.

The second section contains photographs of many of the more commonly used instruments. Many instruments have variable designs (e.g., curved vs. straight, wide vs. narrow, plastic vs. metal, disposable vs. autoclavable). Having an assortment of instruments allows the practitioner to select the most appropriate for the particular patient, thus enhancing safety, comfort, and efficiency.

The third section lists selected suppliers of equipment and instruments commonly used for abortion. Many of these supplies are available to members of the National Abortion Federation (NAF) at discounted prices through NAF's group purchasing program.

The fourth and final section presents a selected list of organizations that offer support for the abortion provider. These organizations include professional societies and research organizations that focus on women's health and abortion; organizations offering abortion-related education and training initiatives and materials; health and safety resources; legal resources; and advocacy groups.

Basic provisions for first-trimester aspiration abortion

Equipment and supplies

- Examination tables, preferably with knee-support crutches and comfortable pillow
- Operator-adjustable stool with castors (at least one per table)
- Vacuum aspiration machine (e.g., Burdick, Berkeley)
- Manual vacuum aspiration syringes or machine with a foot-driven pump (useful in low-resource settings that lack electricity or in the event of a power failure)
- Suction cannulas, rigid (to 14-mm diameter) and flexible (Fig. A-9)
- Light source (may be a floor lamp, head lamp, or mounted on the wall)
- Ultrasonography machine with both vaginal and abdominal probes and image storage or printer
- Autoclave (large enough to sterilize the largest instruments used) and sterile indicators
- Gloves: latex and nonlatex, sterile and nonsterile without talc
- Sterile lubricating jelly
- Heating pads or other source of thermastatically controlled heat (useful in keeping specula, lubricating jelly, and ultrasound gel at or near body temperature)
- Osmotic dilators, individually packaged: *Laminaria* and/or Dilapan-S™ (Fig. A-13)
- Rh(D) antigen testing kit
- Pregnancy tests
- Hematocrit machine and testing supplies
- Disposable paper products (e.g., drape sheets, absorbent pads, table paper)
- Antiseptic solutions: povidone-iodine (Betadine®) and a noniodine substitute for patients allergic to iodine, such as chlorhexidine gluconate (Hibiclens®)
- Intravenous (IV) administration equipment: IV pole or wall hooks, IV tubing, extension sets, needles, intracaths (sizes 18, 20, and 22)
- IV fluids: Ringer's lactate (500- and 1,000-ml units)
- Personal protective equipment, including sharps containers

Instruments

- Cervical dilators (Fig. A-1): Pratt sizes 13 to 43 French (multiple sets) or Denniston sizes 5 to 14; Hanks or Hegars dilators used by some providers

- Cervical tenacula (Fig. A-6): single-toothed Schroeder-Braun (straight), Duplay (curved), Bierer vulsellum, Teale vulsellum or Kelly-type atraumatic jaws with Allis-type tip
- Specula (Figs. A-2, A-3): Graves (small, medium, large), Moore-Graves, and Klopfer
- Foerster (sponge) forceps (Fig. A-6), straight and curved
- Sims uterine dressing forceps or similar
- Uterine curettes (Fig. A-12): Sims sizes 00 through 6
- Medicine cups, 2 oz or larger, autoclavable
- Suction handle, either autoclavable or disposable, and connector tubing
- Safety needles with short bevel, size 21 gauge or smaller × 1.5 inch
- Needle extenders, sizes 3 to 6 inch (Fig. A-8)
- Syringes: 1-, 2-, 5-, 10-, 20-ml
- Cervical os finders (Fig. A-7) and other ultrathin dilators

Medications

- Local anesthetic solutions (e.g., lidocaine 0.5% or 1%)
- Aminophylline, 250 mg, 10-ml ampules
- Atropine, 0.4 mg/ml, 1-ml ampules
- Diazepam, 5 mg/ml, 2-ml ampules or prefilled syringes
- Diphenhydramine (Benadryl®), 50 mg/ml, 1-ml ampules
- Epinephrine, 1:1,000, 1-ml ampules
- Fentanyl, 50 μg/ml, 2-ml vials
- Hydroxyzine hydrochloride, 25 and 50 mg/ml, 1-ml vials
- Meperidine, 50 mg/ml, 2-ml vials
- Midazolam (Versed®), 1 mg/ml, 2-mg ampules
- Naloxone hydrochloride (Narcan®), 0.4 mg/ml, 1-ml ampules
- Phenobarbital, 130 mg/ml, 1-ml ampules
- Supply of D immune globulin, micro dose (50 μg) for ≤ 12 weeks' gestation; full dose (300 μg) for >12 weeks
- Uterotonics: pitocin ampules, 10 units/ml; methylergonovine (Methergine®), 0.2 mg; vasopressin, 200 units/ml; misoprostol, 200-μg tablets; 15-methyl $PGF_{2\alpha}$ (Hemabate®), 250 μg (in hospital settings)
- Silver nitrate or ferferric subsulfate (Monsel's solution)
- Romazicon® (flumazenil), 0.1mg/ml

Emergency equipment

- Oxygen tank (portable) with flowmeter control valve, mask, and tubing
- Resuscitation ventilation bag
- Oropharyngeal plastic airways, curved (small, medium, large)
- Laryngoscope with fully charged batteries
- Cardiac arrest board
- Sterile suture set, including long needle holder, long forceps, long scissors, and 0 chomic or 0 Vicryl suture on a medium needle
- Emergency kit for bleeding, including misoprostol 200-μg tablets, Foley catheters with 30- and 60-cc balloons, and a syringe and sterile saline for inflating Foley
- EKG machine, pulse oximeter, blood pressure cuff
- SOS Bakri Tamponade Balloon Catheter (optional) (Fig. A-14)

Second-trimester instruments and supplies

- Dilators (Fig. A-10): Hern, 45 to 89 French (up to 98 French if needed); Pratt, 41 to 79 French
- Forceps (Fig. A-11): Bierer (small, large), Sopher (small, large, and 15″ for obese patients), Hern (small, medium, and large), Kelly, Van Lith, Finks, and others
- Curettes (Fig. A-12): Bumm sizes 1, 2, 3, and 4; Evans sizes 1–4
- Spinal needles, 20 gauge
- Long Metzenbaum scissors
- Specula (Figs. A-2, A-3, A-4): Weisman-Graves, Moore-Graves, Rolon-Graves, Klopfer, Auvard weighted, Guttmann self-retaining, and Guttmann obstetrical retractor
- Table basin or emesis-type basin
- Medications: digoxin, potassium chloride, 15-methyl $PGF_{2\alpha}$ (Carboprost, Hemabate®)

Photographs of instruments used in abortion care

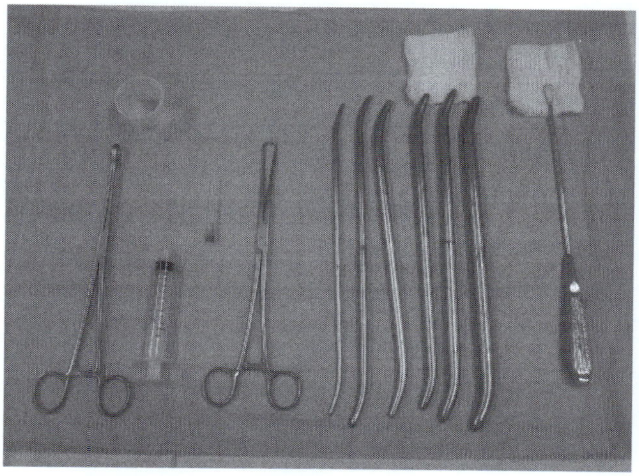

Figure A-1 Sample surgical tray for first-trimester abortion. *Left to right:* Sponge/ring forceps; medicine cup (for anesthetic or antiseptic solutions); syringe; 22-gauge needle (21 to 24 gauge commonly used); single-tooth tenaculum; set of Pratt dilators (sizes 13/15 to 33/35); Sims sharp curette; 4 × 4 cotton sponges. A speculum (see Fig. A-2) would also be included among these standard instruments. Photograph courtesy of Falls Church Health Care Center, LLC.

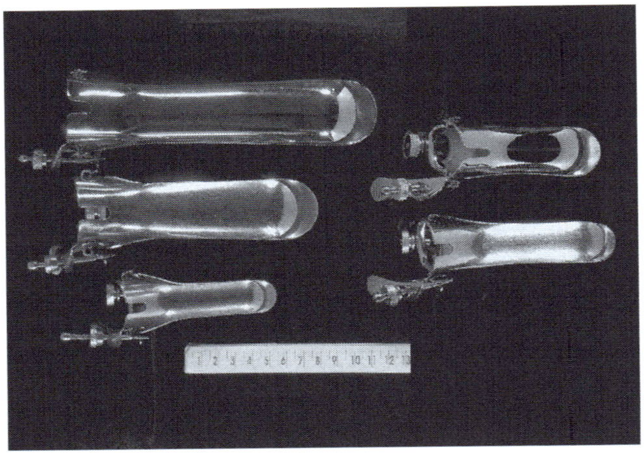

Figure A-2 Assorted vaginal specula, top view. *Left, top to bottom:* Graves' models of various sizes. *Right:* Moore-Graves speculum (top) and a medium Pederson speculum (bottom). Photographer: David Keough, Boston University.

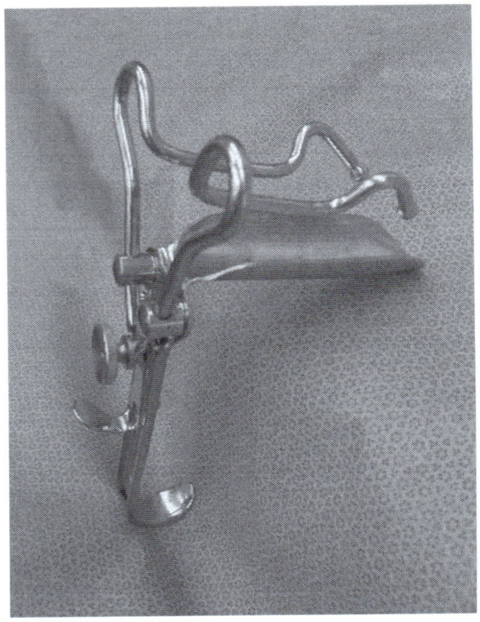

Figure A-4 Guttmann speculum, self-retaining. Photograph courtesy of Dr. Konia J. Trouton.

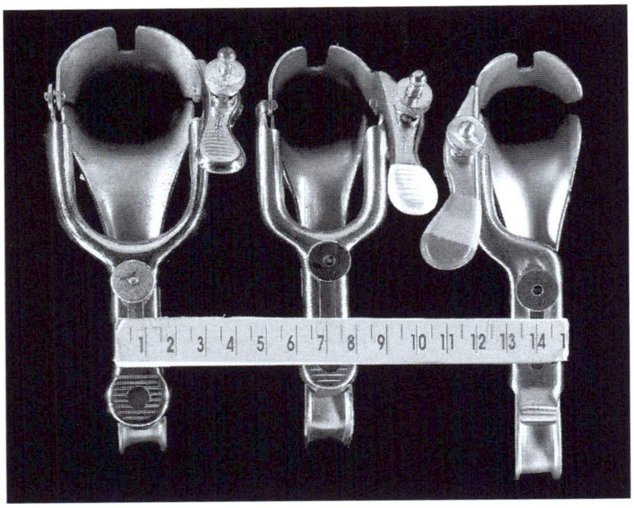

Figure A-3 Vaginal specula, frontal view. Kloepfer model at left has an opening 2 cm wider than the Moore-Graves model pictured center. At right is an open-sided speculum. Photographer: David Keough, Boston University.

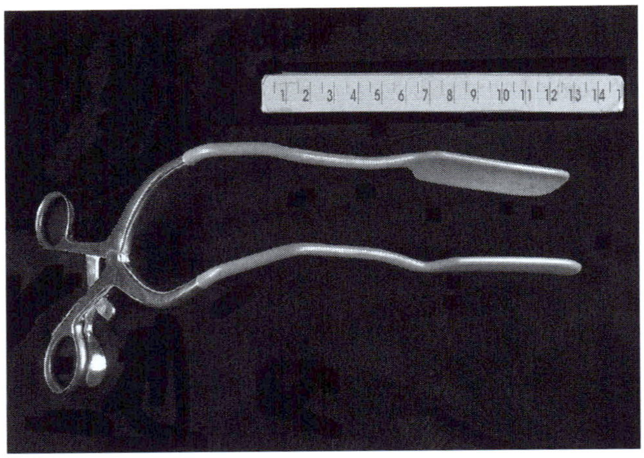

Figure A-5 Self-retaining vaginal wall retractor. Used in conjunction with speculum to retract protruding vaginal sidewalls. Photographer: David Keough, Boston University.

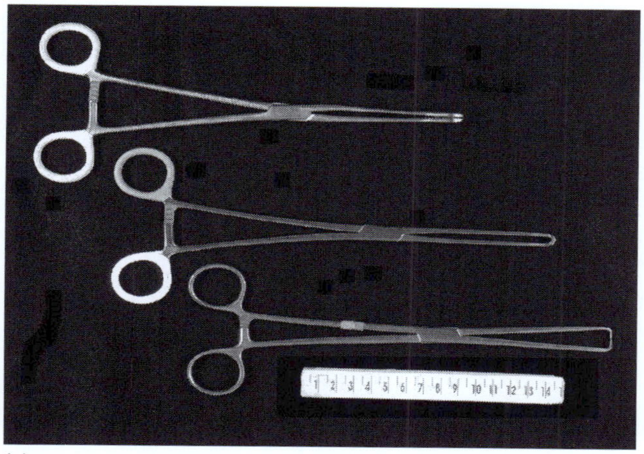

(a)

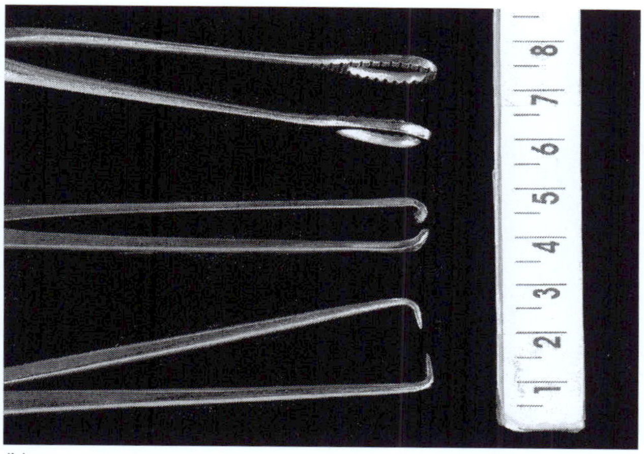

(b)

Figure A-6 Forceps and cervical tenacula. (a) *top to bottom:* Sponge forceps; Allis clamp; single-toothed tenaculum. (b) Close-up views of the three instruments pictured above. Photographer: David Keough, Boston University.

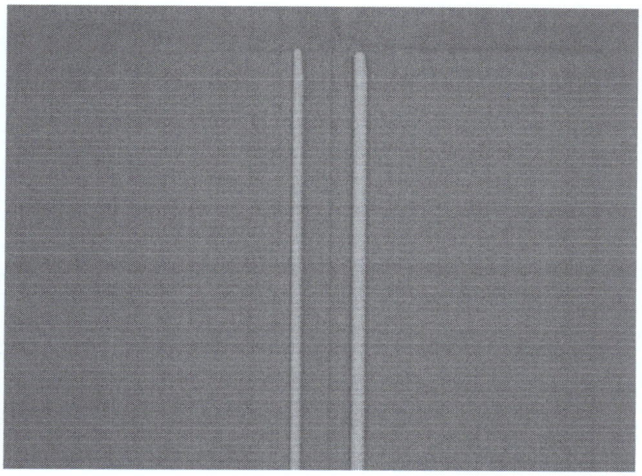

Figure A-7 Flexible, plastic cervical os finders. Photograph courtesy of Falls Church Health Care Center, LLC.

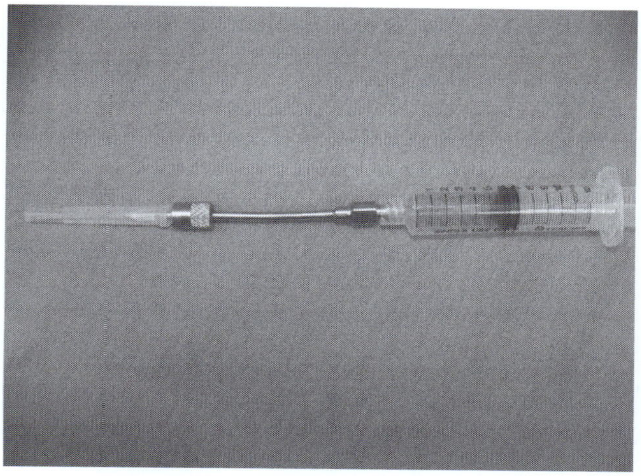

Figure A-8 Needle extender. These are available in a variety of lengths. Photograph courtesy of Dr. Konia J. Trouton.

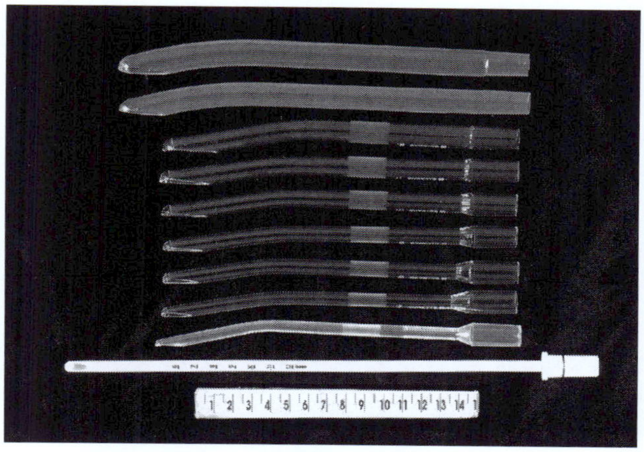

Figure A-9 Disposable suction cannulas. Curved rigid plastic cannulas, ranging in diameter from 6 to 14 mm (16-mm cannulas are also available); *Bottom:* Flexible plastic cannula, 6-mm diameter; these are available up to 12 mm. Photographer: David Keough, Boston University.

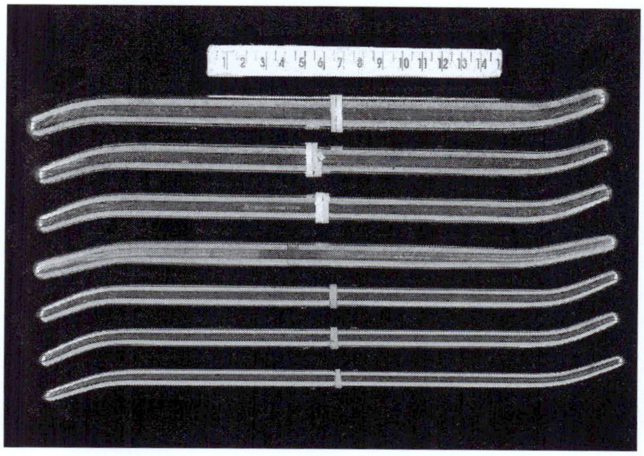

Figure A-10 Pratt cervical dilators used in second-trimester dilation and evacuation procedures. The dilators are shown from size 29/31F up to 53/55F. They are available up to 89 F. Photographer: David Keough, Boston University.

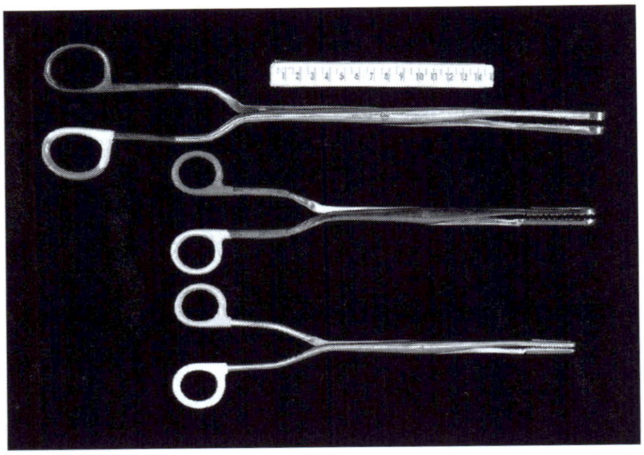

(a)

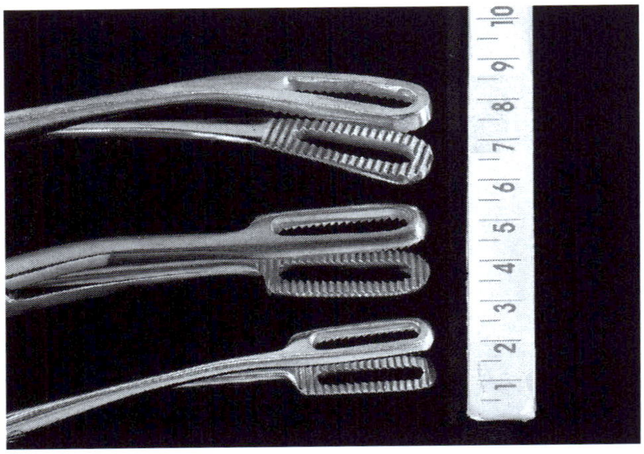

(b)

Figure A-11 (a) Two types of forceps used for second-trimester dilation and evacuation procedures including a Hern forceps (top), and large and small Sopher forceps. (b) Close-up views of the instruments pictured above. Photographer: David Keough, Boston University.

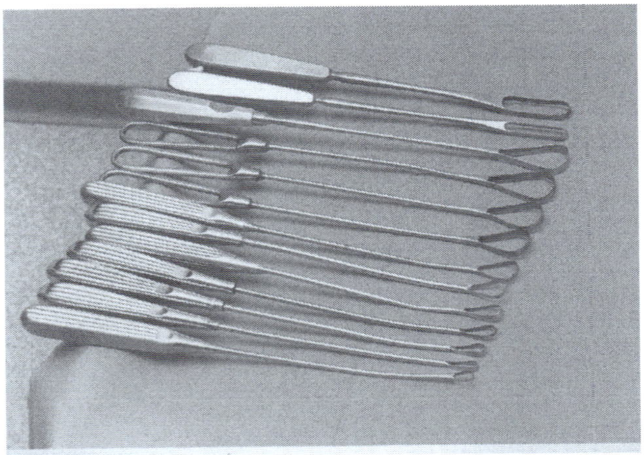

Figure A-12 Metal uterine curettes. *Top to bottom:* Evans curettes with rigid shanks, sizes 4 (12 mm) and 2 (8 mm); Bumm curettes with malleable shanks, sizes 4, 3, 2, and 1; Sims curettes with malleable shanks, sizes 5, 4, 3, 2, 1, 0, and 00.

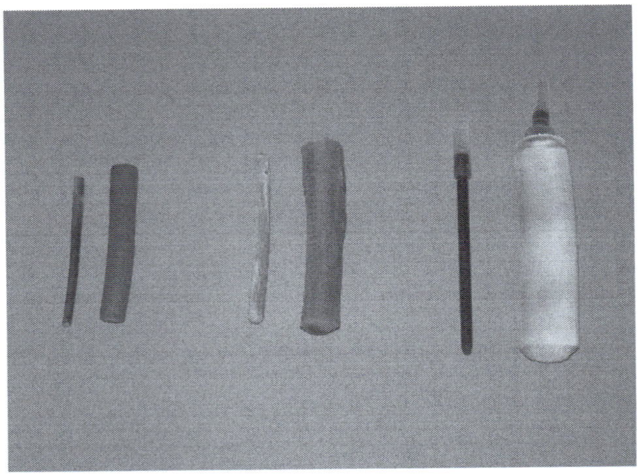

Figure A-13 Osmotic dilators before and after exposure to fluid overnight. *Left to right:* Laminaria, 3 mm, dry and after immersion; laminaria 6 mm, dry and after immersion; and Dilapan-S™, a synthetic polyacrylonitrile rod (hypan), dry and after immersion. See Plate A.1.

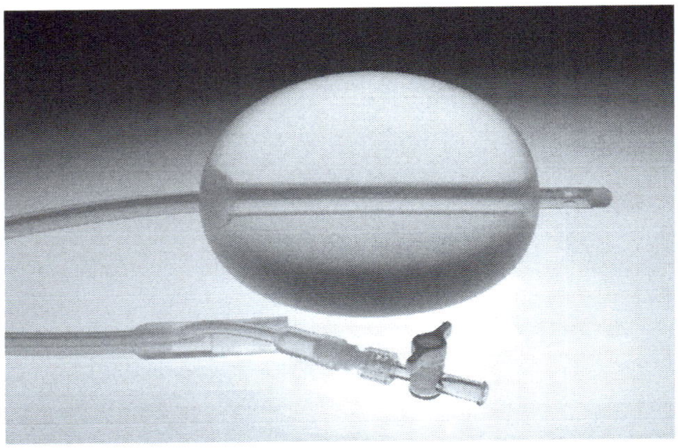

Figure A-14 SOS Bakri Tamponade Balloon Catheter. Used for temporary tamponade of lower uterine segment bleeding. Photograph courtesy of Cook Medical.

Select list of suppliers of medical equipment, supplies, and medications used for abortion

This listing is not comprehensive and does not constitute a recommendation, endorsement, or guarantee of products or services. Members of the NAF can buy supplies at a discount through NAF's group purchasing program.

Allscripts Healthcare Solutions
Pharmaceutical distributor; repackager of medication into smaller units
2401 Commerce Drive
Libertyville, IL 60048
(800) 654-0889
www.allscriptsdirect.com
customerservice@allscriptsdirect.com

Berkeley Medevices, Inc.
Producer and distributor of electric vacuum aspirators; distributor of Laminaria japonicum
1330 South 51st St.
Richmond, CA 94804
(800) 227-2388
In California (510) 231-2474
www.berkeleymedevices.com
contactmedevices@aol.com

Cheshire Medical Specialties, Inc.
OB/GYN instrument vendor
PO Box 894
Cheshire, CT 06410
(800) 243-3020
www.cheshire-medical.com
chesmed@pipeline.com

HPSRx Enterprises
Pharmaceutical distributor; exclusive distributor for Ipas MVAs and cannulas in the USA
1640 Roanoke Boulevard
Salem, VA 24153
(800) 850-1657

MedGyn Products, Inc.
Manufacturer and distributor of ob/gyn supplies, instruments, and equipment
328 North Eisenhower Lane
Lombard, IL 60148
(888) 563-3496
(630) 627-4105
www.medgyn.com
medgyn@medgyn.com

NORSCAN Trading Group
Laminaria distributor
PO Box 3251
Thousand Oaks, CA 91359
(818) 735-0019
www.laminaria.net
norscan@usa.com

PD-RX Pharmaceuticals, Inc.
Pharmaceutical distributor; repackager of medication into smaller units
727 North Ann Arbor
Oklahoma City, OK 73127
(800) 299-7379
(866) 948-5328
www.pdrx.com
pdrx@pdrx.com

Organizational Resources

Included here is a list of organizations that provide support and information to abortion providers. The list is divided into several sections—Medical Professional Organizations, Research Organizations, Legal Resources, Training and Education, Advocacy, Hotlines and Online Referral Services, Occupational Safety and Health, and International Organizations. Please note that some of the organizations listed in this section fall into multiple categories. For example, some medical professional organizations also engage in advocacy activities. Similarly, several organizations engage in both advocacy and research.

Medical professional organizations

American Academy of Family Physicians
The American Academy of Family Physicians is the national association of family doctors. The Academy was founded in 1947 to promote and maintain high-quality standards for family doctors who are providing continuing comprehensive health care to the public.

11400 Tomahawk Creek Parkway
Leawood, KS 66211
(800) 274-2237
www.aafp.org

American Association of Nurse Anesthetists
Founded in 1931, the American Association of Nurse Anesthetists (AANA) is the professional association for more than 37,000 Certified Registered Nurse Anesthetists and student nurse anesthetists.

222 South Prospect Avenue
Park Ridge, IL 60068
(847) 692-7050
www.aana.com

American College of Obstetricians and Gynecologists
Founded in 1951, the American College of Obstetricians and Gynecologists (ACOG) currently has more than 49,000 members. Now based in Washington, DC, it is a private, voluntary, nonprofit membership organization.

409 12th Street SW
PO Box 96920
Washington, DC 20090
(202) 638-5577
www.acog.org

American Institute of Ultrasound in Medicine
The American Institute of Ultrasound in Medicine is a multidisciplinary association dedicated to advancing the safe and effective use of ultrasound in medicine through professional and public education, research, development of guidelines, and accreditation.

14750 Sweitzer Lane, Suite 100
Laurel, MD 20707
(800) 638-5352
www.aium.org

American Medical Women's Association

The American Medical Women's Association (AMWA) is an organization that functions at the local, national, and international level to advance women in medicine and improve women's health. AMWA achieves this by providing and developing leadership, advocacy, education, expertise, mentoring, and strategic alliances.

100 North 20th Street, 4th Floor
Philadelphia, PA 19103
(215) 320-3716
www.amwa-doc.org

American Society of Anesthesiologists

The American Society of Anesthesiologists (ASA) is an educational, research, and scientific association of physicians organized to raise and maintain the standards of the medical practice of anesthesiology and improve the care of the patient.

520 North Northwest Highway
Park Ridge, IL 60068
(847) 825-5586
www.asahq.org

Association of Physician Assistants in Obstetrics and Gynecology

The mission of the Association of Physician Assistants in Obstetrics and Gynecology (APAOG) is to improve the health care of women by supporting physician/PA teams who provide cost-effective, quality care to female patients and by promoting a network of communication and education among providers dedicated to women's health.

702-A Eisenhower Drive
Kimberly, WI 54136
(800) 545-0636
www.paobgyn.org

Association of Reproductive Health Professionals

The Association of Reproductive Health Professionals (ARHP) is a nonprofit membership association comprised of highly qualified and committed experts in reproductive health. Its members are professionals who provide reproductive health services and education, conduct reproductive health research, and influence reproductive health policy. Members include physicians, advanced practice clinicians (nurse practitioners, nurse midwives, and physician assistants), researchers, educators, pharmacists, and other professionals in reproductive health. The organization reaches this broad range of health care professionals both in the USA and abroad with education and information about reproductive health science, practice, and policy.

1901 L Street NW, Suite 300
Washington, DC 20036
(202) 466-3825
www.arhp.org

Consortium of Abortion Providers

The Consortium of Abortion Providers (CAPs), a division of Planned Parenthood Federation of America (PPFA), provides national coordination of technical support, training, and assistance to Planned Parenthood affiliates for starting, expanding, or improving abortion services.

434 West 33rd Street
New York, NY 10001
(212) 541-7800
(727) 896-7499

National Abortion Federation

The National Abortion Federation (NAF) is the professional association of abortion providers in the USA and Canada. NAF members include health care professionals at clinics, doctors' offices, and hospitals, who together care for more than half the women in both countries who choose abortion each year. NAF sets the standard for quality abortion care in North America through evidence-based *Clinical Policy Guidelines* adhered to by all NAF members.

1660 L Street NW, Suite 450
Washington, DC 20036
(202) 667-5881
www.prochoice.org

National Association of Nurse Practitioners in Reproductive Health

The National Association of Nurse Practitioners in Women's Health (NPWH, formerly the National Association of Nurse Practitioners in Reproductive Health) was founded in 1980. NPWH's mission is to assure the provision of quality health care to women of all ages by nurse practitioners. NPWH defines quality health care to be inclusive of an individual's physical, emotional, and spiritual needs.

505 C Street NE
Washington, DC 20002
(202) 543-9693
www.npwh.org

National Family Planning and Reproductive Health Association

The National Family Planning and Reproductive Health Association (NFPRHA) is a vital membership organization representing the nation's dedicated family planning providers—nurses, nurse practitioners, clinic directors, and other key health care providers. NFPRHA serves its members by providing advocacy, education, and training for those in the family planning and reproductive health care field.

1627 K Street NW, 12th Floor
Washington, DC 20006
(202) 293-3114
www.nfprha.org

Physicians for Reproductive Choice and Health
Founded in 1992, Physicians for Reproductive Choice and Health (PRCH) is a national network of pro-choice physicians who are committed to providing and advocating for the best possible care for patients. PRCH exists to ensure that all people have the knowledge, access to quality services, and freedom to make their own reproductive health decisions.

55 West 39th Street, Suite 1001
New York, NY 10018
(646) 366-1890
www.prch.org

Planned Parenthood Federation of America
Planned Parenthood Federation of America (PPFA) is a leading sexual and reproductive health care provider and advocate in the USA, with affiliate health centers offering a wide range of high-quality medical care, including abortion, to millions of clients annually. The Consortium of Abortion Providers (CAPs), a division of PPFA, provides national support for abortion services at Planned Parenthood affiliates. The PPFA website www.planned parenthood.org offers information on reproductive health, including both medication and in-clinic abortion. The website's "Find a Health Center" feature helps users find their nearest Planned Parenthood health center and a list of the services it provides. Website visitors can also search for employment, volunteer, or internship opportunities.

434 West 33rd Street
New York, NY 10001
(212) 541-7800
www.plannedparenthood.org

Society for Maternal-Fetal Medicine
The Society for Maternal-Fetal Medicine was established in 1977 and is the membership organization for obstetricians/gynecologists who have additional formal education and training in maternal-fetal medicine. The Society is also an advocate for improving public policy and expanding research funding and opportunities in the area of maternal-fetal medicine.

409 12th Street SW
Washington, DC 20024
(202) 863-2476
www.smfm.org

Research organizations

Bixby Center for Reproductive Health and Policy, University of California, San Francisco
The Bixby Center for Reproductive Health and Policy's mission is to promote reproductive health, family planning, and the prevention of sexually transmitted infections, including HIV, worldwide through research, training, and policy analysis.

3333 California Street, Suite 335, Box 0744
San Francisco, CA 94143
(415) 502-4086
www.reprohealth.ucsf.edu

Centers for Disease Control and Prevention's Division of Reproductive Health
To better understand the burden of maternal complications and mortality and to decrease disparities among populations at risk of death and complications from pregnancy, the Centers for Disease Control and Prevention's Division of Reproductive Health supports national and state-based surveillance systems to monitor trends and investigate health issues; conducts epidemiologic, behavioral, demographic, and health services research; and works with partners to translate research findings into health care practice, public health policy, and health promotion strategies.

1600 Clifton Road
Atlanta, GA 30333
(800) 232-4636
www.cdc.gov/reproductivehealth

The Guttmacher Institute
The Guttmacher Institute advances sexual and reproductive health through an interrelated program of social science research, policy analysis, and public education designed to generate new ideas, encourage enlightened public debate, promote sound policy and program development and, ultimately, inform individual decision-making.

125 Maiden Lane, 7th Floor
New York, NY 10038
(800) 355-0244
www.guttmacher.org

Gynuity Health Projects
Gynuity Health Projects is a research and technical assistance organization dedicated to the idea that all people should have access to the fruits of medical science and technology development. Gynuity works globally to ensure that reproductive health technologies are widely available

at reasonable cost, provided in the context of high-quality services, and offered in a way that recognizes the dignity and autonomy of each individual. Gynuity's efforts are focused particularly on resource-poor environments, underserved populations, and challenging subject matter.

15 East 26th Street, Suite 801
New York, NY 10010
(212) 448-1230
www.gynuity.org

The Henry J. Kaiser Family Foundation

The Kaiser Family Foundation is a nonprofit, private operating foundation focusing on the major health care issues facing the USA, with a growing role in global health. Unlike grant-making foundations, Kaiser develops and runs its own research and communications programs, sometimes in partnership with other nonprofit research organizations or major media companies.

2400 Sand Hill Road
Menlo Park, CA 94025
(650) 854-9400
www.kff.org

Picker Institute, Inc.

Picker Institute sponsors research and education in the fields of patient-centered care in support of and in cooperation with educational institutions and other interested entities and persons. The institute's mission is to foster a broader understanding of the theoretical and practical implications of patient-centered care by approaching health care with a focus on the concerns of patients and other health care consumers.

PO Box 777
Camden, ME 04843
(888) 680-7500
www.pickerinstitute.org

Sexuality Information and Education Council of the United States

The Sexuality Information and Education Council of the United States (SIECUS) has served as the national voice for sexuality education, sexual health, and sexual rights for more than 40 years. SIECUS affirms that sexuality is a fundamental part of being human, one that is worthy of dignity and respect. SIECUS advocates for the right of all people to accurate information, comprehensive education about sexuality, and sexual health services. SIECUS works to create a world that ensures social justice and sexual rights.

90 John Street, Suite 704
New York, NY 10038
(212) 819-9770
www.siecus.org

Society of Family Planning

The Society of Family Planning (SFP) advances family planning research and education, providing evidence-based insight to improve clinical care in the areas of contraception and abortion. SFP also seeks to cultivate a collaborative and supportive environment to foster scholarly activity and leadership in the areas of reproductive health and family planning.

255 South 17th Street
Philadelphia, PA 19103
(866) 584-6758
www.societyfp.org

Legal resources

American Civil Liberties Union (ACLU) Reproductive Freedom Project

The ACLU's Reproductive Freedom Project protects everyone's right to make informed decisions free from government interference about whether and when to become a parent.

125 Broad Street, 18th Floor
New York, NY 10004
www.aclu.org/reproductiverights

Center for Reproductive Rights

The Center for Reproductive Rights uses the law to advance reproductive freedom as a fundamental right that all governments are legally obligated to protect, respect, and fulfill.

120 Wall Street
New York, NY 10005
(917) 637-3600
www.reproductiverights.org

Law Students for Reproductive Justice

Law Students for Reproductive Justice is a national nonprofit network of law students and lawyers. It educates, organizes, and supports law students to ensure that a new generation of advocates will be prepared to protect and expand reproductive rights as basic civil and human rights.

419 15th Street, Suite 304
Oakland, CA 94612
(510) 622-8134
www.LSRJ.org

National Women's Law Center

Since 1972, the National Women's Law Center has used the law in all its forms: getting new laws on the books and enforced; litigating ground-breaking cases in state and federal courts all the way to the Supreme Court; and educating the public about ways to make the law and public policies work for women and their families.

11 Dupont Circle NW, #800
Washington, DC 20036
(202) 588-5180
www.nwlc.org

Training and education

Clinician Training Initiative of Planned Parenthood of New York City

In 1993, Planned Parenthood of New York City launched the Clinician Training Initiative (CTI) to close the gap between the need for abortion services and the number of clinicians trained to provide abortions. CTI continues to pursue that mission through its partnerships with family medicine and obstetrics/gynecology residency training programs in New York City.

26 Bleecker Street
New York, NY 10012
(212) 274-7255
www.plannedparenthood.org/nyc/clinician-training-initiative-15164-htm

Fellowship in Family Planning

The objective of the Fellowship in Family Planning is to develop specialists focused on research, teaching, and clinical practice in contraception and abortion. Working with respected and innovative leaders in the field, fellows receive training in clinical and epidemiologic research, develop clinical and teaching skills, have opportunities to work internationally, and connect to a rapidly expanding network of family planning experts. During the 2-year program, fellows have the option of pursuing a master's degree in either Public Health or Science.

University of California, San Francisco
Department of Obstetrics, Gynecology, and Reproductive Sciences
Center for Reproductive Health Research and Policy
3333 California Street, Suite 335
San Francisco, CA 94118
www.familyplanningfellowship.org

The Kenneth J. Ryan Residency Training Program in Abortion and Family Planning

The Kenneth J. Ryan Residency Training Program in Abortion and Family Planning was founded in 1999 to provide technical and financial assistance to obstetrics and gynecology departments working to comply with ACGME and other abortion training mandates. The goal of the program is to increase and improve abortion and family planning training opportunities for ob/gyn residents in the USA and Canada. To ensure resident competence, the program offers support in instituting a formal dedicated rotation, either by establishing an outpatient abortion service within the teaching hospital or linking with a freestanding clinic in the community.

The Ryan Residency Training Program
University of California, San Francisco
Center for Reproductive Health Research and Policy
3333 California Street, Suite 335, Box 0744
San Francisco, CA 94143-0744
(415) 502-4091
www.ryanprogram.org

Medical Students for Choice

Medical Students for Choice® (MSFC) is dedicated to ensuring that women receive the full range of reproductive health care choices. MSFC recognizes that one of the greatest obstacles to safe and legal abortion is the absence of trained providers. As medical students and residents, MSFC works to make reproductive health care, including abortion, a part of standard medical education and residency training.

PO Box 40188
Philadelphia, PA 19106
(215) 625-0800
www.ms4c.org

Midwest Access Project

The Midwest Access Project (MAP) exists to increase the provision of full-spectrum reproductive health care in the region, without barriers to access, through education and training of health care providers and the public. MAP is collaborating with the Abortion Access Project to assess the training needs of family medicine residents in the Midwest and to increase the number of abortion providers in the region.

2000 West Armitage Avenue
Chicago, IL 60647
www.midwestaccessproject.org

RHEDI, the Center for Reproductive Health Education In Family Medicine

RHEDI is housed within the Department of Family and Social Medicine at Montefiore Medical Center in the Bronx, New York. RHEDI was established in 2004 to integrate high-quality comprehensive abortion and family planning training into US family medicine residency programs and to expand the definition of the scope of practice of family medicine to include abortion care. Additionally, RHEDI provides funding and expertise to family medicine residency programs to establish required rotations in abortion and family planning.

Department of Family and Social Medicine
Montefiore Medical Center
3544 Jerome Avenue
Bronx, NY 10467
(718) 920-4678
www.rhedi.org

Advocacy

Abortion Access Project

The Abortion Access Project (AAP) is committed to access to safe abortion for all women in the USA. AAP believes that by being clearly focused on abortion within the context of our broader values, we will make a significant contribution to women's health and autonomy.

47 Thorndike Street
Cambridge, MA 02141
(617) 661-1161
www.abortionaccess.org

Boston Women's Health Book Collective

The Boston Women's Health Book Collective (BWHBC), also known as Our Bodies Ourselves (OBOS), is a nonprofit, public interest women's health education, advocacy, and consulting organization.

5 Upland Road #3
Cambridge, MA 02140
(617) 245-0200
www.ourbodiesourselves.org

Catholics for a Free Choice

Catholics for a Free Choice (CFC) shapes and advances sexual and reproductive ethics that are based on justice, reflect a commitment to women's well-being, and respect and affirm the moral capacity of women and men to make sound decisions about their lives. Through discourse, education and advocacy, CFC works in the USA and internationally to infuse these values into public policy, community life, and Catholic social thinking and teaching.

1436 U Street NW, Suite 301
Washington, DC 20009
(202) 986-6093
www.catholicsforchoice.org

Choice USA

As a national pro-choice organization, Choice USA gives emerging leaders the tools they need to organize, network, and exchange ideas to build a youth-centered, pro-choice agenda and mobilize communities for reproductive justice.

1317 F Street NW, Suite 501
Washington, DC 20004
(202) 965-7700
www.choiceusa.org

Civil Liberties and Public Policy Program

The Civil Liberties and Public Policy Program (CLPP), is a reproductive rights organization that trains, educates, and inspires new leaders, organizers, and supporters nationwide. CLP is located at Hampshire College in Amherst, Massachusetts, and works with new generations of activists to advance their leadership and strengthen the reproductive rights movement.

Hampshire College
Amherst, MA 01002
(413) 559-5416
clpp.hampshire.edu

Feminist Majority Foundation

The Feminist Majority Foundation (FMF), which was founded in 1987, is a cutting-edge organization dedicated to women's equality, reproductive health, and nonviolence. In all spheres, FMF utilizes research and action to empower women economically, socially, and politically.

1600 Wilson Boulevard, Suite 801
Arlington, VA 22209
(703) 522-2214
www.feminist.org

Indigenous Women's Reproductive Rights and Pro-Choice Page

The purpose of this page is to provide information concerning indigenous women's reproductive health and their perspectives on pro-choice issues. The Native-American Women's Health Education Resource Center

P.O. Box 572
Lake Andes, South Dakota 57356
(605) 487-7072
www.nativeshop.org/pro-choice.html

NARAL Pro-Choice America

For more than 30 years, NARAL Pro-Choice America has been a leading advocate for privacy and a woman's right to choose. With more than 1 million members and supporters, NARAL Pro-Choice America is fighting to protect the pro-choice values of freedom and privacy.

1156 15th Street NW, Suite 700
Washington, DC 20005
(202) 973-3000
www.prochoiceamerica.org

National Abortion Federation

The National Abortion Federation (NAF) works to ensure safe, legal, and accessible abortion care to promote health and justice for women. NAF's public policy programs provide medical expertise to policy makers and ensure that the voices of abortion providers and patients are heard in policy forums and in the media across the USA and Canada.

1660 L Street NW, Suite 450
Washington, DC 20036
(202) 667-5881
www.prochoice.org

National Advocates for Pregnant Women
National Advocates for Pregnant Women works to secure the human and civil rights, health, and welfare of all women, focusing particularly on pregnant and parenting women, and those who are most vulnerable—low-income women, women of color, and drug-using women.

15 West 36th street, suite 901
New York, NY 10018
(212) 255-9252
www.advocatesforpregnantwomen.org

National Latina Institute for Reproductive Health
The mission of the National Latina Institute for Reproductive Health (NLIRH) is to ensure the fundamental human right to reproductive health for Latinas, their families, and their communities through public education, policy advocacy, and community mobilization.

50 Broad Street, Suite 1825
New York, NY 10004
(212) 422-2553
www.latinainstitute.org

National Network of Abortion Funds
The National Network of Abortion Funds (NNAF) is an affiliation of community-based abortion funds throughout the USA.

42 Seaverns Avenue
Boston, MA 02130
(617) 524-6040
www.nnaf.org

National Women's Health Network
The National Women's Health Network improves the health of all women by developing and promoting a critical analysis of health issues in order to affect policy and support consumer decision-making. The Network aspires to a health care system that is guided by social justice and reflects the needs of diverse women.
514 10th Street NW, Suite 400
Washington, DC 20004
(202) 347-1140
www.nwhn.org

The Pro-Choice Public Education Project
The Pro-Choice Public Education Project (PEP) is dedicated to engaging young women on their terms around the critical issue of reproductive freedom.

PO Box 3952
New York, NY 10163
(212) 977-4266
www.protectchoice.org

Religious Coalition for Reproductive Choice
The Religious Coalition for Reproductive Choice brings the moral power of religious communities to ensure reproductive choice through education and advocacy. The Coalition seeks to give clear voice to the reproductive issues of people of color, those living in poverty, and other underserved populations.

1025 Vermont Avenue NW, Suite 1130
Washington, DC 20005
(202) 628-7700
www.rcrc.org

Reproductive Health Technologies Project
The mission of the Reproductive Health Technologies Project (RHTP) is to advance the ability of every woman to achieve full reproductive freedom with access to the safest, most effective, and preferred methods for controlling her fertility and protecting her health.

1020 19th Street NW, Suite 875
Washington, DC 20036
(202) 530-4401
www.rhtp.org

RH Reality Check
RH Reality Check is an online community and publication serving individuals and organizations committed to advancing sexual and reproductive health and rights. RH Reality Check is guided by the issues and recommendations identified in the Program of Action agreed on at the International Conference on Population and Development at Cairo in 1994.

1800 Massachusetts Avenue, Suite 400
Washington, DC 20036
www.rhrealitycheck.org

SisterSong Women of Color Reproductive Health Collective
The SisterSong Women of Color Reproductive Health Collective is a network of local, regional, and national grassroots agencies representing five primary ethnic populations/

indigenous nations in the USA: African American; Arab American/Middle Eastern; Asian/Pacific Islander; Latina; and Native American/Indigenous. The Collective educates women of color and policy makers on reproductive and sexual health and rights, and works toward the access of health services, information, and resources that are culturally and linguistically appropriate.

1237 Ralph David Abernathy Boulevard, SW
Atlanta, GA 30310
(404) 756-2680
www.sistersong.net

Hotlines and online referral services

Abortion Clinics OnLine

Abortion Clinics OnLine is a directory service comprising websites of more than 400 providers of abortion services and other reproductive health care. They may be private physician's offices, state-licensed abortion clinics, private abortion clinics, or hospital abortion services. Abortion clinics listed are in 40 states, as well as international countries.

PO Box 500788
Atlanta, GA 31150
(770) 350-6161
www.gynpages.com

Backline

Backline is dedicated to addressing the broad range of experiences and emotions surrounding pregnancy, parenting, adoption, and abortion. Backline provides a forum in which women and their loved ones can engage in discussion that goes beyond political rhetoric. Backline envisions a society in which pregnancy options are discussed with openness, honesty, and the deepest respect for reproductive justice.

4934 NE 29th Avenue
Portland, OR 97211
Office phone: (503) 287-4344
Hotline: (888) 493-0092
www.yourbackline.org

Emergency Contraception Hotline and Website, National Women's Health Information Center

The Office on Women's Health (OWH) was established in 1991 within the US Department of Health and Human Services. Its mission is to "provide leadership to promote health equity for women and girls through sex/gender-specific approaches."

Department of Health and Human Services
200 Independence Avenue, SW Room 712E
Washington, DC 20201
Office phone: 202-690-7650
Hotline: (800) 994-9662
Hotline TTD: (888) 220-5446
www.4women.gov/faq/econtracep.htm

Exhale

Exhale creates a social climate where each person's unique experience with abortion is supported, respected, and free from stigma. Exhale provides services, training, and education to empower individuals, families, and communities to achieve postabortion health and well-being.

484 Lake Park Avenue, #63
Oakland, CA 94610
Office phone: (510) 446-7900
Hotline (USA): (866) 439-4253
Hotline (outside USA): (510) 446-7977
www.4exhale.org

National Abortion Federation Hotline and Website

The National Abortion Federation (NAF) Hotline provides callers with unbiased, factual information about abortion in English, Spanish, and French; options counseling; and referrals to providers of quality abortion care. The Hotline also provides case management support and financial assistance to low-income women and underserved women with special needs. Individuals may also use NAF's website to find NAF member clinics by state.

1660 L Street NW, Suite 450
Washington, DC 20036
Office phone: (202) 667-5881
Hotline: (800) 772-9100
www.prochoice.org/pregnant/find/index.html

Not-2-late.com/The Emergency Contraception Website

This website answers frequently asked questions about emergency contraception (EC), and offers tips for obtaining EC in the USA, Canada, and worldwide.

The Office of Population Research at Princeton University
Wallace Hall
Princeton, NJ 08544
(609) 258-4870
ec.princeton.edu

Reproductive Toxicology Center (REPROTOX)

REPROTOX® is a service of the Reproductive Toxicology Center. This resource was developed to provide summary information to health care providers on the effects of chemical and physical agents on fertility, pregnancy, and lactation. Agents include industrial and environmental chemicals, as well as over-the-counter, prescription, and recreational drugs. There are summaries for more than 4,000 agents, along with references for the data included.

7831 Woodmont Avenue #375
Bethesda, MD 20814
(301) 514-3081
www.reprotox.org

Teratogen Information System (TERIS)
TERIS is designed to assist physicians and other health care professionals in assessing the risks of possible teratogenic exposures in pregnant women. The database consists of a series of agent summaries, each of which is based on a thorough review of published clinical and experimental literature. Summaries may be accessed using either generic names or domestic or foreign proprietary names. Each summary includes a risk assessment derived by consensus of an advisory board comprising nationally recognized authorities in clinical teratology.

University of Washington
Box 357920
Seattle, WA 98195
(206) 543-2465
www.depts.washington.edu/terisweb/teris/

Occupational safety and health

National Institute for Occupational Safety and Health
The National Institute for Occupational Safety and Health (NIOSH) is the federal agency responsible for conducting research and making recommendations for the prevention of work-related injury and illness. NIOSH is part of the Centers for Disease Control and Prevention (CDC) in the Department of Health and Human Services.

1600 Clifton Road
Atlanta, GA 30333
(800) 232-4636
www.cdc.gov/niosh

Occupational Safety & Health Administration
The Occupational Safety & Health Administration's (OSHA's) mission is to assure the safety and health of US workers by setting and enforcing standards; providing training, outreach, and education; establishing partnerships; and encouraging continual improvement in workplace safety and health.

200 Constitution Avenue NW
Washington, DC 20210
(800) 321-6742
www.osha.gov

International professional, advocacy, research, and service-delivery organizations

Abortion Rights
Abortion Rights is the national pro-choice campaign working to defend and extend women's abortion rights in the UK.
18 Ashwin Street
London, England E8 3DL
020 7923 9792
www.abortionrights.org.uk

Alliance for Choice
Alliance for Choice is an advocacy organization that campaigns for safe, free, legal abortion in Ireland.

PO Box 8852
Phibsboro, Dublin 7
www.struggle.ws/ireland/allianceforchoice/

British Pregnancy Advisory Service
The British Pregnancy Advisory Service (bpas) is a leading provider of abortion services in the UK, with a national network of consultation centers and clinics.

20 Timothy's Bridge Road
Stratford Enterprise Park
Stratford-upon-Avon
Warwickshire
CV37 9BF
0845 365 5050
www.bpas.org

Canadian Anesthesiologists' Society
The Canadian Anesthesiologists' Society (CAS) is a not-for-profit, voluntary organization that exists for the benefit of its member anesthesiologists. The organization is dedicated to the advancement of the medical practice of anesthesia through research, education, and excellence in patient care.

1 Eglinton Avenue East, Suite 208
Toronto, ON M4P 3A1
CANADA
(416) 480-0602
www.cas.ca

Canadian Medical Protective Association
The Canadian Medical Protective Association is a mutual defense organization for physicians who practice in Canada. They work to protect members' integrity by providing legal defense, indemnification, risk management, educational programs, and general advice.

875 Carling Avenue
Ottawa, ON K1S 5P1
(800) 267-6522
www.cmpa-acpm.ca

Fundación Esar
Fundación Esar aims to expand the coverage of reproductive and sexual health services with an emphasis on the comprehensive management of unwanted pregnancies, ambulatory

treatment of incomplete abortions, and postabortion contraception to the greatest possible number of women in Latin America and the Caribbean while maintaining the highest standards of quality.

Carrera 18 No. 33 A-19
Bogotá Colombia
57 - 1 - 3201013 / 3201029
www.fundacionesar.org

The Grupo de Información en Reproducción Elegida
The Grupo de Información en Reproducción Elegida (GIRE) is a nonprofit, civil organization formed in 1992 to provide objective and current information on reproductive rights to strategic sectors of Mexican society principally, decision makers, opinion leaders, the media, and youth leaders.

PO Box 30782
Seattle, WA 98113
Apartado Postal 21-547
Admón. 21, Coyoacán, C.P. 04021
(52) (55) 5658-6684
www.gire.org.mx

Ibis
Ibis Reproductive Health aims to improve women's reproductive autonomy, choices, and health worldwide. Ibis accomplishes its mission by conducting original clinical and social science research, leveraging existing research, producing educational resources, and promoting policies and practices that support sexual and reproductive rights and health.

17 Dunster Street, Suite 201
Cambridge, MA 02138
(617) 349-0040
www.ibisreproductivehealth.org

International Federation of Gynecology and Obstetrics
The International Federation of Gynecology and Obstetrics (FIGO) is the only organization that brings together professional societies of obstetricians and gynecologists on a global basis. FIGO's mission is to promote the well-being of women and their children and to raise the standard of practice in obstetrics and gynecology around the world.

FIGO Secretariat
FIGO House
Suite 3—Waterloo Court
10 Theed Street
London SE1 8ST
United Kingdom
+44 20 7928 1166
www.figo.org

International Federation of Professional Abortion and Contraception Associates
The International Federation of Professional Abortion and Contraception Associates (FIAPAC) organizes seminars and conferences and publishes a biannual bulletin for those interested in the issue of abortion and contraception and who wish to share ideas and experiences.

Herenweg 211-215
2106 MJ Heemstede
Netherlands
+31 23 528 98 90
www.fiapac.org

International Planned Parenthood Federation
International Planned Parenthood Federation (IPPF) is a global service provider and a leading advocate of sexual and reproductive health and rights for all. IPPF has six regional offices, which are located in Africa (Nairobi, Kenya); Arab World (Tunis, Tunisia); Europe (Brussels, Belgium); South Asia (New Delhi, India); East, South East Asia and Oceania (Kuala Lumpur, Malaysia); and Western Hemisphere (New York, USA).

4 Newhams Row
London
SE1 3UZ
+44 (0)20 7939 8200
www.ippf.org

International Women's Health Coalition
The International Women's Health Coalition (IWHC) envisions a world where women are free from discrimination, sexual coercion, and violence; where they make free and informed choices on sexuality and reproduction; and where health information and services are accessible to all.

333 Seventh Avenue, 6th Floor
New York, NY 10001
(212) 979-8500
www.iwhc.org

Ipas
Ipas is an international organization that works around the world to increase women's ability to exercise their sexual and reproductive rights, and to reduce abortion-related deaths and injuries.

PO Box 5027
Chapel Hill, NC 27514
(800) 334-8446
www.ipas.org

JHPIEGO Corporation

JHPIEGO, an international health organization affiliated with The Johns Hopkins University in Baltimore, Maryland, builds global and local partnerships to enhance the quality of health care services for women and families. JHPIEGO's focus is on training and support for health care providers—including doctors, nurses, midwives, and health educators—working in limited-resource settings throughout Africa, Asia, the Middle East, Latin America, and the Caribbean.

1615 Thames Street
Baltimore, MD 21231, USA
(410) 537-1800
www.jhpiego.org

Marie Stopes International

Marie Stopes International is one of the largest international family planning organizations in the world. In 2006 alone, the organization provided nearly 5 million people in almost 38 countries with high-quality health services, including family planning; safe abortion and postabortion care; maternal and child health care, including safe delivery and obstetrics; diagnosis and treatment of sexually transmitted infections; and HIV/AIDS prevention.

Conway Street
Fitzroy Square
London W1T 6LP
UK
+44 (0)20 7636 6200
www.mariestopes.org

Pacific Institute for Women's Health

The Pacific Institute for Women's Health believes that women's health is a human right, and that access to contraception, reproductive freedom, and gender equality are central to women's empowerment and social justice. Their mission is to increase the ability of women to make informed decisions about their sexuality and reproduction and advance reproductive choice and defend sexual and reproductive rights for women and girls around the world.

614 Grand Avenue, Suite 324
Oakland, California 94610
(510) 272-0150
www.piwh.org

Pathfinder International

Pathfinder International provides women, men, and adolescents throughout the developing world with access to quality family planning and reproductive health information and services. Pathfinder works to halt the spread of HIV/AIDS, to provide care to women suffering from the complications of unsafe abortion, and to advocate for sound reproductive health policies in the USA and abroad.

9 Galen Street, Suite 217
Watertown, MA 02472
(617) 924-7200
www.pathfind.org

The Population Council

The Population Council conducts research worldwide to improve policies, programs, and products in three areas: HIV and AIDS; poverty, gender, and youth; and reproductive health.

One Dag Hammarskjold Plaza
New York, NY 10017
(212) 339-0500
www.popcouncil.org

ProChoix

A French organization that advocates for reproductive rights, ProChoix provides resources, articles, and take-action information on this French-language website.

177 Avenue Ledru-Rollin
75011 Paris
www.prochoix.org

Society of Obstetricians and Gynaecologists of Canada

The mission of the Society of Obstetricians and Gynaecologists of Canada is to promote optimum women's health through leadership, collaboration, education, research, and advocacy in the practice of obstetrics and gynaecology.

780 Echo Drive
Ottawa, ON K1S 5R7
(800) 561-2416
www.sogc.medical.org

Women on Waves

Women on Waves is a Dutch organization working to provide abortions on a medical ship that sails in international waters.

PO Box 15683
1001 ND Amsterdam
The Netherlands
+31 20 465 0004
www.womenonwaves.org

Women's Link Worldwide

Women's Link Worldwide is an international human rights nonprofit organization working to ensure that gender equality is a reality worldwide.

Spain: +34 (91) 185 19 04
Colombia: +57 (1) 346 4179
www.womenslinkworldwide.org/who.html

World Federation for Ultrasound in Medicine and Biology

World Federation for Ultrasound in Medicine and Biology (WFUMB) is a Federation of Affiliated Organisations consisting of Regional Federations. The Regional Federations cover National Societies of Ultrasound in Europe (EFSUMB), Asia (AFSUMB), North America (AIUM), Latin America (FLAUS), Australasia (ASUM), and Africa (MASU).

www.wfumb.org

World Health Organization

The World Health Organization (WHO) is the directing and coordinating authority for health within the United Nations system. It is responsible for providing leadership on global health matters, shaping the health research agenda, setting norms and standards, articulating evidence-based policy options, providing technical support to countries, and monitoring and assessing health trends.

Avenue Appia 20
CH - 1211 Geneva 27
Switzerland
Tel.: +41 22 791 2111
www.who.int/en

Acknowledgment

Special thanks to Dwight Williamson, DO, who wrote the chapter on which this appendix is based:

Chapter 20, "Resources for Abortion Providers," in the 1999 publication *A Clinician's Guide to Medical and Surgical Abortion* (Churchill Livingstone).

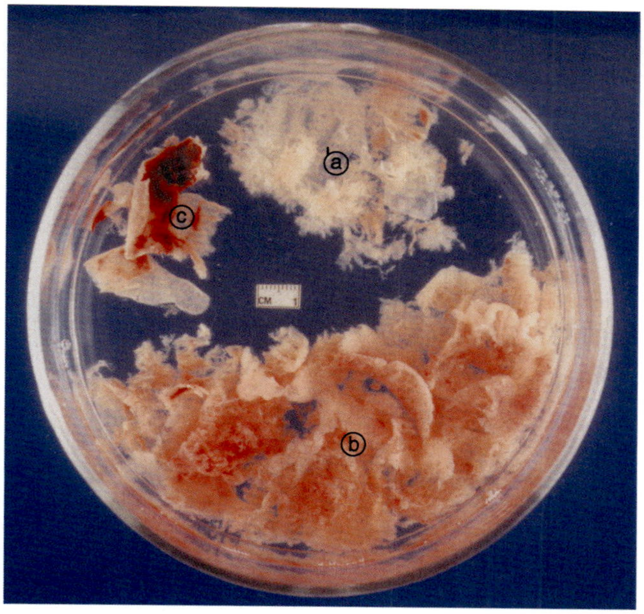

Plate 10.1 Postabortion examination of the uterine aspirate from an 8-week pregnancy. Suspending the tissue in water helps distinguish the various pregnancy elements. Note the thin, transparent gestational sac lined by frond-like villi (a). The decidual tissue is reddish brown or gray and heavier, sinking to the bottom of the dish (b). The decidua capsularis appears as an opaque sheet with hemorrhagic areas (c).

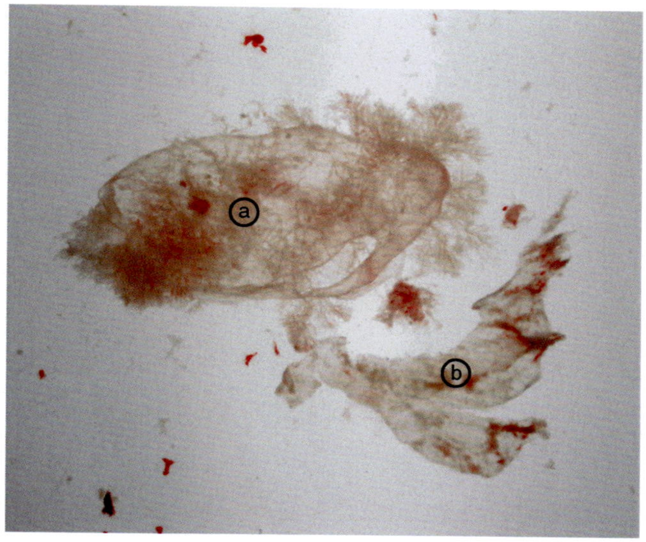

Plate 10.3 Eight week gestational sac (a) adjacent to a sheet of decidua capsularis (b), floated in water. (Courtesy of Dr. Jerry Edwards.)

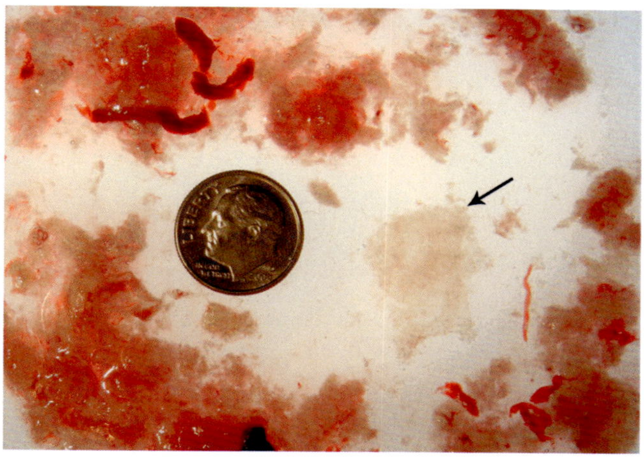

Plate 10.2 Gestational sac (arrow) evacuated from a patient with a 6-week pregnancy is about the size of a dime.

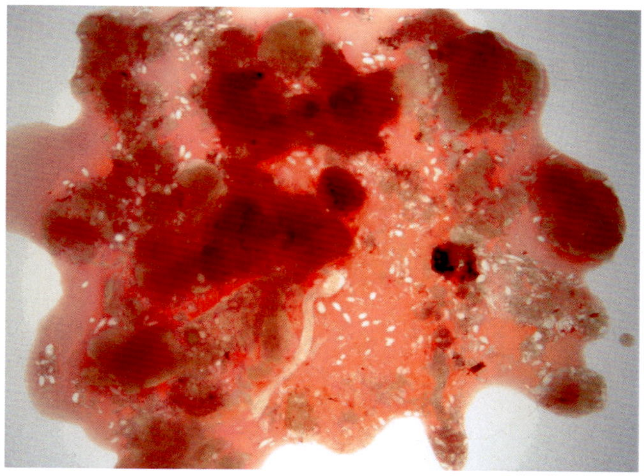

Plate 10.4 Unrinsed hydropic villi from an 11-week pregnancy with trisomy 18.

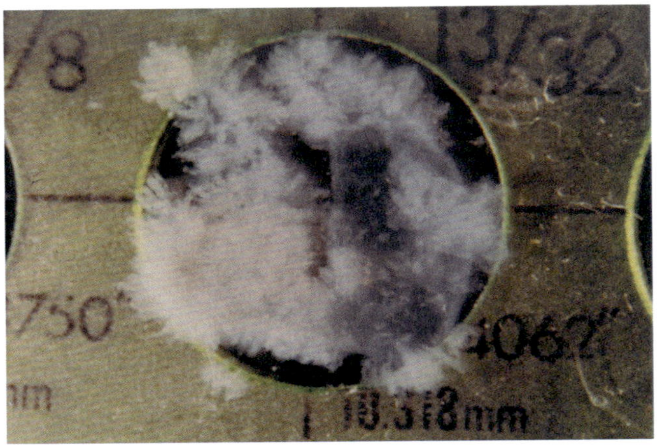

Plate 10.5 Photomicrograph of gestational sac at approximately 4 weeks LMP. Note how delicate and frond-like the villi appear compared to the decidual glands depicted in Plate 10.7. (Courtesy of Dr. Jerry Edwards.)

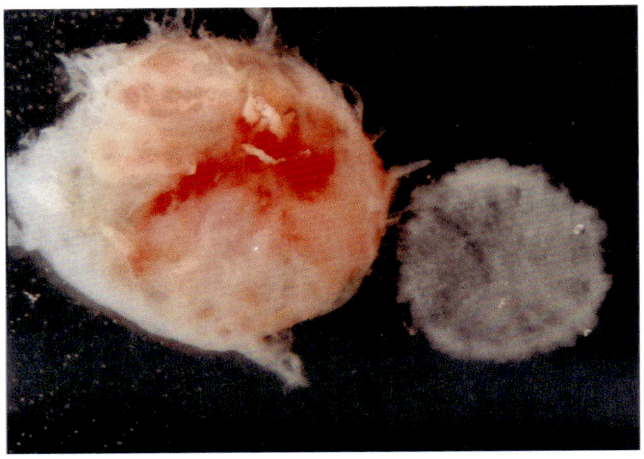

Plate 10.6 Photomicrograph of decidual capsule (left) that has been opened to reveal the early gestational sac, (right). (Courtesy of Dr. Jerry Edwards.)

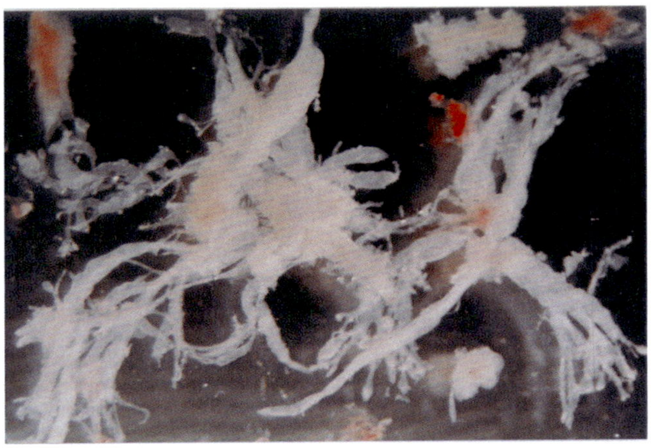

Plate 10.7 Decidual glands as shown in this photomicrograph must not be confused with gestational tissue. (Courtesy of Dr. Jerry Edwards.)

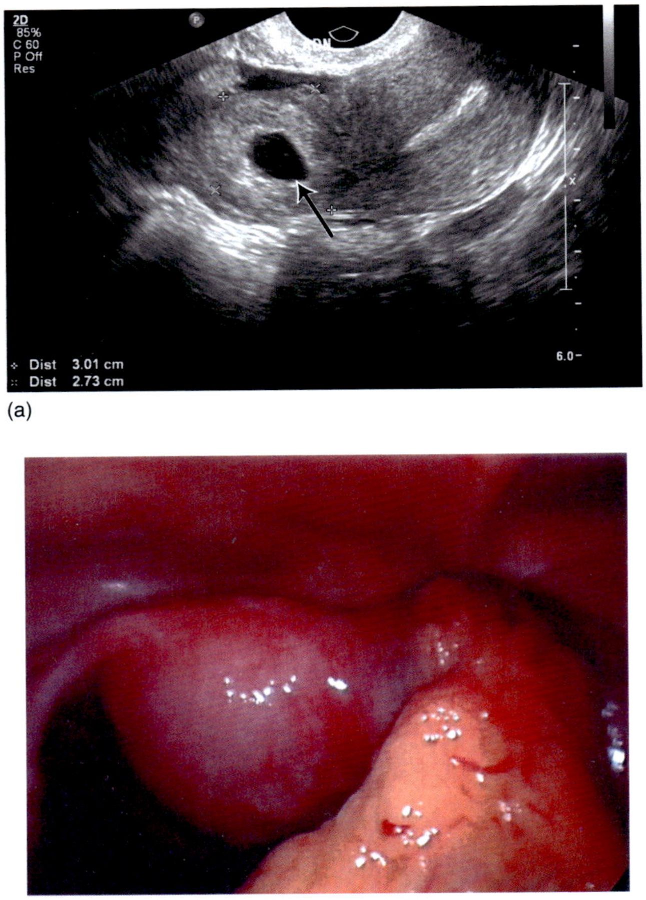

(a)

(b)

Plate 18.1 Patient with a right cornual ectopic pregnancy.
(a) Transvaginal ultrasound image showing a gestational sac with an embryonic pole. The echogenic decidualized endometrium can be seen "pointing" to the gestational sac (arrow). (b) On laparoscopy, a cornual pregnancy was visualized protruding out from the right uterine cornua. The pregnancy was removed without complication. (Courtesy of Dr. Matthew Reeves.)

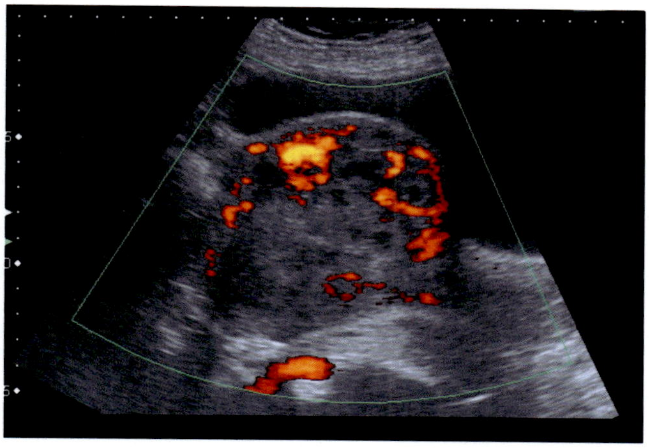

Plate 19.1 Ultrasonographic appearance of an invasive complete hydatidiform mole, showing a localized uterine mass with multiple echolucent cystic spaces and Doppler imaging demonstrating peripheral blood flow.

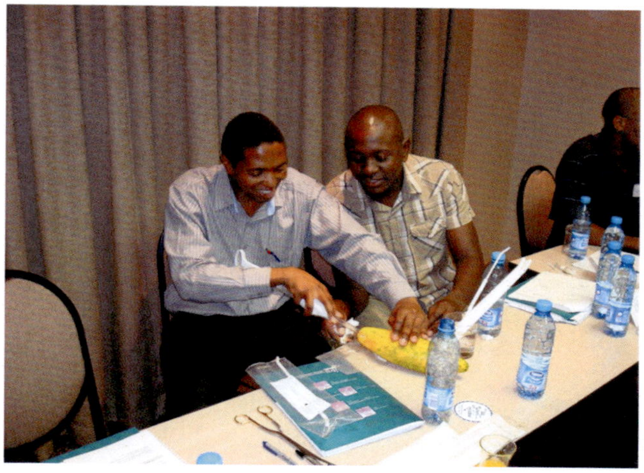

Plate 22.2 Trainees in South Africa learning vacuum aspiration on fruit used as a uterine model. (Courtesy of Alison Edelman MD, MPH.)

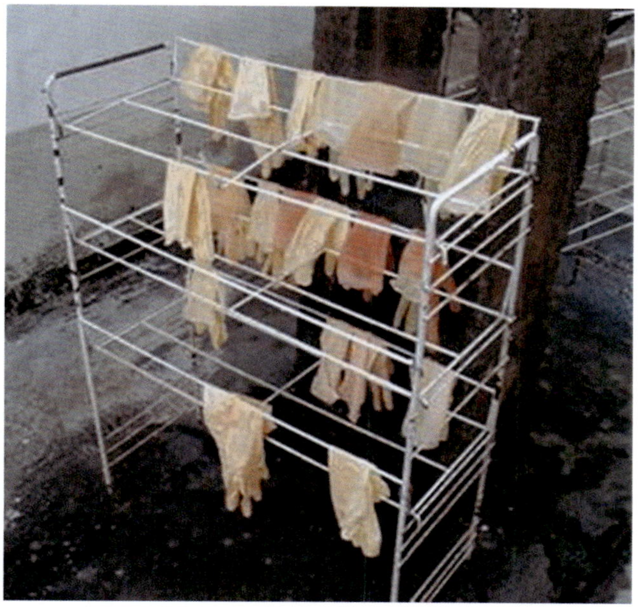

Plate 22.1 Gloves processed for reuse, Viet Nam.

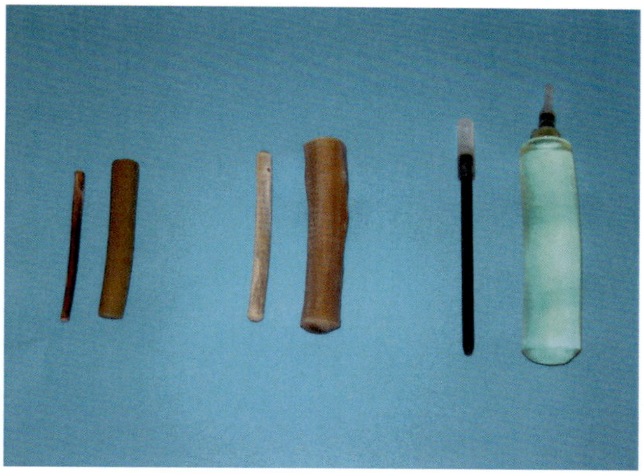

Plate A.1 Osmotic dilators before and after exposure to fluid overnight. *Left to right:* Laminaria, 3 mm, dry and after immersion; laminaria 6 mm, dry and after immersion; and Dilapan-S^{TM}, a synthetic polyacrylonitrile rod (hypan), dry and after immersion.

Index